Register Now for Onli
to Your Bool

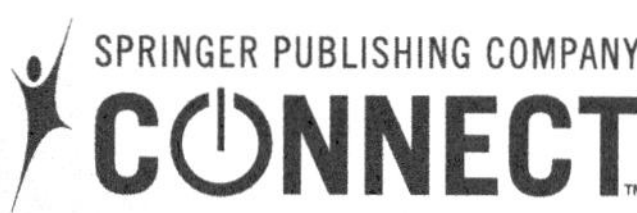

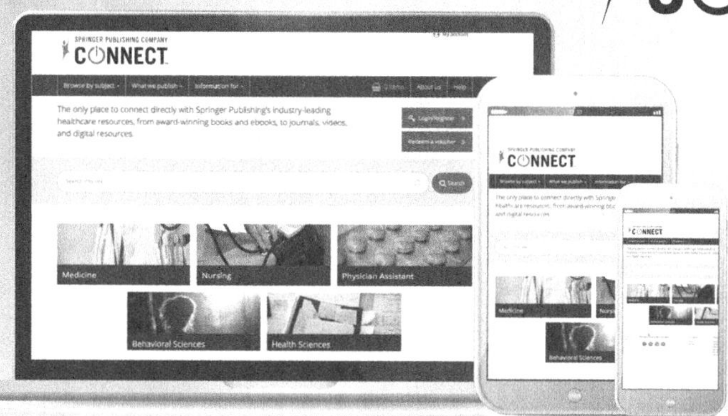

Your print purchase of *Handbook of Gastrointestinal Cancers* **includes online access to the contents of your book—** increasing accessibility, portability, and searchability!

Access today at:
http://connect.springerpub.com/content/book/978-0-8261-3813-2
or scan the QR code at the right with your smartphone
and enter the access code below.

R9051TJJ

Scan here for quick access.

If you are experiencing problems accessing the digital component of this product, please contact our customer service department at cs@springerpub.com

The online access with your print purchase is available at the publisher's discretion and may be removed at any time without notice.

Publisher's Note: New and used products purchased from third-party sellers are not guaranteed for quality, authenticity, or access to any included digital components.

demosMEDICAL
An Imprint of Springer Publishing

View all our products at springerpub.com/demosmedical

Handbook of Gastrointestinal Cancers

Evidence-Based Treatment and Multidisciplinary Patient Care

Editors

Tanios Bekaii-Saab, MD, FACP
Professor, Mayo Clinic College of Medicine and Science
Program Leader, Gastrointestinal Cancer
Mayo Clinic Cancer Center
Phoenix, Arizona

Bassel F. El-Rayes, MD
John Kauffman Family Professor for Pancreatic Cancer Research
Georgia Cancer Coalition Distinguished Scholar
Director of the Gastrointestinal Oncology Program
Vice Chair of Clinical Research, Department of Hematology and Oncology
Associate Cancer Center Director, Winship Cancer Institute
Emory University School of Medicine
Atlanta, Georgia

Timothy M. Pawlik, MD, MPH, MTS, PhD, FACS, FRACS
Professor and Chair, Department of Surgery
The Urban Meyer III and Shelley Meyer Chair for Cancer Research
Professor of Surgery, Oncology, and Health Services Management and Policy
Surgeon-in-Chief, The Ohio State University Wexner Medical Center
The Ohio State University Wexner Medical Center
Columbus, Ohio

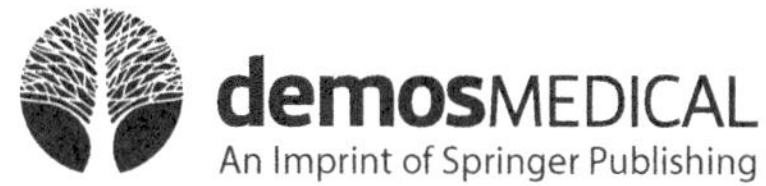

demosMEDICAL
An Imprint of Springer Publishing

Visit www.springerpub.com and http://connect.springerpub.com

ISBN: 978-0-8261-3812-5
ebook ISBN: 978-0-8261-3813-2
DOI: 10.1891/9780826138132

Acquisitions Editor: David D'Addona
Compositor: Exeter Premedia Services Private Ltd.

Medicine is an ever-changing science. Research and clinical experience are continually expanding our knowledge, in particular our understanding of proper treatment and drug therapy. The authors, editors, and publisher have made every effort to ensure that all information in this book is in accordance with the state of knowledge at the time of production of the book. Nevertheless, the authors, editors, and publisher are not responsible for errors or omissions or for any consequences from application of the information in this book and make no warranty, expressed or implied, with respect to the contents of the publication. Every reader should examine carefully the package inserts accompanying each drug and should carefully check whether the dosage schedules mentioned therein or the contraindications stated by the manufacturer differ from the statements made in this book. Such examination is particularly important with drugs that are either rarely used or have been newly released on the market.

Library of Congress Cataloging-in-Publication Data

Names: Bekaii-Saab, Tanios, editor. | El-Rayes, Bassel F., editor. | Pawlik,
    Timothy M., editor.
Title: Handbook of gastrointestinal cancers : evidence-based treatment and
    multidisciplinary patient care / editors, Tanios Bekaii-Saab, Bassel F.
    El-Rayes, Timothy M. Pawlik.
Description: New York : Springer Publishing Company, [2020] | Includes
    bibliographical references and index.
Identifiers: LCCN 2019006499 | ISBN 9780826138125 | ISBN 9780826138132 (eBook)
Subjects: | MESH: Gastrointestinal Neoplasms—therapy | Evidence-Based
    Medicine
Classification: LCC RC280.D5 | NLM WI 195 | DDC 616.99/433—dc23
LC record available at https://lccn.loc.gov/2019006499

Contact us to receive discount rates on bulk purchases.
We can also customize our books to meet your needs.
For more information please contact: sales@springerpub.com

Publisher's Note: New and used products purchased from third-party sellers are not guaranteed for quality, authenticity, or access to any included digital components.

Printed in the United States of America.
19 20 21 22 23 / 5 4 3 2 1

Contents

Contributors   *ix*
Foreword E. Christopher Ellison, MD, FACS   *xv*
Preface   *xvii*

PART I. COLORECTAL CANCER

1. Epidemiology of Colorectal Cancer   *2*
    Amit Surya Narayan, Christina Wu, and Walid L. Shaib

2. Diagnosis and Staging of Colorectal Cancer   *5*
    Amit Surya Narayan, Christina Wu, and Walid L. Shaib

3. Molecular Diagnostic Guidelines for Colorectal Cancer   *7*
    Ibrahim Halil Sahin, Walid L. Shaib, and Christina Wu

4. *How I Treat* Early-Stage Colon Cancer Through Surgery   *15*
    Mark W. Arnold

5. *How I Treat* Early-Stage Colon Cancer With Adjuvant Therapy: Who and
    How Long?   *20*
    Francesca Battaglin and Heinz-Josef Lenz

6. *How I Treat* Early-Stage Rectal Cancer With Neoadjuvant Radiation Therapy   *34*
    Nikhil Sebastian and Terence Williams

7. *How I Treat* Early-Stage Rectal Cancer Through Surgery   *45*
    Nitin Mishra

8. *How I Treat* Early-Stage Rectal Cancer With Adjuvant Therapy   *52*
    Gabriel A. Brooks

9. *How I Treat* Oligometastatic Colorectal Cancer Through Surgery   *57*
    Rory L. Smoot and David M. Nagorney

10. *How I Treat* Oligometastatic Colorectal Cancer With Neoadjuvant Chemotherapy   *62*
    Marwan Fakih

11. *How I Treat* Oligometastatic Colorectal Cancer Through Local
    Nonsurgical Approaches   *70*
    Sadeer Alzubaidi, Alex Wallace, and Rahmi Oklu

12. *How I Treat* Oligometastatic Colorectal Cancer With Adjuvant Chemotherapy   *88*
    Andrea Cercek and Gustavo dos Santos Fernandes

13. *How I Treat* Oligometastatic Colorectal Cancer With Debulking/HIPEC in Limited
    Peritoneal Disease   *95*
    Edward A. Levine

14. *How I Treat* Metastatic Colorectal Cancer With Chemotherapy and Choice
    of Biologics   *106*
    Satya Das and Kristen K. Ciombor

15. *How I Treat* Metastatic Colorectal Cancer With Maintenance Therapies   *116*
    Sakti Chakrabarti and Joleen M. Hubbard

16. *How I Treat* Metastatic Colorectal Cancer With Emerging Therapeutic Strategies   *122*
Niharika B. Mettu and John H. Strickler

17. *How I Treat* Metastatic Colorectal Cancer With Immunotherapy   *132*
Michael Lam and Shubham Pant

PART II. PANCREATIC CANCER

18. Epidemiology of Pancreatic Cancer   *142*
Mehmet Akce, Alexandra G. Lopez-Aguiar, David A. Kooby, Field F. Willingham,
Gregory B. Lesinski, and Shishir K. Maithel

19. Biological Basis for Pancreatic Cancer   *148*
Michael Brandon Ware, Mehmet Akce, Alexandra G. Lopez-Aguiar, David A. Kooby,
Field F. Willingham, Shishir K. Maithel, and Gregory B. Lesinski

20. Diagnosis and Staging of Pancreatic Cancer   *158*
Ramzi Mulki, Parit Mekaroonkamol, Alexandra G. Lopez-Aguiar, Gregory B. Lesinski,
David A. Kooby, Mehmet Akce, Shishir K. Maithel, and Field F. Willingham

21. The Role and Timing of Surgery in Pancreatic Cancer   *169*
Mark J. Truty

22. *How I Treat* Resectable Pancreatic Cancer With Adjuvant Therapy   *184*
Philip A. Philip and Mandana Kamgar

23. *How I Treat* Resectable Pancreatic Cancer With Neoadjuvant Therapy   *192*
Davendra P. S. Sohal

24. *How I Treat* Borderline Resectable and Locally Advanced Pancreatic Cancer   *198*
Hao Xie, Tanios Bekaii-Saab, and Wen Wee Ma

25. *How I Treat* Metastatic Pancreatic Cancer With Chemotherapy   *204*
Benjamin A. Krantz and Eileen M. O'Reilly

26. *How I Treat* Metastatic Pancreatic Cancer With Emerging Therapies   *210*
Benjamin A. Krantz and Eileen M. O'Reilly

PART III. HEPATOCELLULAR CANCER

27. Epidemiology of Hepatocellular Cancer   *224*
Safi Shahda and Bert H. O'Neil

28. Diagnosis and Staging of Hepatocellular Cancer   *229*
Safi Shahda and Bert H. O'Neil

29. Cellular and Molecular Pathology of Hepatocellular Cancer   *233*
Safi Shahda and Bert H. O'Neil

30. *How I Treat* Early-Stage Hepatocellular Cancer Through Transplant   *236*
Emmanouil Giorgakis and Amit K. Mathur

31. *How I Treat* Early-Stage Hepatocellular Cancer Through Surgery   *250*
Rachel M. Lee and Kenneth Cardona

32. *How I Treat* Early-Stage Hepatocellular Cancer With Local Nonsurgical
Approaches (IO)   *259*
Junaid Raja and Hyun S. Kim

33. *How I Treat* Early-Stage Hepatocellular Cancer With Local Nonsurgical
Approaches (Radiation)   *277*
Jonathan B. Ashman

34. *How I Treat* Advanced Hepatocellular Cancer With Multikinase Inhibitors and Other Targeted Therapies   ***287***
Kabir Mody and Ghassan K. Abou-Alfa

35. *How I Treat* Advanced Hepatocellular Cancer With Immunotherapy   ***295***
Olatunji B. Alese and Katerina Zakka

PART IV. GASTRIC AND ESOPHAGEAL CANCER

36. Epidemiology of Gastric and Esophageal Cancer   ***306***
Mohamad Bassam Sonbol and Daniel H. Ahn

37. Diagnosis and Staging of Gastric and Esophageal Cancer   ***309***
Mohamad Bassam Sonbol and Daniel H. Ahn

38. Molecular Diagnostic Guidelines of Gastric and Esophageal Cancer   ***311***
Mohamad Bassam Sonbol and Daniel H. Ahn

39. *How I Treat* Early-Stage Gastric and Esophageal Cancer With Neoadjuvant Therapy   ***313***
William A. Stokes and Karyn A. Goodman

40. *How I Treat* Early-Stage Gastric and Esophageal Cancer With Surgery   ***321***
Sajid A. Khan, Vadim Kurbatov, and Mitchell C. Posner

41. *How I Treat* Metastatic Gastric and Esophageal Cancer With Chemotherapy and Choice of Biologics   ***333***
Mehmet Akce

42. *How I Treat* Metastatic Gastric and Esophageal Cancer With Immunotherapy   ***343***
Curtis R. Chong and Yelena Y. Janjigian

PART V. RARE GASTROINTESTINAL CANCERS

43. Molecular Diagnostic Guidelines of Cancers of the Bile Ducts and Gallbladder   ***350***
Talal Hilal and Mitesh J. Borad

44. Surgery for Early-Stage Cancers of the Bile Ducts and Gallbladder   ***354***
Jordan Cloyd, Charlie Kimbrough, and Timothy M. Pawlik

45. Adjuvant Therapy for Early-Stage Cancers of the Bile Ducts and Gallbladder   ***369***
Flavio G. Rocha

46. Chemotherapy for Advanced Cancers of the Bile Ducts and Gallbladder   ***375***
Jonathan Whisenant

47. Emerging Therapies for Advanced Cancers of the Bile Ducts and Gallbladder   ***382***
Madappa Kundranda and Milind Javle

48. Neuroendocrine Tumors   ***394***
Jonathan Strosberg

49. Early-Stage Anal Cancer   ***407***
Clayton A. Smith, Nitesh Rana, and Lisa A. Kachnic

50. Metastatic Anal Cancer   ***418***
Saivaishnavi Kamatham, Faisal Shahjehan, and Pashtoon M. Kasi

51. Gastrointestinal Stromal Tumors   ***427***
Kantha Ratnam Kolla and Mahesh Seetharam

PART VI. SPECIAL CLINICAL CONSIDERATIONS FOR GASTROINTESTINAL CANCER PATIENTS

52. Nutritional Needs for Gastrointestinal Cancer Patients   *444*
Tiffany Barrett

53. Palliative Care for Gastrointestinal Cancer Patients   *451*
Kimberly Angelia Curseen

54. Care for Elderly Gastrointestinal Cancer Patients   *468*
Grant R. Williams and Hanna K. Sanoff

55. Survivorship Care for Gastrointestinal Cancer Patients   *476*
Nataliya V. Uboha, Mary Mulkerin, Stephanie L. Fricke, and Noelle K. LoConte

Index   485

Contributors

Ghassan K. Abou-Alfa, MD, Medical Oncologist, Gastrointestinal Oncology, Memorial Sloan Kettering Cancer Center, New York, New York

Daniel H. Ahn, DO, Assistant Professor of Medicine, Hematology/Oncology, Department of Internal Medicine, Mayo Clinic, Phoenix, Arizona

Olatunji B. Alese, MD, Assistant Professor, Department of Hematology and Medical Oncology, Winship Cancer Institute of Emory University, Atlanta, Georgia

Sadeer Alzubaidi, MD, Assistant Professor of Radiology, Interventional Radiology, Department of Radiology, Mayo Clinic, Phoenix, Arizona

Mehmet Akce, MD, Assistant Professor, Department of Hematology and Medical Oncology, Winship Cancer Institute of Emory University, Atlanta, Georgia

Mark W. Arnold, MD, Professor of Clinical Surgery, Department of Surgery, The Ohio State University Wexner Medical Center, Columbus, Ohio

Jonathan B. Ashman, MD, PhD, Consultant, Department of Radiation Oncology; Assistant Professor, Mayo College of Medicine and Science, Phoenix, Arizona

Tiffany Barrett, MS, RD, CSO, LD, Clinical Dietitian, Department of Hematology and Medical Oncology, Winship Cancer Institute of Emory University, Atlanta, Georgia

Francesca Battaglin, MD, Post-Doctoral Fellow, Division of Medical Oncology, USC/Norris Comprehensive Cancer Center, Los Angeles, California; Medical Oncologist, Veneto Institute of Oncology IOV-IRCCS, Padua, Italy

Tanios Bekaii-Saab, MD, FACP, Professor, Mayo Clinic College of Medicine and Science; Program Leader, Gastrointestinal Cancer, Mayo Clinic Cancer Center, Phoenix, Arizona

Mitesh J. Borad, MD, Associate Professor of Medicine, Division of Hematology/Oncology, Mayo Clinic, Phoenix, Arizona

Gabriel A. Brooks, MD, MPH, Assistant Professor of Medicine, Division of Medical Oncology, Department of Medicine, Geisel School of Medicine, Hanover, New Hampshire

Kenneth Cardona, MD, FACS, Associate Professor of Surgery, Division of Surgical Oncology, Department of Surgery, Winship Cancer Institute of Emory University, Atlanta, Georgia

Andrea Cercek, MD, Medical Oncologist, Gastrointestinal Oncology Service, Division of Solid Tumor Oncology, Memorial Sloan Kettering Cancer Center, New York, New York

Sakti Chakrabarti, MD, MBBS, Advanced Oncology Fellow, Department of Medical Oncology, Mayo Clinic, Rochester, Minnesota

Curtis R. Chong, MD, PhD, Medical Oncologist, Department of Medical Oncology, Memorial Sloan Kettering Cancer Center, New York, New York

Kristen K. Ciombor, MD, MSCI, Assistant Professor, Division of Hematology/Oncology, Department of Internal Medicine, Vanderbilt University Medical Center, Nashville, Tennessee

Jordan Cloyd, MD, Assistant Professor of Surgery, Division of Surgical Oncology, The Ohio State University Wexner Medical Center, Columbus, Ohio

Kimberly Angelia Curseen, MD, Director of Outpatient Supportive Care Emory Health Care, Emory University School of Medicine, Atlanta, Georgia

Satya Das, MD, Clinical Instructor, Division of Hematology/Oncology, Department of Internal Medicine, Vanderbilt University Medical Center, Nashville, Tennessee

Gustavo dos Santos Fernandes, MD, Fellow, Gastrointestinal Oncology Service, Division of Solid Tumor Oncology, Memorial Sloan Kettering Cancer Center, New York, New York

Marwan Fakih, MD, Professor, Section Head of Gastrointestinal Oncology, City of Hope Comprehensive Cancer Center, Duarte, California

Stephanie L. Fricke, MD, Resident, Department of Medicine, University of Wisconsin, Madison, Wisconsin

Emmanouil Giorgakis, MD, MSc, FEBS, Assistant Professor of Surgery, Division of Transplantation, University of Arkansas for Medical Sciences, Little Rock, Arkansas

Karyn A. Goodman, MD, MS, Professor, Department of Radiation Oncology, University of Colorado Denver, Aurora, Colorado

Talal Hilal, MD, Assistant Professor of Medicine, Division of Hematology/Oncology, Mayo Clinic, Phoenix, Arizona

Joleen M. Hubbard, MD, Associate Professor of Oncology, Department of Medical Oncology, Mayo Clinic, Rochester, Minnesota

Yelena Y. Janjigian, MD, Medical Oncologist, Chief, Gastrointestinal Oncology Service, Department of Medical Oncology, Memorial Sloan Kettering Cancer Center, New York, New York

Milind Javle, MD, Professor, Department of Gastrointestinal Medical Oncology, University of Texas MD Anderson Cancer Center, Houston, Texas

Lisa A. Kachnic, MD, Chair and Professor, Department of Radiation Oncology, Vanderbilt University Medical Center, Nashville, Tennessee

Saivaishnavi Kamatham, MBBS, Visiting Research Fellow, Division of Hematology/Oncology, Mayo Clinic, Jacksonville, Florida

Mandana Kamgar, MD, MPH, Hematology/Oncology Fellow, Department of Oncology, Wayne State University School of Medicine, Barbara Ann Karmanos Cancer Institute, Detroit, Michigan

Pashtoon M. Kasi, MD, MS, Clinical Assistant Professor, Internal Medicine-Hematology/Oncology, Holden Comprehensive Cancer Center, University of Iowa Health Care, Iowa City, Iowa

Sajid A. Khan, MD, FACS, Assistant Professor of Surgery (Oncology), Section of Surgical Oncology, Yale University School of Medicine, New Haven, Connecticut

Hyun S. Kim, MD, Professor of Radiology and Biomedical Imaging, Section Chief of Interventional Radiology; Professor of Internal Medicine (Medical Oncology), Department of Radiology and Biomedical Imaging, Yale Cancer Center, Yale University School of Medicine, New Haven, Connecticut

Charlie Kimbrough, MD, Clinical Fellow, Division of Surgical Oncology, The Ohio State University Wexner Medical Center, Columbus, Ohio

Kantha Ratnam Kolla, MBBS, MPH, Department of Medicine, University of Maryland-Prince George's Hospital, Cheverly, Maryland

David A. Kooby, MD, Professor of Surgery, Department of Surgery, Emory University School of Medicine, Atlanta, Georgia

Benjamin A. Krantz, MD, MBA, Clinical Fellow, Division of Hematology and Medical Oncology, New York University Langone Health, New York, New York

Madappa Kundranda, MD, PhD, Director, Gastrointestinal Oncology Program; Deputy Chief, Division of Medical Oncology; Adjunct Assistant Professor, Department of Gastrointestinal Medical Oncology, University of Texas MD Anderson Cancer Center, Banner MD Anderson, Gilbert, Arizona

Vadim Kurbatov, MD, General Surgery Resident, Research Fellow, Section of Surgical Oncology, Yale University School of Medicine, New Haven, Connecticut

Michael Lam, MBBS, Post-Doctoral Fellow, Department of Gastrointestinal Medical Oncology, University of Texas MD Anderson Cancer Center, Houston, Texas

Rachel M. Lee, MD, MSPH, Resident Physician, Department of Surgery, Emory University School of Medicine, Atlanta, Georgia

Heinz-Josef Lenz, MD, FACP, Professor of Medicine and Preventive Medicine; J. Terrence Lanni Chair for Cancer Research; Associate Director, Adult Oncology; Scientific Director, Cancer Genetics Unit, Division of Medical Oncology, USC/Norris Comprehensive Cancer Center, Los Angeles, California

Gregory B. Lesinski, PhD, MPH, Associate Professor, Department of Hematology and Medical Oncology; Co-Director, Translational GI Malignancy Program, Winship Cancer Institute of Emory University, Atlanta, Georgia

Edward A. Levine, MD, Professor of Surgery, Chief, Surgical Oncology, Wake Forest University, Winston-Salem, North Carolina

Noelle K. LoConte, MD, Associate Professor, Department of Medicine, University of Wisconsin, Madison, Wisconsin

Alexandra G. Lopez-Aguiar, MD, Post-Doctoral Research Fellow, Division of Surgical Oncology, Department of Surgery, Emory University School of Medicine, Atlanta, Georgia

Wen Wee Ma, MBBS, Professor of Oncology, Department of Oncology, Mayo Clinic, Rochester, Minnesota

Shishir K. Maithel, MD, Professor of Surgery, Division of Surgical Oncology, Department of Surgery, Emory University School of Medicine, Atlanta, Georgia

Amit K. Mathur, MD, MS, FACS, Associate Professor of Surgery, Mayo Clinic Alix School of Medicine; Consultant, Division of Transplant Surgery, Mayo Clinic, Phoenix, Arizona

Parit Mekaroonkamol, MD, Assistant Professor, Department of Internal Medicine, Division of Digestive Diseases, Emory University School of Medicine, Atlanta, Georgia; Assistant Professor, Division of Gastroenterology, Faculty of Medicine, Chulalongkorn University and King Chulalongkorn Memorial Hospital, Thai Red Cross Society, Bangkok, Thailand

Niharika B. Mettu, MD, PhD, Assistant Professor, Department of Medicine, Division of Medical Oncology, Duke University Medical Center, Durham, North Carolina

Nitin Mishra, MS, MPH, MBBS, Assistant Professor of Surgery, Department of Colon and Rectal Surgery, Mayo Clinic School of Medicine, Phoenix, Arizona

Kabir Mody, MD, Consultant, Department of Oncology (Medical), Mayo Clinic Cancer Center, Jacksonville, Florida

Mary Mulkerin, MS, RN, OCN, Gastrointestinal Oncology Nurse Coordinator, University of Wisconsin Hospital and Clinics, Madison, Wisconsin

Ramzi Mulki, MD, Clinical Fellow, Department of Internal Medicine, Division of Digestive Diseases, Emory University School of Medicine, Atlanta, Georgia

David M. Nagorney, MD, Professor of Surgery, Division of Hepatobiliary and Pancreas Surgery, Mayo Clinic, Rochester, Minnesota

Amit Surya Narayan, MD, Resident Physician, Department of Internal Medicine, Emory University School of Medicine, Atlanta, Georgia

Rahmi Oklu, MD, PhD, Interventional Radiologist, Senior Associate Consultant, Department of Radiology, Mayo Clinic, Phoenix, Arizona

Bert H. O'Neil, MD, Joseph W. and Jackie J. Cusick Professor of Oncology, Division of Hematology/Oncology, Indiana University School of Medicine, Indianapolis, Indiana

Eileen M. O'Reilly, MD, Attending/Member, Department of Medicine; Professor of Medicine, Memorial Sloan Kettering Cancer Center, New York, New York

Shubham Pant, MD, Associate Medical Director, Associate Professor, Department of Investigational Cancer Therapeutics/Department of Gastrointestinal Medical Oncology, University of Texas MD Anderson Cancer Center, Houston, Texas

Timothy M. Pawlik, MD, MPH, MTS, PhD, FACS, FRACS, Professor and Chair, Department of Surgery, The Urban Meyer III and Shelley Meyer Chair for Cancer Research; Professor of Surgery, Oncology, and Health Services Management and Policy, The Ohio State University Wexner Medical Center, Columbus, Ohio

Philip A. Philip, MD, PhD, FRCP, Professor of Oncology, Department of Oncology, Wayne State University School of Medicine, Barbara Ann Karmanos Cancer Institute, Detroit, Michigan

Mitchell C. Posner, MD, FACS, Professor of Surgery and Vice-Chairman, Chief, Section of General Surgery and Surgical Oncology; Physician-in-Chief, University of Chicago Medicine Comprehensive Cancer Center; Professor, Radiation and Cellular Oncology, University of Chicago Medicine, Chicago, Illinois

Junaid Raja, MD, MSPH, MS, Resident Physician, Section of Interventional Radiology, Department of Radiology and Biomedical Imaging, Yale University School of Medicine, New Haven, Connecticut

Nitesh Rana, MD, MS, Resident Physician, Department of Radiation Oncology, Vanderbilt University Medical Center, Nashville, Tennessee

Flavio G. Rocha, MD, FACS, Associate Medical Director, Cancer Institute, Virginia Mason Medical Center, Seattle, Washington

Ibrahim Halil Sahin, MD, Hematology/Oncology Fellow, Department of Hematology/Oncology, Winship Cancer Institute of Emory University, Atlanta, Georgia

Hanna K. Sanoff, MD, MPH, Associate Professor, Division of Hematology/Oncology, UNC Lineberger Clinical Cancer Center, University of North Carolina at Chapel Hill, Chapel Hill, North Carolina

Nikhil Sebastian, MD, Resident Physician, Department of Radiation Oncology, The Ohio State University Wexner Medical Center, Columbus, Ohio

Mahesh Seetharam, MD, FACP, Assistant Professor, Medical Oncology; Associate Director, Early Cancer Therapeutics Program, Mayo Clinic, Phoenix, Arizona

Safi Shahda, MD, Assistant Professor of Clinical Medicine, Division of Hematology/Oncology, Indiana University School of Medicine, Indianapolis, Indiana

Faisal Shahjehan, MBBS, Research Trainee, Division of Hematology/Oncology, Mayo Clinic, Jacksonville, Florida

Walid L. Shaib, MD, Assistant Professor, Hematology and Oncology Department, Winship Cancer Institute of Emory University, Atlanta, Georgia

Clayton A. Smith, MD, PhD, Assistant Professor, Division of Radiation Oncology, University of South Alabama Mitchell Cancer Institute, Mobile, Alabama

Rory L. Smoot, MD, Assistant Professor of Surgery, Division of Hepatobiliary and Pancreas Surgery, Mayo Clinic, Rochester, Minnesota

Davendra P. S. Sohal, MD, MPH, Associate Professor of Medicine, Staff, Hematology and Medical Oncology; Director, Clinical Genomics Program, Taussig Cancer Institute, Cleveland Clinic, Cleveland, Ohio

Mohamad Bassam Sonbol, MD, Hematology/Oncology Fellow, Department of Internal Medicine, Mayo Clinic, Phoenix, Arizona

William A. Stokes, MD, Resident, Department of Radiation Oncology, University of Colorado Denver, Aurora, Colorado

John H. Strickler, MD, Assistant Professor, Department of Medicine, Division of Medical Oncology, Duke University Medical Center, Durham, North Carolina

Jonathan Strosberg, MD, Associate Professor, Department of Gastrointestinal Oncology, H. Lee Moffitt Cancer Center and Research Institute, Tampa, Florida

Mark J. Truty, MD, MSc, FACS, Practice Chair, Department of Hepatobiliary and Pancreatic Surgery, Mayo Clinic College of Medicine, Rochester, Minnesota

Nataliya V. Uboha, MD, PhD, Assistant Professor (CHS), Department of Medicine, University of Wisconsin, Madison, Wisconsin

Alex Wallace, MD, Radiology Resident, Department of Radiology, Mayo Clinic, Phoenix, Arizona

Michael Brandon Ware, BS, Graduate Researcher, Department of Cancer Biology, Emory University School of Medicine, Atlanta, Georgia

Jonathan Whisenant, MD, Associate Professor, Internal Medical, Huntsman Cancer Institute, Salt Lake City, Utah

Grant R. Williams, MD, Assistant Professor, Divisions of Hematology/Oncology and Gerontology, Geriatrics, and Palliative Care, Institute of Cancer Outcomes and Survivorship, University of Alabama at Birmingham, Birmingham, Alabama

Terence Williams, MD, PhD, Associate Professor, Department of Radiation Oncology, The Ohio State University Wexner Medical Center, Columbus, Ohio

Field F. Willingham, MD, MPH, Associate Professor, Department of Internal Medicine, Division of Digestive Diseases, Emory University School of Medicine, Atlanta, Georgia

Christina Wu, MD, Associate Professor, Hematology and Oncology Department, Winship Cancer Institute of Emory University, Atlanta, Georgia

Hao Xie, MD, PhD, Instructor of Oncology, Department of Oncology, Mayo Clinic, Rochester, Minnesota

Katerina Zakka, MD, Post-Doctoral Research Fellow, Department of Hematology and Medical Oncology, Winship Cancer Institute of Emory University, Atlanta, Georgia

Foreword

Management of gastrointestinal cancers has evolved substantially in the past 30 years. In particular, care today is even more evidence-based and multidisciplinary. No longer is a single physician able to care for these complex cancers. It requires a team of experts in epidemiology, genetics, molecular biology, imaging, chemotherapy, and immunotherapy with access to emerging therapies. Care must focus on the specific biologic and molecular characteristics of the neoplasm. In addition, care must concentrate on the personalized needs of each patient: addressing nutrition during various phases of treatment and managing survivorship in addition to the unique needs of elderly patients with cancer, such as palliative care and end-of-life issues.

The editors and contributors are a team of physicians from top cancer centers and include experts in all facets of care for gastrointestinal cancer. This book is appropriate for physicians in all specialties as well as primary care physicians and other healthcare professionals who are essential members of any team caring for the patient with gastrointestinal cancer. The book begins with the most common of the gastrointestinal cancers, colon and rectal cancer, followed by pancreatic, hepatocellular, esophageal, and gastric cancer, cancer of the bile ducts and gallbladder, and then the more rare and unusual cancers such as gastrointestinal stromal tumors, neuroendocrine tumors, and anal carcinoma. In each of these sections, the authors use evidence-based guidelines for the specific cancer to focus on epidemiology and biologic aspects of the disease, including genetic factors and molecular biology. Chapters also discuss modifiable factors, diagnostic testing, and techniques consisting of the molecular basis of diagnosis and treatment of early and advanced disease, which incorporates the role of surgery, neoadjuvant and adjuvant chemotherapy, radiation therapy, immunotherapy, and biologics and their selection and ablative techniques. The presentation seen here is very helpful and unique in that the authors approach advanced disease as oligometastatic and widely metastatic and account for how these approaches differ. In the last chapters, the clinician will find cogent information on nutrition and survivorship in combination with special considerations for the geriatric patient, palliative care, and end-of-life issues. The latter chapters may be of particular value for primary care physicians or nurse practitioners who coordinate care during various phases of cancer treatment. The book also features representative clinical vignettes that emphasize and illustrate the major points concerning the treatment of each cancer.

In short, this is an excellent resource for inexperienced or experienced medical oncologists, surgeons, and radiation oncologists. I have no doubt that it will be of value for primary care physicians and other members of the care team in the comanagement of the patient with gastrointestinal cancer.

E. Christopher Ellison, MD, FACS
Robert M. Zollinger Professor Emeritus
Department of Surgery
Academy Professor
The Ohio State University
Columbus, Ohio

Preface

The treatment of gastrointestinal cancers involves multiple disciplines, different therapeutic modalities, and emerging novel treatment regimens. In fact, gastrointestinal cancers and their treatment have witnessed many changes in this past decade. In particular, progress in imaging techniques as well as diagnostic tools has improved the manner in which gastrointestinal cancers are identified, characterized, and staged. Innovations in therapeutics—including advances in the field of medical oncology, radiotherapeutics, and operative management—have reshaped the way these diseases are managed. A better understanding of the molecular underpinnings of gastrointestinal cancers has allowed for more targeted therapy, refinements in prognostication, and the ability to target specific mutations to individualize treatment strategies. As systemic therapy for gastrointestinal cancers has expanded, the number of patients who may be candidates for surgical resection has similarly grown. In the face of an ongoing explosion of information around gastrointestinal cancers, medical professionals are constantly challenged to understand how best to apply this knowledge to important clinical questions. As such, the purpose of this handbook is to create a practical guide for trainees, nurse practitioners, physician assistants, and attending physicians to guide them in the treatment of patients with gastrointestinal cancers. The handbook provides key information on diagnosis and treatment, while highlighting the epidemiology, molecular data, and additionally various multimodality treatment options for a broad array of gastrointestinal cancers. It is concise and easy to read, yet broad and practical in its ability to provide for the needs of the medical professional dealing with gastrointestinal cancers. Unique to the book are "How I Treat" vignettes providing not only standards of care but expert recommendations for approaching tough-to-treat disease sites and, in some cases, rare or uncommon patient scenarios. The *Handbook of Gastrointestinal Cancers* represents the hard work and effort of many trainees working with the guidance of faculty physicians at world-renowned cancer centers throughout the country. We would like to thank our colleagues throughout the country and world who contributed their effort and expertise to make this handbook a success. Finally, we extend our sincere appreciation to all of our patients who always teach us some of the most important lessons about the diseases we work so hard to treat.

Tanios Bekaii-Saab
Bassel F. El-Rayes
Timothy M. Pawlik

I

Colorectal Cancer

Epidemiology of Colorectal Cancer

Amit Surya Narayan, Christina Wu, and Walid L. Shaib

Colorectal cancer (CRC) remains one of the most common cancers in both men and women, with an estimated 97,220 colon cancers and 43,030 rectal cancers diagnosed each year in the United States alone (1). The incidence rates for new CRC cases have been dropping by approximately 2.7% per year over the past decade (2). The overall 5-year mortality of CRC is about 35%, and it is currently the second-leading cause of mortality from cancer in the United States (2). The mortality from CRC has, however, declined by about 52% over the past five decades to about 50,630 Americans (about 8% of all cancer-related deaths) (1). The trends of highest increase in incidence happened between 1975 and the mid-80s with a decrease in incidence till 2005. This was attributed to a decrease in smoking. The steep decrease in incidence happened between 2004 and 2013, and that was attributed to the increase in screening rates with the removal of precancerous lesions. In 2009, Kahi et al. showed that colonoscopy screening reduced CRC incidence by 67% over a 15-year average follow-up as compared to the general population (3). The prospective Nurses Heath Study and the Health Professional Follow-Up Study showed a relative risk of 0.32, which equated to a 68% reduction in overall CRC mortality, for patients who received colonoscopy as compared to the general population (4). Another multicenter, long-term, colonoscopy-based cohort study similarly found that the CRC mortality of patients who received colonoscopy screening decreased significantly compared with that of individuals in the general population (5).

The incidence and mortality rates of CRC are higher in men than women; these are at rates of 30% and 40%, respectively. The numbers for colon cancer are essentially equal in men (47,700) and women (47,820), but a larger number of men (23,720) than women (16,190) are diagnosed with rectal cancer. The reason for this gender disparity is unknown (6). Studies relating estrogen levels and exposure have been contradictory with regard to it being protective against CRC (7,8). Other risk factors are attributed to the increase in incidence is smoking, which is higher in men (6).

There is a higher incidence in African Americans (AAs) than in other populations. The risk of CRC for AAs is 20% higher than non-Hispanics and 40% higher than Asians. The mortality rates for AAs are 40% higher than non-Hispanics and are doubled when compared to Asians. This disparity is also not well-studied but has been attributed to socioeconomic status where 25% of AAs live in poverty (9), lower education (10), and a higher prevalence of smoking and obesity in this population (11). This disparity could also be attributed to a lack of utility access to healthcare for the AA population, which is related to other risk factors such as suboptimal screening, poor nutrition (e.g., low-fiber diet), high obesity rates, and higher risk social behaviors such as smoking, alcohol, or drug abuse (12–16).

Other risk factors of CRC include age, genetics, and high-risk behaviors. The median age at diagnosis of CRC is 67 years old with about 24% of new cases diagnosed between ages 65 and 74 (2); however, 37% of cases are diagnosed between ages 45 and 64. Prior to age 40, the incidence of CRC is relatively low but alarmingly rising at approximately 2% annually from 1992 through 2013 (17). The CRC death rates in adults younger than 50 years of age are increasing by about 1% per year from 2005 to 2014 (18). The precise reason for this rise remains under investigation. Speculation of this increase in incidence in the younger age group could be related to the sedentary lifestyle and eating habits in children and young adults (19).

Up to 30% of CRC patients have a family history of the disease, about 5% of whom have an inherited genetic abnormality (20). Familial syndromes represent about 20% of young-onset CRCs (21). The genetics of CRC is a complex field of study that continues to be a topic of research. In addition to syndromes such as familial adenomatous polyposis (FAP) and hereditary nonpolyposis colon cancer (HNPCC), there are several pathogenic mutations (e.g., APC gene, BRCA, CDK) that can predispose patients to CRC (22).

Aside from age, gender, race, and familial cancers, many of the known risk factors for CRC are behavioral and include sedentary lifestyle, Western diet, and smoking. The relationship between CRC and Western diet is strong (23). People living in high-income countries who have a healthy lifestyle have a lower CRC risk. A recent study found a direct reduced risk of CRC to more than a third in people maintaining a healthy weight, physically active, limiting alcohol consumption, and eating healthy diets (24). People who are physically active are at a 25% reduced risk of developing CRC as compared to the least active people (25). Obesity increases the risk of CRC, with a stronger association in men. Obese men have about a 50% higher risk of colon cancer and a 20% higher risk of rectal cancer, whereas obese women have about a 20% increased risk of colon cancer and a 10% increased risk of rectal cancer when compared to their normal weight counterparts (26). There is also a growing interest of the microbiome composition in people with different diets. This has been shown to have a direct effect on the immune and inflammatory responses of the large intestine. This is difficult to account for given the diverse ways of documenting types of food consumed by people (27). Calcium supplementation is associated with decreased risk of adenomas (28). High fiber intake leads to decreased exposure to carcinogens because of high stool volumes and increased transit times, but this remains inconclusive although advisable. Folate consumption is also inconclusive with regard to increased CRC risk (28,29). It is thought to promote growth of preexisting tumors but prevent tumor formation in normal colonic tissue (28). Higher blood levels of vitamin D may be associated with lower risk of CRC, although study results remain inconclusive (28,30). Tobacco smoking causes CRC; risk is higher for rectal than colon cancer (31). Moderate and heavy alcohol use, but not light drinking (<12.5 grams per day, about one drink), is associated with increased risk of CRC (32).

CRC remains one of the most common and lethal cancers today. While the overall incidence and mortality rates have been decreasing over the past several years, it still carries a heavy burden. This decrease in mortality and incidence has been attributed to early screening recommendations at the age of 50 years. The incidence and mortality rates in young adults <50 years of age have been on the rise. This raises the question of whether screening should be initiated before the age of 50. Awareness and lifestyle changes are modifiable factors that should play a significant role in improving the incidence and mortality rates in this disease. There is growing interest in improving methods for screening high-risk individuals and families at risk. This may be a large potential for not only CRC prevention and early detection, but also for other cancers associated with these familial diseases. Screening is very effective in increasing cure rates and decreasing mortality; thus strategies to overcome barriers to screening should be developed for better outcomes.

REFERENCES

1. Siegel RL, Miller KD, Jemal A. Cancer statistics, 2018. *CA Cancer J Clin*. 2018;68(1):7–30. doi:10.3322/caac.21442
2. Howlader N, Noone AM, Krapcho M, et al., eds. *SEER Cancer Statistics Review, 1975-2014*. Bethesda, MD: National Cancer Institute. https://seer.cancer.gov/csr/1975_2014
3. Kahi CJ, Imperiale TF, Juliar BE, et al. Effect of screening colonoscopy on colorectal cancer incidence and mortality. *Clin Gastroenterol Hepatol*. 2009;7(7):770–775; quiz 711. doi:10.1016/j. cgh.2008.12.030
4. Nishihara R, Wu K, Lochhead P, et al. Long-term colorectal-cancer incidence and mortality after lower endoscopy. *N Engl J Med*. 2013;369(12):1095–1105. doi:10.1056/NEJMoa1301969
5. Niikura R, Hirata Y, Suzuki N, et al. Colonoscopy reduces colorectal cancer mortality: a multicenter, long-term, colonoscopy-based cohort. *PLoS One*. 2017;12(9):e0185294. doi:10.1371/journal.pone.0185294. eCollection 2017.
6. Murphy G, Devesa SS, Cross AJ, et al. Sex disparities in colorectal cancer incidence by anatomic subsite, race and age. *Int J Cancer*. 2011;128(7):1668–1675. doi:10.1002/ijc.25481
7. Murphy N, Strickler HD, Stanczyk FZ, et al. A prospective evaluation of endogenous sex hormone levels and colorectal cancer risk in postmenopausal women. *J Natl Cancer Inst*. 2015;107(10):djv210. doi:10.1093/jnci/djv210
8. Gunter MJ, Hoover DR, Yu H, et al. Insulin, insulin-like growth factor-I, endogenous estradiol, and risk of colorectal cancer in postmenopausal women. *Cancer Res*. 2008;68(1):329–337. doi:10.1158/0008-5472.CAN-07-2946
9. Proctor BD, Semega J, Kollar MA. *Income and Poverty in the United States: 2015*. U.S. Government Printing Office, Washington, DC: U.S. Census Bureau, 2016.

10. Doubeni CA, Laiyemo AO, Major JM, et al. Socioeconomic status and the risk of colorectal cancer: an analysis of more than a half million adults in the National Institutes of Health-AARP Diet and Health Study. *Cancer*. 2012;118(14):3636–3644. doi:10.1002/cncr.26677

11. Doubeni, CA, Major JM, Laiyemo AO, et al. Contribution of behavioral risk factors and obesity to socioeconomic differences in colorectal cancer incidence. *J Natl Cancer Inst*. 2012;104(18):1353–1362. doi:10.1093/jnci/djs346

12. Williams R, White P, Nieto J, et al., Colorectal cancer in African Americans: an update. *Clin Transl Gastroenterol*. 2016;7(7):e185. doi:10.1038/ctg.2016.36

13. Jepson C, Kessler LG, Portnoy B, et al. Black-white differences in cancer prevention knowledge and behavior. *Am J Public Health*. 1991;81(4):501–504. doi:10.2105/AJPH.81.4.501

14. Ioannou GN, Chapko MK, Dominitz JA. Predictors of colorectal cancer screening participation in the United States. *Am J Gastroenterol*. 2003;98(9):2082–2091. doi:10.1111/j.1572-0241.2003.07574.x

15. Kauh J, Brawley OW, Berger M. Racial disparities in colorectal cancer. *Curr Probl Cancer*. 2007;31(3):123–133. doi:10.1016/j.currproblcancer.2007.01.002

16. Tammana VS, Laiyemo AO. Colorectal cancer disparities: issues, controversies and solutions. *World J Gastroenterol*. 2014;20(4):869–876. doi:10.3748/wjg.v20.i4.869

17. Surveillance, Epidemiology, and End Results (SEER) Program. *SEER*Stat database: Incidence-SEER 9 Regs Research Data with Delay-adjustment, Malignant Only, Nov 2015 Sub (1975-2013), Katrina/Rita Population Adjustment.-Linked To County Attributes-Total US, 1969-2014 Counties*. Bethesda, MD: National Cancer Institute, Division of Cancer Control and Population Sciences, Surveillance Research Program, Surveillance Systems Branch; 2016. https://seer.cancer.gov/data/seerstat/nov2015

18. Bhandari A, Woodhouse M, Gupta S. Colorectal cancer is a leading cause of cancer incidence and mortality among adults younger than 50 years in the USA: a SEER-based analysis with comparison to other young-onset cancers. *J Investig Med*. 2017;65(2):311–315. doi:10.1136/jim-2016-000229

19. Siegel RL, Jemal A, Ward EM. Increase in incidence of colorectal cancer among young men and women in the United States. *Cancer Epidemiol Biomarkers Prev*. 2009;18(6):1695–1698. doi:10.1158/1055-9965.EPI-09-0186

20. Patel SG, Ahnen DJ. Familial colon cancer syndromes: an update of a rapidly evolving field. *Curr Gastroenterol Rep*. 2012;14(5):428–438. doi:10.1007/s11894-012-0280-6

21. Wender R, Smith R, et al. *Colon Cancer Rising Among Young Adults*. American Cancer Society; 2018. www.cancer.org/cancer/news/news/colon-cancer-cases-rising-among-young-adults

22. Yurgelun MB, Kulke MH, Fuchs CS, et al. Cancer susceptibility gene mutations in individuals with colorectal cancer. *J Clin Oncol*. 2017;35(10):1086–1095. doi:10.1200/JCO.2016.71.0012

23. Arnold M, Sierra MS, Laversanne M, et al. Global patterns and trends in colorectal cancer incidence and mortality. *Gut*. 2017;66(4):683–691. doi:10.1136/gutjnl-2015-310912

24. Aleksandrova K, Pischon T, Jenab M, et al. Combined impact of healthy lifestyle factors on colorectal cancer: a large European cohort study. *BMC Med*. 2014;12:168. doi:10.1186/s12916-014-0168-4

25. Boyle T, Keegel T, Bull F, et al. Physical activity and risks of proximal and distal colon cancers: a systematic review and meta-analysis. *J Natl Cancer Inst*. 2012;104(20):1548–1561. doi:10.1093/jnci/djs354

26. Ma Y, Yang Y, Wang F, et al. Obesity and risk of colorectal cancer: a systematic review of prospective studies. *PLoS One*. 2013;8(1):e53916. doi:10.1371/journal.pone.0053916

27. Brennan CA, Garrett WS. Gut microbiota, inflammation, and colorectal cancer. *Annu Rev Microbiol*. 2016;70:395–411. doi:10.1146/annurev-micro-102215-095513

28. Song M, Garrett WS, Chan AT. Nutrients, foods, and colorectal cancer prevention. *Gastroenterology*. 2015;148(6):1244–1260.e16. doi:10.1053/j.gastro.2014.12.035

29. Velicer CM, Ulrich CM. Vitamin and mineral supplement use among US adults after cancer diagnosis: a systematic review. *J Clin Oncol*. 2008;26(4):665–673. doi:10.1200/JCO.2007.13.5905

30. Baron JA, Barry EL, Mott LA, et al. A trial of calcium and vitamin D for the prevention of colorectal adenomas. *N Engl J Med*. 2015;373(16):1519–1530. doi:10.1056/NEJMoa1500409

31. Secretan B, Straif K, Baan R, et al. A review of human carcinogensPart E: tobacco, areca nut, alcohol, coal smoke, and salted fish. *Lancet Oncol*. 2009;10(11):1033–1034. doi:10.1016/S1470-2045(09)70326-2

32. Bagnardi V, Rota M, Botteri E, et al. Light alcohol drinking and cancer: a meta-analysis. *Ann Oncol*. 2013;24(2):301–308. doi:10.1093/annonc/mds337

Diagnosis and Staging of Colorectal Cancer

Amit Surya Narayan, Christina Wu, and Walid L Shaib

INTRODUCTION

The presenting symptoms of colorectal cancer (CRC) can be the following:

1. Acute symptoms of bleeding, perforation, peritonitis, and/or obstruction
2. No symptoms; diagnosis detected at the time of screening through colonoscopy, fecal occult blood test (FOBT), and other screening modalities
3. Abdominal pain, weakness or fatigue from anemia, change in bowel habits, and change in caliber or color of stools

Once the diagnosis of CRC is established through biopsy, usually obtained at the time of colonoscopy, the local and distant extent of disease must be determined by imaging. For colon cancer, other than T1 disease, the staging is determined after surgical resection to evaluate the status of the T (extent of tumor invasion) and the N (lymph node involvement depends on the number of lymph nodes sampled and cancer involvement) stage. For rectal cancers, staging depends on imaging (MRI or endoscopic rectal ultrasound). Distant metastasis (M) is determined by radiographic imaging of the chest, abdomen, and pelvis.

STAGE DISTRIBUTION AND CANCER SURVIVAL

The relative survival rate for CRC is 65% at 5 years following diagnosis (1). Only 39% of CRC patients are diagnosed with local stage; the 5-year survival rate is 90%. The 5-year survival rate declines to 71% for patients with regional stage and 14% for distant stage disease. More localized stage rectal cancer is diagnosed at presentation than colon cancer (43% vs. 38%). This is likely due to early symptoms of the rectal cancer. Because of this, the overall 5-year relative survival rate is slightly higher for rectal cancer (67%) when compared to colon cancer (64%) (1).

The staging system that is utilized in the United States is the tumor, node, and metastasis (TNM) staging system of American Joint Committee on Cancer (AJCC)/Union for International Cancer Control (UICC; 8th edition, 2017) (2). The T stage is based on tumor invasion into the colonic wall: Tis (carcinoma in situ) is an intramucosal carcinoma (involvement of lamina propria with no extension through muscularis mucosa); T1 is the invasion into the submucosa; T2 involves the muscularis propria; T3 invades into the pericolorectal tissue; T4 is divided into T4a (tumor invades through the visceral peritoneum, including gross perforation of the bowel through tumor and continuous invasion of tumor through areas of inflammation to the surface of the visceral peritoneum) and T4b (tumor directly invades or adheres to adjacent organs or structures). The N stage is the number of lymph nodes invaded by cancer. The N stage separates stage II (N_0) from stage III (N_{1-2}) disease regardless of the T stage. N1 is cancer involvement in 1 to 3 nodes, N2a in 4 to 6 nodes, and N2b in >7 nodes. The M stage is defined by the presence (stage IV) or absence of distant metastasis.

REFERENCES

1. Surveillance, Epidemiology, and End Results (SEER) Program. *SEER*Stat Database: Incidence-SEER 9 Regs Research Data with Delay-Adjustment, Malignant Only, Nov 2015 Sub (1975-2013), Katrina/Rita Population Adjustment.-Linked to County Attributes-Total US, 1969-2014 Counties.*

Bethesda, MD: National Cancer Institute, Division of Cancer Control and Population Sciences, Surveillance Research Program, Surveillance Systems Branch; 2016. https://seer.cancer.gov/data/seerstat/nov2015

2. The American College of Surgeons. *The original source for this information is the AJCC Cancer Staging Manual, Eighth Edition*. New York, NY: Springer International Publishing; 2017.

Molecular Diagnostic Guidelines for Colorectal Cancer

Ibrahim Halil Sahin, Walid L. Shaib, and Christina Wu

INTRODUCTION

Germline and somatic mutations play a key role in the development of cancers. Knowledge of these pathways has created new opportunities for targeted treatments. Precision medicine has helped in the characterization of genetic alterations that are actionable and has resulted in improved clinical responses and survival outcomes for patients with colorectal cancer (CRC). In this section, we discuss the current approach to molecular testing in CRC to identify gene alterations that are targetable and have predictive and prognostic value.

MOLECULAR TESTS FOR EGFR, BRAF, AND HER2 DIRECTED THERAPY

The first targeted therapy discovered in CRC was against epidermal growth factor receptor (EGFR), a transmembrane protein receptor (Figure 3.1). Activation of EGFR upregulates the mitogen-activated protein kinase (MAPK) pathway, which includes well-known oncogenes such as *KRAS*, *NRAS*, and *BRAF*. This signaling pathway has a significant role in colon carcinogenesis, and drives cell growth, invasion, and metastasis (1). Monoclonal antibodies targeting EGFR have led to improved responses and survival. Cetuximab (Erbitux) and panitumumab (Vectibix) are monoclonal antibodies against EGFR that have been shown to be effective as single agents in patients with refractory CRC (CO.17 trial) (2,3) and in the combination with cytotoxic chemotherapy as first-line and second-line treatment in patients (CRYSTAL and PRIME trials) (4–6). The earlier clinical trials investigated the efficacy of these agents in all metastatic CRC patients without biomarker selection (2,3). However, the study investigators observed a lack of objective response and worse overall survival in patients who had tumors harboring a *KRAS* mutation, which could be possibly explained by autonomous and persistent activation of the KRAS driven MAPK pathway despite anti-EGFR therapy (7,8). This discovery led to a retrospective analysis of the CO.17 trial, which showed the absence of clinical response to cetuximab in patients with *KRAS*-mutant tumors and demonstrated the requirement of KRAS wild-type for clinical benefit (9). The efficacy of panitumumab was also found to be confined to CRC patients with tumors that were KRAS wild-type (10). Although initial studies identified *exon 2* (codon 12 [G12D/G12V] and codon 13 [G13D]) mutations as negative predictive biomarkers, non–*exon 2* mutations including *exon 61* and *exon 146* mutations were also found to be predictors of resistance to anti-EGFR directed therapy (11).

The identification of *KRAS* mutations as a negative biomarker has led to the examination of other downstream mediators of the MAPK signaling pathway leading to resistance to anti-EGFR directed therapy. Mutations in *NRAS*, another member of RAS family, have also been found to be predictors of anti-EGFR resistance (12). A retrospective analysis of CRC patients treated with panitumumab or cetuximab identified BRAF mutation as a potentially negative predictive biomarker as well (13). In this study, none of the 11 CRC patients with a *BRAF* mutation responded to anti-EGFR therapy; however, numbers are low. *KRAS* (~45%), *NRAS* (~3%), and *BRAF* (~5%) mutations are known to be mutually exclusive; therefore tumors that are KRAS wild-type warrant further testing for *BRAF* mutation. An analysis of 773 tumor samples from patients treated with cetuximab revealed significantly lower response in patients with tumors that were KRAS wild-type, but had either *NRAS* (2.6%), *BRAF* (4.7%), or *PIK3CA exon 20* (~2.9%) mutations suggesting multiple signal transmitting molecules may indeed create resistance to anti-EGFR therapy (14). Interestingly, the authors reported that *PIK3CA exon 9* (~10%)

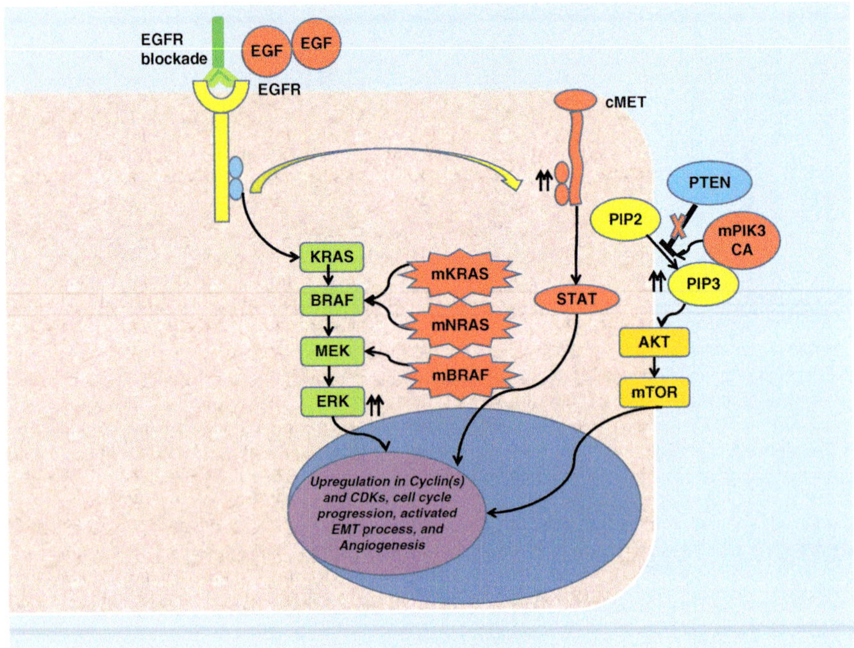

FIGURE 3.1   EGFR signaling with possible resistance pathways, including upregulation in cMET and acquired mutations in the EGFR signaling pathway.

EGFR, epidermal growth factor receptor.

mutations did not have an impact on cetuximab response. A meta-analysis also showed lack of benefit with anti-EGFR therapy in CRC patients carrying *BRAF*, *NRAS*, *PIK2CA*, *PTEN*, and non–*exon 2 KRAS* mutations (15). Further prospective analysis is necessary to confirm the impact of these additional genomic mutations in predicting response to treatment.

There is now an established practice of extended *RAS* mutation (*KRAS* and *NRAS*) testing in all metastatic CRC patients before consideration of monoclonal antibody targeting EGFR. Patients with *BRAF-V600E* mutations will likely not respond to anti-EGFR antibody; however, it is difficult to discern whether this is related to the poor prognosis or to the predictive nature of the biomarker. It is also important to note that the benefit of anti-EGFR directed therapy may be limited to left-sided colon cancer although the underlying molecular mechanism remains to be unclear, which warrants further prospective studies (16).

BRAF V600E mutation is a potentially actionable alteration. Single-agent vemurafenib (BRAF inhibitor) in CRC patients with *BRAF-V600E* mutation, unlike melanoma patients, did not show significant clinical activity. This may be due to rebound MEK activation that has to be simultaneously inhibited in CRC (17). More recently, preliminary results of a phase II study indicated there may be a significantly better response seen in the combining targets of BRAF (vemurafenib) and EGFR (cetuximab) with irinotecan when compared to cetuximab and irino-tecan alone (progression-free survival [PFS] 4.4 vs. 2.0 months hazard ratio [HR] 0.42, 95% confidence interval [CI]: 0.26–0.66, *p* < .001) (18). A recent phase I/II study demonstrated that the combination of dabrafenib (BRAF inhibitor) and trametinib (MEK inhibitor) showed promising responses in 12% of patients achieving a partial response and one patient with complete response for more than 36 months (19). A similar approach is being investigated in an international phase II/III (BEACON trial) in CRC patients with BRAF-V600E randomized to 5-fluorouracil (5-FU)/irinotecan/cetuximab, binimetinib (MEK inhibitor)/encorafenib (BRAF inhibitor)/cetuximab, or encorafenib/cetuximab (NCT02928224). Last, it is important to point out that *BRAF* mutations in CRC have significant prognostic value (20,21). Given the aggressive nature of BRAF-mutant CRC, triplet chemotherapy with FOLFOXIRI rather than doublet chemotherapy should be considered in this select patient population (22).

Human epidermal growth factor receptor 2 (HER2) is an actionable gene for CRC patients (23). Although HER2 amplification constitutes only 3% to 5% metastatic CRC patients, it has been reported to be more frequent in KRAS and BRAF wild-type tumors (24). In the phase II HERACLES trial, the investigators enrolled metastatic CRC patients who had tumors with HER2 overexpression and KRAS codon 12/13 wild-type and treated them with dual HER2 targeted therapy, trastuzumab and lapatinib (25). In this study, one patient achieved complete response, and overall objective response rate (ORR) was 30%; 44% of patients had stable disease after a median follow-up of 94 weeks. A preliminary report of an ongoing phase II clinical trial investigating pertuzumab and trastuzumab in HER2-overexpressed metastatic CRC reported an ORR of 37.5% and durable treatment response (median duration of partial response 11 months) (26). A combination of tucatinib (small molecule inhibitor of HER2) and trastuzumab is currently being investigated in the phase II MOUNTAINEER trial for refractory metastatic CRC patients with HER2 amplification (NCT03043313). Therefore, patients with KRAS and BRAF wild-type tumors should have HER2 testing for potential enrollment for clinical trial.

MISMATCH REPAIR DEFICIENCY SCREENING

Mismatch repair (MMR) genes, which commonly include *MLH1*, *PMS2*, *MSH2*, and *MSH6*, have a crucial role in DNA proofreading. Germline mutations or epigenetic dysregulation of those MMR genes lead to instability in microsatellites, which are repetitive base pairs in certain DNA motifs. Microsatellite instability induced by MMR defect causes frameshift mutations in DNA leading to activation of oncogenes and subsequent development of various microsatellite instability high (MSI-H) or MMR-deficient (MMR-D) tumors (27). The incidence of MSI-H in CRC is approximately 15% (28). A relatively small percentage of MMR-D or MSI-H cases (3% in all CRC cases) are related to germline *MMR* gene mutations or Lynch syndrome. The more common cause of MSI-H CRC is the sporadic loss of MMR function due to hypermethylation of *MLH1* promoter regions, which leads to gene silencing and loss of MLH1 expression. Sporadic MSI-H is strongly associated with *BRAF-V600E* mutations ruling out the possibility of Lynch syndrome (28,29).

MSI-H CRC is phenotypically different from microsatellite stable (MSS) CRC. MSI-H CRC is associated with right-sided tumor, poorly differentiated, and has significantly increased tumor infiltrating lymphocytes (30). A retrospective analysis of resected CRC patients also reported higher T stage and lower N stage in MSI-H patients (31). There is evidence that patients with stage II MSI-H colon cancer patients have better survival when compared to MSS tumors. In addition, patients treated with adjuvant 5-FU based chemotherapy appear to have a worse outcome. This may be due to 5-FU resistance in MSI-H tumors or a better outcome with lack of benefit of adjuvant therapy (32–34).

In the metastatic setting, patients with MSI-H CRC have the option for treatment with immunotherapy. Frameshift mutations induced by MSI lead to accumulation of somatic mutations in DNA, which in turn creates neoantigens and leads to an increase in tumor infiltrating lymphocytes. These features sensitize the tumors to checkpoint inhibitors (28,35). Recently, the Food and Drug Administration (FDA) approved the use of pembrolizumab (Keytruda), an immune checkpoint inhibitor targeting programmed cell death protein 1 (PD-1), in all MSI-H cancer including CRC in the setting of advance stage disease (36,37). The ongoing Checkmate 142 trial of the combination of PD-1 inhibitor, nivolumab (Opdivo), and inhibitor of cytotoxic T-lymphocyte-associated protein 4 (CTLA-4), ipilimumab (Yervoy), shows promising response in MSI-H CRC patients most of whom (76%) were previously treated (ORR, 55%; disease control rate for ≥12 weeks, 80%). Therefore, although the incidence of MSI-H is a relatively small proportion of the CRC population, universal screening in all metastatic CRC patients for MSI-H/MMR-D is the standard of care for oncology practice (38).

Different screening tests have been examined in the clinical studies to identify MSI-H status in CRC patients. Immunohistochemistry (IHC) staining of the tumor specimen for the presence/absence of four MMR proteins is an effective and cost-effective method for screening for MSI-H; it has been widely used in clinical practice (sensitivity, ~92.5%; specificity, 100%) (39). CRC patients with loss of one or more MMR proteins on their tumors are considered to have MMR-D tumors and thereby MSI-H. Identification of PMS2, MSH2, and MSH6 expression loss should trigger germline mutation testing for Lynch syndrome screening (40). However, loss of MLH1 expression will require further testing for BRAF-V600E mutation and MLH-1 promoter hypermethylation analyses, which, when affected, are associated with sporadic MSI-H CRC (41,42). MSI-H can also be detected by using polymerase chain reaction (PCR) that targets certain microsatellites (generally five predetermined regions) (43,44). Currently, PCR is considered a more reliable tool than IHC as it can be conducted with relatively lower quantity and quality matters such as tissue fixation, which is a limitation for IHC staining (45). PCR has been shown to be more sensitive (~100%) and can detect cases not identified by IHC (39). In PCR genotyping, direct analysis of target microsatellites is performed to detect changes in the repeat number created by hypermutational status (46). In patients with very limited tissue samples, next-generation sequencing (NGS) is a very sensitive and specific alternative test to examine MSI status (47). Although a longer turn-around time and higher cost remain to be major limitations for NGS, its use will likely be further extended in the cancer diagnostic field, which may potentially provide additional information for characteristics of MSI-H status such as somatic mutation load. Moreover, genome-wide mutation analysis may shed more light for biomarkers of immunotherapy in MSI-H cancers including CRC as well as for resistance driving genes (48).

MOLECULAR TESTS FOR OTHER POTENTIALLY ACTIONABLE GENES

Recent genome-wide studies have uncovered many valuable molecular targets that provide additional information for clinicians to better identify and tailor treatment for their patients. Caudal type homeobox transcription factor 2 (CDX2), a differentiation marker of colon cancer cells (49), has been found to be a prognostic marker for locally advanced CRC. A study showed that loss of CDX2 expression may predict poorly differentiated tumor with aggressive behavior and worse outcomes (50). Loss of CDX2 expression may be associated with increased risk of recurrence in stage II colon patients, and indeed adjuvant chemotherapy may have potential survival benefit in stage II colon patients with no CDX2 expression (51). This new biomarker discovery should be further studied prospectively in adjuvant treatment of stage II colon cancer patients with high-risk features.

Phosphoinositide 3-kinase (PIK3CA) is another downstream protein of the EGFR pathway and seen in approximately 15% of CRC patients (52). It has been shown to be a marker of poor prognosis in patients who have had surgical resection with stage I–III KRAS wild-type CRC (53). This finding suggests this patient population is at higher risk for cancer-related mortality, and utility of adjuvant chemotherapy in patients with PIK3CA needs to be further investigated. A retrospective analysis of Nurses' Health Study suggested that there may be a survival benefit with the use of aspirin for CRC patients with PIK3CA mutation (54). Another retrospective analysis also suggested there may be clinical benefit of using aspirin to decrease the risk of recurrent disease in CRC patients with PIK3CA mutation who have had curative surgery (55). A subgroup analysis of a study suggested better outcomes in CRC patients carrying PIK3CA mutations treated with yttrium (Y90) radioembolization for their liver metastasis (56). These studies propose that identification of PIK3CA mutation in CRC patients could provide further data to the clinician to practice precision medicine as well as to better stratify patients in future clinical trials.

Mesenchymal–epithelial transition factor (cMET) is a proto-oncogene and a member of receptor tyrosine kinases (RTKs). A study identified frequent cMET amplification particularly in liver metastasis (18%), compared to local disease (2%) (57). This study also suggested poor outcomes in CRC patients with liver metastasis carrying cMET amplification. However, a recent multicohort clinical study of metastatic CRC patients indicated lower incidence of cMET amplification (0%–2%) than the previous study (58). One of the striking findings in this study was the higher incidence of cMET amplification in patients with anti-EGFR refractory disease suggesting cMET amplification could be another biomarker for anti-EGFR resistance or be a pathway for anti-EGFR resistance.

Fibroblast growth factor receptor (FGFR) mutations have been reported in ~5% of CRC patients (59). It functions as RTK and stimulates cell growth. Various multikinase inhibitors (ponatinib, pazopanib, regorafenib, etc.) targeting RTKs including FGFR have been recently approved by the FDA for treatment of various solid tumor. Regorafenib, a multikinase inhibitor, has been recently approved for CRC based on evidence indicating improvement in overall survival as compared to best supportive care (1.4 months). Although the FDA approval of regorafenib is in all chemorefractory metastatic CRC patients, regardless of FGFR status, exploration into selection of FGFR mutation and treatment response should be further investigated.

ALK (anaplastic lymphoma receptor tyrosine kinase) **and** *ROS1* gene rearrangements are two well-established genetic alterations in lung cancer. Although they are relatively uncommon events (~2% of cases) in CRC (60,61), patients identified to have those genetic rearrangements may benefit from ALK/ROS inhibitors (61,62). **ATM** (ataxia telangiectasia mutated) mutation carriers bear an increased risk of various cancers including CRC (63). A study suggested the presence of *ATM* and *BRCA1* mutations may determine outcomes of CRC (64). Although mutations in DNA repair pathways, particularly homologous repair mechanisms, are relatively rare, identification of these genes may yield both prognostic and predictive outcomes as these mutations confer sensitivity to platinum-based chemotherapy and possibly PARP inhibitors (65). Partner and localizer of BRCA2 (PALB2), a protein, binds to BRCA2 for intranuclear recruitment; it also renders susceptibly to DNA targeting agents and has been reported to be mutated in CRC patients although seen relatively rare (<1%) (66). Mutation of this gene leads to genomic instability and hypermutational status that may land an opportunity for the use of PARP inhibitors as well as immune checkpoint inhibitors. *POLE* and *POLD1* genes function in DNA repair pathway and have been associated with increased risk of CRC (67). Whether increased risk of somatic mutations in the defect of these two genes may confer sensitivity to immunotherapy needs to be further investigated in prospective studies (68).

SOURCES OF BIOPSY FOR MOLECULAR ANALYSIS

Genomic analysis discussed thus far has been dedicated to tumor biopsies derived from either the primary tumor or metastatic sites. Dynamic changes in the molecular signature of cancer cells with treatment resistance create a significant challenge for clinicians. The use of liquid biopsies from circulating tumor cells in the blood may yield easier access for clinicians to better characterize disease progression and the mechanism of treatment resistance although they have relatively lower sensitivity compared to direct tumor tissue analysis (69). Easy access to tumor cells and a lack of invasive procedures to obtain relevant genetic information make liquid biopsy a great tool. However, it is important to note that lack of data with regard to the tumor microenvironment remains to be a disadvantage. Moreover, due to tumor heterogeneity, data obtained from liquid tumors may not yield any specific information with regard to the source of tumor cells such as primary disease versus metastatic foci, and conclusion of molecular analysis may not be applicable for all distant sites of tumor.

CONCLUSION

Based on the current evidence, all metastatic CRC patients should undergo MSI status evaluation either using IHC or via PCR to identify patients who may be eligible for immunotherapy-based treatments. Moreover, KRAS, NRAS, and BRAF evaluation should be performed from the tumor samples to determine patients who may benefit from monoclonal antibodies that target the EGFR pathway. Identification of *BRAF V600E* mutations is also necessary as it may change the chemotherapy regimen (triplet vs. doublet), and it may be an actionable gene specifically in clinical trials. HER2 amplification should be examined for metastatic CRC patients with wild-type KRAS for HER2 targeted therapy and clinical trial enrollment. The identification of potential other actionable genes such as *CDX2* and *PI3KCA, FGFR, cMET,* and DNA repair pathway mutations may yield further prognostic and therapeutic information.

REFERENCES

1. Reddy KB, Nabha SM, Atanaskova N. Role of MAP kinase in tumor progression and invasion. *Cancer Metastasis Rev.* 2003;22:395–403. doi:10.1023/A:1023781114568
2. Jonker DJ, O'Callaghan CJ, Karapetis CS, et al. Cetuximab for the treatment of colorectal cancer. *N Engl J Med.* 2007;357:2040–2048. doi:10.1056/NEJMoa071834
3. Van Cutsem E, Peeters M, Siena S, et al. Open-label phase III trial of panitumumab plus best supportive care compared with best supportive care alone in patients with chemotherapy-refractory metastatic colorectal cancer. *J Clin Oncol.* 2007;25:1658–1664. doi:10.1200/JCO.2006.08.1620
4. Van Cutsem E, Köhne C-H, Hitre E, et al. Cetuximab and chemotherapy as initial treatment for metastatic colorectal cancer. *N Engl J Med.* 2009;360:1408–1417. doi:10.1056/nejmoa0805019

5. Douillard J-Y, Siena S, Cassidy J, et al. Randomized, phase III trial of panitumumab with infusional fluorouracil, leucovorin, and oxaliplatin (FOLFOX4) versus FOLFOX4 alone as first-line treatment in patients with previously untreated metastatic colorectal cancer: the PRIME study. *J Clin Oncol.* 2010;28:4697–4705. doi:10.1200/JCO.2009.27.4860

6. Peeters M, Price TJ, Cervantes A, et al. Randomized phase III study of panitumumab with fluorouracil, leucovorin, and irinotecan (FOLFIRI) compared with FOLFIRI alone as second-line treatment in patients with metastatic colorectal cancer. *J Clin Oncol.* 2010;28:4706–4713. doi:10.1200/JCO.2009.27.6055

7. Lievre A, Bachet J-B, Le Corre D, et al. KRAS mutation status is predictive of response to cetuximab therapy in colorectal cancer. *Cancer Res.* 2006;66:3992–3995. doi:10.1158/0008-5472.CAN-06-0191

8. Misale S, Yaeger R, Hobor S, et al. Emergence of KRAS mutations and acquired resistance to anti-EGFR therapy in colorectal cancer. *Nature.* 2012;486:532. doi:10.1038/nature11156

9. Karapetis CS, Khambata-Ford S, Jonker DJ, et al. K-ras mutations and benefit from cetuximab in advanced colorectal cancer. *N Engl J Med.* 2008;359:1757–1765. doi:10.1056/NEJMoa0804385

10. Amado RG, Wolf M, Peeters M, et al. Wild-type KRAS is required for panitumumab efficacy in patients with metastatic colorectal cancer. *J Clin Oncol.* 2008;26:1626–1634. doi:10.1200/JCO.2007.14.7116

11. Loupakis F, Ruzzo A, Cremolini C, et al. KRAS codon 61, 146 and BRAF mutations predict resistance to cetuximab plus irinotecan in KRAS codon 12 and 13 wild-type metastatic colorectal cancer. *Br J Cancer.* 2009;101:715–721. doi:10.1038/sj.bjc.6605177

12. Douillard J-Y, Oliner KS, Siena S, et al. Panitumumab–FOLFOX4 treatment and RAS mutations in colorectal cancer. *N Engl J Med.* 2013;369:1023–1034. doi:10.1056/NEJMoa1305275

13. Di Nicolantonio F, Martini M, Molinari F, et al. Wild-type BRAF is required for response to panitumumab or cetuximab in metastatic colorectal cancer. *J Clin Oncol.* 2008;26:5705–5712. doi:10.1200/JCO.2008.18.0786

14. De Roock W, Claes B, Bernasconi D, et al. Effects of KRAS, BRAF, NRAS, and PIK3CA mutations on the efficacy of cetuximab plus chemotherapy in chemotherapy-refractory metastatic colorectal cancer: a retrospective consortium analysis. *Lancet Oncol.* 2010;11:753–762. doi:10.1016/S1470-2045(10)70130-3

15. Therkildsen C, Bergmann TK, Henrichsen-Schnack T, et al. The predictive value of KRAS, NRAS, BRAF, PIK3CA and PTEN for anti-EGFR treatment in metastatic colorectal cancer: a systematic review and meta-analysis. *Acta Oncol.* 2014;53:852–864. doi:10.3109/0284186X.2014.895036

16. Brule S, Jonker DJ, Karapetis CS, et al. Location of colon cancer (right-sided versus left-sided) as a prognostic factor and a predictor of benefit from cetuximab in NCIC CO.17. *Eur J Cancer.* 2015;51:1405–1414. doi:10.1016/j.ejca.2015.03.015

17. Kopetz S, Desai J, Chan E, et al. Phase II pilot study of vemurafenib in patients with metastatic BRAF-mutated colorectal cancer. *J Clin Oncol.* 2015;33:4032–4038. doi:10.1200/JCO.2015.63.2497

18. Kopetz S, McDonough SL, Morris VK, et al. Randomized trial of irinotecan and cetuximab with or without vemurafenib in BRAF-mutant metastatic colorectal cancer (SWOG 1406). *J Clin Oncol.* 2017;35(4_suppl):520. doi:10.1200/jco.2017.35.4_suppl.520

19. Corcoran RB, Atreya CE, Falchook GS, et al. Combined BRAF and MEK inhibition with dabrafenib and trametinib in BRAF V600–mutant colorectal cancer. *J Clin Oncol.* 2015;33:4023–4031. doi:10.1200/JCO.2015.63.2471

20. Van Cutsem E, Köhne C-H, Láng I, et al. Cetuximab plus irinotecan, fluorouracil, and leucovorin as first-line treatment for metastatic colorectal cancer: updated analysis of overall survival according to tumor KRAS and BRAF mutation status. *J Clin Oncol.* 2011;29:2011–2019. doi:10.1200/JCO.2010.33.5091

21. Roth AD, Tejpar S, Delorenzi M, et al. Prognostic role of KRAS and BRAF in stage II and III resected colon cancer: results of the translational study on the PETACC-3, EORTC 40993, SAKK 60-00 trial. *J Clin Oncol.* 2009;28:466–474. doi:10.1200/JCO.2009.23.3452

22. Loupakis F, Cremolini C, Salvatore L, et al. FOLFOXIRI plus bevacizumab as first-line treatment in BRAF mutant metastatic colorectal cancer. *Eur J Cancer.* 2014;50:57–63. doi:10.1016/j.ejca.2013.08.024

23. Bertotti A, Migliardi G, Galimi F, et al. A molecularly annotated platform of patient-derived xenografts ("xenopatients") identifies HER2 as an effective therapeutic target in cetuximab-resistant colorectal cancer. *Cancer Discov.* 2011;1:508–523. doi:10.1158/2159-8290.CD-11-0109

24. Jeong JH, Kim J, Hong YS, et al. HER2 amplification and cetuximab efficacy in patients with mMetastatic colorectal cancer harboring wild-type RAS and BRAF. *Clin Colorectal Cancer.* 2017;16(3):e147–e152. doi:10.1016/j.clcc.2017.01.005

25. Sartore-Bianchi A, Trusolino L, Martino C, et al. Dual-targeted therapy with trastuzumab and lapatinib in treatment-refractory, KRAS codon 12/13 wild-type, HER2-positive metastatic colorectal cancer (HERACLES): a proof-of-concept, multicentre, open-label, phase 2 trial. *Lancet Oncol.* 2016;17:738–746. doi:10.1016/S1470-2045(16)00150-9

26. Hurwitz H, Raghav KPS, Burris HA, et al. Pertuzumab + trastuzumab for HER2- amplified/over-expressed metastatic colorectal cancer: interim data from MyPathway. *J Clin Oncol.* 2017;35 (4_suppl):676. doi:10.1200/jco.2017.35.4_suppl.676
27. Watson P, Lynch H. The tumor spectrum in HNPCC. *Anticancer Res.* 1994;14:1635–1639.
28. Sinicrope FA, Sargent DJ. Molecular pathways: microsatellite instability in colorectal cancer: prognostic, predictive, and therapeutic implications. *Clin Cancer Res.* 2012;18:1506–1512. doi:10.1158/1078-0432.CCR-11-1469
29. Parsons MT, Buchanan DD, Thompson B, et al. Correlation of tumour BRAF mutations and MLH1 methylation with germline mismatch repair (MMR) gene mutation status: a literature review assessing utility of tumour features for MMR variant classification. *J Med Genet.* 2012;49: 151–157. doi:10.1136/jmedgenet-2011-100714
30. Ward R, Meagher A, Tomlinson I, et al. Microsatellite instability and the clinicopathological features of sporadic colorectal cancer. *Gut.* 2001;48:821–829. doi:10.1136/gut.48.6.821
31. Tejpar S, Bosman F, Delorenzi M, et al. Microsatellite instability (MSI) in stage II and III colon cancer treated with 5FU-LV or 5FU-LV and irinotecan (PETACC 3-EORTC 40993-SAKK 60/00 trial). *J Clin Oncol.* 2009;27:4001.
32. Sargent DJ, Marsoni S, Monges G, et al. Defective mismatch repair as a predictive marker for lack of efficacy of fluorouracil-based adjuvant therapy in colon cancer. *J Clin Oncol.* 2010;28:3219–3226. doi:10.1200/JCO.2009.27.1825
33. Carethers JM, Smith EJ, Behling CA, et al. Use of 5-fluorouracil and survival in patients with microsatellite-unstable colorectal cancer. *Gastroenterology.* 2004;126:394–401. doi:10.1053/j.gastro.2003.12.023
34. Ribic CM, Sargent DJ, Moore MJ, et al. Tumor microsatellite-instability status as a predictor of benefit from fluorouracil-based adjuvant chemotherapy for colon cancer. *N Engl J Med.* 2003;349:247–257. doi:10.1056/NEJMoa022289
35. Schumacher TN, Schreiber RD. Neoantigens in cancer immunotherapy. *Science.* 2015;348: 69–74. doi:10.1126/science.aaa4971
36. Le DT, Uram JN, Wang H, et al. PD-1 blockade in tumors with mismatch-repair deficiency. *N Engl J Med.* 2015;372:2509–2520. doi:10.1056/NEJMoa1500596
37. Lemery S, Keegan P, Pazdur R. First FDA approval agnostic of cancer site--when a biomarker defines the indication. *N Engl J Med.* 2017;377:1409–1411. doi:10.1056/NEJMp1709968
38. Benson AB, Venook AP, Cederquist L, et al. Colon cancer, version 1.2017, NCCN clinical practice guidelines in oncology. *J Natl Compr Cancer Netw.* 2017;15:370–398. doi:10.6004/jnccn.2017.0036
39. Lindor NM, Burgart LJ, Leontovich O, et al. Immunohistochemistry versus microsatellite instability testing in phenotyping colorectal tumors. *J Clin Oncol.* 2002;20:1043–1048. doi:10.1200/JCO.2002.20.4.1043
40. Peltomäki P. Deficient DNA mismatch repair: a common etiologic factor for colon cancer. *Human Mol Genet.* 2001;10:735–740. doi:10.1093/hmg/10.7.735
41. Weisenberger DJ, Siegmund KD, Campan M, et al. CpG island methylator phenotype underlies sporadic microsatellite instability and is tightly associated with BRAF mutation in colorectal cancer. *Nature Genet.* 2006;38:787–793. doi:10.1038/ng1834
42. Esteller M, Levine R, Baylin SB, et al. MLH1 promoter hypermethylation is associated with the microsatellite instability phenotype in sporadic endometrial carcinomas. *Oncogene.* 1998;17:2413–2417. doi:10.1038/sj.onc.1202178
43. Suraweera N, Duval A, Reperant M, et al. Evaluation of tumor microsatellite instability using five quasimonomorphic mononucleotide repeats and pentaplex PCR. *Gastroenterology.* 2002;123:1804–1811. doi:10.1053/gast.2002.37070
44. Sutter C, Gebert J, Bischoff P, et al. Molecular screening of potential HNPCC patients using a multiplex microsatellite PCR system. *Mol Cell Probes.* 1999;13:157–165. doi:10.1006/mcpr.1999.0231
45. Chapusot C, Martin L, Puig L, et al. What is the best way to assess microsatellite instability status in colorectal cancer?: study on a population base of 462 colorectal cancers. *Am J Surg Pathol.* 2004;28:1553–1559. doi:10.1097/00000478-200412000-00002
46. Schlegel J, Bocker T, Hofstädter F, et al. Detection of microsatellite instability in human colorectal carcinomas using a non-radioactive PCR-based screening technique. *Virchows Archiv.* 1995;426:223–227. doi:10.1007/BF00191358
47. Salipante SJ, Scroggins SM, Hampel HL, et al. Microsatellite instability detection by next generation sequencing. *Clin Chem.* 2014;60:1192–1199. doi:10.1373/clinchem.2014.223677
48. Mandelker D, Zhang L, Kemel Y, et al. Mutation detection in patients with advanced cancer by universal sequencing of cancer-related genes in tumor and normal DNA vs guideline-based germline testing. *JAMA.* 2017;318:825–835. doi:10.1001/jama.2017.11137

49. Ricci-Vitiani L, Lombardi DG, Pilozzi E, et al. Identification and expansion of human colon-cancer-initiating cells. *Nature.* 2007;445:111–115. doi:10.1038/nature05384

50. Baba Y, Nosho K, Shima K, et al. Relationship of CDX2 loss with molecular features and prognosis in colorectal cancer. *Clin Cancer Res.* 2009;15:4665–4673. doi:10.1158/1078-0432.CCR-09-0401

51. Dalerba P, Sahoo D, Paik S, et al. CDX2 as a prognostic biomarker in stage II and stage III colon cancer. *N Engl J Med.* 2016;374:211–222. doi:10.1056/NEJMoa1506597

52. Velho S, Oliveira C, Ferreira A, et al. The prevalence of PIK3CA mutations in gastric and colon cancer. *Eur J Cancer.* 2005;41:1649–1654. doi:10.1016/j.ejca.2005.04.022

53. Ogino S, Nosho K, Kirkner GJ, et al. PIK3CA mutation is associated with poor prognosis among patients with curatively resected colon cancer. *J Clin Oncol.* 2009;27:1477–1484. doi:10.1200/JCO.2008.18.6544

54. Liao X, Lochhead P, Nishihara R, et al. Aspirin use, tumor PIK3CA mutation, and colorectal-cancer survival. *N Engl J Med.* 2012;367:1596–1606. doi:10.1056/NEJMoa1207756

55. Domingo E, Church DN, Sieber O, et al. Evaluation of PIK3CA mutation as a predictor of benefit from nonsteroidal anti-inflammatory drug therapy in colorectal cancer. *J Clin Oncol.* 2013;31:4297–4305. doi:10.1200/JCO.2013.50.0322

56. Ziv E, Bergen M, Yarmohammadi H, et al. PI3K pathway mutations are associated with longer time to local progression after radioembolization of colorectal liver metastases. *Oncotarget.* 2017;8:23529–23538. doi:10.18632/oncotarget.15278

57. Zeng Z-S, Weiser MR, Kuntz E, et al. c-Met gene amplification is associated with advanced stage colorectal cancer and liver metastases. *Cancer Letters.* 2008;265:258–269. doi:10.1016/j.canlet.2008.02.049

58. Raghav K, Morris V, Tang C, et al. MET amplification in metastatic colorectal cancer: an acquired response to EGFR inhibition, not a de novo phenomenon. *Oncotarget.* 2016;7:54627–54631. doi:10.18632/oncotarget.10559

59. Jang J-H, Shin K-H, Park J-G. Mutations in fibroblast growth factor receptor 2 and fibroblast growth factor receptor 3 genes associated with human gastric and colorectal cancers. *Cancer Res.* 2001;61:3541–3543.

60. Lipson D, Capelletti M, Yelensky R, et al. Identification of new ALK and RET gene fusions from colorectal and lung cancer biopsies. *Nature Med.* 2012;18:382. doi:10.1038/nm.2673

61. Lin E, Li L, Guan Y, et al. Exon array profiling detects EML4-ALK fusion in breast, colorectal, and non–small cell lung cancers. *Mol Cancer Res.* 2009;7:1466–1476. doi:10.1158/1541-7786.MCR-08-0522

62. Aisner DL, Nguyen TT, Paskulin DD, et al. ROS1 and ALK fusions in colorectal cancer, with evidence of intratumoral heterogeneity for molecular drivers. *Mol Cancer Res.* 2014;12:111–118. doi:10.1158/1541-7786.MCR-13-0479-T

63. Thompson D, Duedal S, Kirner J, et al. Cancer risks and mortality in heterozygous ATM mutation carriers. *J Natl Cancer Inst.* 2005;97:813–822. doi:10.1093/jnci/dji141

64. Grabsch H, Dattani M, Barker L, et al. Expression of DNA double-strand break repair proteins ATM and BRCA1 predicts survival in colorectal cancer. *Clin Cancer Res.* 2006;12:1494–1500. doi:10.1158/1078-0432.CCR-05-2105

65. Farmer H, McCabe N, Lord CJ, et al. Targeting the DNA repair defect in BRCA mutant cells as a therapeutic strategy. *Nature.* 2005;434:917. doi:10.1038/nature03445

66. Yurgelun MB, Kulke MH, Fuchs CS, et al. Cancer susceptibility gene mutations in individuals with colorectal cancer. *J Clin Oncol.* 2017;35:1086–1095. doi:10.1200/JCO.2016.71.0012

67. Buchannan DD, Stewart JR, Clendenning M, et al. Risk of colorectal cancer for carriers of a germline mutation in POLE or POLD1. *Genet Med.* 2018;20(8):890–895. doi:10.1038/gim.2017.185

68. Gargiulo P, Pepa CD, Berardi S, et al. Tumor genotype and immune microenvironment in POLE-ultramutated and MSI-hypermutated endometrial cancers: new candidates for checkpoint blockade immunotherapy? *Cancer Treatment Rev.* 2016;48:61–68. doi:10.1016/j.ctrv.2016.06.008

69. Diaz Jr, LA, Bardelli A. Liquid biopsies: genotyping circulating tumor DNA. *J Clin Oncol.* 2014;32:579–586. doi:10.1200/JCO.2012.45.2011

How I Treat Early-Stage Colon Cancer Through Surgery

Mark W. Arnold

INTRODUCTION

Surgery has been an effective mainstay of therapy for early-stage colon cancers for more than 100 years. While the surgical technique has changed and evolved over time, the goal of extirpation of the bowel containing the primary tumor and the associated mesentery and lymph nodes has remained the same. Dukes and Bussey, in their landmark paper evaluating 25 years of results in 3,596 patients undergoing surgical resection as the definitive therapy, reported a crude 5-year survival rate of 48.3%, with early stages A and B (stages I and II, respectively) doing significantly better than stage C (stage III) (1).

We define early-stage cancers as those that are either stage I or II at the time of the initial diagnosis. Stage I tumors are either T1 or T2 lesions with negative lymph nodes, and stage II tumors are either T3 or T4 lesions with negative lymph nodes. It is often difficult to know the lymph node status prior to surgical resection, so stage III lesions (N1 or N2) are usually treated with surgical extirpation as the initial step. Tumors that are stage IV (M1) and are asymptomatic are usually treated initially with chemotherapy. Surgery in this circumstance is reserved for patients with symptoms (i.e., anemia or impending obstruction) or following a favorable response.

WORKUP

Colon cancers are almost always diagnosed by endoscopy and confirmed by biopsy. Initial workup should include a carcinoembryonic antigen (CEA) draw to determine if the tumor expresses CEA (2) and a CT scan of the chest, abdomen, and pelvis to evaluate for metastatic disease. Most small lesions are nondiagnostic and do not represent metastatic disease. An interval scan is usually sufficient follow-up for these. For larger lesions in the liver or lung, a PET scan may be useful to clarify these or biopsy by interventional radiology. If the patient is found to have metastatic disease, then an evaluation by medical oncology is appropriate to determine if chemotherapy should be initiated. Later stage tumors that are otherwise asymptomatic are best treated by chemotherapy first.

A medical history should be obtained. If the patient, as in our vignette, has a significant history of vascular, cardiac, or chronic obstructive pulmonary disease, a preoperative anesthetic assessment should be obtained to optimize the patient's health and reduce the risk of a perioperative event. We have an outpatient anesthesia clinic (OPAC) for that dedicated purpose.

COLON ENHANCED RECOVERY AFTER SURGERY (CERAS) PROTOCOL

All patients are enrolled in our CERAS protocol. Programs such as this have been shown to be effective in enhancing recovery and reducing hospital stays after colectomy (3). CERAS starts with the presurgery clinic visit. A detailed history including social issues is obtained. Patients with a body mass index (BMI) <18.5 are started in nutritional supplements and undergo dietary counseling. Alcohol and smoking cessation programs are encouraged. Preoperative exercise

---

A Clinical Vignette ("How I Treat") is included at the end of the chapter.

is encouraged and patients with significant deconditioning are referred to Physical Therapy. All the components of the bowel prep, including the mechanical prep and oral antibiotics are given to the patient in the clinic with detailed written instructions that a clinic nurse reviews with the patient prior to leaving. The patient is NPO after the midnight of the day of the procedure except for a small preoperative carbohydrate solution drink that the patient self-administers 2 to 4 hours prior to the scheduled surgery time.

On the day of surgery, most patients receive an epidural for pain control. Also administered are 975 mg of acetaminophen, 800 mg of gabapentin, and 10 mg of oxycodone. For patients undergoing an epidural, deep vein thrombosis (DVT) prophylaxis is given 2 hours after placement. Prophylactic antibiotics are given prior to the incision. An orogastric tube is used during the surgical procedure, but a nasogastric tube is not left in place. Goal-directed fluid management is used to prevent overload, and perioperative glucose management is followed carefully.

Postoperative, the Foley catheter is removed by postoperative day 1 if possible and the patient is started immediately on sips of clears with diet advanced as tolerated. Patients are out of bed on the day of surgery and ambulated on postoperative day 1. Scheduled pain medications are acetaminophen, ibuprofen, and gabapentin. Narcotics are only given for breakthrough pain. The epidural is usually removed by postoperative day 3. This protocol is usually sufficient to manage postoperative pain control. Limiting the use of narcotics has a significant benefit in aiding early return of bowel function. DVT prophylaxis is continued until the patient is sufficiently ambulatory, and postoperative antibiotics are not used. The routine use of CERAS has reduced the length of stay by more than 1 day on average since its initiation.

THE OPERATIVE TECHNIQUE

The basic principle: remove the segment of the bowel containing the tumor and all the associated mesentery, vasculature, and lymph nodes. The National Cancer Institute refers to this as wide surgical resection and anastomosis. This approach enables the surgeon to obtain adequate proximal, distal, and lateral margins and harvest an appropriate number of lymph nodes for accurate staging. For example, a right colon tumor undergoes a right colectomy, a left colon tumor undergoes a left colectomy, and a sigmoid colon tumor undergoes a sigmoid colectomy. A transverse lesion, however, may be best taken with an extended right or left depending on the location to ensure adequate sampling and good blood supply to the two ends of the bowel being anastomosed. A diverting colostomy or ileostomy is almost never necessary and should be avoided if at all possible.

Open Versus Minimally Invasive Surgery

The first reported successful use of minimally invasive surgery (MIS) techniques for operative colectomy was by Jacobs et al. in 1991 (4). They reported on 20 patients undergoing right colectomy (9 patients), sigmoid colectomy (8 patients), low anterior resection (1 patient), Hartmann's procedure (1 patient), and abdominoperineal resection (1 patient). There were no deaths and 70% were discharged within 96 hours of the procedure. This simple feasibility study, showing that MIS techniques could be used for colon cancer resection, revolutionized the operative approach to early colon cancers. As a surgical procedure, its popularity quickly caught on; however, as MIS techniques evolved, the wisdom of using an MIS approach was tested. Was it really as safe? Were enough lymph nodes harvested for adequate staging? Was long-term survival compromised? Did it cost too much? What about port-site recurrences? To answer these and many other questions, two large volume multicenter studies were undertaken in the early 2000s.

The Clinical Outcomes of Surgical Therapy Study Group (COST) trial (5) and the COlon cancer Laparoscopic or Open Resection (COLOR) trial (6) with 872 and 1,248 randomized patients, respectively, showed that laparoscopy was as safe and as effective as open surgery. There were shorter recovery and hospital stays that led to decreased costs with no significant changes in either long-term survival or complications. Lymph node harvest rates were similar also. More recent studies have consistently shown that laparoscopic colectomy is more cost-effective, even considering increased equipment costs, than open colectomy (7). There are, in fact, only three potential contraindications to an MIS approach: a very large primary tumor, which might necessitate using a large extraction incision, rendering the laparoscopic part moot; a large bowel obstruction; an abdomen with extensive previous operative incisions preventing adequate access. If these are absent, there is no real justification for not using a minimally invasive approach to the resection of early-stage colon cancers.

Laparoscopic Versus Robotic Surgery
In 2014, Intuitive Surgical introduced its new Xi robotic platform. This makes docking and undocking easy and has enhanced the usefulness of the robotic approach. While the approach has not yet achieved widespread acceptance, there are some indications of its gaining popularity. It is more useful in low anterior resections for rectal cancer than most early-stage colon cancer. However, it is an acceptable technique for most partial colectomies. As experience with the procedure increases, there is every reason to believe that it will with time become a standard tool in the treatment of early colon cancers (8).

CHEMOTHERAPY

Most early-stage colon cancers do not require adjuvant chemotherapy. There is no evidence to support the use of adjuvant chemotherapy in stage I (T1, T2, and N0) patients (9). For patients with stage II disease, factors associated with increased risk of recurrence are inadequate lymph node sampling, T4 disease, involvement of the visceral peritoneum, and a poorly differentiated histology. In these selected cases, patients may benefit from adjuvant chemotherapy after a full discussion of the risks and benefits.

THE MALIGNANT POLYP

The question sometimes arises whether or not a polyp, whether removed by traditional endoscopic techniques, by endoscopic mucosal resection (EMR), or by endoscopic submucosal resection (ESD), which is found to have a focus of invasive adenocarcinoma, needs wide surgical resection or just close follow-up. A lot depends on the specific circumstances. If the margin is close or positive, wide surgical resection is advisable. Likewise histologic features that favor lymph node metastasis such as poorly differentiated lesions and lymphatic invasion are best treated with surgical resection (10). A well-differentiated lesion, without lymphatic invasion and a clear margin on the stalk, can be safely observed as the risk of spread is low. In general, if the risk of surgery is greater than the risk of recurrence, surgery should be avoided. In all cases, a tattoo should be placed at the lesion to allow for careful follow-up.

FOLLOW-UP

Most early-stage colon cancers will not be treated with adjuvant chemotherapy. However, close follow-up is extremely important as even early-stage tumors can reoccur and many of these patients can be successfully treated with re-excision of the recurrent tumor for cure or chemotherapy. The National Comprehensive Cancer Network Guidelines for Colon Cancer (version 2.2016) are a good place to start.

Typical follow-up includes, at a minimum, 6-month visits for at least the first 3 years postoperative and then yearly visits after this period. These visits should include a detailed history and physical examination as well as a CEA draw. A colonoscopy should be performed at 1 year and then depending on the findings, 1-, 2-, or 3-year intervals. A CT scan should be performed at 1 year and yearly intervals, for the first 3 years, or anytime there is change on examination or elevation of the CEA level. PET scans should not be routinely performed as false positives are common in the postoperative period and should be reserved only for a high suspicion of recurrence. The likelihood of recurrence is greatly reduced after 5 years, but follow-up should continue until 10 years postoperative as there are cases of recurrence within that interval.

Most episodes of tumor recurrence after a curative resection are either at the radial margin of resection, the liver, the lungs, or the retroperitoneal or periaortic lymph nodes. Solitary metastatic disease at these sites can often be re-resected for cure; hence the importance of close postoperative follow-up.

SUMMARY

Early-stage colon cancers have a very favorable prognosis and are best treated with a minimally invasive surgical approach and close follow-up. Patients with stage II lesions that are T4 or have unfavorable histologic characteristics should be offered adjuvant chemotherapy. Malignant polyps can often be observed especially if the margin is clear and the histology is favorable. All patients should be enrolled in CERAS protocols to aid and advance recovery.

Clinical Vignette 4.1

A 47-year-old 70 kg male presents to his primary care physician with a complaint of progressive fatigue and a 10 lb weight loss over the past year. His past medical history is significant for previous stroke. Medications include clopidogrel and aspirin. His family history is significant for a mother who died of breast cancer at age 55 and a father with colon cancer at age 65. A complete blood count (CBC) shows an abnormal finding of hemoglobin of 10.5. He has never had a colonoscopy.

A colonoscopy finds a 3 cm ulcerated mass in the distal ascending colon. A tattoo is placed and biopsies obtained. These are positive for adenocarcinoma of the colon. Microsatellite instability (MSI) testing is negative for mismatch repair gene defects. CT scans of the chest, abdomen, and pelvis are significant only for a few scattered indeterminate nodules in the chest and liver and colonic thickening at the site of the known cancer.

The patient appears to have early-stage colon cancer and is referred to a surgeon for definitive treatment.

After a preoperative assessment, our 47-year-old patient was sent for medical clearance. On their recommendations, clopidogrel was stopped 5 days prior to surgery and aspirin continued to the day of surgery. He underwent a laparoscopic right colectomy using the medial to lateral approach. The ileocolic vessels were divided. The middle colic vessels preserved. The proximal division of the bowel was at the terminal ileum and the distal margin just proximal to the middle colic vessels. The entire mesentery to the right colon was removed. The specimen was extracted through a small incision around the umbilicus using a wound guard. The anastomosis was performed extracorporeally and returned to the abdomen. The fascia was closed with a few interrupted long-term absorbable sutures and the skin was closed with a subcuticular absorbable suture and glued closed.

The CERAS protocol was initiated postoperative and the patient discharged home on postoperative day 3. On pathologic examination of the specimen, a moderately differentiated 2.8 cm T2 lesion was found with 0 of 19 lymph nodes positive for cancer (T2N0M0). The tumor was microsatellite stable. No chemotherapy was offered and close follow-up initiated.

A baseline CEA was 1.8 ng/ml. At 18 months, a follow-up CEA was 4.2 ng/ml. A repeat test 1 month later was 4.8 ng/ml. A CT scan of the chest, abdomen, and pelvis was performed, which showed a new 3.5 cm lesion in segment 3 of the liver. A colonoscopy was performed and identified a healthy anastomosis without evidence of recurrence. On a follow-up PET scan, the liver lesion had increased FDG (2-fluor-2-deoxy-D-glucose) uptake. There were no other areas of nonphysiologic uptake. The patient underwent left lateral lobectomy of the liver with excision of segments 2 and 3 containing the recurrence tumor. A follow-up CEA at 3 months was 2.0 ng/ml, and the patient is currently disease free.

REFERENCES

1. Duke CE, Bussey HJR. The spread of cancer and its effect upon prognosis. *Brt J Cancer.* 1958;12:309–320. doi:10.1038/bjc.1958.37
2. Martin EW Jr, Minton JP, Carey LC. CEA-directed second-look surgery in the asymptomatic patient after primary resection of colorectal carcinoma. *Ann Surg.* 1985;202(3):310–317. doi:10.1097/00000658-198509000-00006

3. Carmichael JC, Keller DS, Baldini G, et al. Clinical practice guidelines for enhanced recovery after colon and rectal surgery from the American Society of Colon and Rectal Surgeons and Society of American Gastrointestinal and Endoscopic Surgeons. *Dis Colon Rectum.* 2017;60:761–784. doi:10.1097/DCR.0000000000000883

4. Jacobs M, Verdega JC, Goldstein HS. Minimally invasive colon resection (laparoscopic colectomy). *Surg Laparosc Endosc.* 1991;1(3):144–150.

5. The Clinical Outcomes of Surgical Therapy Study Group. A comparison of laparoscopically assisted and open colectomy for colon cancer. *N Engl J Med.* 2004;350:2050–2059. doi:10.1056/NEJMoa032651

6. Velkamp R, Kuhry E, Hop WC, et al. COlon cancer Laparoscopic or Open Resection Study Group (COLOR) Laparoscopic surgery versus open surgery for colon cancer: short-term outcome of a randomized trial. *Lancet Oncol.* 2005;6:477–484. doi:10.1016/S1470-2045(05)70221-7

7. Jensen CC, Prasad LM, Abcarian H. Cost-effectiveness of laparoscopic vs open resection of colon and rectal cancer. *Dis Colon Rectum.* 2012;55:1017–1023. doi:10.1097/DCR.0b013e3182656898

8. Yeo HL, Isaacs A, Abelson JS, et.al. Comparison of open, laparoscopic, and robotic colectomies using a large national database: outcomes and trends related to surgery center volume. *Dis Colon Rectum.* 2016;59:535–642. doi:10.1097/DCR.0000000000000580

9. André T, Boni C, Navarro M, et al. Improved overall survival with oxaliplatin, fluorouracil, and leucovorin as adjuvant treatment in stage II or III colon cancer in the MOSAIC trial. *J Clin Oncol.* 2009;27(19):3109–3116. doi:10.1200/JCO.2008.20.6771

10. Robert ME. The malignant colon polyp: Diagnosis and therapeutic recommendations. *Clin Gastro Hepatology.* 2007;5:662–667. doi:10.1016/j.cgh.2007.04.001

How I Treat Early-Stage Colon Cancer With Adjuvant Therapy: Who and How Long?

Francesca Battaglin and Heinz-Josef Lenz

INTRODUCTION

Systemic recurrence of the disease occurs in about 35% of colorectal cancer (CRC) patients following curative surgery and in 80% of cases within 2 to 3 years of primary tumor resection. The 5-year survival after surgery alone varies across different tumor stages with a rate of 85% to 95% for stage I, lowering to 60% to 80% in stage II, and 30% to 65% in stage III.

The administration of adjuvant systemic chemotherapy following surgical resection has been shown to reduce patients' risk of death by an absolute 3% to 5% in stage II and 10% to 15% in stage III with a single agent 5-fluorouracil (5-FU); a further reduction of 4% to 5% can be gained from the use of oxaliplatin-containing regimens in stage III.

ADJUVANT TREATMENT REGIMENS

A summary of common adjuvant treatment regimens can be found in Table 5.1.

Fluoropyrimidine-Based Regimens

Bolus 5-fluorouracil/leucovorin (5-FU/LV) was the first chemotherapy to be established as a standard adjuvant regimen for resected colon cancer based on the results of multiple trials during the 1990s. Different schedules of administration and length of treatment have been tested over the years, showing a more favorable toxicity profile for continuous infusion 5-FU over bolus 5-FU plus LV and indicating 6 months as the standard duration of fluoropyrimidine adjuvant treatment (1,2).

As the administration of infusional FU requires a central venous access, oral fluoropyrimidines can offer an advantage in this aspect. Capecitabine, an orally active fluoropyrimidine, has demonstrated equivalent results in terms of disease-free survival (DFS) compared to intravenous (iv) fluoropyrimidines in the adjuvant treatment of stage III colon cancer in two randomized trials (3,4). Of note, the incidence of adverse events was lower than with 5-FU/LV, except for hand–foot syndrome. Based on these data, capecitabine was approved for the adjuvant treatment of colon cancer in the United States and Europe. It should be noted, however, that the full dose of 1,250 mg/mq twice daily is often poorly tolerated in American patients compared to Europeans and Asians.

Other compounds, S-1 and UFT (uracil and tegafur) plus LV, which have demonstrated a significant benefit in the adjuvant setting and are considered a standard approach for adjuvant chemotherapy of stage III colon cancer in Japan, are not currently available in the United States or in Europe (5,6).

Oxaliplatin-Based Regimens

The survival benefit of adding oxaliplatin to adjuvant fluoropyrimidine-based chemotherapy in node-positive (stage III) colon cancers has been demonstrated in randomized trials and is supported by data from meta-analyses and large observational studies, including data from 12,233 patients in the Adjuvant Colon Cancer End Points (ACCENT) database of adjuvant colon cancer trials (7).

A Clinical Vignette ("How I Treat") is included at the end of the chapter.

TABLE 5.1 Common Adjuvant Treatment Regimens

	Fluoropyrimidine (5-Fluorouracil iv/ Oral Capecitabine)	Leucovorin (iv)	Oxaliplatin (iv)	Treatment Schedule
Simplified 5-FU/LV	5-FU 400 mg/mq bolus day 1, followed by 2,400 mg/mq i.c. over 46–48 hours	400 mg/mq over 2 hours day 1	–	Every 2 weeks
FOLFOX4	5-FU 400 mg/mq bolus + 600 mg/mq i.c. over 22 hours days 1 and 2	400 mg/mq over 2 hours days 1 and 2 before 5-FU	85 mg/mq over 2 hours day 1	Every 2 weeks
Modified FOLFOX6	5-FU 400 mg/mq bolus day 1, followed by 2,400 mg/mq i.c. over 46–48 hours	400 mg/mq over 2 hours day 1	85 mg/mq over 2 hours day 1	Every 2 weeks
Capecitabine	Capecitabine 1,250 mg/mq twice daily on days 1 to 14	–	–	Every 3 weeks
XELOX	Capecitabine 1,000 mg/mq twice daily on days 1 to 14	–	130 mg/mq over 2 hours day 1	Every 3 weeks

5-FU, 5-fluorouracil; i.c., continuous infusion; iv, intravenous; LV, leucovorin.

The European MOSAIC trial was the first to demonstrate the superiority of a 6-month adjuvant treatment with oxaliplatin in combination with 5-FU/LV (FOLFOX regimen) over FU/LV both in terms of DFS and overall survival (OS) in 2,246 patients with resected stage II (40%) or III colon cancer (8). Updated results of this study at a median follow-up of 9.5 years confirmed previous data showing OS rates in the whole population of 71.7% versus 67.1% (hazard ratio [HR]: 0.85, *p* = .043) for the FOLFOX and 5-FU/LV arms, respectively. Notably, the survival advantage was statistically significant in stage III (67.1% vs. 59.0%; HR: 0.80, *p* = .016) but not in stage II (78.4% vs. 79.5%; HR: 1.00, *p* = .980) (9). Peripheral sensory neuropathy (one of the main oxaliplatin-related toxicities) developed in 92% of patients receiving FOLFOX. However, the incidence of grade 3 neuropathy was 12.4% and long-term safety results showed that this toxicity was generally reversible for most patients (15.4% of patients with residual neuropathy at 4 years, mostly grade 1). Based on this study, oxaliplatin was approved in combination with infusional 5-FU/LV for the adjuvant treatment of resected stage III colon cancer. While FOLFOX4 was the regimen used in the registration trial, currently the modified FOLFOX6 regimen, which does not require a day 2 bolus of 5-FU/LV, is the most commonly used regimen.

The NSABP C-07 trial also reported better outcomes with oxaliplatin associated to bolus weekly 5-FU/LV (FLOX regimen) compared to bolus weekly 5-FU/LV alone (10). However, toxicities with this regimen are more severe and it is rarely used in clinical practice in the adjuvant setting.

The combination of capecitabine plus oxaliplatin (XELOX) showed also to be superior to standard iv bolus 5-FU/LV in a phase III trial involving 1,886 patients with stage III colon cancer (11). With a median follow-up of 74 months, DFS was significantly higher in the XELOX arm (HR for DFS 0.80, 95% confidence interval [CI]: 0.69–0.93, 7-year DFS 63% vs. 56%), as well as OS (HR: 0.83, 95% CI: 0.70–0.99, 7-year OS 73% vs. 67%) (12). Overall, toxicity profile for XELOX treatment showed lower incidence of grade 3–4 neutropenia, febrile neutropenia, stomatitis, and alopecia, but higher incidence of neurotoxicity, grade 3 hand–foot syndrome, and grade 3–4 thrombocytopenia when compared to bolus 5-FU/LV.

Of note, data from a pooled analysis of four randomized trials showed that oxaliplatin-based combination therapies consistently improved outcomes irrespective of whether the fluoropyrimidine backbone was capecitabine or 5-FU/LV (13).

Not Recommended Regimens

Based on negative results of randomized trials, irinotecan-containing regimens and the use of anti–vascular epithelial growth factor (VEGF) or anti–epidermal growth factor receptor (EGFR) targeted drugs, such as bevacizumab and cetuximab, are not recommended in the adjuvant setting for resected colon cancer (14–18).

Investigational Treatment: Portal Vein Infusion and Intraperitoneal Chemotherapy

Both prophylactic intrahepatic chemotherapy through portal vein infusion to reduce the risk of liver recurrence and hyperthermic intraperitoneal chemotherapy in patients at high risk for developing peritoneal metastases have been the object of clinical trials. While portal vein infusion mostly failed to show a consistent significant benefit across different studies, preliminary data from a small series of patients treated with prophylactic intraperitoneal chemotherapy seem encouraging, although this approach is burdened by a high risk of severe toxicities (19). These results, however, need further validation and these treatment options remain limited to clinical investigation (e.g., Adjuvant HIPEC in High Risk Colon Cancer, the COLOPEC trial, NCT02231086).

TIMING OF ADJUVANT TREATMENT

Adjuvant chemotherapy is typically started after the patient recovers from primary CRC surgery. The current approach is to begin treatment within 6 to 8 weeks of resection, as soon as patient's conditions are permissive.

Whether a delay in the administration of adjuvant therapy compromises outcomes has been addressed in two large systematic reviews and meta-analyses. Results of these studies showed that a delay of chemotherapy was associated with a significantly higher risk of death (relative risk 1.20, 95% CI: 1.15–1.26) (20), and that each 4-week delay in the time to administer adjuvant chemotherapy beyond 8 weeks was associated with a 14% decrease in OS (HR for death 1.14, 95% CI: 1.10–1.17) and increase in disease relapse (HR: 1.14, 95% CI: 1.10–1.18) (21). Additionally, a retrospective analysis from the National Cancer Database, including 7,794 patients with stage II and III colon cancer, found that a delay greater than 6 weeks between surgery and adjuvant treatment was associated with a reduced survival even after adjustment for clinical-, tumor-, and treatment-related factors (22).

ADJUVANT THERAPY: PATIENT SELECTION AND TREATMENT CHOICE

The evaluation of patients' conditions, age, performance status, comorbidities, disease history, surgery, pathology report, staging, and disease characteristics, alongside patients' opinions and expectations, should be always carefully evaluated and discussed when counseling about the indication to adjuvant treatment after resection of colon cancer.

The main pathological feature determining the indication to adjuvant chemotherapy in CRC is nodal involvement. For stage III patients deemed fit to undergo a combination chemotherapy, an oxaliplatin-based adjuvant treatment (either FOLFOX or XELOX) should be discussed and recommended based on the result of previously discussed trials (see section Oxaliplatin-Based Regimens). In the case of patients unfit for a combination therapy or with contraindications to oxaliplatin, a fluoropyrimidine monotherapy (either 5-FU/LV or capecitabine) should be recommended.

Additional clinicopathological features associated with an increased recurrence risk, beyond the stratification based on the TNM staging (discussed in Chapter 2, Diagnostic and Staging of Colorectal Cancer), are represented by tumor grading, the presence of lymphatic or venous or perineural invasion, lymphoid inflammatory response, and involvement of resection margins. Bowel obstruction and perforation are clinical indicators of a worse prognosis as well as elevated pretreatment serum levels of carcinoembryonic antigen (CEA). A careful risk assessment is particularly important in stage II disease where data on the benefit from adjuvant chemotherapy are not as strong as in stage III, and the current indication to treatment refers to "high-risk" stage II, as further discussed in the next section.

Notably, a global effort is ongoing to integrate comprehensive molecular subtype classifications and/or molecular markers, such as microsatellite instability (MSI) and mutations in

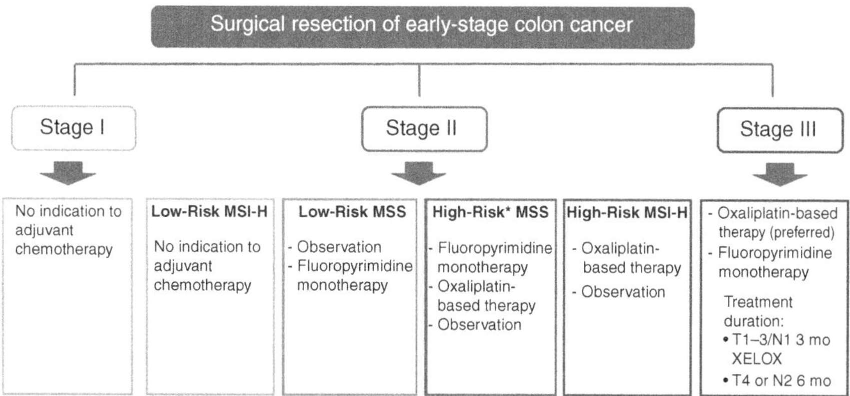

FIGURE 5.1　Proposed algorithm for the adjuvant treatment of early-stage colon cancer.

*see Box 5.1: Recognized High-Risk features in Stage II Colon Cancer.

mo, months; MSI-H, microsatellite instability high; MSS, microsatellite stable.

BRAF or *KRAS,* into multivariable models that include detailed clinicopathological annotation to improve prognostic estimation and aid patient selection for adjuvant treatment in stage II and III colon cancer (23–25).

Adjuvant chemotherapy is not indicated in patients with stage I colon cancer.

A summary of adjuvant treatment recommendations according to disease stage can be found in Figure 5.1.

Recent evidence from observational studies suggests that the use of low-dose aspirin may improve survival among patients with early-stage colon cancer whose tumors harbor mutations in the *PIK3CA* gene (26–28). This topic has been highly debated and results from ongoing prospective randomized trials (NCT00565708, NCT01150045, NCT02945033) are warranted in order to confirm the benefit of aspirin in the adjuvant setting and the clinical utility of a possible molecular selection of patients based on PIK3CA status or other biomarkers.

Finally, physical exercise and several dietary factors, such as coffee, fiber, and nut intake, have been associated with prognosis in early-stage CRC in large observational studies (29–32). Higher vitamin D levels have been associated with a better prognosis as well (33); however, whether vitamin D supplementation can improve prognosis if combined with adjuvant chemotherapy is still under investigation.

Treatment of Stage II Disease and Risk Stratification

Multiple adjuvant trials have enrolled patients with both stage II and III colon cancer showing an OS and DFS benefit in the combined population compared to surgery alone. In most cases, however, results were clinically and statistically significant only in the stage III subgroup.

The QUASAR study specifically addressed the issue of the benefit of a fluoropyrimidine-based chemotherapy in 3,238 patients with resected colon (71%) or rectal cancer with an "uncertain indication for adjuvant therapy" (91% stage II) (34). Overall, adjuvant chemotherapy was associated with a significant lower risk of disease recurrence and reduction in death, translating into a 3% to 4% absolute benefit in 5-year OS. However, results in the subgroup of patients with stage II colon cancer were not statistically significant (HR: 0.86, 95% CI: 0.54–1.19).

Results of two large meta-analyses of early adjuvant trials evaluating the benefit of a fluoropyrimidine-based chemotherapy in stage II colon cancer showed, on the one hand, a small but not statistically significant benefit in 5-year OS favoring the adjuvant treatment and, on the other hand, a small but significant absolute improvement in DFS (about 5%) (35,36). Similar results came from an intergroup analysis based on pooled individual data from 3,302 patients with stage II or III colon cancer enrolled in seven randomized fluoropyrimidine-based adjuvant trials (37). For patients with stage II disease, adjuvant chemotherapy showed a significant benefit in terms of 5-year DFS (76% vs. 72%), but the benefit in OS was not statistically significant. However, in a follow-up analysis of long-term outcomes by the ACCENT collaboration, including nearly 6,900 patients with stage II cancer, adjuvant 5-FU-based treatment was associated with a 5% absolute survival benefit at 8 years (72% vs. 66.8%, p = .026) (38).

Long-term results from both the MOSAIC and the NSABP C-07 trials did not show a significant benefit from the addition of oxaliplatin to adjuvant 5-FU/LV for patients with stage II colon cancer (40% of patients in the MOSAIC trial and 29% in the NSABP C-07 trial, respectively), either in terms of DFS or OS (10,39). Similar results were confirmed by a subsequent analysis of data from patients in the ACCENT database (7). Of note, in an exploratory analysis of the MOSAIC trial, patients with high-risk stage II disease showed a trend toward a benefit from adjuvant oxaliplatin-based treatment with a 7% improvement in DFS and a small improvement in OS although not statistically significant.

Finally, a 2016 retrospective analysis of data from the National Cancer Database, including 153,110 patients diagnosed with stage II colon cancer between 1998 and 2011, reported that adjuvant treatment (irrespective of monotherapy or combined treatment) was associated with improved survival (HR: 0.76, $p < .001$) (40).

Based on these data, adjuvant chemotherapy is not considered as a standard of care for all patients with resected stage II disease. However, it should be discussed as an option especially for patients with multiple high-risk features. Patients with low-risk stage II should generally be observed without treatment; nevertheless, potential benefit and risk of an adjuvant fluoropyrimidine monotherapy (either 5-FU/LV or capecitabine) can be discussed in an individualized approach; enrollment in a clinical trial may be an additional option. Patients with stage II colon cancer with high-risk features should be considered for adjuvant chemotherapy with either an oxaliplatin-based regimen (either FOLFOX or XELOX) or a fluoropyrimidine monotherapy (either 5-FU/LV or capecitabine). A careful risk assessment and an extensive discussion on expected benefit and risk from adjuvant treatment are mandatory to inform individual patient's ohoiooo in thic cotting.

The clinicopathological features that have been associated with a worse prognosis in patients with stage II disease and the presence of which define a "high-risk stage II" are summarized in Box 5.1. They include a T4 primary tumor (41), a high-grade/poorly differentiated histology (except for microsatellite instability high [MSI-H] tumors) (42), lymphovascular invasion (LVI) (43), perineural invasion (PNI) (44), bowel obstruction or perforation (45), inadequate lymph node sampling (<12 resected nodes) (46), and close/undetermined/positive margins.

A crucial molecular biomarker for risk stratification in stage II colon cancer is MSI (see Chapter 3, Molecular Diagnostic Guidelines for Colorectal Cancer). Approximately 20% of CRCs in stage I and II and 12% in stage III are deficient in one or more DNA mismatch repair (MMR) proteins in one quarter of cases due to hereditary Lynch syndrome. Up to 80% to 90% of sporadic MSI cases are due to promoter hypermethylation of the MLH1 gene, associated with a high CpG island methylation phenotype, and about 30% of cases harbor a *BRAF V600E* mutation (47,48). MSI-H CRCs are characterized by distinct pathological features such as prominent lymphocytic infiltrate, poor differentiation, and mucinous histology (49). MSI status provides important prognostic and predictive information in stage II colon cancer with MMR deficiency being associated with both a good prognosis (significantly lower recurrence risk) and apparently a lack of efficacy or even possibly a detrimental effect from fluoropyrimidine adjuvant treatment (25,50,51). The most solid data have been derived from an analysis of the ACCENT database investigating the impact of MSI on adjuvant treatment benefit in patients

BOX 5.1 Recognized High-Risk Features in Stage II Colon Cancer

T4 primary tumor
Poorly differentiated tumor (G3–4)*
Lymphovascular invasion
Perineural invasion
Inadequate lymph node sampling (<12)
Close/indeterminate or positive resection margins
Perforation
Obstruction

*Excluding microsatellite instability (MSI) high tumors.

with stage II and III colon cancer enrolled in 17 trials. MSI-H stage II and III patients showed better outcome with surgery alone compared to those with microsatellite stable (MSS) tumors (HR for OS in stage II patients 0.27, p = .01). Nevertheless, stage III patients showed a significant survival benefit from 5-FU adjuvant therapy regardless of MSI status, while no benefit and a trend toward a worse survival were observed in MSI-H stage II patients (51). In contrast, a subgroup analysis of the QUASAR study confirmed the prognostic significance of MSI but not its predictive value (52). Of note, MSI etiology (germline vs. sporadic) might affect the benefit from fluoropyrimidine treatment, as a retrospective evaluation of stage II and III patients who received either adjuvant 5-FU or placebo showed that individuals with MSI-H due to germline mutations had an improved DFS with 5-FU compared to those with sporadic MSI-H tumors (53). Conversely, despite the lack of randomized prospective trials, data from retrospective analyses consistently suggest that the benefit from oxaliplatin-based adjuvant chemotherapy seems to be independent of MSI status (9,54,55).

To date, adjuvant chemotherapy is not recommended for patients with low-risk stage II MSI-H colon cancer due to their excellent prognosis, while stage III patients should receive adjuvant treatment irrespective of MSI status. An oxaliplatin-based adjuvant treatment should be preferred for MSI-H tumors.

The use of additional molecular markers for risk stratification such as *RAS* and *BRAF* mutations, chromosome 18q deletion, *TP53* mutations, CDX2 expression, epigenetic alterations (e.g., aberrant DNA methylation, CpG island methylation phenotype), gene expression arrays (e.g., the 12-gene recurrence score assay Oncotype DX Colon Cancer Assay, the 18-gene classifier ColoPrint, or the 13-gene classifier ColoGuideEx), as well as classifiers based on the Immunoscore, microRNA expression, and presence of circulating tumor cells by molecular methods, has been the object of study but has not been implemented in the current practice yet (see also Chapter 3, Molecular Diagnostic Guidelines for Colorectal Cancer).

Adjuvant Treatment of Elderly Patients

The basic principles of adjuvant treatment for colon cancer remain the same in the elderly population as in younger adult patients. However, safety and efficacy of adjuvant chemotherapy in elderly patients may be difficult to evaluate as patients older than 65 years with comorbidities and poorer functional status are underrepresented in clinical trials. A careful assessment of patients' performance status, comorbidities, age-related organ function, life expectancy, potential treatment-related toxicity, and quality-of-life issues has to be performed in order to select those patients who could benefit from treatment.

The comprehensive geriatric assessment (CGA), a multidisciplinary evaluation covering domains such as cognitive and psychological status, physical function, comorbidities, social support, nutrition, and polypharmacy, has been shown to provide important information related to prognosis and likelihood of toxicity from chemotherapy in elderly cancer patients (56,57). Additionally, several multidimensional geriatric assessment scores are available in order to aid patient selection and estimate the life expectancy and risk of severe chemotherapy-related toxicities in this complex population of patients (58,59). The use of these tools should be implemented in the decision making when evaluating older cancer patients (see also Chapter 54, Care for Elderly Gastrointestinal Cancer Patients).

Adjuvant chemotherapy is not recommended in frail elderly patients with severe comorbidities, geriatric syndromes, significant functional impairment, or a compromised performance status (Eastern Cooperative Oncology Group [ECOG], <2). Conversely, an adjuvant treatment should be generally offered to active and independent older patients without relevant comorbidities (fit patients). In the case of vulnerable patients (neither frail nor fit), a personalized decision should be made after a careful evaluation of each single case and a geriatric assessment to plan adequate interventions to improve a patient's conditions and likelihood to tolerate treatment.

Evidence on the benefit of adjuvant chemotherapy in the elderly population comes from pooled analyses of randomized clinical trials, population-based retrospective analyses, and systematic reviews of available data. Overall, the advantage from 5-FU/LV appears similar between older and younger patients. Large retrospective analyses of data from the SEER-Medicare Database and NCCN Outcome Database confirmed a survival benefit in patients with stage III colon cancer older than 65 years (HR: 0.70, p < .001) and aged 75 years or older (HR: 0.60, 95% CI: 0.53–0.68), respectively (60,61). The benefit from the addition of oxaliplatin in this setting, however, does not appear to be clearly significant. A retrospective analysis of 12,000 patients from the ACCENT database, in fact, highlighted a reduced benefit from the addition of oxaliplatin to fluoropyrimidines in stage III patients aged 70 years or older (62). Similarly, subgroup analyses from the MOSAIC and NSABP C-07 trials showed no benefit from the addition of oxaliplatin to 5-FU/LV in stage II or III patients aged 70 years or older (HR: 1.10, 95% CI: 0.73–1.65 and HR: 1.18, 95% CI: 0.86–1.62, respectively) (10,39). On the other hand, a pooled analyses of data from four other randomized trials (including the XELOXA and X-ACT trial) reported an improvement in DFS and OS with adjuvant XELOX or FOLFOX over 5-FU/LV in patients aged 70 years or older (HR for DFS 0.77, 95% CI: 0.62–0.95, *p* = .014 and HR for OS 0.78, 95% CI: 0.61–0.99, *p* = .045) (63).

In terms of risks of treatment-related toxicities, the majority of evidence from adjuvant trials suggests a similar safety profile for patients older than 65 years when compared to younger patients, with limited data reporting a higher toxicity rate of grade 3–4 adverse events among elderly patients for cardiac disorders, neutropenia, infection, dehydration, diarrhea, and fatigue (64). However, a pooled analysis of 37,568 patients from the ACCENT database showed that the risk of early mortality (within 1 to 6 months of adjuvant treatment start), although infrequent, was significantly higher in older patients, particularly for those over 70 years of age (65). If an oxaliplatin-based regimen is considered, the risk of neurotoxicity and its potential impact on patient quality of life should be carefully weighted.

Capecitabine should be used with caution in patients with reduced renal function. A 25% dose reduction is recommended for glomerular filtration rates (GFRs) between 30 and 50 mL/min, and the drug should be avoided with GFR <30 mL/min. Additionally, in elderly patients it appears reasonable to start treatment at a lower dose (i.e., 1,000 mg/mq twice daily) and subsequently evaluate a dose escalation based on treatment tolerability.

Web-Based Tools for Risk Stratification

Recently, several web-based tools have been developed to assist clinicians in assessing disease recurrence and mortality risk and to calculate the relative benefit of adjuvant chemotherapy. One of these tools, the ACCENT-based web calculator (available online) (66), has been approved for predicting prognosis of patients with resected colon cancer by the American Joint Committee on Cancer (AJCC). This calculator uses clinical and pathologic information as well as treatment information (oxaliplatin vs. non-oxaliplatin-based adjuvant regimen) to estimate the recurrence-free probability at 3 years and the 5-year survival after adjuvant treatment.

Future Perspectives for Patient Selection: The Role of Liquid Biopsy

A novel promising approach to the evaluation of residual disease and risk stratification of patients after surgery in early-stage colon cancer is the analysis of circulating tumor DNA (ctDNA). This technology, commonly referred to as liquid biopsy, has been rapidly developing in the past few years as a less invasive and more comprehensive approach to pharmacogenomic profiling and dynamic monitoring in CRC patients (67). The analysis of ctDNA allows large-scale genomic testing and is able to capture the molecular heterogeneity of different tumor subclones in the same patient; additionally, it has been demonstrated that seriated analyses over time can allow an early detection of the emergence of treatment resistance to targeted therapies in the metastatic setting, and thus guide a personalized treatment strategy through a dynamic molecular profiling (68,69). In the adjuvant setting, growing evidence suggests that the analysis of ctDNA after radical surgical resection represents an innovative tool to evaluate the presence of minimal residual disease and consequently identify patients at a high risk of recurrence to receive a more aggressive adjuvant treatment (70). Moreover, monitoring the levels of ctDNA after adjuvant treatment in previously positive patients may represent both a prognostic biomarker and a tool for early detection of disease recurrence during follow-up (71).

Although still needing extensive investigations and validation before entering clinical practice (72), liquid biopsy approaches to profile and monitor patients after surgery in the adjuvant setting in colon cancer are currently already under investigation in several clinical trials (e.g., NCT02842203, NCT03284684, NCT01198743, NCT02997241, NCT03312374, NCT03416478).

OPTIMAL DURATION OF TREATMENT

The consensus on the optimal duration of adjuvant chemotherapy for patients with stage III colon cancer has been the object of an intense debate. To date, 6 months of adjuvant oxaliplatin-based chemotherapy following surgery has been considered the standard of care for stage III patients. However, oxaliplatin is associated with a cumulative and dose-limiting peripheral neurotoxicity, and a high percentage of patients are not able to conclude the full treatment course without reducing or omitting this drug during the last cycles. The International Duration Evaluation of Adjuvant Chemotherapy (IDEA) collaborative study evaluated the possibility of shortening the duration of adjuvant treatment without compromising its efficacy, testing the noninferiority of 3 months of adjuvant chemotherapy with either FOLFOX or XELOX compared to 6 months of either regimen in stage III colon cancer. Initial results of this prospective pre-planned pooled analysis of data from six randomized phase III trials of 3 versus 6 months of adjuvant therapy (TOSCA, SCOT, Alliance/SWOG 80702, IDEA France, ACHIEVE, and HORG), involving 12,834 patients in 12 countries, have been presented at the American Society of Clinical Oncology (ASCO) Annual Meeting in 2017 and recently published (73). The primary end point of the study was 3-year DFS, setting to 1.12 the predefined upper limit for noninferiority of the two-sided 95% CI for the HR for DFS. Patients were accrued between June 2007 and December 2015, and data presented at a median follow-up of 39 months. Three-year DFS was 75.5% in the 6-month arm and 74.6% in the 3-month arm (HR: 1.07, 95% CI: 1.00–1.15). From a statistical point of view, noninferiority was not established; however, the DFS curves of the two treatment arms overlap, and the absolute gain in efficacy with 6 months of adjuvant treatment is <1%. Additionally, the risk of severe (grade $\geq$3) neurotoxicity was significantly higher in the 6-month arm compared to the 3-month arm (16% vs. 3% with FOLFOX and 9% vs. 3% with XELOX, respectively, $p < .0001$). Notably, in the preplanned subgroup analysis according to the treatment regimen, noninferiority of 3 months of treatment versus 6 months was proved in the overall population of patients treated with XELOX, comprising about 40% of the analyzed patients (HR: 0.95, 95% CI: 0.85–1.06), while 3 months of FOLFOX was inferior to 6 months (HR: 1.16, 95% CI: 1.06–1.26). When data were analyzed according to risk group (classifying T1–3/N1 tumors as low risk and T4 and/or N2 tumors as high risk), 3 months of XELOX confirmed to be noninferior to 6 months in the low-risk group, comprising about 60% of the analyzed patients (HR: 0.85, 95% CI: 0.71–1.01), while 3 months of FOLFOX was inferior to 6 months in the high-risk group (HR: 1.20, 95% CI: 1.07–1.35). Noninferiority of 3 months of XELOX in the high-risk group was not proven, as well as noninferiority of 3 months of FOLFOX in the low-risk group. Overall, combining the two regimens, 3 months was noninferior to 6 months in the treatment of low-risk patients (3-year DFS 83.1% vs. 83.3%; HR: 1.01, 95% CI: 0.90–1.12), while 6 months was superior to 3 months in high-risk patients (3-year DFS 64.4% vs. 62.7%; HR: 1.12, 95% CI: 1.03–1.23, $p = .01$ for superiority) (73). Thus, both adjuvant chemotherapy regimen selection and disease characteristics appear to be crucial in determining the best treatment choice in individual patients. Although still debated, these data support a practice changing approach in treatment selection and modulation of adjuvant treatment duration in stage III colon cancer, as 3 months of adjuvant treatment with the XELOX regimen emerges as the best option for low-risk T1–3/N1 stage III patients, while at present no evidence supports a shorter duration of treatment in high-risk T4 and/or N2 patients.

Overall, based on the MOSAIC and NSABP C-07 trials and the discussed initial results from the IDEA trial, 6 months of oxaliplatin-based chemotherapy remains the standard for individuals with high-risk stage III tumors (T4 or N2). On the other hand, given the small predicted loss of DFS benefit and the significantly lower rates of oxaliplatin-related neurotoxicity, alongside the results of the preplanned subgroup analysis, 3 months of adjuvant oxaliplatin-based therapy should be considered the new standard in patients with low-risk disease (T1–3/N1) favoring the administration of XELOX over FOLFOX.

For patients receiving a fluoropyrimidine monotherapy, 6 months of adjuvant treatment remains the standard (1).

Clinical Vignette 5.1

CASE SCENARIO: A 36-year-old woman presents to your oncology clinic for consultation 3 weeks post a right hemicolectomy for a colon cancer. She has researched her disease thoroughly and states that she would like to be treated aggressively. **Patient clinical details:** No history of previous diseases. No family history of cancer. Married, no children. Office worker. **Disease presentation and surgical treatment:** The patient presented to the ED with symptoms of acute bowel obstruction. CT imaging of the chest, abdomen, and pelvis showed an obstructing mass in the right-sided colon with no evidence of other sites of disease. An emergency right hemicolectomy was performed. **Pathology report:** Grade 3 poorly differentiated adenocarcinoma of the ascending colon perforating the serosa without direct invasion of other organs, with presence of lymphovascular and perineural invasion and extensive lymphoid infiltrate; no regional node involved out of 24 resected nodes.

QUESTION 1: Disease stage? **Answer:** Stage IIb (pT4aN0M0, G3).

QUESTION 2: Clinicopathological risk factors? **Answer:** Presentation of disease with acute obstruction and emergency surgery. T4 primary. Poorly differentiated histology. Lymphovascular and perineural invasion.

QUESTION 3: Are we missing something? **Answer:** Young woman with stage II poorly differentiated right-sided primary tumor with extensive lymphoid infiltrate. Indication to MSI testing for Lynch syndrome screening and risk stratification.

Additional Information: Molecular testing positive for MSI-H and *BRAF V600E* mutation.

Discussion: This case requires counseling for the indication to an adjuvant treatment of a young patient with MSI-H stage II colon cancer with multiple high-risk factors (of note, considering the presence of an MSI-H status, poor differentiation of primary tumor is not considered a risk factor in this patient).

- The benefit of adjuvant treatment for stage II colon cancer has been discussed in the section Treatment of Stage II Disease and Risk Stratification; although data in stage II disease are sometimes contradictory and mainly derive from retrospective subgroup analyses and pooled meta-analyses, adjuvant chemotherapy in stage II colon cancer, particularly in the presence of high-risk factors, appears to confer an absolute improvement in 5-year survival up to 4% to 5%. Additionally, an exploratory analysis of the MOSAIC trial showed a trend toward an improvement in 5-year DFS favoring an oxaliplatin-based regimen in the subgroup of stage II patients with high-risk tumors. As an example of the impact of high-risk features on prognosis, the presence of a T4 primary is associated with a 5-year relative survival after surgery alone around 71% in stage II, which is lower than the survival rates of stage IIIA, versus a 5-year relative survival around 87% for stage IIA (T3N0) tumors (74). Based on available data and treatment guidelines, patients presenting with a high-risk stage II colon cancer, particularly in the presence of a T4 primary tumor or multiple high-risk features, should be considered for 6 months of adjuvant chemotherapy with either a fluoropyrimidine-based or an oxaliplatin-based treatment. Risk of recurrence, expected treatment benefit, and treatment-related toxicities should be discussed to inform patient's choice. In our case, considering the presence of multiple high-risk factors and the patient's request for treatment, in the absence of contraindications, a 6-month adjuvant oxaliplatin-based regimen should be the recommendation of choice.
- **Do tumor molecular features change our approach in this case scenario?** MSI-H is a recognized good prognostic factor in stage II colon cancer. The excellent survival outcome of MSI-H stage II patients, even in the absence of postsurgical treatment, has been demonstrated in retrospective subgroup analyses of several trials, both for T3 and T4 tumors. However, the combined impact of MSI-H and different risk factors in high-risk stage II, particularly in the presence of multiple risk factors as in our case, has not been extensively investigated and remains unclear. The presence of a *BRAF V600E* mutation, diagnostic of sporadic MSI-H, does not appear to confer a negative prognostic impact in early-stage MSI-H tumors, contrarily to MSS tumors, and does not affect treatment choices in this setting (75). In the case of disease recurrence, on the other hand, *BRAF V600E* mutation has been associated with worse postrelapse survival (54), and particular attention to distinctive recurrence patterns related to MSI-H and *BRAF* mutations (i.e., peritoneal and lymph nodal recurrence) should be paid in these patients. Finally, as mentioned earlier, stage II MSI-H tumors appear not to derive any benefit from a fluoropyrimidine-based adjuvant treatment, while oxaliplatin efficacy has been shown to be independent of MSI status. Altogether, in our case scenario, the evaluation of tumor molecular features supports the recommendation of an oxaliplatin-based chemotherapy to our patient.

Summary of Recommendations

- Adjuvant chemotherapy has been proven to reduce the risk of disease recurrence and risk of death in stage III (node-positive) colon cancer after potentially curative resection.
- Patients with stage I and MSI-H low-risk stage II colon cancer do not require adjuvant treatment.
- Patients with low-risk MSS stage II disease should generally be observed without treatment. However, potential benefit and risk of an adjuvant fluoropyrimidine monotherapy can be discussed as an individualized option. Patients with stage II colon cancer with high-risk features (T4, poorly differentiated histology [except MSI-H tumors], LVI, PNI, bowel obstruction/perforation, inadequate nodal sampling, or close/undetermined/positive margins) should be considered for adjuvant chemotherapy with either an oxaliplatin-based regimen or a fluoropyrimidine monotherapy. A detailed discussion on risk assessment, treatment options, treatment-related toxicities, and expected benefit should be conducted to inform the patient and personalize the treatment choice.
- A fluoropyrimidine monotherapy is not recommended in stage II MSI-H colon cancer as MSI-H appears to be associated with lack of efficacy from 5-FU in this setting. For patients with high-risk MSI-H stage II disease, the use of an oxaliplatin-based regimen can be an option.
- Adjuvant chemotherapy with an oxaliplatin-based regimen rather than a fluoropyrimidine monotherapy is recommended for stage III patients who are likely to tolerate oxaliplatin. A fluoropyrimidine monotherapy is an acceptable option for patients with a contraindication to oxaliplatin or for those not considered candidates to a combination regimen.
- Adjuvant chemotherapy should be recommended to fit older ($\geq$70 years) patients with stage III and high-risk stage II colon cancer, considering treatment-related risks and individual preferences and values. Risks and benefits of chemotherapy should be discussed and treatment choice individualized on single-case bases for vulnerable patients. Frail elderly patients are not appropriate candidates for an adjuvant treatment. A CGA should be implemented in the evaluation of elderly patients to aid patient selection and formulate an individualized treatment plan, when appropriate.
- A fluoropyrimidine monotherapy is generally the preferred adjuvant treatment in elderly patients. However, for selected fit patients with stage III disease, an oxaliplatin-based regimen can be discussed as an option.
- If possible, adjuvant chemotherapy should be initiated within 6 to 8 weeks of surgery.
- The optimal duration of adjuvant oxaliplatin-based chemotherapy for patients with high-risk stage III (T4 and/or N2) colon cancer is 6 months. For patients with low-risk stage III (T1-3/N1) 3 months, favoring XELOX over FOLFOX appears to be the new standard of treatment based on the results of the IDEA trial.
- The optimal duration of adjuvant fluoropyrimidine monotherapy is 6 months.
- Irinotecan-based treatment and targeted treatments with anti-VEGFs and anti-EGFRs are not recommended in the adjuvant setting.

ADDITIONAL READINGS

Labianca R, Nordlinger B, Beretta GD, et al. Early colon cancer: ESMO clinical practice guidelines. *Ann Oncol.* 2013;24(Suppl 6):vi64–vi72. doi:10.1093/annonc/mdt354

NCCN Guidelines v 2.2018. Colorectal Cancer. Retrieved from https://www.nccn.org/professionals/physician_gls/pdf/colon.pdf

REFERENCES

1. Des Guetz G, Uzzan B, Morere JF, et al. Duration of adjuvant chemotherapy for patients with non-metastatic colorectal cancer. *Cochrane Database Syst Rev.* 2010;(1):Cd007046. doi:10.1002/14651858.CD007046.pub2

2. Kohne CH, Bedenne L, Carrato A, et al. A randomised phase III intergroup trial comparing high-dose infusional 5-fluorouracil with or without folinic acid with standard bolus 5-fluorouracil/folinic acid in the adjuvant treatment of stage III colon cancer: the Pan-European Trial in Adjuvant Colon Cancer 2 study. *Eur J Cancer (Oxford, England: 1990)*. 2013;49(8):1868–1875. doi:10.1016/j.ejca.2013.01.030

3. Pectasides D, Karavasilis V, Papaxoinis G, et al. Randomized phase III clinical trial comparing the combination of capecitabine and oxaliplatin (CAPOX) with the combination of 5-fluorouracil, leucovorin and oxaliplatin (modified FOLFOX6) as adjuvant therapy in patients with operated high-risk stage II or stage III colorectal cancer. *BMC Cancer*. 2015;15:384. doi:10.1186/s12885-015-1406-7

4. Twelves C, Scheithauer W, McKendrick J, et al. Capecitabine versus 5-fluorouracil/folinic acid as adjuvant therapy for stage III colon cancer: final results from the X-ACT trial with analysis by age and preliminary evidence of a pharmacodynamic marker of efficacy. *Ann Oncol*. 2012;23(5):1190–1197. doi:10.1093/annonc/mdr366

5. Sadahiro S, Tsuchiya T, Sasaki K, et al. Randomized phase III trial of treatment duration for oral uracil and tegafur plus leucovorin as adjuvant chemotherapy for patients with stage IIB/III colon cancer: final results of JFMC33-0502. *Ann Oncol*. 2015;26(11):2274–2280. doi:10.1093/annonc/mdv358

6. Yoshida M, Ishiguro M, Ikejiri K, et al. S-1 as adjuvant chemotherapy for stage III colon cancer: a randomized phase III study (ACTS-CC trial). *Ann Oncol*. 2014;25(9):1743–1749. doi:10.1093/annonc/mdu232

7. Shah MA, Renfro LA, Allegra CJ, et al. Impact of patient factors on recurrence risk and time dependency of oxaliplatin benefit in patients with colon cancer: analysis from modern-era adjuvant studies in the Adjuvant Colon Cancer End Points (ACCENT) database. *J Clin Oncol*. 2016;34(8):843–853. doi:10.1200/JCO.2015.63.0558

8. Andre T, Boni C, Navarro M, et al. Improved overall survival with oxaliplatin, fluorouracil, and leucovorin as adjuvant treatment in stage II or III colon cancer in the MOSAIC trial. *J Clin Oncol*. 2009;27(19):3109–3116. doi:10.1200/JCO.2008.20.6771

9. Andre T, de Gramont A, Vernerey D, et al. Adjuvant fluorouracil, leucovorin, and oxaliplatin in stage II to III colon cancer: updated 10-year survival and outcomes according to braf mutation and mismatch repair status of the MOSAIC study. *J Clin Oncol*. 2015;33(35):4176–4187. doi:10.1200/JCO.2015.63.4238

10. Yothers G, O'Connell MJ, Allegra CJ, et al. Oxaliplatin as adjuvant therapy for colon cancer: updated results of NSABP C-07 trial, including survival and subset analyses. *J Clin Oncol*. 2011;29(28):3768–3774. doi:10.1200/JCO.2011.36.4539

11. Haller DG, Tabernero J, Maroun J, et al. Capecitabine plus oxaliplatin compared with fluorouracil and folinic acid as adjuvant therapy for stage III colon cancer. *J Clin Oncol*. 2011;29(11):1465–1471. doi:10.1200/JCO.2010.33.6297

12. Schmoll HJ, Tabernero J, Maroun J, et al. Capecitabine plus oxaliplatin compared with fluorouracil/folinic acid as adjuvant therapy for stage III colon cancer: final results of the NO16968 randomized controlled phase III trial. *J Clin Oncol*. 2015;33(32):3733–3740. doi:10.1200/JCO.2015.60.9107

13. Schmoll HJ, Twelves C, Sun W, et al. Effect of adjuvant capecitabine or fluorouracil, with or without oxaliplatin, on survival outcomes in stage III colon cancer and the effect of oxaliplatin on post-relapse survival: a pooled analysis of individual patient data from four randomised controlled trials. *Lancet Oncol*. 2014;15(13):1481–1492. doi:10.1016/S1470-2045(14)70486-3

14. Van Cutsem E, Labianca R, Bodoky G, et al. Randomized phase III trial comparing biweekly infusional fluorouracil/leucovorin alone or with irinotecan in the adjuvant treatment of stage III colon cancer: PETACC-3. *J Clin Oncol*. 2009;27(19):3117–3125. doi:10.1200/JCO.2008.21.6663

15. de Gramont A, Van Cutsem E, Schmoll HJ, et al. Bevacizumab plus oxaliplatin-based chemotherapy as adjuvant treatment for colon cancer (AVANT): a phase 3 randomised controlled trial. *Lancet Oncol*. 2012;13(12):1225–1233. doi:10.1016/S1470-2045(12)70509-0

16. Allegra CJ, Yothers G, O'Connell MJ, et al. Bevacizumab in stage II-III colon cancer: 5-year update of the National Surgical Adjuvant Breast and Bowel Project C-08 trial. *J Clin Oncol*. 2013;31(3):359–364. doi:10.1200/JCO.2012.44.4711

17. Kerr RS, Love S, Segelov E, et al. Adjuvant capecitabine plus bevacizumab versus capecitabine alone in patients with colorectal cancer (QUASAR 2): an open-label, randomised phase 3 trial. *Lancet Oncol*. 2016;17(11):1543–1557. doi:10.1016/S1470-2045(16)30172-3

18. Taieb J, Balogoun R, Le Malicot K, et al. Adjuvant FOLFOX +/− cetuximab in full RAS and BRAF wildtype stage III colon cancer patients. *Ann Oncol*. 2017;28(4):824–830. doi:10.1093/annonc/mdw687

19. Sammartino P, Sibio S, Biacchi D, et al. Prevention of peritoneal metastases from colon cancer in high-risk patients: preliminary results of surgery plus prophylactic HIPEC. *Gastroenterol Res Pract.* 2012;2012:141585. doi:10.1155/2012/141585

20. Des Guetz G, Nicolas P, Perret GY, et al. Does delaying adjuvant chemotherapy after curative surgery for colorectal cancer impair survival? A meta-analysis. *Eur J Cancer (Oxford, England: 1990).* 2010;46(6):1049–1055. doi:10.1016/j.ejca.2010.01.020

21. Biagi JJ, Raphael MJ, Mackillop WJ, et al. Association between time to initiation of adjuvant chemotherapy and survival in colorectal cancer: a systematic review and meta-analysis. *JAMA.* 2011;305(22):2335–2342. doi:10.1001/jama.2011.749

22. Sun Z, Adam MA, Kim J, et al. Determining the optimal timing for initiation of adjuvant chemotherapy after resection for stage II and III colon cancer. *Dis Colon Rectum.* 2016;59(2):87–93. doi:10.1097/DCR.0000000000000518

23. Roth AD, Delorenzi M, Tejpar S, et al. Integrated analysis of molecular and clinical prognostic factors in stage II/III colon cancer. *J Natl Cancer Inst.* 2012;104(21):1635–1646. doi:10.1093/jnci/djs427

24. Song N, Pogue-Geile KL, Gavin PG, et al. Clinical outcome from oxaliplatin treatment in stage II/III colon cancer according to intrinsic subtypes: secondary analysis of NSABP C-07/NRG oncology randomized clinical trial. *JAMA Oncol.* 2016;2(9):1162–1169. doi:10.1001/jamaoncol.2016.2314

25. Dienstmann R, Mason MJ, Sinicrope FA, et al. Prediction of overall survival in stage II and III colon cancer beyond TNM system: a retrospective, pooled biomarker study. *Ann Oncol.* 2017;28(5):1023–1031. doi:10.1093/annonc/mdx052

26. Liao X, Lochhead P, Nishihara R, et al. Aspirin use, tumor PIK3CA mutation, and colorectal-cancer survival. *N Engl J Med.* 2012;367(17):1596–1606. doi:10.1056/NEJMoa1207756

27. Domingo E, Church DN, Sieber O, et al. Evaluation of PIK3CA mutation as a predictor of benefit from nonsteroidal anti-inflammatory drug therapy in colorectal cancer. *J Clin Oncol.* 2013;31(34):4297–4305. doi:10.1200/JCO.2013.50.0322

28. Paleari L, Puntoni M, Clavarezza M, et al. PIK3CA mutation, aspirin use after diagnosis and survival of colorectal cancer: a systematic review and meta-analysis of epidemiological studies. *Clin Oncol.* 2016;28(5):317–326. doi:10.1016/j.clon.2015.11.008

29. Guercio BJ, Sato K, Niedzwiecki D, et al. Coffee intake, recurrence, and mortality in stage III colon cancer: results from CALGB 89803 (Alliance). *J Clin Oncol.* 2015;33(31):3598–3607. doi:10.1200/JCO.2015.61.5062

30. Hu Y, Ding M, Yuan C, et al. Association between coffee intake after diagnosis of colorectal cancer and reduced mortality. *Gastroenterology.* 2018;154(4):916.e919–926.e919. doi:10.1053/j.gastro.2017.11.010

31. Song M, Wu K, Meyerhardt JA, et al. Fiber intake and survival after colorectal cancer diagnosis. *JAMA Oncol.* 2018;4(1):71–79. doi:10.1001/jamaoncol.2017.3684

32. Fadelu T, Zhang S, Niedzwiecki D, et al. Nut consumption and survival in patients with stage III colon cancer: results from CALGB 89803 (Alliance). *J Clin Oncol.* 2018;36(11):1112–1120. doi:10.1200/jco.2017.75.5413

33. Mohr SB, Gorham ED, Kim J, et al. Could vitamin D sufficiency improve the survival of colorectal cancer patients? *J Steroid Biochem Mol Biol.* 2015;148:239–244. doi:10.1016/j.jsbmb.2014.12.010

34. Gray R, Barnwell J, McConkey C, et al. Adjuvant chemotherapy versus observation in patients with colorectal cancer: a randomised study. *Lancet.* 2007;370(9604):2020–2029. doi:10.1016/S0140-6736(07)61866-2

35. Efficacy of adjuvant fluorouracil and folinic acid in B2 colon cancer. International Multicentre Pooled Analysis of B2 Colon Cancer Trials (IMPACT B2) Investigators. *J Clin Oncol.* 1999;17(5):1356–1363. doi:10.1200/JCO.1999.17.5.1356

36. Figueredo A, Charette ML, Maroun J, et al. Adjuvant therapy for stage II colon cancer: a systematic review from the Cancer Care Ontario Program in evidence-based care's gastrointestinal cancer disease site group. *J Clin Oncol.* 2004;22(16):3395–3407. doi:10.1200/JCO.2004.03.087

37. Gill S, Loprinzi CL, Sargent DJ, et al. Pooled analysis of fluorouracil-based adjuvant therapy for stage II and III colon cancer: who benefits and by how much? *J Clin Oncol.* 2004;22(10):1797–1806. doi:10.1200/JCO.2004.09.059

38. Sargent D, Sobrero A, Grothey A, et al. Evidence for cure by adjuvant therapy in colon cancer: observations based on individual patient data from 20,898 patients on 18 randomized trials. *J Clin Oncol.* 2009;27(6):872–877. doi:10.1200/JCO.2008.19.5362

39. Tournigand C, Andre T, Bonnetain F, et al. Adjuvant therapy with fluorouracil and oxaliplatin in stage II and elderly patients (between ages 70 and 75 years) with colon cancer: subgroup analyses of the Multicenter International Study of Oxaliplatin, Fluorouracil, and Leucovorin in the Adjuvant Treatment of Colon Cancer trial. *J Clin Oncol.* 2012;30(27):3353–3360. doi:10.1200/JCO.2012.42.5645

40. Casadaban L, Rauscher G, Aklilu M, et al. Adjuvant chemotherapy is associated with improved survival in patients with stage II colon cancer. *Cancer.* 2016;122(21):3277–3287. doi:10.1002/cncr.30181

41. Quah HM, Chou JF, Gonen M, et al. Identification of patients with high-risk stage II colon cancer for adjuvant therapy. *Dis Colon Rectum.* 2008;51(5):503–507. doi:10.1007/s10350-008-9246-z

42. Amri R, Bordeianou LG, Berger D. Effect of high-grade disease on outcomes of surgically treated colon cancer. *Ann Surg Oncol.* 2016;23:1157. doi:10.1245/s10434-015-4983-4

43. Yuan H, Dong Q, Zheng Ba, et al. Lymphovascular invasion is a high risk factor for stage I/II colorectal cancer: a systematic review and meta-analysis. *Oncotarget.* 2017;8(28):46565–46579. doi:10.18632/oncotarget.15425

44. Cienfuegos JA, Martinez P, Baixauli J, et al. Perineural invasion is a major prognostic and predictive factor of response to adjuvant chemotherapy in stage I-II colon cancer. *Ann Surg Oncol.* 2017;24(4):1077–1084. doi:10.1245/s10434-016-5561-0

45. Chen HS, Sheen-Chen SM. Obstruction and perforation in colorectal adenocarcinoma: an analysis of prognosis and current trends. *Surgery.* 2000;127(4):370–376. doi:10.1067/msy.2000.104674

46. Chang GJ, Rodriguez-Bigas MA, Skibber JM, et al. Lymph node evaluation and survival after curative resection of colon cancer: systematic review. *J Natl Cancer Inst.* 2007;99(6):433–441. doi:10.1093/jnci/djk092

47. Lynch HT, Lynch JF, Lynch PM. Toward a consensus in molecular diagnosis of hereditary nonpolyposis colorectal cancer (Lynch syndrome). *J Natl Cancer Inst.* 2007;99(4):261–263. doi:10.1093/jnci/djk077

48. Dienstmann R, Vermeulen L, Guinney J, et al. Consensus molecular subtypes and the evolution of precision medicine in colorectal cancer. *Nature Rev Cancer.* 2017;17(2):79–92. doi:10.1038/nrc.2016.126

49. Raut CP, Pawlik TM, Rodriguez-Bigas MA. Clinicopathologic features in colorectal cancer patients with microsatellite instability. *Mutat Res.* 2004;568(2):275–282. doi:10.1016/j.mrfmmm.2004.05.025

50. Sargent DJ, Marsoni S, Monges G, et al. Defective mismatch repair as a predictive marker for lack of efficacy of fluorouracil-based adjuvant therapy in colon cancer. *J Clin Oncol.* 2010;28(20):3219–3226. doi:10.1200/JCO.2009.27.1825

51. Sargent DJ, Shi Q, Yothers G, et al. Prognostic impact of deficient mismatch repair (dMMR) in 7,803 stage II/III colon cancer (CC) patients (pts): a pooled individual pt data analysis of 17 adjuvant trials in the ACCENT database. *J Clin Oncol.* 2014;32(15_suppl):3507. doi:10.1200/jco.2014.32.15_suppl.3507

52. Hutchins G, Southward K, Handley K, et al. Value of mismatch repair, KRAS, and BRAF mutations in predicting recurrence and benefits from chemotherapy in colorectal cancer. *J Clin Oncol.* 2011;29(10):1261–1270. doi:10.1200/JCO.2010.30.1366

53. Sinicrope FA, Foster NR, Thibodeau SN, et al. DNA mismatch repair status and colon cancer recurrence and survival in clinical trials of 5-fluorouracil-based adjuvant therapy. *J Natl Cancer Inst.* 2011;103(11):863–875. doi:10.1093/jnci/djr153

54. Gavin PG, Colangelo LH, Fumagalli D, et al. Mutation profiling and microsatellite instability in stage II and III colon cancer: an assessment of their prognostic and oxaliplatin predictive value. *Clin Cancer Res.* 2012;18(23):6531–6541. doi:10.1158/1078-0432.CCR-12-0605

55. Tougeron D, Mouillet G, Trouilloud I, et al. Efficacy of adjuvant chemotherapy in colon cancer with microsatellite instability: a large multicenter AGEO study. *J Natl Cancer Inst.* 2016;108(7):djv438. doi:10.1093/jnci/djv438

56. Hamaker ME, Vos AG, Smorenburg CH, et al. The value of geriatric assessments in predicting treatment tolerance and all-cause mortality in older patients with cancer. *Oncologist.* 2012;17(11):1439–1449. doi:10.1634/theoncologist.2012-0186

57. Puts MT, Santos B, Hardt J, et al. An update on a systematic review of the use of geriatric assessment for older adults in oncology. *Ann Oncol.* 2014;25(2):307–315. doi:10.1093/annonc/mdt386

58. Decoster L, Van Puyvelde K, Mohile S, et al. Screening tools for multidimensional health problems warranting a geriatric assessment in older cancer patients: an update on SIOG recommendations. *Ann Oncol.* 2015;26(2):288–300. doi:10.1093/annonc/mdu210

59. Extermann M, Boler I, Reich RR, et al. Predicting the risk of chemotherapy toxicity in older patients: the Chemotherapy Risk Assessment Scale for High-Age Patients (CRASH) score. *Cancer.* 2012;118(13):3377–3386. doi:10.1002/cncr.26646

60. Hanna NN, Onukwugha E, Choti MA, et al. Comparative analysis of various prognostic nodal factors, adjuvant chemotherapy and survival among stage III colon cancer patients over 65 years: an analysis using surveillance, epidemiology and end results (SEER)-Medicare data. *Colorectal Dis.* 2012;14(1):48–55. doi:10.1111/j.1463-1318.2011.02545.x

61. Sanoff HK, Carpenter WR, Sturmer T, et al. Effect of adjuvant chemotherapy on survival of patients with stage III colon cancer diagnosed after age 75 years. *J Clin Oncol.* 2012;30(21):2624–2634. doi:10.1200/JCO.2011.41.1140

62. McCleary NJ, Meyerhardt JA, Green E, et al. Impact of age on the efficacy of newer adjuvant therapies in patients with stage II/III colon cancer: findings from the ACCENT database. *J Clin Oncol.* 2013;31(20):2600–2606. doi:10.1200/JCO.2013.49.6638

63. Haller DG, O'Connell MJ, Cartwright TH, et al. Impact of age and medical comorbidity on adjuvant treatment outcomes for stage III colon cancer: a pooled analysis of individual patient data from four randomized, controlled trials. *Ann Oncol.* 2015;26(4):715–724. doi:10.1093/annonc/mdv003

64. Hung A, Mullins CD. Relative effectiveness and safety of chemotherapy in elderly and nonelderly patients with stage III colon cancer: a systematic review. *Oncologist.* 2013;18(1):54–63. doi:10.1634/theoncologist.2012-0050

65. Cheung WY, Renfro LA, Kerr D, et al. Determinants of early mortality among 37,568 patients with colon cancer who participated in 25 clinical trials from the adjuvant colon cancer endpoints database. *J Clin Oncol.* 2016;34(11):1182–1189. doi:10.1200/JCO.2015.65.1158

66. Renfro LA, Grothey A, Xue Y, et al. ACCENT-based web calculators to predict recurrence and overall survival in stage III colon cancer. *J Natl Cancer Inst.* 2014;106(12). doi:10.1093/jnci/dju333

67. Bettegowda C, Sausen M, Leary RJ, et al. Detection of circulating tumor DNA in early- and late-stage human malignancies. *Sci Transl Med.* 2014;6(224):224ra24. doi:10.1126/scitranslmed.3007094

68. Siravegna G, Mussolin B, Buscarino M, et al. Clonal evolution and resistance to EGFR blockade in the blood of colorectal cancer patients. *Nature Med.* 2015;21(7):795–801. doi:10.1038/nm.3870

69. Strickler JH, Loree JM, Ahronian LG, et al. Genomic landscape of cell-free DNA in patients with colorectal cancer. *Cancer Discov.* 2017;8(2):164–173. doi:10.1158/2159-8290.cd-17-1009

70. Tie J, Wang Y, Tomasetti C, et al. Circulating tumor DNA analysis detects minimal residual disease and predicts recurrence in patients with stage II colon cancer. *Sci Transl Med.* 2016;8(346):346ra392. doi:10.1126/scitranslmed.aaf6219

71. Reinert T, Scholer LV, Thomsen R, et al. Analysis of circulating tumour DNA to monitor disease burden following colorectal cancer surgery. *Gut.* 2016;65(4):625–634. doi:10.1136/gutjnl-2014-308859

72. Merker JD, Oxnard GR, Compton C, et al. Circulating tumor DNA analysis in patients with cancer: American Society of Clinical Oncology and College of American Pathologists joint review. *J Clin Oncol.* 2018;36:16:1631–1641. doi:10.1200/jco.2017.76.8671

73. Grothey A, Sobrero AF, Shields AF, et al. Duration of adjuvant chemotherapy for stage III colon cancer. *N Engl J Med.* 2018;378(13):1177–1188. doi:10.1056/NEJMoa1713709

74. Gunderson LL, Jessup JM, Sargent DJ, et al. Revised TN categorization for colon cancer based on national survival outcomes data. *J Clin Oncol.* 2010;28(2):264–271. doi:10.1200/JCO.2009.24.0952

75. Sanz-Garcia E, Argiles G, Elez E, et al. BRAF mutant colorectal cancer: prognosis, treatment, and new perspectives. *Ann Oncol.* 2017;28(11):2648–2657. doi:10.1093/annonc/mdx401

How I Treat Early-Stage Rectal Cancer With Neoadjuvant Radiation Therapy

Nikhil Sebastian and Terence Williams

INTRODUCTION

Prior to 1990, standard-of-care treatment for locally advanced (stage T3–4 and/or N1–2) rectal cancer (adenocarcinoma) in the United States consisted of surgery with as-needed postoperative radiotherapy. Historical results from surgical series for rectal cancer in this era were marked by unacceptably high local failure in patients with T3–4 or node-positive disease, ranging from 15% to 40% (1–3). These suboptimal outcomes in locally advanced rectal cancer, particularly in light of the morbidity of local recurrence, prompted more than 20 randomized trials conducted between 1963 and 1984 that compared surgery alone to surgery with perioperative irradiation. Aggregated, the results of these trials showed decreased local failure with the use of radiotherapy (at biologically effective doses ≥30 Gy), with no significant benefit in overall survival (4). These outcomes, in tandem with those from studies identifying the benefit of systemic therapy on overall survival (5–8), prompted the National Institutes of Health (NIH) consensus that postoperative chemoradiation is the optimal treatment in patients with stage II and III rectal cancer in 1990 (9). Soon after, results of randomized trials revealing improved local control, disease-free survival, toxicity rates, and potential for sphincter preservation with preoperative therapy (10,11) led to the establishment of neoadjuvant therapy as the standard of care.

SHORT-COURSE PREOPERATIVE RADIOTHERAPY

Of the >20 randomized trials evaluating preoperative radiation therapy, all showed improved local control (4). Only one of these, the Swedish Rectal Cancer Trial, showed a survival benefit. In this trial, 1,168 patients with resectable rectal cancer were randomized to surgery and preoperative radiotherapy arms, the latter of which used a short-course 5 Gy × 5-fraction regimen popularized in Northern European countries, delivered 1 week prior to surgery. After a minimum follow-up of 5 years, radiation was shown to improve 5-year overall survival (58% vs. 48%; p = .004) and local recurrence (11% vs. 27%; p < .001), as well as 9-year cancer-specific survival (74% vs. 65%; p = .002) (12). With a long-term follow-up of 13 years, all end points continued to favor the irradiated group, including overall survival (38% vs. 30%; p = .008), cancer-specific survival (72% vs. 62%; p = .03), and local recurrence (9% vs. 26%; p < .001) (13).

A subsequent meta-analysis of 14 randomized controlled trials comparing preoperative radiation and surgery with surgery alone showed significantly reduced 5-year overall mortality (odds ratio [OR] 0.84; p = .03), cancer-related mortality (OR 0.71; p < .001), and local recurrence (OR 0.49; p < .001) (14). Another meta-analysis showed a 46% reduction in local recurrence with the addition of preoperative radiation (p < .0001) with a trend toward improved survival (62% mortality vs. 63%; p = .06) (4).

Soon after the advent of trials evaluating adjuvant radiotherapy, total mesorectal excision (TME), introduced by Heald in 1979 (15), gained widespread popularity. In recognition of the role of perirectal lymph nodes as the initial basin of tumor drainage, this technique, which entails circumferential, sharp dissection of the mesentery surrounding the rectum, was found to improve local control in several retrospective series (16–18). Thus, it was postulated that

---

A Clinical Vignette ("How I Treat") is included at the end of the chapter.

preoperative radiation was potentially compensating for suboptimal surgery. This premise was evaluated in the Dutch CKVO 95-04 trial, in which 1,805 patients were randomized to preoperative radiation (5 Gy × 5) and TME. More than half (58%) of these patients had T1 or T2 disease. Initial 2-year outcomes showed improved local recurrence in the preoperative radiotherapy group (2.4% vs. 8.2%; $p < .001$) and no difference in overall survival (82% vs. 81.8%; $p = .84$) (3). Five-year local recurrence remained improved at 5.6% and 10.9% ($p < .001$) for preoperative radiotherapy and TME alone groups, respectively, and overall survival was 64.2% and 63.5%, respectively (19). Ten-year outcomes showed persistently improved local control (5.1% vs. 11.1%; $p < .001$) for the radiotherapy–surgery versus the surgery-alone group, with no statistical difference in overall survival (48% vs. 49%; $p = .86$) or cancer-specific mortality (28% vs. 31%; $p = .20$). Interestingly, in a post hoc subgroup analysis of stage III cancer with negative circumferential resection margins, preoperative radiation was found to be associated with improved survival (50% vs. 40%; $p = .032$) (20).

STANDARD-COURSE PREOPERATIVE CHEMORADIOTHERAPY

Given the aforementioned European studies showing improved local control with preoperative radiation versus surgery alone, and the results of synchronous U.S. trials showing survival benefit with the addition of chemotherapy to postoperative radiotherapy (7,21), it was inevitable these approaches would converge in the evaluation of preoperative chemoradiation. Two U.S. trials, RTOG 94-01/Intergroup 0417 and NSABP R-03, sought to evaluate the role of preoperative chemoradiation but closed due to poor accrual. Data are available for the 267 patients of the intended 900 accrued to NSABP R-03 (1993–1999), albeit underpowered for the trial's primary end points—overall survival and disease-free survival. In this trial, patients with clinical T3/T4 or node-positive rectal cancer were randomized to preoperative or postoperative chemoradiation arms consisting of fluorouracil and leucovorin with 45 Gy in 25 fractions with a 5.4 Gy boost. Five-year disease-free survival was 64.7% and 53.4% ($p = .011$) for pre- and postoperative patients, respectively. There was a trend toward improved overall survival (74.5% vs. 65.6%; $p = .065$) and improved sphincter-preservation rate (33.9% vs. 24.2%; $p = .13$), but no difference in locoregional recurrence (10.7% in both groups; $p = .693$) (22). This rate of 5-year locoregional recurrence is notably higher than that seen in the preoperative arm of the Dutch CKVO 95-04 trial, likely a function of mandatory TME and high frequency of stage I cancers in the Dutch trial (19).

The role of preoperative chemoradiotherapy was definitively established in the German Rectal Study Group CAO/ARO/AIO-94 trial (1994–2002). In this trial, patients with uT3–4 and/or lymph node-positive resectable rectal cancer less than 16 cm from the anal verge were randomized to pre- (n = 405) and postoperative (n = 394) chemoradiotherapy arms, respectively, consisting of 50.4 Gy in 28 fractions with continuous infusion fluorouracil and consolidation bolus fluorouracil for four cycles (after surgery in the preoperative arm and after chemoradiation in the postoperative arm). Postoperative patients also received a 5.4 Gy boost to the tumor bed. TME was performed 6 weeks after preoperative chemoradiation. There was no difference between preoperative and postoperative treatment groups with regard to 5-year overall survival (76% vs. 74%; $p = .80$), disease-free survival (68% vs. 65%; $p = .32$), or distant recurrence (36% vs. 38%; $p = .84$). However, there was a statistically significant improvement in local control with preoperative chemoradiation (6% vs. 13%; $p = .006$) (10). Of note, 18% of patients randomized to the postoperative therapy were found to have T1-2N0 disease, suggesting that clinical staging overestimates true surgical staging, resulting in overtreatment. Despite this, at 10 years, a local control benefit still remained (7.1% vs. 10.1%; $p = .048$), with no difference in overall survival (29.8% vs. 29.6%; $p = .9$) (23). Other end points in the German trial favored preoperative treatment. First, the rate of sphincter-preserving surgery was significantly increased (39% vs. 19%; $p = .004$) in the group of patients deemed to require abdominoperineal resection (APR) prior to initiation of treatment. Notably, preoperative therapy was associated with pathologic downstaging, with complete response in 8% of patients and more stage I tumors (25% vs. 18%) and fewer stage III tumors (25% vs. 40%) when compared to the postoperative therapy group ($p < .001$) (10). A subsequent unplanned analysis revealed that the extent of tumor regression after preoperative chemoradiation, as determined by tumor regression grading, is prognostic for disease-free survival (24). Additionally, preoperative therapy was also favored with regard to toxicity. Rates of grade 3 or 4 toxicity were improved in the preoperative group (acute 27% vs. 40%; $p = .001$; late 14% vs. 24%; $p = .01$), particularly with regard to acute diarrhea (12% vs. 18%; p = .04), chronic diarrhea or small bowel obstruction (9% vs. 15%; p = .07), and strictures at the anastomotic site (4% vs. 12%; p = .003) (10).

PREOPERATIVE VERSUS SELECTIVE POSTOPERATIVE RADIATION

A trial from Uppsala University in Sweden randomized 471 patients between preoperative irradiation (25.5 Gy in 5 fractions) and split-course postoperative irradiation (40 Gy in 20 fractions followed by additional 20 Gy 1–1.5 weeks later). In the patients randomized to the postoperative radiotherapy group, postoperative radiation was given only to patients with pathologic Duke Stage B or C, while patients with Duke A cancer were observed. Surgery was performed within a week of preoperative radiation and within 5 to 8 weeks prior to postoperative radiation. Five-year local recurrence was 13% and 22% in the pre- and postoperative groups, respectively (p = .02), with no difference in overall survival (60% for both groups; p = .5). Rates of small bowel obstruction were higher in patients who received postoperative radiation compared to those who received preoperative radiation (11% vs. 5%; p < .01); those patients who received surgery alone had a 6% rate of late bowel obstruction. The overall rates of late side effects related to bowel, urinary tract, and skin/nerve toxicity were 20% in the preoperative group, 41% in the postoperative group, and 23% in the surgery-alone group. Thus, preoperative radiotherapy was effectively able to nearly halve the risk of local recurrence without significantly increasing late toxicity (25).

A more modern trial, MRC CR07/NCIC C016 (1998–2005), randomized 1,350 patients from 80 centers to short-course preoperative radiation (25 Gy in 5 fractions) followed by surgery within a week or surgery with selective postoperative chemoradiation for patients with involvement of the circumferential resection margin (≤1 mm) consisting of 45 Gy in 25 fractions with concurrent 5-fluorouracil (5-FU; either continuous infusion 200 mg/m^2 or weekly bolus 300 mg/m^2). TME was encouraged and performed in the majority (92%) of patients. Of the patients with positive circumferential resection margins in the postoperative chemoradiation group, 12% had positive circumferential resection margins and of these patients 69% received chemoradiotherapy as intended. Of the patients with negative resection margin in this group, the majority (91%) received no radiotherapy. Adjuvant chemotherapy, which was permitted as per the local policy of the treating center, was given in 40% of preoperative and 45% of postoperative patients. Three-year local recurrence was 4.4% in the preoperative radiotherapy group and 10.6% in the selective postoperative radiotherapy group (p < .0001). This translated into a similar absolute difference in disease-free survival (77.5% vs. 71.5%; p = .013). There was no difference in 3-year overall survival (80.3% vs. 78.6%; p = .40) (26). Patient-reported quality-of-life data show preoperative radiation negatively affects male sexual dysfunction (although to a much smaller extent than surgery) persisting at least 3 years after surgery. Although overall bowel dysfunction was similar between preoperative and postoperative cohorts, there was an apparent increase in patient-reported incontinence in preoperative patients (27).

SHORT-COURSE PREOPERATIVE RADIOTHERAPY VERSUS STANDARD-COURSE PREOPERATIVE CHEMORADIOTHERAPY

In a multi-institutional Polish trial (1999–2002), 316 patients with cT3–T4 rectal cancer were randomized to preoperative short-course (5 Gy × 5) radiation or 50.4 Gy in 1.8 Gy fractions with two courses of bolus 5-FU (325 mg/m^2/day for 5 days) with leucovorin. TME was performed within 1 week and 4 to 6 weeks, respectively, for the two treatment groups. Chemoradiation patients had higher rates of pathologic complete response (16% vs. 1%; p < .001), fewer positive radial margins (4% vs. 13%; p = .017), and an average of 1.9 cm shorter tumor diameter along the bowel axis (p < .001). Despite this, there was no statistical difference in the rate of sphincter preservation between the 5 Gy × 5 arm (61%) and chemoradiation arm (58%; p = .57) (28). There was no statistical difference between radiation-alone and chemoradiation groups with regard to 4-year overall survival (67.2% vs. 66.2%; p = .960), disease-free survival (58.4% vs. 55.6%; p = .820), local recurrence (9.0% vs. 14.2%; p = .17), or late toxicity (28.3% vs. 27.0%; p = .81) (29).

The Trans-Tasman Radiation Oncology Group (TROG) trial 01.04 (2001–2006) randomized 326 patients with T3N0-2M0 (per ultrasound or MRI) rectal adenocarcinoma between short-course radiotherapy and 50.4 Gy in 1.8 fractions with continuous infusional fluorouracil 225 mg/m^2/day. Both arms received 6 monthly courses of fluorouracil (425 mg/m^2) and folinic acid (20 mg/m^2) daily for 5 days starting 4 to 6 weeks after surgery. There was no statistical difference in 5-year local recurrence between short- and long-course groups (7.5% vs. 5.7%; p = .51), as well as no difference in distant recurrence (27% vs. 30%; p = .89), overall survival (74% vs. 70%; p = .62), or late grade 3 to 4 toxicity (5.8% vs. 8.2%; p = .53). There was more pathologic downstaging with long-course treatment (45% vs. 28%; p = .002); however, this did not translate to a difference in rates of APR in patients with distal (<5 cm from anal verge) tumors (79% vs. 77%; p = .87). Overall, these results parallel those of the Polish trial. Of note, in the TROG study, there was a large (albeit not statistically significant) difference in local recurrence in favor of long-course treatment for the specific subset of patients with distal tumors (12.5% vs. 0%; p = .21) (30).

RADIOTHERAPY-TO-SURGERY INTERVAL

The premise that a longer interval from radiation to surgery could cause improved downstaging and consequent sphincter preservation was evaluated in Lyon R90-01 (1991–1995). This trial randomized 201 patients with T1-3N1-3M0 rectal cancer accessible to digital rectal examination receiving 39 Gy in 13 fractions of preoperative radiation to short- and long-interval arms for which surgery was required to be performed within 2 and 6 to 8 weeks of completing radiotherapy, respectively. Patients assigned to a long interval more often had pathologic complete response (26% vs. 10.3%; p = .0054) and findings of pT0/1 tumor (28.7% vs. 15.2%; p = .026) as well as decreased likelihood of pN2–3 disease (5% vs. 16%; p = .011) with no statistical difference in rates of pN0–1 disease. These findings translated into higher rates of sphincter-preserving surgery in the long-interval group (75.5% vs. 67.7%), although this did not reach statistical significance (p = .27). There was no difference between short- and long-interval cohorts with regard to overall survival (78% vs. 73%) or local recurrence (9% in both groups). Of note, the interval between radiotherapy and surgery did not increase postoperative complications or mortality (31).

In the Stockholm III trial (1998–2013), 840 patients with resectable rectal adenocarcinoma less than 15 cm from the anal verge were randomized to short-course radiotherapy (5 x 5 Gy) with surgery within 1 week, short-course radiotherapy with surgery after 4 to 8 weeks (short course with delay), or long-course radiotherapy (50 Gy in 2 Gy fractions) with surgery after 4 to 8 weeks. No concomitant chemotherapy was given. Adjuvant radiotherapy was given in 13% of short-course treatments and 19% of patients receiving long-course radiotherapy. After approximately a year, a protocol amendment permitted hospitals to choose to randomize patients to just the short-course radiotherapy arms or all three arms. Consequently, analysis was performed separately for patients in the three-arm randomization and those in the two-arm randomization. In a preplanned interim analysis of 462 patients in short-course arms, there was statistically significant tumor downstaging in the short course with delay, including pathologic complete response of 11.8% versus 1.7% (p < .001) (32). There was no significant difference in local recurrence, distant metastasis, or overall survival in the three treatment cohorts. Five-year overall survival was 73% for short-course radiotherapy, 76% for short-course radiotherapy with delay, and 78% for long-course radiotherapy with delay (p = .62). In the three-arm randomization, there was no statistical difference in the rate of postoperative complications for short-course (50%), short-course with delay (38%), and long-course (39%) radiotherapy arms (p = .075). Interestingly, in a pooled analysis of the short-course arms in the two-arm and three-arm randomizations, the group of patients receiving short-course radiotherapy had a higher rate of postoperative complications compared to those patients receiving short-course radiotherapy with delay (53% vs. 41%; p = .001) (33).

SELECTIVE NONOPERATIVE MANAGEMENT

The concept of nonoperative management was pioneered in São Paolo, Brazil, by Habr-Gama and colleagues on the basis that up to one-third of patients treated with chemoradiotherapy achieve clinical complete response and could thus potentially be spared from significant operative mortality and morbidity by using an organ-preservation strategy (34). In their first large institutional series, 265 patients with distal rectal adenocarcinoma were treated with concurrent 50.4 Gy with 5-FU and leucovorin. Of these, 71 patients (~27%) achieved a clinical complete response. Patients with incomplete clinical response were referred to surgery and those patients with pathologic stage 0 (resection group) were compared to patients who achieved clinical complete response with chemoradiation and did not have surgery (observation group). Five-year overall survival was 88% versus 100% in the resection and observation groups ($p = .01$), respectively, and disease-free survival was 83% versus 92% ($p = .09$) (35). In a subsequent analysis of 183 patients treated with 50.4 to 54 Gy with concurrent 5-FU based chemotherapy, 31% of patients who achieved clinical complete response (and thus received no surgery) developed local recurrence within a year. Of these, 93% were successfully salvaged, yielding an overall 5-year local (first) recurrence-free survival of 69% and unresectable local recurrence-free survival (including prior salvage) of 94%. This translated into a 78% rate of organ preservation. Five-year cancer-specific overall survival and disease-free survival were 91% and 68%, respectively. Thus, while a "wait-and-see" approach was associated with high local recurrence, the majority of these were successfully salvaged to offer good long-term local control and organ preservation (36).

Several such retrospective studies have been performed, many of which have been unsuccessful in reproducing the results of Habr-Gama and colleagues (37). Consequently, a prospective observational Danish trial (2009–2013) of 55 patients with T2-3N0-1 rectal cancer in the lower 6 cm of the rectum evaluated a "wait-and-see" approach in patients receiving a complete response after chemoradiation. Treatment consisted of concurrent oral tegafur–uracil and a radiotherapy regimen of 60 Gy in 30 fractions to the tumor, 50 Gy in 30 fractions to elective lymph nodes, and a 5 Gy endorectal brachytherapy boost. Seventy-eight percent of patients achieved complete response, and in this observation group, 1- and 2-year local recurrence was 15.5% and 25.9%, respectively. The most common late toxicity was rectal bleeding, present in 7% of patients at 1 year and 6% at 2 years (38). The high complete response rate achieved in this study is likely in part due to the intensity of the chemoradiation used, and longer follow-up is required to assess the durability of local control and the long-term comorbidity associated with this intensive treatment regimen.

Another prospective study by Renehan and colleagues reported a local regrowth rate of 34% after 33 months of follow-up in 129 patients (39), while a similar study by Martens and colleagues showed a local regrowth rate of only 15% and 3-year colostomy-free survival of 95% (40). The impressive results of the latter study may be a function of the strict selection process used to determine appropriate candidates for evaluation, with clinical examination, endoscopy, and MRI (including diffusion-weighted sequences), all used to verify treatment response.

While it is tempting to envision treatment of rectal cancer undergoing the same shift in paradigm from trimodality therapy to definitive chemoradiotherapy as in the treatment of anal cancer (41), ultimately more long-term prospective, observational studies with uniform inclusion criteria are needed to verify the safety and efficacy of an organ-preservation approach (37).

Additionally, it is worth noting here that local excision after neoadjuvant chemoradiotherapy is another means of organ preservation that is currently being evaluated, in particular for T2N0 cancer. At present, local excision after neoadjuvant therapy, particularly in patients who refuse or are otherwise not candidates for transabdominal resection, appears to be a feasible option, although longer follow-up is needed (42).

INTENSITY-MODULATED RADIATION THERAPY

Given relatively high rates (36%–44%) of acute grade ≥ 3 gastrointestinal (GI) toxicity reported in patients treated with concurrent pelvic radiation and concurrent 5-FU (11), the role of intensity-modulated radiation therapy (IMRT), which entails improved dose conformality and normal tissue sparing compared to traditional techniques, has been evaluated in the context of chemoradiotherapy for rectal cancer, particularly given its demonstrated benefit in other pelvic malignancies (43,44). Due to its ability to create concave dose distributions, IMRT can hypothetically reduce GI and genitourinary (GU) toxicity related to decreased radiation dose to bowel and urinary structures.

NRG Oncology Radiation Therapy Oncology Group (RTOG) 0822 (2008–2009) prospectively evaluated GI toxicity by preoperative chemoradiation using IMRT and capecitabine and oxaliplatin in 79 patients with locally advanced rectal cancer. Treatment consisted of 45 Gy in

1.8 Gy fractions to the rectum and regional lymph nodes followed by a three-dimensional (3D) boost of 5.4 Gy in 1.8 Gy fractions to the gross disease with a 2 cm margin including the pre-sacral space. Small bowel dose constraints were V35 <180 cc, V40 <100 cc, and V45 <65 cc. Chemotherapy was capecitabine 825 mg/m^2 twice daily orally and oxaliplatin 50 mg/m^2 intravenous (IV) weekly for five doses (CAPOX). Postoperative chemotherapy consisted of oxaliplatin, leucovorin, and 5-FU (FOLFOX) for nine cycles. Surgery was performed 4 to 8 weeks after completing radiation therapy. The primary end point of grade ≥2 GI adverse events (AEs) was compared to the rates found in RTOG 0247, a preceding phase II trial that was suspended due to unacceptable rates of grade 3/4 toxicity and compared CAPOX with capecitabine and irinotecan (CAPIRI) using traditional two-dimensional (2D)/3D radiotherapy techniques (45). Interestingly, 51.5% of patients on RTOG 0822 developed a grade ≥2 GI AE, higher than the observed 40% of patients in RTOG 0247 (p = .93), and 17.6% developed grade ≥3 diarrhea. There was no statistically significant correlation of GI toxicity with small bowel dose–volume histogram parameters (46).

A potential criticism of RTOG 0822 is its use of oxaliplatin, which is still considered nonstandard and is known to worsen GI toxicity, which IMRT may not be able to nullify. All randomized prospective trials evaluating the addition of oxaliplatin to preoperative chemoradiation demonstrate a significant increase in GI side effects, most of which do not demonstrate improvement in pathologic complete response and/or disease-free survival (47–49), but two that do (50,51). A retrospective study evaluating IMRT compared to conventional pelvic radiation in the setting of standard 5-FU concurrent chemotherapy showed significant improvement in grade 2+ toxicity with IMRT (48% vs. 62%; p = .006) (52). Typically, 3D conformal treatment is sufficient in meeting dose constraints; however, IMRT can be considered in select instances, for example, with low-lying rectal tumors or T4 tumors, when inguinal and external iliac chains are at risk, respectively, in order to limit the toxicity associated with inclusion of these volumes.

REIRRADIATION

The combination of preoperative radiotherapy and TME has significantly decreased local recurrence in rectal cancer. Nevertheless, recurrences in this setting entail significant morbidity (53) and unique challenges in the setting of prior irradiation (54). In a retrospective study, Mohiuddin and colleagues evaluated 103 patients with locally recurrent rectal cancer after surgery and pre- or postoperative radiotherapy to a median dose of 50.4 Gy. For retreatment, patients were treated to the recurrent tumor with a 2 to 4 cm margin with either 30 Gy in 1.2 Gy twice-daily fractions or 30.6 Gy in 1.8 Gy daily fractions with a 6 to 20 Gy boost to the gross tumor with a 2 cm margin with concurrent continuous infusion 5-FU. The median time from initial treatment was 19 months. Twenty-two percent of patients required significant treatment interruption or discontinuation due to acute toxicity. Late toxicity was seen in 21.4% of patients and predominantly chronic grade 3 diarrhea (17%) and small bowel obstruction (15%), the latter likely multifactorial and at least partially attributable to tumor. Twice-daily irradiation was associated with decreased late toxicity compared to once-daily treatment (p < .05). In the 21 patients who presented with bleeding, all achieved palliation. Five-year survival was 22% for patients who underwent surgical resection after reirradiation and 15% for patients who received reirradiation alone (p = .001) (55).

In a prospective phase II Italian study, 59 patients with recurrent disease were treated to 40 Gy with a 10.8 Gy boost in 1.2 Gy twice-daily fractions and concomitant 5-FU IV 225 mg/m^2/day. If feasible, surgery was performed 6 to 8 weeks after chemoradiation. This was followed by postoperative raltitrexed for five cycles. Most (86.4%) patients completed chemoradiation, 66.1% received surgery, and half completed adjuvant chemotherapy. Overall 5-year survival was 39.3% and in the subset of 21 patients in whom complete resection was feasible, survival was 66.8%. Late toxicity was noted in 11.8% of patients and bowel obstruction, in particular, occurred in only 1.7% of patients. Despite the nonstandard adjuvant chemotherapy regimen and short follow-up (median 36 months), this trial demonstrated the feasibility and relative safety of reirradiation with a hyperfractionated regimen (56).

Other retrospective studies have corroborated the safety and efficacy of hyperfractionated reirradiation followed by surgery in carefully selected patients (57). Additionally, other techniques, such as intraoperative radiotherapy, may also be beneficial in the setting of retreatment (58,59).

TREATMENT TECHNIQUES

The whole-pelvic radiation field is designed with regard to patterns of failure informed by seminal surgical series (60). At-risk sites include the presacral space, primary tumor site, and, in patients who have undergone APR, the perineum. The first basin for lymphatic spread is the mesorectal lymph nodes that are removed during TME. Spread occurs either in the upward direction along the superior rectal and inferior mesenteric arteries or laterally, particularly seen in tumors at or below the peritoneal reflection, along the middle rectal, obturator, and internal iliac drainage (61,62). Coverage of external iliac nodes should be considered in the case of T4 tumors with invasion of gynecologic or GU organs. Coverage of inguinal lymph nodes should be considered for involvement of the anal canal or lower third of the vagina. Para-aortic nodes are not included due to the low risk of spread and potential morbidity from treatment (63).

Patients are simulated prone, with arms above the head, and a belly board for displacement of the small bowel. Oral and IV contrast for simulation should be administered for delineation of the small bowel and tumor/lymph nodes, respectively. Use of an anal marker, for delineation of the anus, and barium enema, for tumor delineation, can also be considered. If possible, simulation and treatment should be performed with a full bladder for maximal small bowel displacement.

Treatment is generally delivered via a 3-field or 4-field technique. For the anterior–posterior/posterior–anterior (AP/PA) fields, the superior field edge is placed at the L5/S1 interspace. The distal field edge should be 3 to 5 cm below the palpable tumor for patients receiving preoperative irradiation. Postoperatively, the distal field edge should be placed 2 to 3 cm below the surgical anastomosis; if the surgery was an APR, the perineum and perineal scar must be included. The lateral border should be placed 1.5 cm lateral to the widest bony margin of the true pelvic wall (to cover any lateral extension of disease and the internal iliac chain). The posterior border of the lateral fields should be placed at least 1.5 cm behind the anterior margin of the sacrum to adequately cover the presacral space. The anterior border should be approximately 4 cm anterior to the rectum, and often the posterior pubic symphysis is used as an anterior landmark for T1–T3 tumors (anterior pubic symphysis for T4 tumors). Fields are expanded accordingly for significant extrarectal extension or to include the external iliac or inguinal nodes. Boost fields should include the primary tumor or tumor bed with a 3 cm margin and potentially include the presacral space. Modern radiation planning has evolved away from setting borders based on osseous landmarks on digitally reconstructed radiographs to using gross, clinical, and planning target volume (GTV/CTV/PTV)-based planning. A recently published atlas from members of RTOG provides helpful contouring guidelines to establish the CTV for anorectal tumors (63). Typically, standard dosing is 45 Gy in 25 fractions of 1.8 Gy/fraction to the whole-pelvic fields with a 5.4 to 9 Gy boost (excluding the small bowel after 50 Gy to limit toxicity).

CONCLUSIONS

For locally advanced rectal cancer, preoperative short-course radiation (5 Gy × 5) and long-course chemoradiation (typically 50.4 Gy) with infusional 5-FU or capecitabine are the standard approaches, as opposed to postoperative or selective postoperative radiation/chemoradiation. Longer time intervals after completion of radiation may improve tumor response rates at the time of surgery, and the recent Stockholm III trial showed that a longer delay (4–8 weeks) is also reasonable for short-course radiation, with an acceptable toxicity/complication profile. Nonoperative management can be considered for select patients with distal tumors who wish to avoid an APR, but further study on optimal patient and treatment factors for this approach is

Clinical Vignette 6.1

Patient "K" noticed rectal bleeding for several weeks that prompted a colonoscopy showing a low-lying rectal tumor, biopsy-positive for adenocarcinoma. MRI showed diffuse thickening and enhancement of the rectal wall without focal mass and bilateral pelvic lymphadenopathy. He was staged as IIIC (T3N2b).

The patient received 45 Gy in 25 fractions with 6 MV photons and IMRT with a boost to the primary tumor of 5.4 Gy in 3 fractions using 18 MV photons with a conformal technique. The cumulative dose was 50.4 Gy in 28 fractions. The volumes of the small bowel receiving 35 Gy, 40 Gy, and 45 Gy were 57 cc, 24 cc, and 2 cc, respectively, and the maximum point dose was 47 Gy. Chemotherapy was 5-fluorouracil 225 mg/m²/day continuous infusion for 120 hours. The patient experienced moist desquamation of the perianal skin and nausea during treatment but overall tolerated treatment well. Six weeks after completing chemoradiation, the patient had an APR. The pathologic stage was ypT3N2 with a positive radial margin. Because of this, roughly 4 weeks after surgery the patient received a postoperative radiotherapy boost of 16.2 Gy in nine fractions with concurrent capecitabine, and this was followed by four cycles of adjuvant FOLFOX.

Unfortunately, 7 months after the patient's APR, he was found to have hypermetabolic liver lesions as well as a hypermetabolic presacral focus. He subsequently underwent ablation of the liver lesions followed by systemic therapy with irinotecan, panitumumab, FOLFIRI/bevacizumab, and multiple phase I trial drugs over the next 3 years. He ultimately developed pelvic pain and light hematuria and was found to have a recurrent pelvic mass with anterior bladder invasion and associated hydronephrosis, but no other evidence of disease progression. The presacral recurrence was deemed not to be surgically resectable (Figure 6.1).

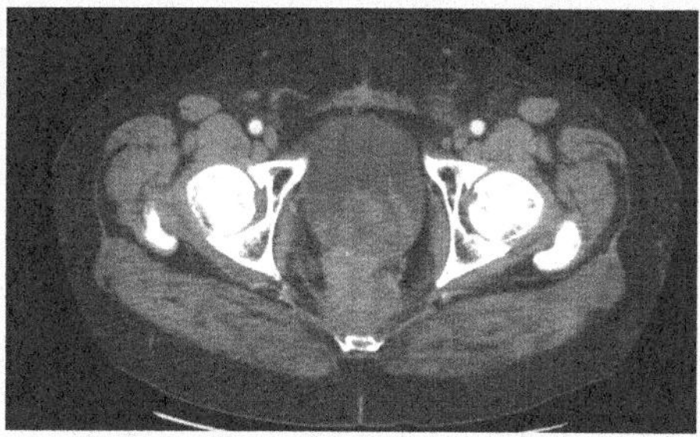

FIGURE 6.1   This patient experienced pelvic pain and light hematuria secondary to a presacral recurrence 3 years after definitive chemoradiation and surgery for T3N2b rectal cancer. Note the tumor involves the presacral space with posterior bladder wall invasion.

Questions

* What radiation regimen would be appropriate for palliation in this setting?
* Would concurrent systemic therapy be indicated?
* For what toxicities is this patient at risk?

Based on the published literature (55–57), this patient underwent reirradiation with 30 Gy to the pelvis with a boost of 9.6 Gy to the gross disease (total 39.6 Gy) in 1.2 Gy twice-daily fractions using an IMRT plan with 6 MV photons. The patient received concurrent capecitabine with treatment. He tolerated treatment, although he did have nausea, dysuria, dermatitis, and proctitis during treatment. He experienced significant improvement in his symptoms.

certainly needed. IMRT may have utility in select circumstances, but additional data is needed before this technique should be applied to all patients with rectal cancer. For patients who develop pelvic recurrence in the setting of prior pelvic radiation, reirradiation can be considered in select patients for palliation and/or maximizing pelvic control.

REFERENCES

1. Phillips RK, Hittinger R, Blesovsky L, et al. Local recurrence following "curative" surgery for large bowel cancer: I. The overall picture. *Br J Surg*. 1984;71:12–16. doi:10.1002/bjs.1800710104

2. Harnsberger JR, Vernava VM, Longo WE. Radical abdominopelvic lymphadenectomy: historic perspective and current role in the surgical management of rectal cancer. *Dis Colon Rectum*. 1994;37:73–87. doi:10.1007/BF02047218

3. Kapiteijn E, Marijnen CA, Nagtegaal ID, et al. Preoperative radiotherapy combined with total mesorectal excision for resectable rectal cancer. *N Engl J Med*. 2001;345:638–646. doi:10.1056/NEJMoa010580

4. Colorectal Cancer Collaborative Group. Adjuvant radiotherapy for rectal cancer: a systematic overview of 8,507 patients from 22 randomised trials. *Lancet Lond Engl*. 2001;358:1291–1304. doi:10.1016/S0140-6736(01)06409-1

5. Gastrointestinal Tumor Study Group. Radiation therapy and fluorouracil with or without semustine for the treatment of patients with surgical adjuvant adenocarcinoma of the rectum. *J Clin Oncol Off J Am Soc Clin Oncol*. 1992;10:549–557. doi:10.1200/JCO.1992.10.4.549

6. Thomas PR, Lindblad AS. Adjuvant postoperative radiotherapy and chemotherapy in rectal carcinoma: a review of the Gastrointestinal Tumor Study Group experience. *Radiother Oncol J Eur Soc Ther Radiol Oncol*. 1988;13:245–252. doi:10.1016/0167-8140(88)90219-8

7. Krook JE, Moertel CG, Gunderson LL, et al: Effective surgical adjuvant therapy for high-risk rectal carcinoma. *N Engl J Med*. 1991;324:709–715. doi:10.1056/NEJM199103143241101

8. Fisher B, Wolmark N, Rockette H, et al. Postoperative adjuvant chemotherapy or radiation therapy for rectal cancer: results from NSABP protocol R-01. *J Natl Cancer Inst*. 1988;80:21–29. doi:10.1093/jnci/80.1.21

9. NIC consensus conference. Adjuvant therapy for patients with colon and rectal cancer. *JAMA*. 1990;264:1444–1450. doi:10.1001/jama.1990.03450110090034

10. Sauer R, Becker H, Hohenberger W, et al. Preoperative versus postoperative chemoradiotherapy for rectal cancer. *N Engl J Med*. 2004;351:1731–1740. doi:10.1056/NEJMoa040694

11. Roh MS, Colangelo LH, O'Connell MJ, et al. Preoperative multimodality therapy improves disease-free survival in patients with carcinoma of the rectum: NSABP R-03. *J Clin Oncol Off J Am Soc Clin Oncol*. 2009;27:5124–5130. doi:10.1200/JCO.2009.22.0467

12. Swedish Rectal Cancer Trial, Cedermark B, Dahlberg M, et al. Improved survival with preoperative radiotherapy in resectable rectal cancer. *N Engl J Med*. 1997;336:980–987. doi:10.1056/NEJM199704033361402

13. Folkesson J, Birgisson H, Pahlman L, et al. Swedish Rectal Cancer Trial: long lasting benefits from radiotherapy on survival and local recurrence rate. *J Clin Oncol Off J Am Soc Clin Oncol*. 2005;23:5644–5650. doi:10.1200/JCO.2005.08.144

14. Cammà C, Giunta M, Fiorica F, et al. Preoperative radiotherapy for resectable rectal cancer: a meta-analysis. *JAMA*. 2000;284:1008–1015. doi:10.1001/jama.284.8.1008

15. Heald RJ. A new approach to rectal cancer. *Br J Hosp Med*. 1979;22:277–281.

16. MacFarlane JK, Ryall RDH, Heald RJ. Mesorectal excision for rectal cancer. *Lancet*. 1993;341:457–460. doi:10.1016/0140-6736(93)90207-W

17. Enker WE, Thaler HT, Cranor ML, et al. Total mesorectal excision in the operative treatment of carcinoma of the rectum. *J Am Coll Surg*. 1995;181:335–346.

18. Aitken RJ. Mesorectal excision for rectal cancer. *Br J Surg*. 1996;83:214–216. doi:10.1002/bjs.1800830218

19. Peeters KCMJ, Marijnen CAM, Nagtegaal ID, et al. The TME trial after a median follow-up of 6 years: increased local control but no survival benefit in irradiated patients with resectable rectal carcinoma. *Ann Surg*. 2007;246:693–701. doi:10.1097/01.sla.0000257358.56863.ce

20. van Gijn W, Marijnen CA, Nagtegaal ID, et al. Preoperative radiotherapy combined with total mesorectal excision for resectable rectal cancer: 12-year follow-up of the multicentre, randomised controlled TME trial. *Lancet Oncol*. 2011;12:575–582. doi:10.1016/S1470-2045(11)70097-3

21. Gastrointestinal Tumor Study Group. Prolongation of the disease-free interval in surgically treated rectal carcinoma. *N Engl J Med*. 1985;312:1465–1472. doi:10.1056/NEJM198506063122301

22. Hyams DM, Mamounas EP, Petrelli N, et al. A clinical trial to evaluate the worth of preoperative multimodality therapy in patients with operable carcinoma of the rectum: a progress report of National Surgical Breast and Bowel Project Protocol R-03. *Dis Colon Rectum*. 1997;40:131–139. doi:10.1007/BF02054976

23. Sauer R, Liersch T, Merkel S, et al. Preoperative versus postoperative chemoradiotherapy for locally advanced rectal cancer: results of the German CAO/ARO/AIO-94 randomized phase III trial after a median follow-up of 11 years. *J Clin Oncol Off J Am Soc Clin Oncol*. 2012;30:1926–1933. doi:10.1200/JCO.2011.40.1836

24. Rödel C, Martus P, Papadoupolos T, et al. Prognostic Significance of Tumor Regression After Preoperative Chemoradiotherapy for Rectal Cancer. *J Clin Oncol*. 2005;23:8688–8696. doi:10.1200/JCO.2005.02.1329

25. Frykholm GJ, Glimelius B, Påhlman L. Preoperative or postoperative irradiation in adenocarcinoma of the rectum: final treatment results of a randomized trial and an evaluation of late secondary effects. *Dis Colon Rectum*. 1993;36:564–572. doi:10.1007/BF02049863
26. Sebag-Montefiore D, Stephens RJ, Steele R, et al. Preoperative radiotherapy versus selective postoperative chemoradiotherapy in patients with rectal cancer (MRC CR07 and NCIC-CTG C016): a multicentre, randomised trial. *Lancet*. 2009;373:811–820. doi:10.1016/S0140-6736(09)60484-0
27. Stephens RJ, Thompson LC, Quirke P, et al. Impact of short-course preoperative radiotherapy for rectal cancer on patients' quality of life: data from the Medical Research Council CR07/National Cancer Institute of Canada Clinical Trials Group C016 randomized clinical trial. *J Clin Oncol Off J Am Soc Clin Oncol*. 2010;28:4233–4239. doi:10.1200/JCO.2009.26.5264
28. Bujko K, Nowacki MP, Nasierowska-Guttmejer A, et al. Sphincter preservation following preoperative radiotherapy for rectal cancer: report of a randomised trial comparing short-term radiotherapy vs. conventionally fractionated radiochemotherapy. *Radiother Oncol*. 2004;72:15–24. doi:10.1016/j.radonc.2003.12.006
29. Bujko K, Nowacki MP, Nasierowska-Guttmejer A, et al. Long-term results of a randomized trial comparing preoperative short-course radiotherapy with preoperative conventionally fractionated chemoradiation for rectal cancer. *Br J Surg*. 2006;93:1215–1223. doi:10.1002/bjs.5506
30. Ngan SY, Burmeister B, Fisher RJ, et al. Randomized Trial of Short-Course Radiotherapy Versus Long-Course Chemoradiation Comparing Rates of Local Recurrence in Patients With T3 Rectal Cancer: Trans-Tasman Radiation Oncology Group Trial 01.04. *J Clin Oncol*. 2012;30:3827–3833. doi:10.1200/JCO.2012.42.9597
31. Francois Y, Nemoz CJ, Baulieux J, et al. Influence of the interval between preoperative radiation therapy and surgery on downstaging and on the rate of sphincter-sparing surgery for rectal cancer: the Lyon R90-01 randomized trial. *J Clin Oncol Off J Am Soc Clin Oncol*. 1999;17:2396. doi:10.1200/JCO.1999.17.8.2396
32. Pettersson D, Lörinc E, Holm T, et al. Tumour regression in the randomized Stockholm III Trial of radiotherapy regimens for rectal cancer. *Br J Surg*. 2015;102:972–978. doi:10.1002/bjs.9811
33. Erlandsson J, Holm T, Pettersson D, et al. Optimal fractionation of preoperative radiotherapy and timing to surgery for rectal cancer (Stockholm III): a multicentre, randomised, non-blinded, phase 3, non-inferiority trial. *Lancet Oncol*. 2017;18:336–346. doi:10.1016/S1470-2045(17)30086-4
34. Habr-Gama A, de Souza PM, Ribeiro U, et al. Low rectal cancer: impact of radiation and chemotherapy on surgical treatment. *Dis Colon Rectum*. 1998;41:1087–1096. doi:10.1007/BF02239429
35. Habr-Gama A, Perez RO, Nadalin W, et al. Operative versus nonoperative treatment for stage 0 distal rectal cancer following chemoradiation therapy: long-term results. *Trans Meet Am Surg Assoc*. 2004;CXXII:309–316. doi:10.1097/01.sla.0000141194.27992.32
36. Habr-Gama A, Gama-Rodrigues J, São Julião GP, et al. Local recurrence after complete clinical response and watch and wait in rectal cancer after neoadjuvant chemoradiation: impact of salvage therapy on local disease control. *Int J Radiat Oncol*. 2014;88:822–828. doi:10.1016/j.ijrobp.2013.12.012
37. Glynne-Jones R, Hughes R. Critical appraisal of the "wait and see" approach in rectal cancer for clinical complete responders after chemoradiation. *Br J Surg*. 2012;99:897–909. doi:10.1002/bjs.8732
38. Appelt AL, Pløen J, Harling H, et al. High-dose chemoradiotherapy and watchful waiting for distal rectal cancer: a prospective observational study. *Lancet Oncol*. 2015;16:919–927. doi:10.1016/S1470-2045(15)00120-5
39. Renehan AG, Malcomson L, Emsley R, et al. Watch-and-wait approach versus surgical resection after chemoradiotherapy for patients with rectal cancer (the OnCoRe project): a propensity-score matched cohort analysis. *Lancet Oncol*. 2016;17:174–183. doi:10.1016/S1470-2045(15)00467-2
40. Martens MH, Maas M, Heijnen LA, et al. Long-term outcome of an organ preservation program after neoadjuvant treatment for rectal cancer. *J Natl Cancer Inst*. 2016;108:djw171. doi:10.1093/jnci/djw171
41. Ryan DP, Compton CC, Mayer RJ. Carcinoma of the anal canal. *N Engl J Med*. 2000;342:792–800. doi:10.1056/NEJM200003163421107
42. Garcia-Aguilar J, Renfro LA, Chow OS, et al. Organ preservation for clinical T2N0 distal rectal cancer using neoadjuvant chemoradiotherapy and local excision (ACOSOG Z6041): results of an open-label, single-arm, multi-institutional, phase 2 trial. *Lancet Oncol*. 2015;16:1537–1546. doi:10.1016/S1470-2045(15)00215-6
43. Vieillot S, Fenoglietto P, Lemanski C, et al. IMRT for locally advanced anal cancer: clinical experience of the Montpellier Cancer Center. *Radiat Oncol Lond Engl*. 2012;7:45. doi:10.1186/1748-717X-7-45

44. Mundt AJ, Lujan AE, Rotmensch J, et al. Intensity-modulated whole pelvic radiotherapy in women with gynecologic malignancies. *Int J Radiat Oncol*. 2002;52:1330–1337. doi:10.1016/S0360-3016(01)02785-7

45. Wong SJ, Winter K, Meropol NJ, et al. Radiation therapy oncology group 0247: a randomized phase II study of neoadjuvant capecitabine and irinotecan or capecitabine and oxaliplatin with concurrent radiotherapy for patients with locally advanced rectal cancer. *Int J Radiat Oncol*. 2012;82:1367–1375. doi:10.1016/j.ijrobp.2011.05.027

46. Hong TS, Moughan J, Garofalo MC, et al. NRG oncology radiation therapy oncology group 0822: a phase 2 study of preoperative chemoradiation therapy using intensity modulated radiation therapy in combination with capecitabine and oxaliplatin for patients with locally advanced rectal cancer. *Int J Radiat Oncol*. 2015;93:29–36. doi:10.1016/j.ijrobp.2015.05.005

47. O'Connell MJ, Colangelo LH, Beart RW, et al. Capecitabine and oxaliplatin in the preoperative multimodality treatment of rectal cancer: surgical end points from National Surgical Adjuvant Breast and Bowel Project trial R-04. *J Clin Oncol Off J Am Soc Clin Oncol*. 2014;32:1927–1934. doi:10.1200/JCO.2013.53.7753

48. Aschele C, Cionini L, Lonardi S, et al. Primary tumor response to preoperative chemoradiation with or without oxaliplatin in locally advanced rectal cancer: pathologic results of the STAR-01 randomized phase III trial. *J Clin Oncol*. 2011;29:2773–2780. doi:10.1200/JCO.2010.34.4911

49. Gérard J-P, Azria D, Gourgou-Bourgade S, et al. Comparison of two neoadjuvant chemora-diotherapy regimens for locally advanced rectal cancer: results of the phase III trial ACCORD 12/0405-Prodige 2. *J Clin Oncol*. 2010;28:1638–1644. doi:10.1200/JCO.2009.25.8376

50. Rödel C, Graeven U, Fietkau R, et al. Oxaliplatin added to fluorouracil-based preoperative chemoradiotherapy and postoperative chemotherapy of locally advanced rectal cancer (the German CAO/ARO/AIO-04 study): final results of the multicentre, open-label, randomised, phase 3 trial. *Lancet Oncol*. 2015;16:979–989. doi:10.1016/S1470-2045(15)00159-X

51. Deng Y, Chi P, Lan P, et al. Modified FOLFOX6 with or without radiation versus fluorouracil and leucovorin with radiation in neoadjuvant treatment of locally advanced rectal cancer: initial results of the Chinese FOWARC multicenter, Open-label, Randomized three-arm phase III trial. *J Clin Oncol Off J Am Soc Clin Oncol*. 2016;34:3300–3307. doi:10.1200/JCO.2016.66.6198

52. Samuelian JM, Callister MD, Ashman JB, et al. Reduced acute bowel toxicity in patients treated with intensity-modulated radiotherapy for rectal cancer. *Int J Radiat Oncol*. 2012;82:1981–1987. doi:10.1016/j.ijrobp.2011.01.051

53. Camilleri-Brennan J, Steele RJ. The impact of recurrent rectal cancer on quality of life. *Eur J Surg Oncol EJSO*. 2001;27:349–353. doi:10.1053/ejso.2001.1115

54. Glimelius B. Recurrent rectal cancer. The pre-irradiated primary tumour: can more radiotherapy be given? *Colorectal Dis*. 2003;5:501–503. doi:10.1046/j.1463-1318.2003.00501.x

55. Mohiuddin M, Marks G, Marks J. Long-term results of reirradiation for patients with recurrent rectal carcinoma. *Cancer*. 2002;95:1144–1150. doi:10.1002/cncr.10799

56. Valentini V, Morganti AG, Gambacorta MA, et al. Preoperative hyperfractionated chemoradiation for locally recurrent rectal cancer in patients previously irradiated to the pelvis: a multicentric phase II study. *Int J Radiat Oncol*. 2006;64:1129–1139. doi:10.1016/j.ijrobp.2005.09.017

57. Das P, Delclos ME, Skibber JM, et al. Hyperfractionated accelerated radiotherapy for rectal cancer in patients with prior pelvic irradiation. *Int J Radiat Oncol*. 2010;77:60–65. doi:10.1016/j.ijrobp.2009.04.056

58. Haddock MG, Gunderson LL, Nelson H, et al. Intraoperative irradiation for locally recurrent colorectal cancer in previously irradiated patients. *Int J Radiat Oncol Biol Phys*. 2001;49:1267–1274. doi:10.1016/S0360-3016(00)01528-5

59. Vermaas M, Nuyttens JJME, Ferenschild FTJ, et al. Reirradiation, surgery and IORT for recurrent rectal cancer in previously irradiated patients. *Radiother Oncol J Eur Soc Ther Radiol Oncol*. 2008;87:357–360. doi:10.1016/j.radonc.2008.02.021

60. Gunderson LL, Sosin H. Areas of failure found at reoperation (second or symptomatic look) following "curative surgery" for adenocarcinoma of the rectum: Clinicopathologic correlation and implications for adjuvant therapy. *Cancer*. 1974;34:1278–1292. doi:10.1002/1097-0142(197410)34:4<1278::AID-CNCR2820340440>3.0.CO;2-F

61. Steup WH, Moriya Y, van de Velde CJH. Patterns of lymphatic spread in rectal cancer. A topographical analysis on lymph node metastases. *Eur J Cancer*. 2002;38:911–918. doi:10.1016/S0959-8049(02)00046-1

62. Wang C, Zhou Z-G, Yu Y-Y, et al. Patterns of lateral pelvic lymph node metastases and micrometastases for patients with lower rectal cancer. *Eur J Surg Oncol EJSO*. 2007;33:463–467. doi:10.1016/j.ejso.2006.09.015

63. Myerson RJ, Garofalo MC, El Naqa I, et al. Elective clinical target volumes for conformal therapy in anorectal cancer: a radiation therapy oncology group consensus panel contouring atlas. *Int J Radiat Oncol*. 2009;74:824–830. doi:10.1016/j.ijrobp.2008.08.070

How I Treat Early-Stage Rectal Cancer Through Surgery

Nitin Mishra

INTRODUCTION

Early-stage rectal cancer refers to patients with stage 0 or stage I rectal cancer. This includes patients with carcinoma in situ and invasive cancer confined to a polyp. The goal of treatment for early-stage rectal cancer is to achieve cure. Depending on the anatomical location of the cancer, surgical resection may lead to the formation of an end colostomy or a very low anastomosis. This leads to alteration of function, changes in body image, alteration of lifestyle, and may lead to short- and long-term morbidity with the need for additional procedures. In the past three decades, several modalities have been used to perform transanal excisions of early-stage rectal cancers, namely, transanal endoscopic microsurgery (TEM), transanal minimally invasive surgery (TAMIS), and transanal robotic surgery. These procedures avoid the morbidity from radical surgery and, hence, are an appealing alternative for patients with early-stage rectal cancer, however, these procedures do not come with this certainty of addressing the local lymphatics that radical surgery provides. Thus, the surgeon has to weigh the risks and benefits of local excision versus radical surgery for every individual patient diagnosed with early-stage rectal cancer. This need to balance the potential for achieving oncological cure with the potential for causing short- and long-term morbidity is what makes treating early-stage rectal cancer uniquely challenging. In this chapter, we review the presentation, diagnosis, and workup of early-stage rectal cancer patients followed by the treatment options for patients with the following scenarios:

1. A patient with cancer confined to a polyp in the rectum
2. A patient with suspected T1 N0 M0 rectal cancer
3. A patient with suspected T2 N0 M0 rectal cancer

PRESENTATION

Most patients with early-stage rectal cancer are asymptomatic and may be diagnosed on screening colonoscopy or via a rectal exam performed as a part of routine medical examination. A fraction of patients present with complaints of anal bleeding, mucus discharge, tenesmus, and, rarely, with the sensation of a prolapsing mass.

DIAGNOSIS

Diagnosis is dependent on the level of the tumor. Most tumors are diagnosed during endoluminal examination either during a colonoscopy, proctoscopy, or a digital rectal examination. Early-stage rectal cancer may rarely be diagnosed as an incidental finding on imaging. A biopsy is necessary to confirm the diagnosis.

WORKUP

A standard workup for stage I rectal cancer includes a complete colonoscopy, baseline serum carcinoembryonic antigen (CEA) level, CT scan of chest and abdomen with intravenous (IV)

A Clinical Vignette ("How I Treat") is included at the end of the chapter.

contrast, and MRI of the pelvis with rectal cancer protocol using rectal gel with 3-T magnetic resonance scanner, small field of view, and high-resolution images in three orthogonal planes (sagittal, axial, and coronal) by a dedicated gastrointestinal (GI) radiologist. In our institution, MRI has substituted endoscopic ultrasound (EUS) as the imaging modality of choice for these patients. We use EUS only in those patients where MRI is contraindicated or MRI reveals a suspicious lymph node that needs to be biopsied or MRI cannot accurately delineate the tumor depth (mostly secondary to motion artifact or the presence of pelvic hardware). Any outside pathology slides need to be reviewed by a dedicated GI pathologist. For patients with carcinoma in situ confined to a completely excised polyp, the workup is limited to a complete colonoscopy.

TREATMENT

A Patient With Cancer Confined to a Polyp in the Rectum

Patients with cancer confined to a polyp in the rectum may have carcinoma in situ or invasive cancer. Those patients who have carcinoma in situ in a polyp that has been completely excised with negative margins can be safely observed with serial colonoscopies and do not need surgery. Invasive cancer in a polyp may arise in a pedunculated polyp or a sessile polyp. Treatment of these patients depends on the risk of local recurrence and the risk of regional (lymph node) disease. Local recurrence is dependent on the polyp resection margin. With resection margins more than 1 mm, the risk of local recurrence is less than 2% and increases to 33% with positive margins (1). The risk of nodal involvement is dependent on the depth of invasion of the cancer. Depth of cancer invasion has been categorized by the Haggitt classification and the Japanese S M calcification (2–4) (Figure 7.1). Usually the level of invasion into the submucosa of cancer arising in a sessile polyp is deeper than a pedunculated polyp. Any invasion into the submucosa of a sessile polyp corresponds to the level of Haggitt 3 in a pedunculated polyp. The risk of lymph node involvement by the tumor invading the submucosa varies from 0% to 27% (5). It is dependent on the depth of submucosal involvement, the level of the tumor in the rectum, tumor differentiation, the presence or absence of tumor budding, and the presence or absence of lymphovascular invasion.

It is very important to have a detailed discussion with the patient about the fact that accurate prediction of the risk of lymph node involvement is impossible with our current understanding of rectal cancer. However, we can make an educated guess and risk-stratify these patients in terms of the likelihood of lymph node involvement. In addition to this, the level of the polyp in the rectum is a very important factor in planning the treatment. A polyp very low in the rectum has a higher likelihood of lymph node involvement compared to a polyp higher up in the rectum, and radical excision of such a polyp leads to higher short- and long-term morbidity including the possibility of an end colostomy. If the polyp is excised en bloc, it is possible to accurately assess the depth of submucosal invasion and margins. When this excision is piecemeal, it makes it impossible to assess the margins of the excision.

We offer radical surgical resection in the form of anterior resection, low anterior resection, or abdominoperineal resection to patients who are good surgical candidates and have any of the following:

- Poorly differentiated cancer
- Presence of lymphovascular invasion
- Submucosal invasion more than 1 mm
- Tumor budding
- Positive, indeterminate or margin less than 1 mm, or piecemeal resection

Patients who have *all* of the following features are offered the choice of surgical resection versus observation with colonoscopy at 3 months and pelvic MRI with rectal cancer protocol at 6 months:

- Pedunculated (Haggitt level 1–3) polyp
- Well-differentiated cancer
- No lymphovascular invasion
- Submucosal invasion less than 1 mm
- En bloc resection with 2 mm or more margin.

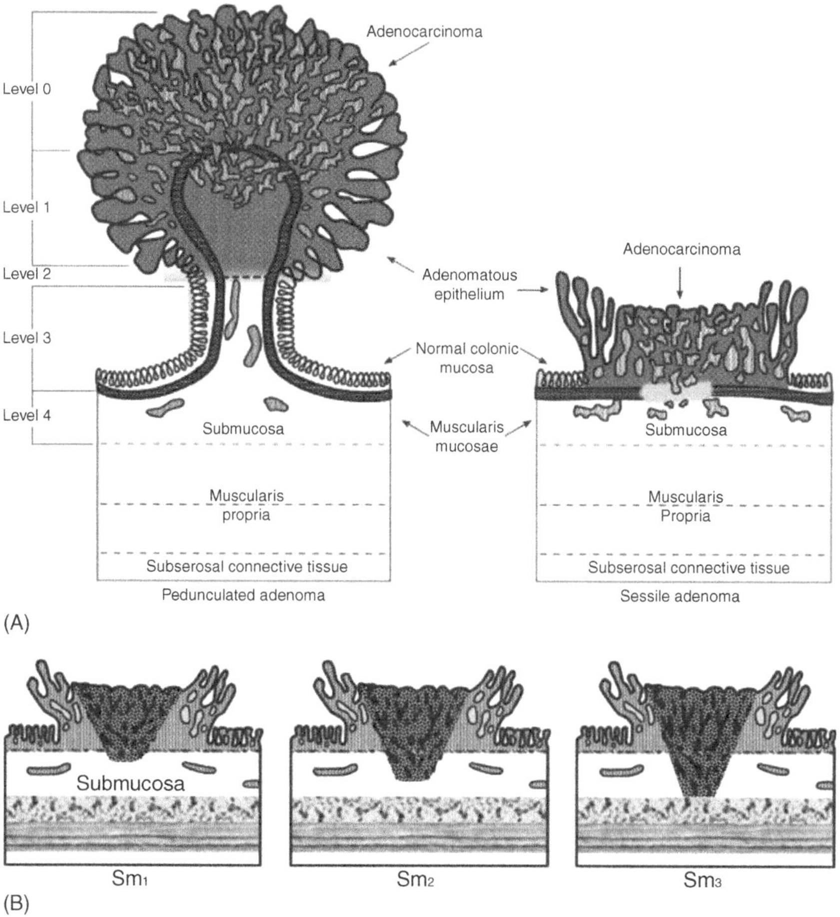

FIGURE 7.1   (A) Haggitt classification of pedunculated and sessile polyps. (B) Classification of Sm invasion of malignant polyps.

Sm, submucosal.

Patients who are poor candidates for surgery are offered transanal excision and close observation if the initial margin was positive. Adjuvant radiation treatment can be considered in these patients.

A Patient With Suspected T1 N0 M0 Rectal Cancer Not Arising in a Polyp

T1 rectal cancer not arising in a polyp can be treated like those arising in a sessile polyp with the understanding that these tumors are more likely to have deeper invasion of the submucosa. Because of the low likelihood of lymph node involvement, these patients can be treated by a transanal excision and observation. However, the safest oncological approach is to resect the tumor along with its draining lymphatics, that is, anterior resection, low anterior resection, or abdominoperineal resection, depending on the location of the tumor.

A Patient With Suspected T2 N0 M0 Rectal Cancer

Patients with T2 rectal cancer (i.e., tumor invasion into the muscularis propria) have a substantial risk of regional lymph node involvement. The risk of local recurrence following transanal excision of T2 tumors is estimated to be 26% to 47%. The current standard of care is to offer these patients radical surgical resection. Patients with T2 cancer, as a rule, get offered radical surgical resection in our practice. The exceptions are those who were not a candidate for surgery or those who refused radical surgical resection. Such patients can be offered transanal excision with, or without, chemoradiation.

TECHNICAL DETAILS

Transanal Excision

Transanal excisions for rectal cancer should be full-thickness, with at least a 10 millimeter circumferential margin. It is very important to correctly orient the specimen for proper pathological evaluation and accurate determination of positive margin.

Indications
- Benign polyp or T1 tumor with favorable features (submucosal 1 [Sm1], well differentiated, no lymphovascular invasion, no perineural invasion, no tumor budding)

Relative Contraindications
- T1 tumor with high-risk features (Sm2 deeper, moderately or poorly differentiated, lymphovascular invasion, perineural invasion, tumor budding)
- T2 tumor (should be limited to trial settings)
- Lesion size more than 3 cm or involving 30% of rectal circumference

Types
1. Conventional transanal excision: This is performed using standard anorectal instruments and retractors, and is optimal for lesions 8 to 10 cm from the anal verge.
2. TEM: This technique was introduced in the 1980s and is performed by using specialized instruments and an operating proctoscope, which is 4 cm in diameter and varies in length from 12 to 20 cm (6). This is ideal for lesions in the mid to upper rectum. Successful resections have been reported up to 20 cm from the anal verge. This platform has a stable CO_2 insufflating mechanism and specialized instruments. The visualization and pneumorectum tend to be excellent (Figure 7.2).
3. TAMIS: This technique was introduced in 2009 and is performed using a special transanal single incision laparoscopic port and conventional laparoscopic instruments (7). This is used for lesions up to 15 cm from the anal verge. A conventional CO_2 insufflator can be used but a high flow insufflator with constant smoke evacuation capabilities is preferred and provides a more stable platform. The outcomes with TAMIS and TEM are comparable; however, long-term oncological data is lacking with TAMIS as it is a newer procedure. The choice of technique is dependent on the distance of the tumor from the anal verge and the surgeon's experience and preference.

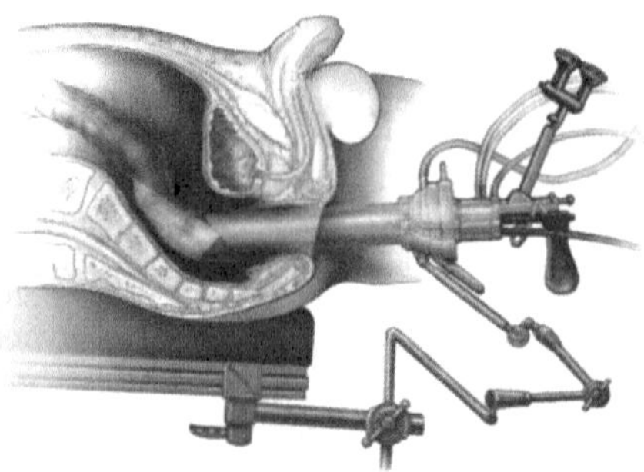

FIGURE 7.2   Transanal endoscopic microsurgery.

Source: From Sacharides TJ. Transanal endoscopic microsurgery. *Oper Tech Gen Surg.* 2005;7(3):107.

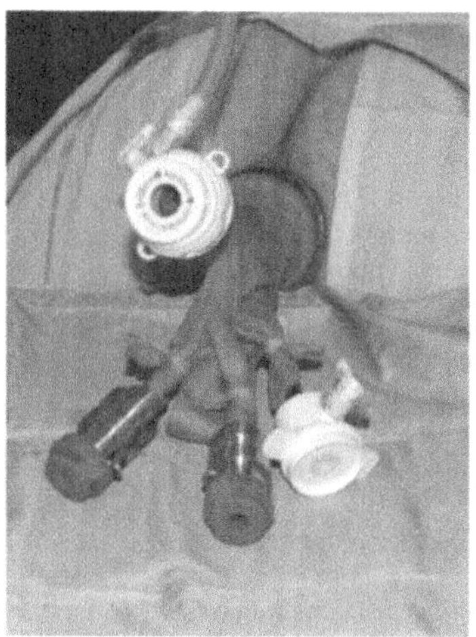
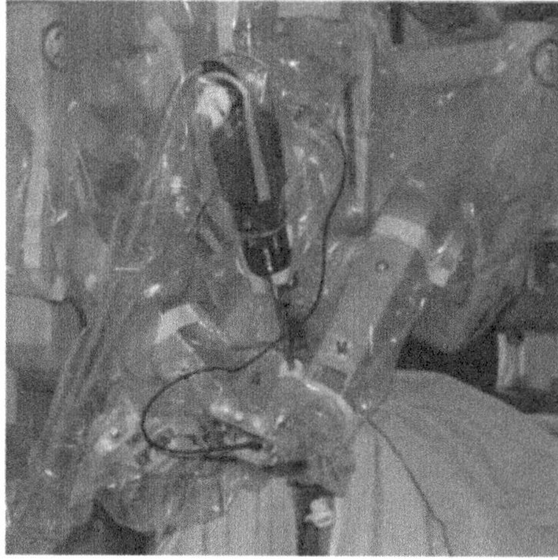

(A) Set-up of transanal glove port   (B) Completed docking procedure

FIGURE 7.3   Robotic transanal minimally invasive surgery.

Source: From Hompers R, Rauh SM, Ris F, et al. Robotic transanal minimally invasive surgery for local excision of rectal neoplasms. *Br J Surg.* 2014;101(5):579. doi:10.1002/bjs.9454

4. Robotic TAMIS: This technique was introduced in 2012 (8). The reach is comparable to conventional TAMIS; the reported benefits are that of three-dimensional (3D) visualization and better range of movement. Although early results are promising, the long-term outcomes are awaited (Figure 7.3).

RADICAL SURGICAL RESECTION

Types

1. Anterior resection: This is carried out for rectosigmoid or low sigmoid tumors. The affected portion of the rectosigmoid is removed along with the draining lymphatics and an end-to-end anastomosis is fashioned between the colon and the rectum at the level of, or above, the peritoneal reflection.
2. Low anterior resection: This is carried out for rectal cancer with the lower border being at least 0.5 cm above the anorectal ring. Resection is similar to anterior resection; however, the anastomosis is fashioned below the peritoneal reflection. Such anastomoses have a higher risk of leak and so these patients are typically diverted with a loop ileostomy.
3. Abdominal perineal resection: This is performed for tumors involving the anal sphincter or those tumors where it is impossible to get a negative margin without removing a portion of the sphincter. An abdominal perineal resection is also likely to provide better quality of life for patients with mid to low rectal cancer who have baseline sphincter dysfunction. In this surgery, the entire rectum, anus, and a portion of the sigmoid colon are removed with a permanent colostomy.

All of the aforementioned procedures can be carried out in an open, laparoscopic or robotic fashion. The key is to follow standard oncological principles such as high ligation of the inferior mesenteric artery and total mesorectal excision. Open and laparoscopic approaches are comparable in terms of oncological outcomes. Further long-term data is awaited for the robotic approach. A newer technique has recently been introduced—transanal total mesorectal excision for low rectal cancer. The early results from this approach have shown some concerning complications such as urethral injuries. Short- and long-term data are lacking, and currently the use of this technique is limited to selected centers.

In our practice, the robotic approach is preferred because of superior visualization, more stable operating platform, greater range of movement within a narrow operating field, and the surgeon's ability to control three operating arms.

Clinical Vignette 7.1

A 58-year-old female patient with a history of deep venous thrombosis and pulmonary embolism 4 months ago, a body mass index (BMI) of 54, history of well-controlled chronic obstructive pulmonary disease (COPD), hypertension, and diabetes presented to the office after a colonoscopy was performed for rectal bleeding. The gastroenterologist found a 2 cm polyp 2 cm from the anorectal ring and removed it in a piecemeal fashion. Pathology was found to be T1 invasive rectal cancer with less than 1 mm invasion into the submucosa, a 2 mm margin, no lymphovascular invasion, no tumor budding, and no perineural invasion. Should this patient have the surgical treatment or adjuvant radiation or can she be observed?

Discussion

This patient has one high-risk feature, namely the piecemeal removal of this lesion. All other pathological pattern meters are favorable. She is a high-risk surgical candidate with a BMI of 54 and comorbidities. In balancing the risk and benefit of a radical surgical resection versus observation, our multidisciplinary tumor board recommended observation and the patient agreed with that approach.

Note: The morbidity and quality-of-life impact after total mesorectal excision is significant and considerably higher than an anterior resection. Rectal preservation for early rectal cancer patients in the subgroup who would need removal of the entire rectum is especially appealing. Whether such an approach is oncologically safe is currently not known. A phase 3 multicentered randomized controlled trial to answer this question is currently under way in Europe. Details of this trial protocol are available at www.clinicaltrials.gov. The trial is labeled "Rectal Preserving Treatment for Early Rectal Cancer. A Multi-Centred Randomised Trial of Radical Surgery Versus Adjuvant Chemoradiotherapy After Local Excision for Early Rectal Cancers (TESAR)."

SUGGESTED READINGS

Monson JR, Weiser MR, Buie WD, et al. Standards Practice Task Force of the American Society of Colon and Rectal Surgeons. Practice parameters for the management of rectal cancer (revised). *Dis Colon Rectum*. 2013;56(5):535–550.
NCCN Clinical practice guidelines in oncology rectal cancer, Version I.2018-March 14, 2018.

REFERENCES

1. Butte JM, Tang P, Gonen M, et al. Rate of residual disease after complete endoscopic resection of malignant colonic polyp. *Dis Colon Rectum*. 2012;55(2):122–127. doi:10.1097/DCR.0b013e3182336c38
2. Haggitt RC, Glotzbach RE, Soffer EE, et al. Prognostic factors in colorectal carcinomas arising in adenomas: implications for lesions removed by endoscopic polypectomy. *Gastroenterology*. 1985;89(2):328–336. doi:10.1016/0016-5085(85)90333-6
3. Kikuchi R, Takano M, Takagi K, et al. Management of early invasive colorectal cancer. Risk of recurrence and clinical guidelines. *Dis Colon Rectum*. 1995;38(12):1286–1295. doi:10.1007/BF02049154
4. Kudo S. Endoscopic mucosal resection of flat and depressed types of early colorectal cancer. *Endoscopy*. 1993;25(7):455–461. doi:10.1055/s-2007-1010367
5. Nivatvongs S, Rojanasakul A, Reiman HM, et al. The risk of lymph node metastasis in colorectal polyps with invasive adenocarcinoma. *Dis Colon Rectum*. 1991;34(4):323–328. doi:10.1007/BF02050592
6. Buess G, Theiss R, Hutterer F, et al. Transanal endoscopic surgery of the rectum—testing a new method in animal experiments. *Leber, Magen, Darm*. 1983;13(2):73–77.

7. Atallah S, Albert M, Larach S. Transanal minimally invasive surgery: a giant leap forward. *Surg Endosc.* 2010;24(9):2200–2205. doi:10.1007/s00464-010-0927-z

8. Atallah S, Parra-Davila E, DeBeche-Adams T, et al. Excision of a rectal neoplasm using robotic transanal surgery (RTS): a description of the technique. *Tech Coloproctol.* 2012;16(5):389–392. doi:10.1007/s10151-012-0833-6

How I Treat Early-Stage Rectal Cancer With Adjuvant Therapy

Gabriel A. Brooks

INTRODUCTION

The primary goal of adjuvant therapy for rectal cancer is to reduce the risk of cancer recurrence after definitive surgical therapy and thereby to improve long-term survival. Combination chemotherapy and radiation are critical for the prevention of local recurrences, and chemotherapy serves the additional purpose of preventing distant recurrences. For patients with distal rectal cancers, neoadjuvant chemoradiation may also facilitate sphincter-sparing surgery. Chemoradiation is most commonly employed in the neoadjuvant setting (i.e., preoperatively), and adjuvant chemotherapy is generally delivered postoperatively.

PATIENT SELECTION

The role of rectal cancer adjuvant therapy is best established for patients with clinical T3/4 disease (for neoadjuvant chemoradiation) or pathologic stage II/III (for patients not receiving neoadjuvant therapy). Neoadjuvant chemoradiation may also be used in patients with clinical T1–2, node-positive disease, or in patients with distal, early-stage rectal cancer where abdominoperineal resection is planned (when preoperative therapy may allow for sphincter preservation). Additional criteria for the use of adjuvant chemotherapy include an adequate performance status (generally, Eastern Cooperative Oncology Group [ECOG] 2 or better) and the absence of other known contraindications to chemotherapy. Notably, impaired renal or hepatic functions are not contraindications to adjuvant therapy in most cases, as the chemotherapy agents used in adjuvant therapy (fluoropyrimidines and oxaliplatin) are tolerated even with moderate to severe renal and hepatic dysfunction.

Because fluoropyrimidines (5-fluorouracil [5-FU] and capecitabine) are the backbone of adjuvant chemotherapy for rectal cancer, it is my practice to obtain mutation analysis of the *DPYD* gene prior to initiating adjuvant chemotherapy. The 2% to 3% of patients who carry a deleterious polymorphism of the *DPYD* gene are at substantially increased risk for severe toxicity with standard doses of fluoropyrimidine chemotherapy; however, toxicity risk can be mitigated with genotype-directed dosing (1).

NEOADJUVANT THERAPY

For most patients with clinical stage II or III rectal cancer, the first component of cancer treatment is neoadjuvant chemoradiation. While adjuvant therapy for rectal cancer was first developed in the postoperative setting (both radiation and chemotherapy), the benefits of a neoadjuvant (preoperative) approach became apparent in the early 2000s, with the first reporting of the pivotal German Rectal Cancer Study Group trial (2,3). This study compared preoperative versus postoperative adjuvant chemoradiation for patients with T3/4 and/or node-positive rectal cancer. Chemotherapy in both neoadjuvant and postoperative therapy groups consisted of 5-FU delivered as a 5-day infusion during weeks 1 and 5 of radiation, with four additional cycles of postoperative chemotherapy (also in both groups). Though overall survival did not differ between neoadjuvant and postoperative therapy groups (10-year overall survival 59.6%

A Clinical Vignette ("How I Treat") is included at the end of the chapter.

vs. 59.9%, $p = .80$), neoadjuvant therapy was associated with a clinically significant reduction in local relapse (10-year local recurrence 7.1% vs. 10.1%, $p = .048$). Rates of acute and long-term toxic effects were also reduced with preoperative treatment. The critical contribution of chemotherapy in combination with long-course neoadjuvant radiation has been confirmed in multiple randomized trials, with neoadjuvant chemoradiation cutting local recurrence rates by approximately half compared with radiation alone (4,5).

Although neoadjuvant combined chemoradiation is the most widely used form of neoadjuvant therapy for rectal cancer, alternative approaches include short-course radiotherapy and the so-called total neoadjuvant therapy (TNT). The TNT approach involves neoadjuvant treatment starting with chemotherapy first (generally 3–4 months of modified FOLFOX or CAPOX), followed by chemoradiation (6,7). While the disease control outcomes of these treatments appear to be roughly similar (7), purported advantages of the TNT approach include maximal preoperative downstaging and better chemotherapy tolerance in the neoadjuvant setting. These hypothetical benefits of the TNT approach have yet to be confirmed in comparative trials, however.

In current practice, chemotherapy during neoadjuvant chemoradiation is most often delivered throughout the course of radiation rather than only in weeks 1 and 5 of radiation (as was done in the German Rectal Cancer Study Group trial). Chemotherapy may be given as a continuous infusion of 5-FU (either 5 or 7 days per week during radiation therapy) or as capecitabine, dosed at 825 mg/m^2 taken orally twice daily on radiation treatment days (8–10). In my practice, I prefer capecitabine for most patients; capecitabine monotherapy is effective and well-tolerated, and the logistics of the 5-week ambulatory 5-FU infusion are challenging for many patients.

ADJUVANT THERAPY

For patients who received neoadjuvant chemoradiation, additional postoperative adjuvant chemotherapy is generally recommended. The pathologic stage is not used to identify candidates for adjuvant therapy after neoadjuvant chemoradiation and surgery, as the downstaging effects of chemoradiation can obscure the "true" pathologic stage (e.g., the pathologic stage that would have been detected had surgery been the initial treatment). For patients who did not receive neoadjuvant chemoradiation, postoperative chemoradiation and chemotherapy are recommended for T3/4 or pathologically node-positive disease. Despite the inclusion of postoperative adjuvant chemotherapy in most rectal cancer treatment guidelines, evidence of survival improvement from adjuvant chemotherapy in rectal cancer is limited and mixed at best (11,12). Benefit from adjuvant chemotherapy in rectal cancer is inferred from the inclusion of 4 months of postoperative chemotherapy in key studies of neoadjuvant chemoradiation (3), as well as from the benefit observed in colon cancer adjuvant therapy trials.

With limited evidence for the benefit from postoperative adjuvant chemotherapy in rectal cancer, the optimal chemotherapy regimen for use in this setting is also uncertain. The German Rectal Cancer Study Group trial used 5 days of bolus 5-FU, repeated every 4 weeks for four cycles; however, this regimen is both more toxic and less effective than more modern regimens. Commonly used regimens include capecitabine, biweekly infusional 5-FU and leucovorin, modified FOLFOX, and CAPOX. The use of oxaliplatin in rectal cancer adjuvant chemotherapy is supported by the observation of improved 3-year disease-free survival in the phase II ADORE study (13), as well as by extrapolation from improved survival outcomes in stage III colon cancer (14,15). However, the chemotherapy regimen used in the comparator arm of the ADORE study was a bolus regimen, leading to the uncertainty of whether the disease-free survival improvement in that study is best attributed to the difference in 5-FU administration or the inclusion of oxaliplatin.

In my practice, I recommend 3 to 4 months of postoperative adjuvant chemotherapy for patients who meet eligibility criteria (e.g., receipt of neoadjuvant chemoradiation, or pathologic stage II/III disease in patients who did not have neoadjuvant chemoradiation). For patients with clinical or pathologic T4 or node-positive rectal cancer, I generally use FOLFOX (or CAPOX) chemotherapy. However, given the substantial uncertainty about the benefit of oxaliplatin, I am quick to discontinue oxaliplatin in patients who experience bothersome and persistent neuropathy. For patients with clinical T3N0 rectal cancer where staging is either confirmed or downstaged at surgery, I generally use capecitabine adjuvant chemotherapy (or biweekly infusional 5-FU with leucovorin). I sometimes use TNT for patients with bulky, distal rectal cancers, especially in patients considering an attempt at nonoperative therapy. However, more data are needed before a wider role for TNT is adopted. Last, it is not unreasonable to omit adjuvant chemotherapy for well-informed patients who remain averse to treatment after a discussion of the potential benefits and risks of therapy (and after completion of either neoadjuvant or adjuvant chemoradiation).

FUTURE DIRECTIONS

Total mesorectal excision and neoadjuvant chemoradiation represent the critical innovations in rectal cancer management over the past three decades. Critical innovations of the next decade are unknown, but one candidate is the development of better prognostic and predictive biomarkers for rectal cancer treatment. Biomarkers hold promise for helping to tailor risk-stratified treatment strategies based on patient and tumor characteristics. The PROSPECT study is one example of a study that uses a biomarker (radiographic response to neoadjuvant FOLFOX) to identify patients who may be able to safely forego neoadjuvant radiation. The case presentation highlights another potentially useful biomarker, pathologic complete response. Pathologic complete response to neoadjuvant chemoradiation predicts a substantially improved disease-free survival, compared to a less than complete response (16), and further study is needed to evaluate whether pathologic complete response identifies patients who can safely forego some or all components of postoperative adjuvant chemotherapy. While immunotherapies have yet to arrive in rectal cancer treatment, microsatellite instability status may serve as a biomarker to investigate immune-based rectal cancer adjuvant treatments.

Clinical Vignette 8.1

JB is a 53-year-old woman without significant past medical history who presented with 2 months of bright red blood in her stool. Her primary care physician ordered a diagnostic colonoscopy, which showed an anterior, nonobstructing rectal mass starting at 6 cm from the anal verge. Pathologic review of the colonoscopic biopsy showed invasive adenocarcinoma with intact expression of mismatch repair proteins. Pelvic MRI showed a T3 primary tumor, with two suspicious-appearing mesorectal lymph nodes (pT3N1b). CT of the chest, abdomen, and pelvis showed no evidence of distant metastasis in the lungs, liver, or elsewhere. Pharmacogenomic testing showed no deleterious polymorphisms of *DPYD* gene, including negative testing for the following alleles: c. 1679T>G, c. 1905+1G>A, and c. 2846A>T.

The location of the primary tumor at 6 cm from the anal verge was confirmed during preoperative surgical evaluation, and the surgeon documented that a low anterior resection was feasible without downstaging. JB's case was discussed at the institutional multidisciplinary tumor board, and she was identified as a potential candidate for the PROSPECT study (NCT01515787). PROSPECT is a randomized, controlled trial evaluating an adaptive approach to neoadjuvant therapy that omits chemoradiation in patients with greater than 20% response to induction chemotherapy. She consented to participate in PROSPECT, and she was randomized to the standard therapy arm (neoadjuvant chemoradiation, followed by surgery, followed by recommended adjuvant chemotherapy).

She received 50.4 Gray of radiation over 28 fractions, with concurrent capecitabine dosed at 825 mg/m2 twice daily on radiation treatment days. Neoadjuvant chemoradiation was complicated by fatigue and irregular bowel movements, and JB began medical leave from work partway through this treatment. She completed chemoradiation without complications, and 10 weeks later she had a low anterior resection with total mesorectal excision, with formation of a temporary ileostomy. Sigmoidoscopy before the surgery showed a flat scar at the site of the primary tumor. Operative pathology showed a complete pathologic response to neoadjuvant chemoradiation, without evidence of residual adenocarcinoma (ypT0N0).

Four weeks after her surgery, I met with JB to discuss postoperative adjuvant chemotherapy. We reviewed her baseline staging (cT3N1M0), as well as the operative finding of complete pathologic response (no residual cancer in the surgical specimen). I explained that complete pathologic response likely indicated an excellent prognosis, with a low risk for local or distant recurrence. Based on the initial clinical staging findings, I recommended that we proceed with planned adjuvant chemotherapy. FOLFOX was recommended but not mandated by the PROSPECT study protocol, and we discussed the possible alternative of capecitabine monotherapy. Ultimately, we made the decision together to proceed with FOLFOX, with a plan for eight cycles of treatment.

Adjuvant chemotherapy with FOLFOX began 6 weeks after her surgery. Oxaliplatin was dose-reduced to 65 mg/m^2 starting in cycle 3 due to bothersome and persistent acute neuropathy symptoms. She elected to discontinue adjuvant chemotherapy after completing six cycles, due to increasing difficulties with treatment tolerance. Her ileostomy was reversed 1 month after her last chemotherapy treatment.

REFERENCES

1. Deenen MJ, Meulendijks D, Cats A, et al. Upfront genotyping of DPYD*2A to individualize fluoro-pyrimidine therapy: a safety and cost analysis. *J Clin Oncol.* 2016;34(3), 227–234. doi: 10.1200/jco.2015.63.1325
2. Sauer R, Becker H, Hohenberger W, et al. Preoperative versus postoperative chemoradiotherapy for rectal cancer. *N Engl J Med.* 2004;351(17):1731–1740. doi:10.1056/NEJMoa040694
3. Sauer R, Liersch T, Merkel S, et al. Preoperative versus postoperative chemoradiotherapy for locally advanced rectal cancer: results of the German CAO/ARO/AIO-94 randomized phase III trial after a median follow-up of 11 years. *J Clin Oncol.* 2012;30(16), 1926–1933. doi: 10.1200/JCO.2011.40.1836
4. Bosset JF, Collette L, Calais G, et al. Chemotherapy with preoperative radiotherapy in rectal cancer. *N Engl J Med.* 2006;355(11):1114–1123. doi:10.1056/NEJMoa060829
5. Gerard JP, Conroy T, Bonnetain F, et al. Preoperative radiotherapy with or without concurrent fluorouracil and leucovorin in T3-4 rectal cancers: results of FFCD 9203. *J Clin Oncol.* 2006;24(28):4620–4625. doi:10.1200/jco.2006.06.7629
6. Cercek A, Roxburgh CSD, Strombom P, et al. Adoption of Total Neoadjuvant Therapy for Locally Advanced Rectal Cancer. *JAMA Oncol.* 2018;4(6):e180071. doi:10.1001/jamaoncol.2018.0071
7. Fernandez-Martos C, Garcia-Albeniz X, Pericay C, et al. Chemoradiation, surgery and adjuvant chemotherapy versus induction chemotherapy followed by chemoradiation and surgery: long-term results of the Spanish GCR-3 phase II randomized trial dagger. *Ann Oncol.* 2015;26(8):1722–1728. doi:10.1093/annonc/mdv223
8. Hofheinz RD, Wenz F, Post S, et al. Chemoradiotherapy with capecitabine versus fluorouracil for locally advanced rectal cancer: a randomised, multicentre, non-inferiority, phase 3 trial. *Lancet Oncol.* 2012;13(6), 579–588. doi:10.1016/s1470-2045(12)70116-x
9. O'Connell MJ, Colangelo LH, Beart RW, et al. Capecitabine and oxaliplatin in the preoperative multimodality treatment of rectal cancer: surgical end points from National Surgical Adjuvant Breast and Bowel Project trial R-04. *J Clin Oncol.* 2014;32(18):1927–1934. doi:10.1200/jco.2013.53.7753
10. O'Connell MJ, Lavery I, Yothers G, et al. Relationship between tumor gene expression and recurrence in four independent studies of patients with stage II/III colon cancer treated with surgery alone or surgery plus adjuvant fluorouracil plus leucovorin. *J Clin Oncol.* 2010;28(25):3937–3944. doi:10.1200/JCO.2010.28.9538
11. Breugom AJ, Swets M, Bosset JF, et al. Adjuvant chemotherapy after preoperative (chemo)radiotherapy and surgery for patients with rectal cancer: a systematic review and meta-analysis of individual patient data. *Lancet Oncol.* 2015;16(2):200–207. doi:10.1016/s1470-2045(14)71199-4
12. Petersen SH, Harling H, Kirkeby LT, et al. Postoperative adjuvant chemotherapy in rectal cancer operated for cure. *Cochrane Database Syst Rev.* 2012;(3):CD004078. doi:10.1002/14651858.CD004078.pub2
13. Hong YS, Nam BH, Kim KP, et al. Oxaliplatin, fluorouracil, and leucovorin versus fluorouracil and leucovorin as adjuvant chemotherapy for locally advanced rectal cancer after preoperative chemoradiotherapy (ADORE): an open-label, multicentre, phase 2, randomised controlled trial. *Lancet Oncol.* 2014;15(11):1245–1253. doi:10.1016/s1470-2045(14)70377-8

14. Andre T, Boni C, Mounedji-Boudiaf L, et al. Oxaliplatin, fluorouracil, and leucovorin as adjuvant treatment for colon cancer. *N Engl J Med.* 2004;350(23):2343–2351. doi:10.1056/NEJMoa032709
15. Andre T, Boni C, Navarro M, et al. Improved overall survival with oxaliplatin, fluorouracil, and leucovorin as adjuvant treatment in stage II or III colon cancer in the MOSAIC trial. *J Clin Oncol.* 2009;27(19):3109–3116. doi:10.1200/JCO.2008.20.6771
16. Maas M, Nelemans PJ, Valentini V, et al. Long-term outcome in patients with a pathological complete response after chemoradiation for rectal cancer: a pooled analysis of individual patient data. *Lancet Oncol.* 2010;11(9):835–844. doi: 10.1016/S1470-2045(10)70172-8

How I Treat Oligometastatic Colorectal Cancer Through Surgery

Rory L. Smoot and David M. Nagorney

INTRODUCTION

Surgical resection remains the most definitive therapy for resectable colorectal liver metastases. Patient selection is paramount, and long-term durable responses are contingent on patient and disease risk factors. When evaluating patients for resection of oligometastatic liver disease, we utilize an "ABC" (anatomy, biology, conditional) paradigm (Table 9.1). Meeting resection criteria for all three categories in this paradigm is necessary, and optimization strategies may be employed to meet criteria.

ANATOMIC CONSIDERATIONS

Anatomic resectability criteria mandate a sufficient future liver remnant (FLR) for an R0 resection. Traditionally, the minimum FLR considered for liver resection has been 20%, which practically speaking entails a minimum of two contiguous liver segments with vascular inflow, vascular outflow, and biliary drainage intact. This 20% threshold is seldom applicable because of chemotherapy associated liver disease, and underlying liver steatosis and/or fibrosis. In the setting of neoadjuvant chemotherapy or significant steatosis a minimal FLR of 30% is recommended, and in the setting of significant fibrosis or cirrhosis a minimal FLR of 40% is recommended. In practice, these considerations come into play in several ways. First, accurate determination of all disease present within the liver is necessary. Traditionally, contrast-enhanced CT scan (portal phase scanning) has been utilized for lesion identification. Given the superior resolution of MRI, especially in the setting of steatosis and/or neoadjuvant therapy, we now employ MR with gadoxetic acid based contrast routinely (1–3). Ultrasound evaluation is reserved for intraoperative lesion identification and localization; in the preoperative setting, ultrasound is utilized only for image directed biopsies if indicated. PET scanning may have utility in the overall disease evaluation/staging, but in terms of directing liver resection the utility has been demonstrated to be limited in a large randomized trial and we do not employ it for evaluation of the liver specifically (4). Accurate lesion identification allows both risk stratification based on the total number of lesions and informed discussions with the patient regarding operative strategies and risks (5). Planning for a margin negative resection is the standard approach, and more commonly, parenchymal-sparing techniques are favored. Although a 1 cm margin is considered standard, large studies have demonstrated no significant detriment to closer margins in patients who have demonstrable response to neoadjuvant therapy (6–9). Based on these reports, we do not limit the determination of anatomic resectability to 1 cm margins in patients who have responded to neoadjuvant therapy. Allowing marginal resections in patients who respond to therapy increases the number of patients who are candidates for resection without significantly impacting patient outcomes. Finally, we do not routinely obtain volumetry in patients unless significant underlying liver steatosis/fibrosis is suggested on MRI or extended resections are necessary to clear disease, if so, then we do compute FLR volumes from CT and/or MRI. FLR volumes below the threshold values necessitate optimization strategies, and subsequent volumetry is normalized to body surface area for comparison. Functional assays such as indocyanine green (ICG) clearance are not routinely used.

A Clinical Vignette ("How I Treat") is included at the end of the chapter.

TABLE 9.1 Criteria for Selection of Patients for Liver Resection

	Resectable	Borderline (Optimization Needed)	Unresectable
Anatomy	Adequate FLR	FLR too small	FLR fails hypertrophy
	Unilobar disease	Bilobar disease	Extrahepatic disease
	No vascular issues	FLR vascular involvement	Unreconstructable vascular involvement
Biology	3 or fewer lesions	4 or more lesions	Progression on systemic therapy
	>12 months since primary	<12 months since primary	
Condition	ECOG 1 or less	ECOG 2	ECOG >1 without possible improvement

ECOG, Eastern Cooperative Oncology Group; FLR: future liver remnant.

ANATOMIC OPTIMIZATION STRATEGIES

Parenchymal-sparing techniques, including the combination of resection and intraoperative ablation, can increase the FLR for patients with either solitary or multiple metastases and often allow single stage resections. However, for those patients with bilobar metastases and an FLR below resection thresholds, we most commonly employ portal vein embolization (PVE) to drive FLR growth. The remnant liver is most commonly cleared of metastases prior to embolization and the embolized liver resected in a second stage if appropriate hypertrophy is obtained. In practice, embolization is completed during the index hospitalization following first stage resection if the patient is convalescing well, and in a delayed fashion (1–2 weeks after discharge) if the recovery is complicated. Evaluation of hypertrophy is undertaken 4 to 6 weeks following PVE. Previous studies have demonstrated the effectiveness of PVE and validated that the response to embolization predicts liver functional outcomes (10–13). Growth beyond the threshold FLR percentage is needed; however, additionally a kinetic growth rate of greater than 2% and a total response of greater than 7.5% denote an optimal response (14). Another approach to optimize FLR is the variants of associating liver partition with portal vein ligation (ALPPS). This approach carries significant morbidity, and we employ ALPPS only in patients who have failed to hypertrophy following PVE (15). In patients in whom vascular outflow involvement limits the anatomic resectability, resection and reconstruction of the hepatic veins and inferior vena cava through various techniques of vascular isolation (ex vivo resection and in vitro perfusion) are possible. However, these techniques have steep learning curves and high morbidity (16). We do not routinely employ these techniques given the morbidity and would consider patients in these situations for combinatorial therapy with resection and radiation. Moreover, hepatic veins can be preserved despite tumor involvement depending on the response of metastases to neoadjuvant chemotherapy (17).

BIOLOGIC CONSIDERATIONS

Biologic resectability criteria mandate that the metastases either fit a "low-risk" category (5), most typically based on the timing of presentation (metachronous) and the number of lesions (3 or fewer), serum carcinoembryonic antigen (CEA) level, or demonstrable response to neoadjuvant therapy. In patients undergoing neoadjuvant therapy, we consider progressive disease to preclude resection based on biology, regardless of anatomic considerations. Response to therapy defines the necessary margin of resection and stratifies expected patient outcomes; however, neoadjuvant therapy often causes some degree of liver injury and the total number of cycles must be limited prior to attempted resection. Previous studies have defined less than nine cycles as a threshold for the number of preoperative cycles (18); however, in practice, we routinely simply "test" the biologic sensitivity of the disease to first-line therapy with four cycles prior to resection. For patients requiring an attempt at downsizing of lesions to optimize FLR and/or anatomic resectability, extended cycles and/or triplet therapy may be needed and subsequent risk of liver injury and postoperative liver insufficiency may be increased. A further consideration is that anti-VEGF therapy requires cessation for a minimum of 4 weeks but more typically, 6 weeks prior to any operative attempt secondary to increased bleeding risk. Finally, an emerging factor regarding biology includes molecular characterization. Currently, tumor mutational status is used as a surrogate factor to define biologic resectability. These markers clearly affect type and response to neoadjuvant therapy, and response to such therapy affects the decision for resection by the multidisciplinary team (19–23).

CONDITIONAL CONSIDERATIONS

Underlying patient comorbidity may preclude liver resection. We consider patients with an Eastern Cooperative Oncology Group (ECOG) performance status of 1 or better to be suitable for liver resection. Patients with extensive comorbidity that cannot be corrected are considered for less invasive liver-directed therapy or palliative nonsurgical approaches.

Synchronous Disease

For patients with synchronous liver metastases that meet our ABC resectability criteria, we routinely employ concurrent resection of the primary colorectal cancer and liver metastases. The advantage of this approach is a single surgical recovery and theoretically a faster return to systemic therapy. We and others have demonstrated acceptable morbidity combining liver and colon resection, including with major hepatectomy. The combination of major hepatectomy with rectal resection carries a higher risk and, although feasible, must be approached with more caution (24). It is possible to combine colon resection with the first stage of two-stage liver approaches in order to expedite completion of surgical therapy and return to systemic therapy; however, any bowel related complication may delay the second-stage liver resection. Due to these concerns, in those patients with extensive liver disease requiring a two-stage approach, and/or extended resections in patients with rectal cancer, a liver-first approach is considered.

Clinical Vignette 9.1

A 48-year-old, otherwise healthy male, ECOG 0, has synchronous, liver-only metastasis from a sigmoid cancer. There are multiple, bilobar lesions with sparing of segment 2/3 and the caudate. He initiates systemic therapy and following four cycles has had an objective response with shrinkage of the lesions and no new metastases on interval MRI. Liver volumetry demonstrates an anticipated future liver remnant (FLR) of 19%. What maneuvers are available to increase FLR prior to resection? What entails an optimal response to PVE? What approaches are available for the primary tumor?

The most common approach in this scenario would be PVE of the right portal vein and segment four branches, followed by repeat imaging with volume calculations in 4 to 6 weeks. Optimal response would include an increase in FLR by at least 7.5%, a kinetic growth rate of greater than 2%, and, ideally, an FLR of 30% or greater given his previous chemotherapy. ALPPS would be another option, less routinely employed. Assuming optimal liver hypertrophy, the primary tumor could be resected at the time of liver resection in a combined approach. However, given the extended nature of the resection (right trisectionectomy), it would be reasonable to pursue a liver-first approach with colon resection following 6 to 8 weeks, if recovery is uncomplicated.

REFERENCES

1. Berger-Kulemann V, Schima W, Baroud S, et al. Gadoxetic acid-enhanced 3.0 T MR imaging versus multidetector-row CT in the detection of colorectal metastases in fatty liver using intraoperative ultrasound and histopathology as a standard of reference. *Eur J Surg Oncol.* 2012;38:670–676. doi:10.1016/j.ejso.2012.05.004

2. Floriani I, Torri V, Rulli E, et al. Performance of imaging modalities in diagnosis of liver metastases from colorectal cancer: a systematic review and meta-analysis. *J Magn Reson Imaging.* 2010;31:19–31. doi:10.1002/jmri.22010

3. Kulemann V, Schima W, Tamandl D, et al. Preoperative detection of colorectal liver metastases in fatty liver: MDCT or MRI? *Eur J Radiol.* 2011;79:e1–e6. doi:10.1016/j.ejrad.2010.03.004

4. Moulton CA, Gu CS, Law CH, et al. Effect of PET before liver resection on surgical management for colorectal adenocarcinoma metastases: a randomized clinical trial. *JAMA.* 2014;311: 1863–1869. doi:10.1001/jama.2014.3740

5. Fong Y, Fortner J, Sun RL, et al. Clinical score for predicting recurrence after hepatic resection for metastatic colorectal cancer: analysis of 1001 consecutive cases. *Ann Surg.* 1999;230: 309–318; discussion 318–321. doi:10.1097/00000658-199909000-00004

6. Andreou A, Aloia TA, Brouquet A, et al. Margin status remains an important determinant of survival after surgical resection of colorectal liver metastases in the era of modern chemotherapy. *Ann Surg.* 2013;257:1079–1088. doi:10.1097/SLA.0b013e318283a4d1

7. de Haas RJ, Wicherts DA, Flores E, et al. R1 resection by necessity for colorectal liver metastases: is it still a contraindication to surgery? *Ann Surg.* 2008;248:626–637. doi:10.1097/SLA.0b013e31818a07f1

8. Hamady ZZ, Cameron IC, Wyatt J, et al. Resection margin in patients undergoing hepatectomy for colorectal liver metastasis: a critical appraisal of the 1 cm rule. *Eur J Surg Oncol.* 2006;32:557–563. doi:10.1016/j.ejso.2006.02.001

9. Memeo R, French Colorectal Liver Metastases Working Group, Association Française de Chirurgie (AFC), et al. Margin status is still an important prognostic factor in hepatectomies for colorectal liver metastases: a propensity score matching analysis. *World J Surg.* 2018;42: 892–901. doi:10.1007/s00268-017-4229-7

10. Huang SY, Aloia TA, Shindoh J, et al. Efficacy and safety of portal vein embolization for two-stage hepatectomy in patients with colorectal liver metastasis. *J Vasc Interv Radiol.* 2014;25:608–617. doi:10.1016/j.jvir.2013.10.028

11. Omichi K, Yamashita S, Cloyd JM, et al. Portal vein embolization reduces postoperative hepatic insufficiency associated with postchemotherapy hepatic atrophy. *J Gastrointest Surg.* 2018;22:60–67. doi:10.1007/s11605-017-3467-1

12. Passot G, Chun YS, Kopetz SE, et al. Predictors of safety and efficacy of 2-stage hepatectomy for bilateral colorectal liver metastases. *J Am Coll Surg.* 2016;223:99–108. doi:10.1016/j.jamcollsurg.2015.12.057

13. Shindoh J, Tzeng C-WD, Aloia TA, et al. Portal vein embolization improves rate of resection of extensive colorectal liver metastases without worsening survival. *Br J Surg.* 2013;100:1777–1783. doi:10.1002/bjs.9317

14. Shindoh J, Truty MJ, Aloia TA, et al. Kinetic growth rate after portal vein embolization predicts posthepatectomy outcomes: toward zero liver-related mortality in patients with colorectal liver metastases and small future liver remnant. *J Am Coll Surg.* 2013;216:201–209. doi:10.1016/j.jamcollsurg.2012.10.018

15. Moris D, Ronnekleiv-Kelly S, Kostakis ID, et al. Operative results and oncologic outcomes of associating liver partition and portal vein ligation for staged hepatectomy (ALPPS) versus two-stage hepatectomy (TSH) in patients with unresectable colorectal liver metastases: a systematic review and meta-analysis. *World J Surg.* 2018;42:806–815. doi:10.1007/s00268-017-4181-6

16. Hemming AW, Reed AI, Langham MR, et al. Hepatic vein reconstruction for resection of hepatic tumors. *Ann Surg.* 2002;235:850–858. doi:10.1097/00000658-200206000-00013

17. Torzilli G, Procopio F, Viganò L, et al. Hepatic vein management in a parenchyma-sparing policy for resecting colorectal liver metastases at the caval confluence. *Surgery.* 2018;163:277–284. doi:10.1016/j.surg.2017.09.003

18. Kishi Y, Zorzi D, Contreras CM, et al. Extended preoperative chemotherapy does not improve pathologic response and increases postoperative liver insufficiency after hepatic resection for colorectal liver metastases. *Ann Surg Oncol.* 2010;17:2870–2876. doi:10.1245/s10434-010-1166-1

19. Barbon C, Margonis GA, Andreatos N, et al. Colorectal liver metastases: does the future of precision medicine lie in genetic testing? *J Gastrointest Surg.* 2018. doi:10.1007/s11605-018-3766-1

20. Brudvik KW, Kopetz SE, Li L, et al. Meta-analysis of KRAS mutations and survival after resection of colorectal liver metastases. *Br J Surg.* 2015;102:1175–1183. doi:10.1002/bjs.9870

21. Brudvik KW, Vauthey JN. Surgery: KRAS mutations and hepatic recurrence after treatment of colorectal liver metastases. *Nat Rev Gastroenterol Hepatol.* 2017;14:638–639. doi:10.1038/nrgastro.2017.129

22. Johnson B, Jin Z, Truty MJ, et al. Impact of metastasectomy in the multimodality approach for BRAF V600E metastatic colorectal cancer: the Mayo Clinic experience. *Oncologist.* 2018;23: 128–134. doi:10.1634/theoncologist.2017-0230

23. Margonis GA, Buettner S, Andreatos N, et al. Prognostic factors change over time after hepatectomy for colorectal liver metastases: a multi-institutional, International analysis of 1099 patients. *Ann Surg*. 2019;269(6):1129–1137. doi:10.1097/SLA.0000000000002664
24. Shubert CR, Habermann EB, Bergquist JR, et al. A NSQIP review of major morbidity and mortality of synchronous liver resection for colorectal metastasis stratified by extent of liver resection and type of colorectal resection. *J Gastrointest Surg*. 2015;19:1982–1994. doi:10.1007/s11605-015-2895-z

How I Treat Oligometastatic Colorectal Cancer With Neoadjuvant Chemotherapy

Marwan Fakih

INTRODUCTION

When considering neoadjuvant treatment in the management of oligometastatic colorectal cancer, one must define the goal of neoadjuvant therapy. In general, the role of neoadjuvant therapy for metastatic oligometastatic disease boils down to two main objectives: (a) ensuring that subsequent planned surgical intervention becomes feasible and is associated with an R0 surgical resection and (b) decreasing the risk of disease recurrence following subsequent curative-intent surgical intervention. Numerous neoadjuvant clinical trials have been conducted in patients with oligometastatic colorectal cancer to the liver, which are reviewed in this chapter. Unfortunately, no randomized or large prospective studies have been conducted in patients with oligometastatic extrahepatic colorectal cancers to support firm recommendations in such settings.

NEOADJUVANT CHEMOTHERAPY FOR OLIGOMETASTATIC RESECTABLE LIVER METASTASES

FOLFOX Chemotherapy

The European Organisation for Research and Treatment of Cancer (EORTC) 40983 study randomized patients with 4 or less resettable hepatic colorectal metastases to perioperative folinic acid, fluorouracil, and oxaliplatin (FOLFOX) chemotherapy or observation (1). Patients randomized to perioperative FOLFOX chemotherapy received six cycles (3 months) of chemotherapy, followed by hepatic resection, and then an additional six cycles of chemotherapy. The progression-free survival (PFS) in the overall population trended in favor of the chemotherapy arm: 3-year PFS 35.4% versus 28.1% (hazard ratio [HR] 0·79 [0·62–1·02]; $p = .058$). This reached statistical significance in the treatment eligible population (36.2% vs. 28.1%; HR = 0.77, $p = .041$) (1). Treatment translated in a statistically insignificant trend in improvement in overall survival (OS) on the FOLFOX arm (5-year OS = 51.2%) versus observation (5-year OS = 47.8%) (2). While this study confirms a modest clinical advantage for perioperative FOLFOX chemotherapy in resectable hepatic colorectal metastases, it does not provide any guidance to the additional benefits of FOLFOX in comparison to 5-fluorouracil/leucovorin (5-FU/LV) nor does it confirm a definitive benefit for a neoadjuvant strategy versus an adjuvant strategy. Despite the lack of comparative studies for neoadjuvant versus adjuvant FOLFOX in resectable metastatic disease, several advantages can be cited in favor of the neoadjuvant approach: (a) no randomized studies have been conducted to support posthepatectomy FOLFOX adjuvant therapy; (b) neoadjuvant strategies have the advantage of immediately addressing micrometastatic disease; (c) neoadjuvant approaches provide an in vivo assessment of chemotherapy activity, which can guide further postoperative chemotherapy choice; (d) neoadjuvant therapy ensures the administration of adjuvant treatments, which otherwise may not be possible in patients with significant postsurgical morbidities.

Of note, the EORTC 40983 study excluded patients who received prior oxaliplatin-based adjuvant therapy (prior to the occurrence of hepatic metastatic disease). Therefore, a perioperative FOLFOX strategy cannot be recommended in patients who have previously received FOLFOX or CAPOX (capecitabine plus oxaliplatin) chemotherapy for stage II or stage III colorectal cancers.

A Clinical Vignette ("How I Treat") is included at the end of the chapter.

FOLFIRI Chemotherapy

Several studies investigated folinic acid, fluorouracil, and irinotecan (FOLFIRI) chemotherapy in patients with metastatic colorectal cancer with resectable or resectable/potentially resectable metastatic colorectal cancer. These studies confirm a high response rate (>50%) with FOLFIRI as well as the feasibility and safety of this approach in a neoadjuvant setting (3,4). No randomized studies have been conducted to support the use of neoadjuvant FOLFIRI over FOLFOX in oxaliplatin-naïve colorectal cancers. In addition, a randomized phase III clinical trial of FOLFIRI versus 5-FU/LV failed to show any disease-free survival (DFS) or OS benefit from the addition of irinotecan to 5-FU in the adjuvant treatment of resected colorectal cancer metastases (5). These findings are in line with other adjuvant clinical trials in stage III disease where irinotecan did not improve the disease outcome in comparison to 5-FU/LV (6–8). These data question the effectiveness of irinotecan in reducing disease recurrence in metastasectomy settings. Given such, we favor FOLFOX over FOLFIRI as a neoadjuvant strategy in oxaliplatin-naïve patients with resectable hepatic metastatic disease (Figure 10.1). In patients with limited hepatic resectable metastatic disease who received prior adjuvant oxaliplatin-based therapy, we favor proceeding with upfront surgical intervention. In patients with high-risk, resectable, multifocal metastatic disease who received prior adjuvant oxaliplatin-based therapy, we do consider neoadjuvant FOLFIRI chemotherapy to achieve disease control and to allow for adequate patient selection prior to surgical intervention (Figure 10.1).

Biological Therapy in the Neoadjuvant Setting

Bevacizumab addition to neoadjuvant CAPOX, FOLFOX, FOLFIRI, and FOLFOXIRI (folinic acid, fluorouracil, oxaliplatin, and irinotecan) has been shown to be feasible in patients with resectable liver metastatic colorectal cancer (9–11). Retrospective analyses suggest an increased likelihood of complete pathological responses of liver metastases and a lower incidence of sinusoidal damage with the integration of bevacizumab in the preoperative chemotherapy treatment of metastatic colorectal cancer to the liver (12–15). However, there is no strong evidence to date to support an improvement in DFS or OS with the addition of bevacizumab to preoperative chemotherapy in these settings. Given the discouraging DFS and OS data with bevacizumab in stage III colorectal clinical trials, there is no strong rationale to incorporate bevacizumab in the neoadjuvant or postoperative therapy in patients with resectable metastatic colorectal cancer (16,17). Indeed, a retrospective analysis of patients undergoing hepatectomy with adjuvant chemotherapy with or without bevacizumab failed to show any additional benefit in the bevacizumab arm (18).

The role of cetuximab as part of a neoadjuvant chemotherapy regimen in resectable metastatic colorectal cancer to the liver was investigated through the New EPOC trial (19). In this randomized phase III clinical trial, patients with resectable or suboptimally resectable *KRAS* wild-type metastatic colorectal cancer to the liver were randomized to perioperative chemotherapy with or without cetuximab. The PFS was significantly shorter in the chemotherapy plus cetuximab versus the chemotherapy arm (14.1 vs. 20.5 months; HR = 1.48 with a 95% CI: 1.04–2.12). Chemotherapy consisted predominantly of oxaliplatin-based therapy (FOLFOX or CAPOX), while 11% of the patient population received FOLFIRI. Given the small number of patients on the irinotecan arm, no definitive conclusions can be extrapolated for this subgroup (19). An updated analysis that excluded *BRAF, NRAS,* and *KRAS* mutations continued to favor

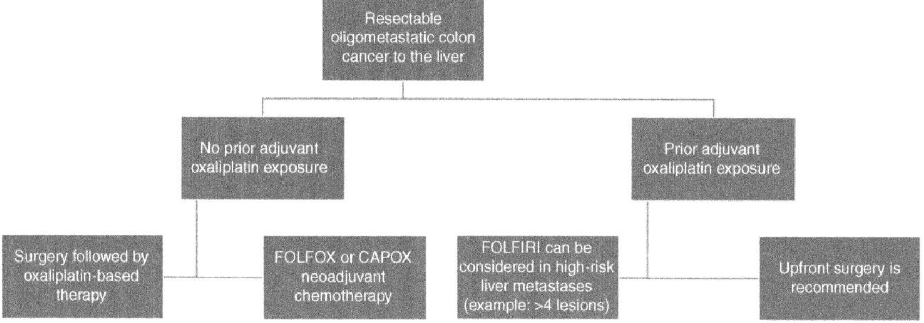

FIGURE 10.1 Neoadjuvant strategy for resectable colorectal liver metastases.

the non-cetuximab arm over the cetuximab arm (20). This study was criticized for lack of adequate surgical quality control, imbalance in patient characteristics, variations in chemotherapy backbones, and increased rate of early death without clear attribution (21).

The detrimental impact of cetuximab on the New EPOC trial and the lack of benefit from adjuvant cetuximab treatment in stage III disease suggest that the addition of cetuximab to chemotherapy in *RAS* wild-type colon cancer does not improve the rate of microscopic disease eradication and hence does not decrease the risk of disease relapse (19,22,23). This strategy should be avoided in patients with resectable liver metastases.

NEOADJUVANT THERAPY FOR OLIGOMETASTATIC POTENTIALLY RESECTABLE LIVER METASTASES

Downstaging for resection in the setting of metastatic disease that is deemed unresectable at the time of presentation but potentially resectable following a major clinical response should be considered a standard approach. Patients who are converted to resectable disease with chemotherapy achieve a 5-year OS of 30% to 50%, far exceeding any 5-year survival reported with palliative chemotherapy (24,25). It is therefore imperative that the most effective combination chemotherapy is considered in patients with advanced, potentially resectable, metastatic colorectal cancer (26).

FOLFOXIRI Plus Bevacizumab

Since no randomized studies have evaluated the combination cytotoxic chemotherapy versus cytotoxic chemotherapy plus bevacizumab in such settings, one cannot conclusively determine the role of angiogenesis inhibition in downstaging for resection. However, since many of the potentially resectable patients do not achieve a resectable status and given the positive impact of bevacizumab on PFS and OS, the routine implementation of bevacizumab in this setting is considered an acceptable practice, particularly when anti-EGFR (epidermal growth factor receptor) therapy is not considered or advisable. Additional support for the addition of bevacizumab in this setting includes retrospective analyses suggesting increased complete pathological responses and decreased sinusoidal liver damage with the addition of bevacizumab to chemotherapy (12–15).

When considering bevacizumab in the management of potentially resectable metastatic colorectal cancer, it is important to consider the most effective chemotherapy backbones (26). To that end, the OLIVIA clinical trial randomized patients with initially unresectable colorectal liver metastases to FOLFOX plus bevacizumab or FOLFOXIRI plus bevacizumab (11). The FOLFOXIRI bevacizumab was associated with an improved response rate, a higher resection rate, higher R0 resection rate and improved PFS (Table 10.1). The contribution of bevacizumab to downstaging when added to FOLFOXIRI is unknown given the lack of a FOLFOXIRI control arm. In addition, bevacizumab has not been associated with improvements in response rate when combined to oxaliplatin-based combinations in prior phase III first-line metastatic colorectal cancer studies (27,28).

Anti-EGFR and Chemotherapy Combinations

While the addition of cetuximab to chemotherapy in the setting of resectable hepatic metastatic disease has resulted in disappointing results, the value of cetuximab in unresectable/potentially resectable hepatic metastases has been demonstrated in several studies. A phase III clinical trial randomized patients with *KRAS*-WT tumors with unresectable hepatic metastatic colorectal cancer to receive first-line FOLFOX or FOLFOX plus cetuximab (29). Patients on the cetuximab arm achieved a higher response rate, R0 hepatic resection rates, and OS (Table 10.1). Additional support to this strategy comes from several other phase II clinical trials describing a high response rate and resection rates with cetuximab and panitumumab-based combinations (30–33) (Table 10.1). In addition, a recent update from CALGB 80405 reported that 15.7% of 1137 *KRAS*-WT patients underwent resection following 1:1 randomization to chemotherapy with bevacizumab or chemotherapy plus cetuximab (34). A higher percentage of patients underwent resection on the cetuximab arm in comparison to bevacizumab (62% vs. 38% of the resected patients). No OS difference in outcome was noted between arms following resection, suggesting that preoperative cetuximab does not worsen postoperative outlook when compared with a bevacizumab backbone. Additional evidence as to the role of anti-EGFR downstaging on resection was demonstrated on the VOLFI trial (35). In this study,

TABLE 10.1 Key Published Prospective Neoadjuvant Clinical Trials in Unresectable but Potentially Resectable Metastatic Colorectal Cancer to the Liver

	Study Design	Treatment Arms	RR	R0 Resection Rate	PFS and/or OS
Gruenberger (11) N = 80	Randomized phase II clinical trial	FOLFOX + bevacizumab vs. FOLFOXIRI bevacizumab	82% vs. 62% in favor of FOLFOXIRI bevacizumab	49% vs. 23% in favor of FOLFOXIRI bevacizumab	PFS = 18.6 vs. 11.9 m in favor of FOLFOXIRI bevacizumab
Ye (29) N = 138	Randomized phase II clinical trial (*KRAS* wild-type CRC)	FOLFOX vs. FOLFOX + cetuximab	57% vs. 29% in favor of cetuximab arm	26% vs. 7% in favor of cetuximab arm	OS = 30.9 vs. 21 m in favor of cetuximab arm
Folprecht (30,31) N = 111 (*KRAS* wild-type = 70)	Randomized phase II	FOLFOX cetuximab vs. FOLFIRI cetuximab	RR = 70% in *KRAS* wild-type patients	36% in overall population	5-year OS for R0 resection = 46.2%
Carrato (32) N = 77	Randomized phase II (*KRAS* wild-type CRC)	FOLFOX panitumumab vs. FOLFIRI panitumumab	RR = 74% on FOLFOX arm and 67% on FOLFIRI arm	R0/1 34% on FOLFOX arm and 46% in FOLFIRI arm	Median OS for resected patients = 52 m

FOLFIRI, folinic acid, fluorouracil, and irinotecan; FOLFOX, folinic acid, fluorouracil, and oxaliplatin; FOLFOXIRI, folinic acid, fluorouracil, oxaliplatin, and irinotecan; OS, overall survival; PFS, progression-free survival; RR, response rate.

96 patients with potentially resectable and unresectable *RAS* wild-type colorectal cancer were randomized to receive FOLFOXIRI plus panitumumab versus FOLFOXIRI (2:1 randomization). Panitumumab led to higher response rates, which translated in a higher R0 resection rate in the potentially resectable population (50% vs. 27%). However, the addition of anti-EGFR therapy to FOLFOXIRI led to higher grade 3 to 4 toxicity rates, particularly gastrointestinal. There are no mature data yet on the DFS and OS on these two arms to support the routine integration of anti-EGFR with a FOLFOXIRI backbone in potentially resectable metastatic colorectal cancers.

Sidedness, RAS/BRAF Status, and Treatment Selection

Both bevacizumab and cetuximab are justified in the setting of unresectable, potentially resectable metastatic colorectal cancer. Since most of these patients do not attain resectable disease, the integration of biological therapy in the first-line setting is recommended in view of its positive impact on PFS and OS. In the setting of *RAS*-MT or *BRAF*-MT tumors, one should favor the use of FOLFOXIRI plus bevacizumab in younger, good performance status, cases (36,37). Anti-EGFR agents combined with FOLFOX or FOLFIRI in *RAS/BRAF* wild-type left colon cancer have comparable response rates to FOLFOXIRI and can be considered as a standard option in this patient population. For right-sided *RAS* wild-type cancer, and in view of the lack of anti-EGFR benefits in frontline settings on the FIRE-3 and CALGB 80405 studies, FOLFOXIRI plus bevacizumab should be considered as the combination of choice (38,39). In lesser fit patients and elderly patients, FOLFOXIRI (with or without bevacizumab) is often contraindicated due to potential toxicities; in such instances, one should resort to doublet cytotoxics with the biologic of choice being guided by *RAS/BRAF* status and sidedness (Table 10.2).

SPECIAL CONSIDERATIONS: EXTRAHEPATIC OLIGOMETASTATIC DISEASE

Lung Metastases

There is a paucity of prospective data on the value of neoadjuvant systemic chemotherapy in patients with curative-intent lung metastasectomy. Retrospective series suggest that the

TABLE 10.2 Neoadjuvant Strategy for Potentially Resectable Colorectal Liver Metastases

	Left Colon Cancer			Right Colon Cancer		
	RAS/BRAF wild-type	**RAS mutant**	**BRAF mutant**	**RAS/BRAF wild-type**	**RAS mutant**	**BRAF mutant**
Good performance status and younger	FOLFOXIRI (+/− bevacizumab) FOLFOX + anti-EGFR FOLFIRI + anti-EGFR	FOLFOXIRI (+/− bevacizumab)	FOLFOXIRI (+/− bevacizumab)	FOLFOXIRI (+/− bevacizumab)	FOLFOXIRI (+/− bevacizumab)	FOLFOXIRI (+/− bevacizumab)
Limited performance status and older	FOLFOX + anti-EGFR FOLFIRI + anti-EGFR	FOLFOX (+/− bevacizumab) FOLFIRI (+/− bevacizumab)	FOLFOX (+/− bevacizumab) FOLFIRI (+/− bevacizumab)	FOLFOX (+/− bevacizumab) FOLFIRI (+/− bevacizumab)	FOLFOX (+/− bevacizumab) FOLFIRI (+/− bevacizumab)	FOLFOX (+/− bevacizumab) FOLFIRI (+/− bevacizumab)

FOLFIRI, folinic acid, fluorouracil, and irinotecan; FOLFOX, folinic acid, fluorouracil, and oxaliplatin; FOLFOXIRI, folinic acid, fluorouracil, oxaliplatin, and irinotecan; EGFR, epidermal growth factor receptor.

outcome of patients with resection of pulmonary metastases has a favorable OS with median survival exceeding 5 years (40). Several small retrospective studies and a large meta analysis did not support a benefit from adjuvant chemotherapy post pulmonary colorectal metastases resection (40–43). Other studies reported an improvement in DFS but no improvement in associated OS (44). Given the limited data in support of adjuvant therapy in resected pulmonary metastases, the administration of neoadjuvant therapy in resectable lung-only disease cannot be routinely recommended.

Synchronous metastatic disease to the liver and lung can also benefit from curative-intent surgical intervention. When completely resected, these patients have 5-year survival rates that neighbor those achieved with liver-only or lung-only resected metastatic disease (45). In general, we approach these patients in a similar fashion and with the same algorithm that we have defined earlier for patients with metastatic liver disease.

Ovarian Metastases and Peritoneal Metastases

Ovarian colorectal metastases are considered relatively chemoresistant and often exhibit lower response rates from chemotherapy than extraovarian metastases (46). Given the relative chemoresistance of ovarian metastases, we advocate upfront resection without any neoadjuvant therapy. Similarly, lower responses are noted in peritoneal metastases (47). Patients with oligometastatic peritoneal carcinomatosis with a favorable peritoneal carcinomatosis index should therefore undergo upfront surgery without consideration for neoadjuvant therapy.

Clinical Vignette 10.1

A 60-year-old female was diagnosed on her second screening colonoscopy to have a sigmoid colon adenocarcinoma. Imaging studies did not show any evidence of metastatic disease. She underwent a low anterior resection. Her pathological staging was T3N2aM0. She received 6 months of adjuvant chemotherapy with FOLFOX and enrolled in a surveillance program. One year after completion of adjuvant therapy, imaging studies confirmed five hepatic lesions in the right lobe of the liver, and a single lesion in the left lobe, abutting the inferior vena cava. The patient was evaluated by the hepatobiliary service and was deemed unresectable. Downstaging for possible resection with or without ablation was recommended. The patient's performance status is an Eastern Cooperative Oncology Group (ECOG) score of 0. The tumor was RAS-WT, BRAF-WT, HER-2 negative, microsatellite stable (MSS). What chemotherapy combination do you recommend?

Answer: In this case, maximum downstaging would be recommended. The patient is technically unresectable and therefore should be treated similarly to metastatic unresectable colorectal cancer while shooting for maximum response rate. Since she has progressed 1 year after completion of adjuvant FOLFOX, there would be some concern regarding the use of oxaliplatin-based regimens, including the OLIVIA FOLFOXIRI bevacizumab regimen. The regimen of choice here would be FOLFIRI + cetuximab or FOLFIRI + panitumumab, both of which have been associated with response rates of approximately 70% in first-line treatment of metastatic disease. While recent data suggest that FOLFOXIRI + panitumumab may provide better downstaging over FOLFOXIRI (VOLFI trial), there are no data comparing FOLFOXIRI + anti-EGFR to a doublet chemotherapy + anti-EGFR. In addition, FOLFOXIRI plus anti-EGFR therapy is considered a toxic regimen with a high rate of gastrointestinal adverse events. There may be some concerns regarding a potential increased risk of relapse with neoadjuvant anti-EGFR based therapy based on the New EPOC trial. However, New EPOC was performed in the setting of resectable metastatic disease and was not designed to investigate the benefit of anti-EGFR therapy in left-sided RAS-WT cancers. Given the advantage of anti-EGFR therapy + chemotherapy over bevacizumab + chemotherapy in tumor downstaging (RAS-WT, left colon), FOLFIRI + anti-EGFR will be favored over FOLFIRI + bevacizumab.

REFERENCES

1. Nordlinger B, Sorbye H, Glimelius B, et al. Perioperative chemotherapy with FOLFOX4 and surgery versus surgery alone for resectable liver metastases from colorectal cancer (EORTC Intergroup trial 40983): a randomised controlled trial. *Lancet*. 2008;371:1007–1016. doi:10.1016/S0140-6736(08)60455-9
2. Nordlinger B, Sorbye H, Glimelius B, et al. Perioperative FOLFOX4 chemotherapy and surgery versus surgery alone for resectable liver metastases from colorectal cancer (EORTC 40983): long-term results of a randomised, controlled, phase 3 trial. *Lancet Oncol*. 2013;14:1208–1215. doi:10.1016/S1470-2045(13)70447-9
3. Ychou M, Rivoire M, Thezenas S, et al. A randomized phase II trial of three intensified chemotherapy regimens in first-line treatment of colorectal cancer patients with initially unresectable or not optimally resectable liver metastases. The METHEP trial. *Ann Surg Oncol*. 2013;20:4289–4297. doi:10.1245/s10434-013-3217-x
4. Kim JY, Kim JS, Baek MJ, et al. Prospective multicenter phase II clinical trial of FOLFIRI chemotherapy as a neoadjuvant treatment for colorectal cancer with multiple liver metastases. *J Korean Surg Soc*. 2013;85:154–160. doi:10.4174/jkss.2013.85.4.154
5. Ychou M, Hohenberger W, Thezenas S, et al. A randomized phase III study comparing adjuvant 5-fluorouracil/folinic acid with FOLFIRI in patients following complete resection of liver metastases from colorectal cancer. *Ann Oncol*. 2009;20:1964–1970. doi:10.1093/annonc/mdp236
6. Saltz LB, Niedzwiecki D, Hollis D, et al. Irinotecan fluorouracil plus leucovorin is not superior to fluorouracil plus leucovorin alone as adjuvant treatment for stage III colon cancer: Results of CALGB 89803. *J Clin Oncol*. 2007;25:3456–3461. doi:10.1200/JCO.2007.11.2144
7. Van Cutsem E, Labianca R, Bodoky G, et al. Randomized phase III trial comparing biweekly infusional fluorouracil/leucovorin alone or with irinotecan in the adjuvant treatment of stage III colon cancer: PETACC-3. *J Clin Oncol*. 2009;27:3117–3125. doi:10.1200/JCO.2008.21.6663
8. Ychou M, Raoul JL, Douillard JY, et al. A phase III randomised trial of LV5FU2 + irinotecan versus LV5FU2 alone in adjuvant high-risk colon cancer (FNCLCC Accord02/FFCD9802). *Ann Oncol*. 2009;20:674–680. doi:10.1093/annonc/mdn680
9. Nasti G, Piccirillo MC, Izzo F, et al. Neoadjuvant FOLFIRI+bevacizumab in patients with resectable liver metastases from colorectal cancer: a phase 2 trial. *Br J Cancer*. 2013;108:1566–1570. doi:10.1038/bjc.2013.140
10. Gruenberger B, Tamandl D, Schueller J, et al. Bevacizumab, capecitabine, and oxaliplatin as neoadjuvant therapy for patients with potentially curable metastatic colorectal cancer. *J Clin Oncol*. 2008;26:1830–1835. doi:10.1200/JCO.2007.13.7679
11. Gruenberger T, Bridgewater J, Chau I, et al. Bevacizumab plus mFOLFOX-6 or FOLFOXIRI in patients with initially unresectable liver metastases from colorectal cancer: the OLIVIA multinational randomized phase II trial. *Ann Oncol*. 2014;26(4): 702-708. doi:10.1093/annonc/mdu580

12. Ribero D, Wang H, Donadon M, et al. Bevacizumab improves pathologic response and protects against hepatic injury in patients treated with oxaliplatin-based chemotherapy for colorectal liver metastases. *Cancer*. 2007;110:2761–2767. doi:10.1002/cncr.23099
13. Gruenberger T, Arnold D, Rubbia-Brandt L. Pathologic response to bevacizumab-containing chemotherapy in patients with colorectal liver metastases and its correlation with survival. *Surg Oncol*. 2012;21:309–315. doi:10.1016/j.suronc.2012.07.003
14. Klinger M, Eipeldauer S, Hacker S, et al. Bevacizumab protects against sinusoidal obstruction syndrome and does not increase response rate in neoadjuvant XELOX/FOLFOX therapy of colorectal cancer liver metastases. *Eur J Surg Oncol*. 2009;35:515–520. doi:10.1016/j.ejso.2008.12.013
15. Overman MJ, Ferrarotto R, Raghav K, et al. The addition of bevacizumab to oxaliplatin-based chemotherapy: impact upon hepatic sinusoidal injury and thrombocytopenia. *J Natl Cancer Inst*. 2018;110(8):888–894. doi:10.1093/jnci/djx288
16. Allegra CJ, Yothers G, O'Connell MJ, et al. Phase III trial assessing bevacizumab in stages II and III carcinoma of the colon: results of NSABP protocol C-08. *J Clin Oncol*. 2011;29:11–16. doi:10.1200/JCO.2010.30.0855
17. de Gramont A, Van Cutsem E, Schmoll HJ, et al. Bevacizumab plus oxaliplatin-based chemotherapy as adjuvant treatment for colon cancer (AVANT): a phase 3 randomised controlled trial. *Lancet Oncol*. 2012;13:1225–1233. doi:10.1016/S1470-2045(12)70509-0
18. Turan N, Benekli M, Koca D, et al. Adjuvant systemic chemotherapy with or without bevacizumab in patients with resected liver metastases from colorectal cancer. *Oncology*. 2013;84:14–21. doi:10.1159/000342429
19. Primrose J, Falk S, Finch-Jones M, et al. Systemic chemotherapy with or without cetuximab in patients with resectable colorectal liver metastasis: the New EPOC randomised controlled trial. *Lancet Oncol*. 2014;15:601–611. doi:10.1016/S1470-2045(14)70105-6
20. Bridgewater J, Pugh S, Moutasim K, et al. Analysis of progression-free survival in the new EPOC study in an "all wild-type" population. *J Clin Oncol*. 2014;32(15_suppl):3566. doi:10.1200/jco.2014.32.15_suppl.3566
21. Nordlinger B, Poston GJ, Goldberg RM. Should the results of the new EPOC trial change practice in the management of patients with resectable metastatic colorectal cancer confined to the liver? *J Clin Oncol*. 2015;33:241–243. doi:10.1200/JCO.2014.58.3989
22. Taieb J, Tabernero J, Mini E, et al. Oxaliplatin, fluorouracil, and leucovorin with or without cetuximab in patients with resected stage III colon cancer (PETACC-8): an open-label, randomised phase 3 trial. *Lancet Oncol*. 2014;15:862–873. doi:10.1016/S1470-2045(14)70227-X
23. Alberts SR, Sargent DJ, Nair S, et al. Effect of oxaliplatin, fluorouracil, and leucovorin with or without cetuximab on survival among patients with resected stage III colon cancer: a randomized trial. *JAMA*. 2012;307:1383–1393. doi:10.1001/jama.2012.385
24. Adam R, Avisar E, Ariche A, et al. Five-year survival following hepatic resection after neoadjuvant therapy for nonresectable colorectal. *Ann Surg Oncol*. 2001;8:347–353. doi:10.1007/s10434-001-0347-3
25. Adam R, Delvart V, Pascal G, et al. Rescue surgery for unresectable colorectal liver metastases downstaged by chemotherapy: a model to predict long-term survival. *Ann Surg*. 2004;240:644–657; discussion 657–658.
26. Folprecht G, Grothey A, Alberts S, et al. Neoadjuvant treatment of unresectable colorectal liver metastases: correlation between tumour response and resection rates. *Ann Oncol*. 2005;16:1311–1319. doi:10.1093/annonc/mdi246
27. Saltz LB, Clarke S, Diaz-Rubio E, et al. Bevacizumab in combination with oxaliplatin-based chemotherapy as first-line therapy in metastatic colorectal cancer: a randomized phase III study. *J Clin Oncol*. 2008;26:2013–2019. doi:10.1200/JCO.2007.14.9930
28. Passardi A, Nanni O, Tassinari D, et al. Effectiveness of bevacizumab added to standard chemotherapy in metastatic colorectal cancer: final results for first-line treatment from the ITACa randomized clinical trial. *Ann Oncol*. 2015;26:1201–1207. doi:10.1093/annonc/mdv130
29. Ye LC, Liu TS, Ren L, et al. Randomized controlled trial of cetuximab plus chemotherapy for patients with KRAS wild-type unresectable colorectal liver-limited metastases. *J Clin Oncol*. 2013;31:1931–1938. doi:10.1200/JCO.2012.44.8308
30. Folprecht G, Gruenberger T, Bechstein WO, et al. Tumour response and secondary resectability of colorectal liver metastases following neoadjuvant chemotherapy with cetuximab: the CELIM randomised phase 2 trial. *Lancet Oncol*. 2010;11:38–47. doi:10.1016/S1470-2045(09)70330-4
31. Folprecht G, Gruenberger T, Bechstein W, et al. Survival of patients with initially unresectable colorectal liver metastases treated with FOLFOX/cetuximab or FOLFIRI/cetuximab in a multidisciplinary concept (CELIM study). *Ann Oncol*. 2014;25:1018–1025. doi:10.1093/annonc/mdu088
32. Carrato A, Abad A, Massuti B, et al. First-line panitumumab plus FOLFOX4 or FOLFIRI in colorectal cancer with multiple or unresectable liver metastases: a randomised, phase II trial (PLANET-TTD). *Eur J Cancer*. 2017;81:191–202. doi:10.1016/j.ejca.2017.04.024

33. Garufi C, Torsello A, Tumolo S, et al. Cetuximab plus chronomodulated irinotecan, 5-fluorouracil, leucovorin and oxaliplatin as neoadjuvant chemotherapy in colorectal liver metastases: POCHER trial. *Br J Cancer*. 2010;103:1542–1547. doi:10.1038/sj.bjc.6605940
34. Venook A, Niedzwiecki D, Lenz H, et al. CALGB/SWOG 80405: analysis of patients undergoing surgery as part of treatment strategy. *Ann Oncol*. 2014;25(5):1–41.
35. Geissler M, Martens U, Knorrenschield R, et al. mFOLFOXIRI + Panitumumab versus FOLFOXIRI as first-line treatment in patients with RAS wild-type metastatic colorectal cancer (mCRC): a randomized phase II trial of the AIO (AIO-KRK-0109) *Ann Oncol*. 2017;28(suppl_5):v158–v208.
36. Falcone A, Ricci S, Brunetti I, et al. Phase III trial of infusional fluorouracil, leucovorin, oxaliplatin, and irinotecan (FOLFOXIRI) compared with infusional fluorouracil, leucovorin, and irinotecan (FOLFIRI) as first-line treatment for metastatic colorectal cancer: the Gruppo Oncologico Nord Ovest. *J Clin Oncol*. 2007;25:1670–1676. doi:10.1200/JCO.2006.09.0928
37. Loupakis F, Cremolini C, Masi G, et al. Initial therapy with FOLFOXIRI and bevacizumab for metastatic colorectal cancer. *N Engl J Med*. 2014;371:1609–1618. doi:10.1056/NEJMoa1403108
38. Tejpar S, Stintzing S, Ciardiello F, et al. Prognostic and predictive relevance of primary tumor location in patients with RAS wild-type metastatic colorectal cancer: retrospective analyses of the CRYSTAL and FIRE-3 trials. *JAMA Oncol*. 2016;3(2):194-201. doi:10.1001/jamaoncol.2016.3797
39. Venook AP, Niedzwiecki D, Lenz HJ, et al. Effect of first-line chemotherapy combined with cetuximab or bevacizumab on overall survival in patients with KRAS wild-type advanced or metastatic colorectal cancer: a randomized clinical trial. *JAMA*. 2017;317:2392–2401. doi:10.1001/jama.2017.7105
40. Salah S, Watanabe K, Welter S, et al. Colorectal cancer pulmonary oligometastases: pooled analysis and construction of a clinical lung metastasectomy prognostic model. *Ann Oncol*. 2012;23:2649–2655. doi:10.1093/annonc/mds100
41. Saito Y, Omiya H, Kohno K, et al. Pulmonary metastasectomy for 165 patients with colorectal carcinoma: a prognostic assessment. *J Thorac Cardiovasc Surg*. 2002;124:1007–1013. doi:10.1067/mtc.2002.125165
42. Hawkes EA, Ladas G, Cunningham D, et al. Peri-operative chemotherapy in the management of resectable colorectal cancer pulmonary metastases. *BMC Cancer*. 2012;12:326. doi:10.1186/1471-2407-12-326
43. Onaitis MW, Petersen RP, Haney JC, et al. Prognostic factors for recurrence after pulmonary resection of colorectal cancer metastases. *Ann Thorac Surg*. 2009;87:1684–1688. doi:10.1016/j.athoracsur.2009.03.034
44. Park HS, Jung M, Shin SJ, et al. Benefit of adjuvant chemotherapy after curative resection of lung metastasis in colorectal cancer. *Ann Surg Oncol*. 2016;23:928–935. doi:10.1245/s10434-015-4951-z
45. Neeff H, Horth W, Makowiec F, et al. Outcome after resection of hepatic and pulmonary metastases of colorectal cancer. *J Gastrointest Surg*. 2009;13:1813–1820. doi:10.1007/s11605-009-0960-1
46. Ganesh K, Shah RH, Vakiani E, et al. Clinical and genetic determinants of ovarian metastases from colorectal cancer. *Cancer*. 2017;123:1134–1143. doi:10.1002/cncr.30424
47. Franko J, Shi Q, Goldman CD, et al. Treatment of colorectal peritoneal carcinomatosis with systemic chemotherapy: a pooled analysis of north central cancer treatment group phase III trials N9741 and N9841. *J Clin Oncol*. 2012;30:263–267. doi:10.1200/JCO.2011.37.1039

How I Treat Oligometastatic Colorectal Cancer Through Local Nonsurgical Approaches

Sadeer Alzubaidi, Alex Wallace, and Rahmi Oklu

INTRODUCTION

Colorectal cancer is the third most common cancer diagnosis in the United States (1). It is the third leading cause of cancer deaths (1). Twenty to thirty percent of patients have hepatic metastasis and 60% of patients will have liver metastasis at some point during their disease course (2). The first line of treatment for liver metastasis is surgery; however, only 10% to 25% of patients with metastasis have resectable disease (2). The 5-year survival with resectable disease ranges between 39% and 58% (3) while liver transplant for unresectable disease is near 56% (4). However, 5-year survival in unresectable disease is less than 11% (3). Systemic chemotherapy can help downstage these patients and increase the candidacy for resection; but only 10% to 25% of patients benefit from this approach (5). In the setting of poor response to systemic chemotherapy, patients may receive local-regional therapy performed by an interventional radiologist. Locoregional therapy may include percutaneous or transarterial ablative therapies. Percutaneous techniques include thermal (radiofrequency, microwave, and cryoablation) and nonthermal techniques (irreversible electroporation [IRE]). Transarterial therapies include hepatic arterial infusion (HAI), bland embolization, chemotherapy embolization (transarterial chemoembolization [TACE]), and selective internal radiation therapy (SIRT). Here, we review the role of interventional radiology in the management of colorectal cancer with liver metastasis (CRLM).

INTERVENTIONAL RADIOLOGY'S ROLE IN COLORECTAL CANCER WITH LIVER METASTASIS

Interventional oncology (IO), an emerging field within interventional radiology, is at the forefront of specialties directing the treatment of patients with cancer. IO primarily employs two distinct modalities: ablation and transarterial therapy. Ablation is the direct deposition of energy into a volume of tissue to eradicate tumor cells within that volume. Ablation therapy is often used with the intent to cure (6), similar to surgery and transplantation, but can also be performed for cytoreduction or as a bridge to transplant. Transarterial therapy is the delivery of an agent via the arterial system to the vasculature of the tumor in order to limit the distribution of that agent while minimizing collateral injury. Transarterial therapies can be employed with high precision narrowing the treatment field to a single hepatic segment or used in a broad lobar treatment field. Agents that may be delivered transarterially include particles bound with chemotherapeutic agents, biologic agents, or radiopharmaceuticals, and can be combined with particles meant to occlude vessels of varying sizes. In the setting of CRLM, the burden of the tumor in the liver usually affects the survival and these strategies can reduce that tumor burden with minimal side effects. IO approaches are an effective alternative with the added benefit of its minimally invasive nature with decreased recovery time and significantly improved quality of life especially because the approach often requires a single administration.

A few concepts are crucial to the effective management of CRLM. These include the test of time, the chemotherapy holiday, and progression-free survival (PFS).

A Clinical Vignette ("How I Treat") is included at the end of the chapter.

The test of time concept, as described by Livraghi et al. in 2003, can be used to effectively avoid unnecessary surgery (7). The premise of this concept stems from ablating resectable lesions prior to surgical removal and asks: If a lesion is ablated and observed for a period of time and no residual disease is found, does the lesion still need to be resected? In a study by Livraghi et al., 88 patients with colorectal cancer liver metastases were treated with radiofrequency ablation (RFA) and 53 patients achieved complete necrosis. Of the patients who achieved complete necrosis, 98% (52/53) of these patients did not require surgery, 23/53 (44%) patients remained disease free, and 29/53 (56%) patients manifested with widespread disease. After these findings, ablation therapy correctly can be thought of as similar in fashion to surgical resection.

The chemotherapy holiday concept is applied in settings where induction chemotherapy has failed in the treatment of liver metastasis. IO approaches can be used in this setting to allow the patient to take time off from chemotherapy saving the patient multiple hospital visits for chemotherapy administration, unpleasant drug side effects, and expense. This strategy may improve the patient's quality of life substantially.

PERCUTANEOUS ABLATION

Percutaneous ablation is the focused delivery of energy into tissue in order to cause tissue necrosis. Ablations can be performed with thermal or nonthermal techniques and under a variety of conditions. When ablation is used with curative intent, success can be measured similar to surgical outcomes. As with surgical margins with the goal of an R0 resection (microscopically margin negative), ablations will destroy a margin of tissue to achieve an A0 ablation. Multiple technical factors need to be addressed prior to ablation that will determine patient eligibility. These include:

1. Number of tumors. Less than 4 lesions is usually permissible.
2. Tumor size. Usually less than 3 cm, but less than 5 cm is often acceptable. The most recent approaches for lesions between 3 and 5 cm in size use a combination therapy to achieve better control.
3. Location. Tumor location is important in deciding the number and positions of the probes in order to achieve a safe and effective margin. Tumor location near vital structures may preclude thermal ablation as an option if positioning the patient and temporary organ displacement techniques are not enough to ensure a reasonable level of safety. IRE is a nonthermal based ablation technique that can be used in these situations.

The location of the lesions to be ablated and their features determine the ablation technique to be used. Thermal ablative techniques include RFA, microwave ablation (MWA), and cryoablation. Currently, the only nonthermal ablation technique is IRE, which utilizes electrical potentials to cause cell death. The imaging findings before and after ablation can be seen in Figure 11.1.

ABLATIVE THERAPIES

Radiofrequency Ablation
RFA employs a probe, placed under real-time ultrasound and/or CT guidance, that emits radiofrequency waves within the target mass. This can be done percutaneously in an outpatient setting or intraoperatively. The probe is then used to deliver energy with a frequency less than 900 kHz. This energy agitates ions that heat the local tissue resulting in rapid temperature elevations of 50°C to 100°C. At 60°C, coagulation necrosis occurs. At 100°C, carbonization or charring of the surrounding tissue limits the expanding ablation zone by causing a sharp rise in tissue impedance to heat conduction. The ablation zone can be expanded by using specially designed electrodes with internal cooling by saline, which prevents charring (8). Rapidly flowing fluids such as medium- to large-sized blood vessels can alter the effects of ablations by rapidly drawing heat away from the ablation zone, an effect known as "heat sink." This effect can prevent cellular death if the heat sink is strong enough. While this is often considered a limitation, it can also be used to advantage.

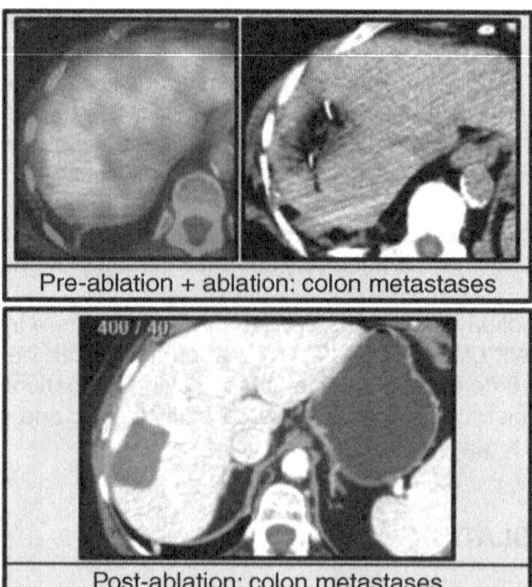

Pre-ablation + ablation: colon metastases

Post-ablation: colon metastases

FIGURE 11.1   Pre-ablation PET CT demonstrates a large right liver lobe lesion. Post-ablation contrast-enhanced CT study demonstrates successful treatment of the tumor without any viable tumor remaining.

The criterion for treatment of liver lesions with RFA is usually defined as five or fewer lesions each 3 cm or less. Contraindications for ablation include:

1. Inability to access the targeted lesion and ablate without injury to vital surrounding tissue even with the use of protective measures such as hydro or balloon dissection
2. Bleeding diathesis that has not been corrected
3. Diffuse metastatic disease

To achieve A0 ablation (complete elimination of tumor at microscopic assessment), at least a 5 mm margin of normal tissue should be included in the ablation zone although a 10 mm margin is preferred in all directions to ensure good results (9,10). After ablating the targeted lesions, the probe is removed while still activated in order to eliminate tumor seeding along the tract.

No definitive guidelines have been released on the use of RFA for treating metastatic colorectal cancer (mCRC). RFA is used to treat oligometastatic lung metastases from mCRC. Ferguson demonstrated in 157 patients with 434 lung lesions a tumor-free survival rate at 12 months, 3 years, and 5 years, of 60.5%, 14.4%, and 7%, respectively (11). Ociai et al. showed that in lung tumor patients, lung RFA provided local tumor control and survival that were similar to those achieved using stereotactic body radiation therapy (SBRT) with equal safety (12). Table 11.1 lists a collection of studies describing outcomes of RFA in the setting of mCRC to the liver.

Adverse effects of RFA may include biliary tract damage, liver failure, refractory pleural effusions, and local recurrence. Retroperitoneal hemorrhage can be a severe complication. Limitations to RFA include the heat sink effect, the inability to distinguish normal tissue from tumor while ablating, injuring heat sensitive normal tissues before causing tumor necrosis, and difficulties eradicating large tumor masses (13).

Microwave Ablation

MWA has developed over the past decade to improve on the limitations of RFA (14), particularly addressing the heat sink effect and charring. This technique uses high-frequency electromagnetic waves from 900 MHz to 2.4 GHz to oscillate water molecules and rapidly creating heat by friction causing tissue destruction by coagulative necrosis. MWA, compared to RFA, produces a larger ablation zone, higher intratumoral temperatures, reduced treatment times, and less pain. The ablation zone is significantly less affected by heat sink of the surrounding tissues (15) and can be used to successfully ablate larger tumors up to 6 cm in diameter (8).

TABLE 11.1 A Summary Collection of the Literature Describing RFA Outcomes in the Setting of Colorectal Metastasis to the Liver

Study	Year	Cohort	Findings
Gillams et al.	2004	167 patients Percutaneous Mean 4 lesions Mean 4 cm max diameter	Median OS 38 mo and 5 y OS 25%
Hildebrand et al.	2006	88 pts/420 lesions Percutaneous Mean 3.5 lesions	3 y OS 42%
Berber et al.	2008	68 pts/68 lesions Laparoscopic All solitary lesions Median 3.7 cm max diameter	5 y OS 30%, median OS 20.5 m
Sofocleous et al.	2011	56 pts/71 lesions Percutaneous Mean 1.4 lesions Median 1.9 cm max diameter	3 y OS 41%, median OS 31 m Procedure related complications 4%
Hamada et al.	2012	84 pts/141 lesions Percutaneous Mean 1.7 lesions Mean 2.3 cm max diameter +/− 1.4 cm	5 y OS 20.8%, median OS 34.9 mo Procedure related complications 2.2%
Kim et al.	2016	Cost analysis	RFA vs. SBRT is not cost-effective compared with RFA for inoperable colorectal liver metastases
Cirocchi et al.	2012	Comparing 60 patients receiving RFA plus CT versus 59 patients receiving CT alone	PFS was significantly higher in the group that received RFA; however, not able to provide information on OS
Lee et al.	2015	51 RFA vs. 102 hepatectomy	RFA is suitable for patients with single, ≤2 cm CRLM
Veltri et al,	2012	262 patients with CRLM treated with RFA	Largest lesion diameter ≤3 cm is the most favorable Prognostic factor for survival in CRLM treated with RFA

CRLM, colorectal cancer with liver metastasis; OS, overall survival; PFS, progression-free survival; SBRT, stereotactic body radiation therapy; RFA, radiofrequency ablation.

Similar to RFA, the microwave probes are placed under ultrasound or CT guidance. High-power MWA (100 W versus 45 W) is less effected by heat sink (16). MWA does not utilize electricity for its thermal effects and is thus renitent to the increased resistance of charring that hinders treatment by RFA (17).

A recent study in 2018 by Vietti Violi et al. (18) compared treatment between MWA and RFA treated HCC lesions. In this study, there was decreased local recurrence in the MWA treatment group although the findings were not significantly different (*p* value of .27). The complications in the study were low but included two grade 4 complications of arterial bleeding that required embolization.

MWA is relatively safe with low complication rates reported by studies such as those listed in Table 11.2. Given the nonelectrical nature of the treatment, grounding pads are not required for safety concerns as with some other types of ablation techniques. MWA has demonstrated safety and efficacy when used on lesions near the heart (19). In this study, lesions (primary and metastatic lesions) with a mean distance from the myocardium of 1.1 cm were treated by

TABLE 11.2 A Summary Collection of the Literature Describing MWA Outcomes in the Setting of Colorectal Metastasis to the Liver

Study	Year	Cohort	Findings	Complications
Liang et al. (20)	2003	74 patients, 149 lesions Laparotomy Mean 2 lesions Mean 0.8 cm max diameter	5 y OS 29%, median OS 20.5 m	4%
Tanaka et al. (21)	2006	16 patients, 35 lesions Laparotomy Mean 2 lesions Mean 0.8 cm max diameter	5 y OS 17%, median OS 28 m	19%
Wang et al. (22)	2014	115 patients with CRLM	Local progression rate = 11.82%; recurrence rates were 27.8%, 48.4%, and 59.3%, and the cumulative survival rates were 98.1%, 87.1%, and 78.7% in years 1, 2, and 3 posttreatment, respectively	
Correa-Gallego et al. (23)	2014	RFA vs. MWA 254 tumors (127 per group) from 134 patients	MWA has lower ablation-site recurrence rates (6% vs. 20%; $p < .01$)	
Song et al. (17)	2017	62 patients with liver mCRC treated with MWA (28) or surgical resection (34)	No statistical difference between MWA and surgical resection at median follow-up of 55 months	No severe complications in the MWA group
Vietti Violi et al. (18)	2018	144 patients with HCC, 71 received MWA, 73 received RFA	6% of lesions with local progression in MWA, 12% in RFA group although there was no statistically significant difference	Two grade 4 bleeding events requiring embolization; three grade 3 events

CRLM, colorectal cancer with liver metastasis; HCC, hepatocellular carcinoma; mCRC, metastatic colorectal cancer; MWA, microwave ablation; OS, overall survival; RFA, radiofrequency ablation.

MWA and compared to safety and efficacy outcomes of peripheral liver tumors. No cardiac arrhythmias occurred during the procedure or afterward in follow-up (19). Additionally, there were similar rates of local progression (19).

MWA complications include pain, ascites, fever, bile duct injury, and pleural effusion. Lesions less than 3 cm and those remote from blood vessels treated with MWA have a lower recurrence rate (23).

Cryoablation

Cryoablation freezes tissue to cause tumor destruction. The technique was popularized in the early 2000s and is the oldest technique for ablation. Argon is used to first freeze the tumor after being injected through specialized probes. Liquid oxygen or nitrogen has been previously used. After freezing the desired area, the tissue temperature may reach $-30°C$. The tissue is then thawed and the process is repeated as needed. The thawing process can use helium, but other methods are available. The crystallization and subsequent expansion of water, as well as the repeated freeze and thaw cycle, destroys the tissue selected for ablation. There are some unique advantages to this technique; one that is particularly beneficial is the well-delineated "ice ball" created through the freezing process that can be easily distinguished from normal tissue on CT imaging. This allows for precisely selected ablation zones. Other benefits include the preservation of protein structures and soft tissue planes leading to less injury of treated and adjacent organs. This can reduce the amount of scar tissue after treatment. Table 11.3 lists a summary of studies investigating the outcomes of cryoablation in mCRC to the liver.

TABLE 11.3 A Summary Collection of the Literature Describing Cryoablation Outcomes in the Setting of Colorectal Metastasis to the Liver

Study	Year	Cohort	Findings	Complications
Zhou et al.	2009	124 primary HCC patients divided into 3 categories: early stage, middle stage, and advanced stage	Median survival 31.25 in early stage, 17.41 months in middle stage, 6.82 months in advanced stage. AFP reduced 82.6% of patients and 92.3% of lesions.	
Chen et al.	2011	40 patients with unresectable HCC and 26 patients with recurrent HCC. 76 treated lesions, mean size 2.8 +/− 1.7 cm	Unresectable HCC group: Disease-free survival at 1 year 67.6%, 3 years 20.8%, and OS 81.4% and 60.3%. Recurrent HCC group: Disease-free survival at 1 year 53.8% and 3 years 7.7%, OS of 70.2% and 28.8%.	Overall rate 12.1%.
Li et al.	2013	82 patients with solitary HCC, 24 received cryoablation, and 58 received surgical resection	Cryoablation OS at 1, 3, and 5 years was 100%, 75%, and 66%, and surgical resection OS was 100%, 78%, and 71%. Recurrence-free survival respectively was 83%, 46%, and 29%, and 84%, 48%, and 33%. No statistically significant difference.	Major adverse events and duration of hospital stay was significantly increased in the surgical resection group.
Qian et al.	2003	34 patients with primary or metastatic liver lesions previously treated with TACE. Subsequent treatment with cryoablation at 1 month.	Curative rate at 15 months was 41.1%. Effective treatment rate of 44.1% at 15 months.	
Xu et al.	2009	420 patients with unresectable HCC, divided into TACE/cryoablation (290) and cryoablation (130)	Mean follow-up 42 +/− 17 months. Local recurrence 11% and 23% in sequential versus cryoablation groups. OS at 1, 2, 3, 4, and 5 years was 72%, 57%, 47%, 39%, and 31%. Sequential 4- and 5-year OS was 49% and 39% versus 29% and 23% of cryoablation group.	Overall complications 24%. 21% and 26% in sequential and cryoablation group, not statistically significantly different.
Glazer et al.	2017	186 patients with 299 liver lesions (243 metastases and 56 primary), mean diameter of 2.5 cm ranging from 0.3 to 7.8 cm	Efficacy rate 98.5%, greater for tumors smaller than 4 cm (93.4%) than for larger (60%). Local progression greater for larger than 4 cm tumors (63.3%) compared to smaller (18%).	Overall complication rate 33.8%, major complications after 10.6%, and more likely to follow larger tumors (19.5% vs. 8.7%).
Littrup et al.	2016	212 patients (176 metastases, 36 primary) with 342 procedures for 443 masses. Average tumor diameter 2.8 cm, average cryoprobes 4–5. Followed for 24 months.	Local recurrence rates at average 1.8-year follow-up were 5.5%, 11.1%, and 9.4% for HCC, CRC, and non-CRC metastases. No significant difference for larger tumors or near blood vessels.	Major complication rate was 5.8% and primarily hematologic.

AFP, alpha fetoprotein; CRC, colorectal cancer; HCC, hepatocellular carcinoma; OS, overall survival; TACE, transarterial chemoembolization.

A unique complication of cryoablation is cryoshock. After freezing and thawing, various cellular components from normal tissue and tumoral cells are released into the bloodstream. This rapid release of factors can stimulate a swift and aggressive inflammatory response and cause multiorgan failure. Bleeding is a significant risk with cryoablation, particularly as treatment zones increase in size, because there is no charring and thermal coagulation effect.

A study by Bhardwaj et al. compared the complete killing of tumor cells within ablated lesions between RFA, MWA, and cryotherapy, and found that MWA had the most complete tumoricidal effect (24). It was postulated that this was due to the heat sink effect, of which MWA is relatively resistant.

Irreversible Electroporation

Irreversible electroporation (IRE) is a relatively new ablative technique that has been used in nonclinical fields for decades. High-frequency electrical pulses induce temporary permeability of cellular membranes. This permeability can move ions across the wall to generate a sufficient transmembrane electrical potential to cause apoptosis. Comparatively, this ablative technique uses a much lower amount of energy to induce cellular death and does not cause thermal injury, which can help prevent injury to the surrounding blood vessels, ducts, and nerves. Multiple studies have demonstrated well-preserved biliary and vascular structures after treatment with IRE despite the proximity to the treated area (25).

After introducing at least two probes around the target lesions under ultrasound or CT guidance, IRE ablation produces approximately 90 pulses of 1,500 to 3,000 volts across the probes. This technique creates well-defined ablation margins and usually with a shorter treatment period compared to thermal-based ablations.

Limitations of IRE include requiring general anesthesia and sufficient neuromuscular blockade to prevent muscular contractions during treatment, difficulty with ablating large lesions (typically greater than 5 cm) necessitating multiple probes or repositioning, and cardiac arrhythmia induced by electrical current in close proximity to the heart. Ventricular bigeminy, ventricular tachycardia, and atrial fibrillation have all been reported in the setting of IRE treatment (25). Some of these limitations can be reduced with careful planning of probe positioning, patient selection, and cardiac monitoring with treatment synchronization.

INTRA-ARTERIAL THERAPIES

Hepatic Artery Chemotherapy

HAI of chemotherapy was first studied in the 1950s by Sullivan et al. (26). HAI is performed by placing a catheter into the hepatic artery selective to the desired location, delivering the chemotherapeutic agent over the desired time, and then removing the catheter. The technique of an implantable pump (hepatic artery infusion pump [HAIP]) delivering continuous chemotherapy was evaluated in 1980 (27). HAI is based on the premise that primary liver and liver metastases derive their blood supply primarily from the hepatic arterial system. It follows then that focal delivery of chemotherapeutic agents directly through the hepatic artery will selectively affect mCRC. With localized delivery, dramatically higher doses can be used on the tumor while reducing the overall systemic dose. With 5-fluoro-2-deoxyuridine (FUDR), intratumoral concentrations can reach 400 times the value when introduced intra-arterially compared to systemically (28). Unfortunately, the biliary tree is also primarily supplied by the hepatic artery and suffers from the higher local dose.

Relative contraindications to HAIP include portal vein occlusion as these patients have been shown to have poorer response rates. Complications of the device are somewhat common having been reported to be in the range of 12% to 41%. These include technical issues with the pump device, implant pocket complications, vascular injury and thrombosis, and biliary injury from chemotherapy. Biliary toxicity is closely monitored throughout chemotherapy administration and is often managed with dose reduction. Using catheters without an implanted pump removes the complications associated with the pump but requires repeated placement of a catheter when infusions are needed.

Bland Embolization

Bland embolization uses temporary or permanent embolic agents delivered via the hepatic arterial system to occlude the vasculature, resulting in ischemia and necrosis. Temporary embolic agents include gelatin sponges, autologous blood clots, and degradable microspheres. Other permanent agents include polyvinyl alcohol, metallic coils, and permanent microspheres. Multiple embolization procedures are usually required in order to achieve the desired effect as the tumor and surrounding tissue recruit collaterals during ischemic events. Additional embolizations target these collateral systems in order to maintain sufficient ischemia to cause necrosis. Distal embolization is important during these procedures to reduce the effective blood flow that collateral circulation can provide to the tumor by occluding the vessels as close to the capillaries as possible. Lipiodol and smaller sized microspheres are advantageous in this regard.

Chemoembolization

TACE was developed in 1983 by Yamada et al. (29). This treatment method delivers embolic material with chemotherapy drugs locally via the hepatic artery. This can be done broadly across both lobes of the liver or selectively to individual segments. Currently, TACE is a second-line therapy after systemic chemotherapy has failed. Table 11.4 lists a summary collection of studies investigating outcomes of TACE in mCRC of the liver.

After introduction of the catheter into the hepatic artery, the vasculature associated with the tumor is identified and selected. The chemoembolic agent is then delivered and the catheter and kit are removed. The embolic agent used is variable based on provider preference and the desired effect. Agents can include temporary or permanent embolics. Temporary agents include starch microspheres, collagen, and gelatin sponges. Permanent agents include polyvinyl alcohol and lipiodol. A common practice is to inject the combination of a chemotherapeutic agent with lipiodol which, given its lipophilic nature, delivers the chemotherapeutic agent localized to the cells of the tumor. After this mixture is delivered, the area is then embolized with particles until there is stagnant blood flow or reflux is noted to ensure some ischemic effect. Cisplatin and doxorubicin are common chemotherapeutic agents used in injection. Irinotecan-loaded drug-eluting beads (DEBIRIs) are newer agents that combine microspheres and a slowly released chemotherapeutic agent (Figure 11.2). With this combination, irinotecan is delivered locally at high concentrations while keeping systemic effects to a minimum.

Complications from TACE are rare but include postembolization syndrome and nontarget embolization. Postembolization syndrome is the combination of pain, nausea, vomiting, and fatigue, and is generally self-limited. Intra-arterial lidocaine injection may reduce postembolization pain (30,31) while corticosteroids do not appear to have any benefit (31). Oral analgesics are often sufficient to control postprocedural pain.

A strong benefit of TACE therapy is the simple postprocedural course. Often, therapy can be performed as an outpatient with minimal recovery time in the postprocedural area (32,33). Less often, a single recovery night spent in the hospital is used for observation.

Radioembolization

SIRT is a similar technique to chemoembolization but uses radiation for the tumoricidal effects (Figure 11.3). Similar to chemoembolization, the radiation effects are delivered locally and thus

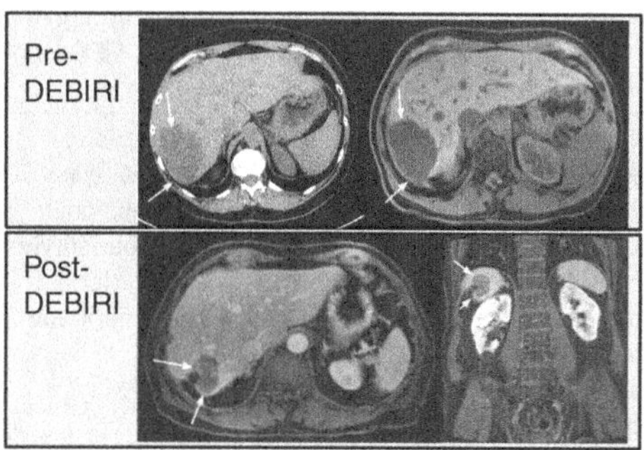

FIGURE 11.2 CT and MRI images of a large liver metastasis before and after treatment with DEBIRI.

DEBIRI, irinotecan-loaded drug-eluting bead.

TABLE 11.4 A Summary Collection of the Literature Describing TACE Outcomes in the Setting of Colorectal Metastasis to the Liver

Study	Year	Cohort	Findings	Complications
Huppert et al.	2014	29 patients with 71 procedures of liver mCRC who failed systemic chemotherapy. 200 mg of irinotecan on SAP microspheres. Selective administration.	At 3, 6, and 12 months, there was partial response in 72%, 32%, and 0% (by EASL criteria) with stable disease in 86%, 48%, and 8% (no complete or partial response by RECIST). Median OS was 8 months after first TACE. Median time to progression was 5 months. Median OS better with limited versus extensive intrahepatic disease.	No major complications.
Tellez et al.	2000	30 patients undergoing chemoembolization with bovine collagen material, cisplatin, doxorubicin, and mitomycin C. Repeat treatments at 6–8 week intervals.	Radiologic response in 63% of cases, CEA decrease in 95% of cases. All responses were transient. Median survival 8.6 months after chemoembolization, 29 months after initial metastatic liver disease.	
Martin et al.	2010	55 patients who failed systemic chemotherapy underwent 99 DEBIRI treatments (median 2 treatments), 86% as lobar infusions, 30% treated with concurrent chemotherapy.	Response rates of 66% at 6 months and 75% at 12 months. OS was 19 months. PFS 11 months.	28% with major adverse events. No deaths at 30 days post procedure.
Fiorentini et al.	2013	74 patients assigned DEBIRI (36) versus FOLFIRI (38).	Median survival 22 months for DEBIRI and 15 months for FOLFIRI. PFS was 7 months for DEBIRI versus 4 with FOLFIRI. Extrahepatic progression in all patients with median time of 13 months DEBIRI versus 9 months FOLFIRI. Statistically significant improved OS, PFS, and quality of life.	
Gruber-Rouh et al.	2014	564 patients with liver mCRC treated with TACE using lipiodol and starch microspheres and combinations of mitomycin C, gemcitabine, irinotecan, and cisplatin. 3,384 TACE procedures performed, average of 6 per patient.	Partial response rates of 16.7%, stable disease in 48.2%, and progression in 16.7%. 2- and 3-year survival was 28% and 7%. Median survival from treatment start was 14.3 months.	

(continued)

TABLE 11.4 A Summary Collection of the Literature Describing TACE Outcomes in the Setting of Colorectal Metastasis to the Liver (*continued*)

Study	Year	Cohort	Findings	Complications
Zacharias, et al.	2015	90 studies (52 HAI, 24 radioemboliza-tion, and 14 TACE) were selected for comparison for meta-analysis after searching PubMed for 2003–2013	Median OS for 21.4 for HAI, 29.4 for RE, 15.2 for TACE. Failing at least one prior systemic therapy median OS was 13.2 HAI, 10.7 RE, and 21.3 TACE.	Overall major adverse events were 40% in HAI, 19% in RE, and 18% in TACE, all of which were increased com-pared to systemic chemotherapy.
Sanz-Altamira et al.	1997	40 patients undergo-ing chemoemboliza-tion for liver mCRC using lipiodol, 5-FU, and mitomycin C.	Median OS from first chemo-embolization was 10 months.	

5-FU, 5-fluorouracil; CEA, carcinoembryonic antigen; DEBIRI, irinotecan-loaded drug-eluting bead; HAI, hepatic arterial infusion; HCC, hepatocellular carcinoma; mCRC, metastatic colorectal cancer; OS, overall survival; PFS, progression-free survival; RE, Radioembolization; SAP, superabsorbent polymer; TACE, transarterial chemoembolization.

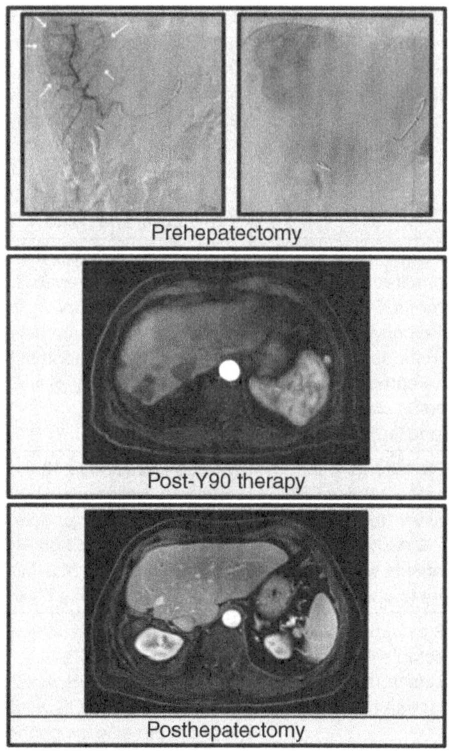

FIGURE 11.3   Fluoroscopic and MRI images of a large hepatic mass before and after Y-90 therapy and hepatectomy.

have significantly reduced systemic effects if any at all. The radiation travels only very short distances, which limits the radioactive effect on people or objects near the patient. An additional benefit of such local administration of radiation is the ability to deliver very high doses of radiation. This can cause complete obliteration of the treated area. Table 11.5 provides a summary collection of studies investigating outcomes of radioembolization with mCRCC of the liver.

The radioisotope used in SIRT is yttrium-90 (Y-90). The isotope undergoes beta minus decay with a long half-life (64.2 hours) and a short effective radiation distance (2.4 mm). The Y-90 is bound to treatment spheres made of resin or glass. These microspheres are smaller than the spheres used in TACE and provide some embolic effect. The amount of ischemia should be limited unlike in other arterial therapies in order to deliver oxygen to the tumor cells and enhance the tumoricidal effects.

Delivery of the radioembolic material should be closely monitored under fluoroscopy in order to monitor for reflux and nontarget embolization and delivery. The delivery system should be closed circuit and the area surveyed for radiation spills or ineffective delivery. Following the procedure, the delivered dose is detected under a gamma camera to ensure proper administration. The area is also monitored with cross-sectional imaging (contrast enhanced CT or MRI) in order to observe the complete elimination of the tumor, segment or lobe, and to monitor for recurrence particularly along the ablated margins. Additionally, the arteriovenous shunting through the liver should be assessed prior to therapy to limit the embolization and radiation exposure to the lungs (34).

TABLE 11.5 A Summary Collection of the Literature Describing Y90 Therapy Outcomes in the Setting of Colorectal Metastasis to the Liver

Study	Year	Cohort	Findings	Complications
Gray et al.	2001	74 patients with nonresectable liver metastases from mCRC undergoing SIR-Spheres and chemotherapy versus chemotherapy alone.	Partial and complete response rates of 44% (combined) versus 17.6% (chemotherapy). TTP (median) 15.9 months (combined) versus 9.7 months (chemotherapy). 1-, 2-, 3-, and 5-year survival for combined was 72%, 39%, 17%, and 3.5% versus 68%, 29%, 6.5%, and 0%.	No increase in major adverse events or loss of quality of life with combined therapy.
Hazel et al.	2004	21 patients with untreated advanced liver mCRC treated with combination SIR-Spheres and chemotherapy (11) versus chemotherapy alone (10).	TTP increased with combination therapy 18.6 versus 3.6 months. Median survival longer with combination therapy, 29.4 versus 12.8 months. No difference in quality of life over 3 months.	Increased major adverse events in combination therapy.
Kennedy et al.	2006	208 patients with unresectable mCRC to liver treated with Y-90 microspheres. Patients were refractory to chemotherapy.	Median survival was 10.5 months for responders but 4.5 months for nonresponders. Partial response rate 35%, PET response rate of 91%, and CEA reduction in 70%.	No treatment-related deaths or veno-occlusive liver failure.
Kosmider et al.	2011	19 patients with unresectable liver metastases from CRC, first-line treatment.	Response rate was 84%. Median PFS was 10.4 months. Median OS was 29.4 months. PFS and OS were improved in disease confined to the liver compared to extrahepatic disease.	Major adverse events included febrile neutropenia, perforated duodenal ulcer, and one death from hepatic toxicity.

(continued)

TABLE 11.5 A Summary Collection of the Literature Describing Y90 Therapy Outcomes in the Setting of Colorectal Metastasis to the Liver (*continued*)

Study	Year	Cohort	Findings	Complications
Cortesi et al.	2016	68 patients, retrospective analysis, with metastatic colorectal cancer treated with SIR-Spheres using the body surface model.	Median PFS was 9 months and 3 months for treatments used after one or more than two lines of chemotherapy.	No major adverse events were identified. GI adverse events were usually mild as well as hepatobiliary events.
Janowski et al.	2017	58 patients with chemorefractory mCRC with liver metastases treated with resin-based Y-90 therapy.	Median survival was 6 months, 12-month survival rate of 33%. KRAS wild-type patient survival was not significantly different than KRAS mutants.	
Rosenbaum et al.	2016	42 patients with unresectable chemorefractory mCRC to the liver. Angiogenic factors VEGF, HGF, and Ang-2 were collected at 0, 1, 3, 7, and 30 days follow-up as well as 1- and 3-month imaging follow-up.	Median OS was 9.2 months. Nonresponders had increase in Ang-2 and HGF at 3 and 7 days compared to responders, who had little to no changes.	
Hazel et al.	2016	530 chemotherapy-naive patients with liver mCRC received FOLFOX or mFOLFOX6 plus SIRT with or without bevacizumab.	Median PFS was 10.2 versus 10.7 months in control versus SIRT groups. ORRs were similar at 68.1% versus 76.4% in control versus SIRT. ORR was improved with SIRT at 68.8% versus 78.7% in control versus SIRT.	Major adverse events were reported in 73.4% versus 85.4% in control versus SIRT groups.
Wasan et al.	2017	Meta-analysis of FOXFIRE, SIFLOX, and FOXFIRE-Global trials. 549 patients assigned to FOLFOX alone and 554 patients to FOLFOX plus SIRT.	OS hazard ratio was 1.04 between the groups. Median survival time was 22.6 months (SIRT) versus 23.3 months (FOLFOX).	Neutropenia most common major adverse event with 24% in FOLFOX versus 37% in SIRT group. All major adverse events in 43% versus 54% of FOLFOX versus SIRT.
Salem et al. (35)	2016	179 HCC patients with BCLC stage A or B compared cTACE or Y-90 therapy.	TTP of Y-90 group was >26 months while that of cTACE group was 6.8 months. Median survival time was 18.6 months for Y-90 and 17.7 months for cTACE.	More patients experienced diarrhea or hypoalbuminemia in the cTACE group compared to the Y-90 group.

BCLC, Barcelona Clinic Liver Cancer; CEA, carcinoembryonic antigen; CRC, colorectal cancer; cTACE, conventional transarterial chemoembolization; GI, gastrointestinal; HGF, hepatocyte growth factor; mCRC, metastatic colorectal cancer; ORR, objective response rate; OS, overall survival; PFS, progression-free survival; SIRT, selective internal radiation therapy; TTP, time to progression; VEGF, vascular endothelial growth factor.

Complications from SIRT are rare. Minor complications include fever, nausea, fatigue, pain, and anorexia. Major complications include nontarget embolization with particular concern for excess embolization of normal liver parenchyma or spillage into the gastrointestinal system. Radiation liver disease occurs in 4% and can manifest as ascites, jaundice, and hepatic dysfunction (36). If the stomach is affected, this can cause local inflammation and ulceration to varying degrees. Ulceration or radiation gastritis occurs in 5% to 10% of cases (37) while pancreatitis and cholecystitis are much less common, less than 1% (37). Excess embolization or profound nontarget embolization of the liver can be life-threatening although this is very rare.

MANAGEMENT OF CONCURRENT COLORECTAL METASTASIS IN THE LUNGS

The lung is the second most common site of metastasis. Treatment options have previously included medical, surgical, and radiation therapy with SBRT. Surgical options include lobectomy, segmentectomy, and video-assisted thoracoscopic surgery (VATS). Metastasectomy has been shown to be beneficial with median survival rates of 35 to 50 months and 5-year survival rates ranging from 36% to 67.8% (38–42). Repeat treatments with surgical resections of new metastatic lesions have also been shown to improve survival (43,44). Smaller resections offer similar outcomes when comparing wedge resection, lobar resection, and pneumonectomy. These findings suggest ablation techniques would be ideal for treatment of metastatic disease in the lung. Median survival ranges when using thermal ablative techniques have similar outcomes to surgical metastasectomy of 33 to 46 months (45–47). With similar outcomes, the benefits of the minimally invasive technique become more influential. These include improvements in quality of life and recovery time (48), better preservation of vital lung parenchyma (40,49), repeatability for new or incompletely treated lesions, and reduced cost compared to surgical intervention. Thermal ablation techniques do not require extended hospitalizations or recovery, and studies have shown improved lung function scores compared to surgical techniques (49). Because of these promising results, the number of lung ablations has been increasing.

ABLATIVE THERAPIES

Indications for ablation include metastatic lesions in the lungs that are less than 3 cm in size following the Cardiovascular and Interventional Radiological Society of Europe (CIRSE) guidelines (59). Although there are no clear guidelines on the number of lesions to treat at one time, most centers treat 5 or fewer at a time (60). Treating multiple lesions over 3 cm in size should be avoided as per these guidelines (59). Table 11.6 summarizes outcomes by treatment modality of non-small cell lung cancer including RFA and cryoablation.

TABLE 11.6 Summary of Outcomes After Various Treatment Modalities Including RFA and Cryoablation in the Setting of NSCLC

Modality	5-Year Survival Stage I NSCLC	Local Recurrence (Most Within 2 Years)
Lobar resection (50)	60%–80%	6.40%
Sublobar resection (50,51)	60%–74%	17.20%
Lobar resection in octogenarians (52)	60%	
Radiofrequency ablation (53,54)	27%–55.7%	22.20%
SBRT (55,56)	41.2%–42%	14%
External beam radiation (57)	10%–27%	50%–55%
Cryoablation (58)	67.80%	36.20%

NSCLC, non–small cell lung cancer; SBRT, stereotactic body radiation therapy.

The test of time, chemotherapy holiday, and PFS concepts applied to liver lesions may also apply to the lungs. These specific treatments can allow the disease process to be better elucidated and then targeted with the appropriate treatment, possibly avoiding unnecessary surgical interventions.

Contraindications to ablation therapy in the lungs relate to complications from reduced lung capacity, bleeding, and injury to surrounding structures. Severe underlying interstitial disease with FEV1 less than 500 mL, or pulmonary arterial hypertension greater than 40 mmHg, predisposes the patient to severe pulmonary failure and should be carefully considered. Coagulopathy, as with ablations performed anywhere, predisposes to severe bleeding complications. The proximity of the lesion to critical structures such as the trachea, main bronchi, esophagus, or major vessels must be accurately determined. If the lesion is within 1 cm of these structures, the lesion may be incompletely ablated to preserve these structures if other methods of preservation cannot be performed.

Complications of thermal ablations in the lung are rare occurring after 9.8% of procedures (61) and can be minimized with appropriate patient selection. Serious risks of ablation may involve bronchopleural fistula, seeding of the needle tracts, and diaphragm or nerve injury. These, fortunately, are particularly rare occurring only 0.3% of the time (62). Other risks of the procedure include skin burns, pneumonia, abscess, bleeding, and pneumothorax. Risk factors for complications include emphysema, thrombocytopenia, and previous chemotherapy, which predispose to pneumonia, bleeding, and pleuritis, respectively (63). Prior radiotherapy also has an association with pneumonia (63).

The majority of studies have reported on outcomes related to RFA ablation in the lungs. Outcomes for survival in the ablation literature are generally measured on the order of 1 to 3 years while the surgical literature tends to measure 5-year survival rates. While 1- to 3-year ablation survival data is comparable with 3-year surgical survival data of 46% to 59.6%, 5-year survival favors surgery. This may reflect the differences in patient selection. Ablation is generally reserved for patients with multiple comorbidities and who are unable to undergo surgical options.

Cryoablation is a promising treatment tool for treating lung metastasis. The ECLIPSE trial interim analysis at 1 year assessed 60 treated lesions in 40 patients with lung metastasis, the majority being colorectal cancer primary, and found 94.6% local tumor control at 12 months (64). There are multiple distinct advantages of cryoablation over RFA. None of the patients experienced significant pain after the procedure. Cryoablation offers clearly defined margins on CT imaging, allowing for easy monitoring and control of the ablation zone. The ablation zone is not limited by the high electrical resistance of air and creates its own medium during the process to extending the ice ball in a predictable manner. Finally, cryoablation preserves the collagenous structure of the ablation zone, which enables preservation of the tracheobronchial tree (65).

Post-ablation management in the lungs generally involves follow-up imaging in 2 months after ablation with CT or PET–CT. Inflammatory uptake from the ablation procedure can exist from 24 hours to 1 month after ablation and should resolve by 3 months (66). Surveillance imaging is recommended every 3 months until 1 year, after which yearly surveillance is sufficient (60). The ablation zone may appear larger on initial follow-up imaging compared to pre-ablation size; however, after this, it should decrease in size modestly. There may be surrounding atelectasis or fibrosis with central cavitation. The treated nodule or mass rarely disappears completely (60). On PET, the ablated area should show a uniform ring of low level activity that generally improves at 1 year (67). As with follow-up of other ablation zones in the body, nodule growth at the periphery, solid areas of enhancement, or increased metabolic activity in a nodular or central pattern, is concerning for recurrence.

Clinical Vignette 11.1

Case 1: Refer to Figure 11.1

A 63-year-old woman has left side colon cancer status post resection with end-to-end anastomosis on follow-up imaging; a single biopsy proven colorectal metastatic lesion in the right hepatic lobe is noted. The patient has an Eastern Cooperative Oncology Group (ECOG) performance status of 0.

Patient's lab

Serum albumin 3.4 g/dl, serum Cr 1.4 mg/dl, total bilirubin 1.5 mg/dl, and international normalized ratio (INR) 1.6.

The patient was offered surgical resection; however, she preferred percutaneous ablation as her treatment option. Microwave ablation was performed and post-ablation images demonstrated no residual disease.

Case 2: Refer to Figure 11.2

A 74-year-old man has an ECOG performance status of 0 with metastatic lesion measuring 5.4 × 3.8 cm in segment VI of the liver biopsy proven colorectal cancer with liver metastasis (CRLM). Status post colon resection 2 years ago. No other evidence of disease outside the liver. The liver tumor burden progressed on two lines of treatment. Surgical resection was not offered.

Patient's lab

Serum albumin 4.1 g/dl, serum Cr 1.1 mg/dl, total bilirubin 1.01 mg/dl, and INR 1.3.

Transarterial embolization using drug-eluting beads with irinotecan was performed. Significant tumor reduction was noted on follow-up images with no evidence of active disease seen.

REFERENCES

1. American Cancer Society. *Cancer Facts & Figures 2017*. Atlanta: American Cancer Society; 2017.
2. Sasson AR, Sigurdson ER. Surgical treatment of liver metastases. *Semin Oncol*. 2002;29:107–118. doi:10.1053/sonc.2002.31676
3. Valderrama-Treviño AI, Barrera-Mera B, Ceballos-Villalva J, et al. Hepatic metastasis from colorectal cancer. *Euroasian J Hepatogastroenterol*. 2017;7:166–175. doi:10.5005/jp-journals-10018-1241
4. Dueland S, Guren TK, Hagness M, et al. Chemotherapy or liver transplantation for nonresectable liver metastases from colorectal cancer? *Ann Surg*. 2015;261:956–960. doi:10.1097/SLA.0000000000000786
5. Xing M, Kooby DA, El-Rayes BF, et al. Locoregional therapies for metastatic colorectal carcinoma to the liver—an evidence-based review. *J Surg Oncol*. 2014;110:182–196. doi:10.1002/jso.23619
6. Liccioni A, Reig M, Bruix J. Treatment of hepatocellular carcinoma. *Dig Dis*. 2014;32:554–563. doi:10.1159/000360501
7. Livraghi T, Solbiati L, Meloni F, et al. Percutaneous radiofrequency ablation of liver metastases in potential candidates for resection: the "test-of-time" approach. *Cancer*. 2003;97:3027–3035. doi:10.1002/cncr.11426
8. Gruber-Rouh T, Naguib NNN, Eichler K, et al. Transarterial chemoembolization of unresectable systemic chemotherapy-refractory liver metastases from colorectal cancer: long-term results over a 10-year period. *Int J Cancer*. 2014;134:1225–1231. doi:10.1002/ijc.28443
9. Petre EN, Sofocleous C. Thermal ablation in the management of colorectal cancer patients with oligometastatic liver disease. *Visceral Med*. 2017;33;62–68. doi:10.1159/000454697
10. Veltri A, Guarnieri T, Gazzera C, et al. Long-term outcome of radiofrequency thermal ablation (RFA) of liver metastases from colorectal cancer (CRC): size as the leading prognostic factor for survival. *La Radiologia Medica*. 2012;117:1139–1151. doi:10.1007/s11547-012-0803-3
11. Ferguson J, Alzahrani N, Zhao J, et al. Long term results of RFA to lung metastases from colorectal cancer in 157 patients. *Eur J Surg Oncol*. 2015;41:690–695. doi:10.1016/j.ejso.2015.01.024
12. Ochiai S, Yamakado K, Kodama H, et al. Comparison of therapeutic results from radiofrequency ablation and stereotactic body radiotherapy in solitary lung tumors measuring 5 cm or smaller. *Int J Clin Oncol*. 2015;20:499–507. doi:10.1007/s10147-014-0741-z
13. Kunzli BM, Abitabile P, Maurer CA. Radiofrequency ablation of liver tumors: actual limitations and potential solutions in the future. *World J Hepatol*. 2011;3:8–14. doi:10.4254/wjh.v3.i1.8
14. Solbiati L, Ahmed M, Cova L, et al. Small liver colorectal metastases treated with percutaneous radiofrequency ablation: local response rate and long-term survival with up to 10-year follow-up. *Radiology*. 2012;265:958–968. doi:10.1148/radiol.12111851

15. Pillai K, Akhter J, Chua TC, et al. Heat sink effect on tumor ablation characteristics as observed in monopolar radiofrequency, bipolar radiofrequency, and microwave, using ex vivo calf liver model. *Medicine.* 2015;94:e580. doi:10.1097/MD.0000000000000580
16. Valdix R, Wacker F, Hans-Juergen R, et al. High power microwave ablation of liver tissue – is the heat sink effect negligible? *J Vasc Interv Radiol.* 2015;26:S118. doi:10.1016/j.jvir.2014.12.319
17. Song P, Sheng L, Sun Y, et al. The clinical utility and outcomes of microwave ablation for colorectal cancer liver metastases. *Oncotarget.* 2017;8:51792–51799. doi:10.18632/oncotarget.15244
18. Violi NV, Duran R, Guiu B, et al. Efficacy of microwave ablation versus radiofrequency ablation for the treatment of hepatocellular carcinoma in patients with chronic liver disease: a randomised controlled phase 2 trial. *Lancet Gastroenterol Hepatol.* 2018;3:317–325. doi:10.1016/S2468-1253(18)30029-3
19. Carberry G, Smolock A, Cristescu M, et al. Percutaneous microwave ablation of liver tumors near the heart: safety and efficacy. *J Vasc Interv Radiol.* 2016;27:S80. doi:10.1016/j.jvir.2015.12.214
20. Liang P, Dong B, Yu X, et al. Prognostic factors for percutaneous microwave coagulation therapy of hepatic metastases. *Am J Roentgenol.* 2003;181:1319–1325. doi:10.2214/ajr.181.5.1811319
21. Tanaka K, Shimada H, Nagano Y, et al. Outcome after hepatic resection versus combined resection and microwave ablation for multiple bilobar colorectal metastases to the liver. *Surgery.* 2006;139:263–273. doi:10.1016/j.surg.2005.07.036
22. Wang J, Liang P, Yu J, et al. Clinical outcome of ultrasound-guided percutaneous microwave ablation on colorectal liver metastases. *Oncol Lett.* 2014;8:323–326. doi:10.3892/ol.2014.2106
23. Correa-Gallego C, Fong Y, Gonen M, et al. A retrospective comparison of microwave ablation vs. radiofrequency ablation for colorectal cancer hepatic metastases. *Ann Surg Oncol.* 2014;21:4278–4283. doi:10.1245/s10434-014-3817-0
24. Bhardwaj N, Strickland AD, Ahmad F, et al. A comparative histological evaluation of the ablations produced by microwave, cryotherapy and radiofrequency in the liver. *Pathology.* 2009;41:168–172. doi:10.1080/00313020802579292
25. Lyu T, Wang X, Su Z, et al. Irreversible electroporation in primary and metastatic hepatic malignancies. *Medicine.* 2017;96:1–7. doi:10.1097/md.0000000000006386
26. Sullivan RD, Zurek WZ. Chemotherapy for liver cancer by protracted ambulatory infusion. *JAMA.* 1965;194:481–486. doi:10.1001/jama.1965.03090180005001
27. Buchwald H, Grage TB, Vassilopoulos PP, et al. Intraarterial infusion chemotherapy for hepatic carcinoma using a totally implantable infusion pump. *Cancer.* 1980;45:866–869. doi:10.1002/1097-0142(19800301)45:5<866::AID-CNCR2820450507>3.0.CO;2-3
28. Lewis HL, Bloomston M. Hepatic artery infusional chemotherapy. *Surg Clin North Am.* 2016;96:341–355. doi:10.1016/j.suc.2015.11.002
29. Yamada R, Sato M, Kawabata M, et al. Hepatic artery embolization in 120 patients with unresectable hepatoma. *Radiology.* 1983;148:397–401. doi:10.1148/radiology.148.2.6306721
30. Hartnell GG, Gates J, Stuart K, et al. Hepatic chemoembolization: effect of intraarterial lidocaine on pain and postprocedure recovery. *Cardiovasc Interv Radiol.* 1999;22:293–297. doi:10.1007/s002709900391
31. Romano M, Giojelli A, Tamburrini O, et al. Chemoembolization for hepatocellular carcinoma: effect of intraarterial lidocaine in peri- and post-procedural pain and hospitalization. *Radiol Med.* 2003;105:350–355.
32. Mitchell JW, O'Connell WG, Kisza P, et al. Safety and feasibility of outpatient transcatheter hepatic arterial embolization for hepatocellular carcinoma. *J Vasc Interv Radiol.* 2009;20:203–208. doi:10.1016/j.jvir.2008.10.027
33. Nasser F, Cavalcante RN, Galastri FL, et al. Safety and feasibility of same-day discharge of patients with hepatocellular carcinoma treated with transarterial chemoembolization with drug-eluting beads in a liver transplantation program. *J Vasc Interv Radiol.* 2014;25:1012–1017. doi:10.1016/j.jvir.2014.02.025
34. Murthy R, Nunez R, Szklaruk J, et al. Yttrium-90 microsphere therapy for hepatic malignancy: devices, indications, technical considerations, and potential complications. *RadioGraphics.* 2005;25:S41–S55. doi:10.1148/rg.25si055515
35. Salem R, Gordon AC, Mouli S, et al. Y90 Radioembolization significantly prolongs time to progression compared with chemoembolization in patients with hepatocellular carcinoma. *Gastroenterology.* 2016;151:1155–1163.e1152. doi:10.1053/j.gastro.2016.08.029
36. de Baere T, Tselikas L, Pearson E, et al. Interventional oncology for liver and lung metastases from colorectal cancer: the current state of the art. *Diagn Interv Imaging.* 2015;96:647–654. doi:10.1016/j.diii.2015.04.004
37. Nicolay NH, Berry DP, Sharma RA. Liver metastases from colorectal cancer: radioembolization with systemic therapy. *Nat Rev Clin Oncol.* 2009;6:687–697. doi:10.1038/nrclinonc.2009.165

38. Meimarakis G, Spelsberg F, Angele M, et al. Resection of pulmonary metastases from colon and rectal cancer: factors to predict survival differ regarding to the origin of the primary tumor. *Ann Surg Oncol.* 2014;21:2563–2572. doi:10.1245/s10434-014-3646-1

39. Zampino MG, Maisonneuve P, Ravenda PS, et al. Lung metastases from colorectal cancer: analysis of prognostic factors in a single institution study. *Ann Thorac Surg.* 2014;98:1238–1245. doi:10.1016/j.athoracsur.2014.05.048

40. Watanabe I, Arai T, Ono M, et al. Prognostic factors in resection of pulmonary metastasis from colorectal cancer. *Br J Surg.* 2003;90:1436–1440. doi:10.1002/bjs.4331

41. Mori M, Tomoda H, Ishida T, et al. Surgical resection of pulmonary metastases from colorectal adenocarcinoma: special reference to repeated pulmonary resections. *Arch Surg.* 1991;126:1297–1302. doi:10.1001/archsurg.1991.01410340139020

42. Saito Y, Omiya H, Kohno K, et al. Pulmonary metastasectomy for 165 patients with colorectal carcinoma: a prognostic assessment. *J Thorac Cardiovasc Surg.* 2002;124:1007–1013. doi:10.1067/mtc.2002.125165

43. Pastorino U. Lung metastasectomy: why, when, how. *Crit Rev Oncol Hematol.* 1997;26:137–145. doi:10.1016/S1040-8428(97)00017-6

44. Casiraghi M, De Pas T, Maisonneuve P, et al. A 10-year single-center experience on 708 lung metastasectomies: the evidence of the "international registry of lung metastases". *J Thorac Oncol.* 2011;6:1373–1378. doi:10.1097/JTO.0b013e3182208e58

45. Yamakado K, Inoue Y, Takao M, et al. Long-term results of radiofrequency ablation in colorectal lung metastases: single center experience. *Oncol Rep.* 2009;22:885–891. doi:10.3892/or_00000513

46. Gillams A, Khan Z, Osborn P, et al. Survival after radiofrequency ablation in 122 patients with inoperable colorectal lung metastases. *Cardiovasc Interv Radiol.* 2013;36:724–730. doi:10.1007/s00270-012-0500-3

47. Yamauchi Y, Izumi Y, Hashimoto K, et al. Percutaneous cryoablation for the treatment of medically inoperable stage I non-small cell lung cancer. *PloS One.* 2012;7:e33223. doi:10.1371/journal.pone.0033223

48. Suh RD, Wallace AB, Sheehan RE, et al. Unresectable pulmonary malignancies: CT-guided percutaneous radiofrequency ablation—preliminary results. *Radiology.* 2003;229:821–829. doi:10.1148/radiol.2293021756

49. Lencioni R, Crocetti L, Cioni R, et al. Response to radiofrequency ablation of pulmonary tumours: a prospective, intention-to-treat, multicentre clinical trial (the RAPTURE study). *Lancet Oncol.* 2008;9:621–628. doi:10.1016/S1470-2045(08)70155-4

50. Mery CM, Pappas AN, Bueno R, et al. Similar long-term survival of elderly patients with non-small cell lung cancer treated with lobectomy or wedge resection within the surveillance, epidemiology, and end results database. *Chest.* 2005;128:237–245. doi:10.1378/chest.128.1.237

51. Ghosh S, Sujendran V, Alexiou C, et al. Long term results of surgery versus continuous hyperfractionated accelerated radiotherapy (CHART) in patients aged >70 years with stage 1 non-small cell lung cancer. *Eur J Cardiothorac Surg.* 2003;24:1002–1007. doi:10.1016/S1010-7940(03)00474-3

52. Dell'Amore A, Monteverde M, Martucci N, et al. Lobar and sub-lobar lung resection in octogenarians with early stage non-small cell lung cancer: factors affecting surgical outcomes and long-term results. *Gen Thorac Cardiovasc Surg.* 2015;63:222–230. doi:10.1007/s11748-014-0493-8

53. Simon CJ, Dupuy DE, DiPetrillo TA, et al. Pulmonary radiofrequency ablation: long-term safety and efficacy in 153 patients. *Radiology.* 2007;243:268–275. doi:10.1148/radiol.2431060088

54. Kodama H, Yamakado K, Takaki H, et al. Lung radiofrequency ablation for the treatment of unresectable recurrent non-small-cell lung cancer after surgical intervention. *Cardiovasc Intervent Radiol.* 2012;35:563–569. doi:10.1007/s00270-011-0220-0

55. Grutters JP, Kessels AGH, Pijls-Johannesma M, et al. Comparison of the effectiveness of radiotherapy with photons, protons and carbon-ions for non-small cell lung cancer: a meta-analysis. *Radiother Oncol.* 2010;95:32–40. doi:10.1016/j.radonc.2009.08.003

56. Zheng X, Schipper M, Kidwell K, et al. Survival outcome after stereotactic body radiation therapy and surgery for stage I non-small cell lung cancer: a meta-analysis. *Int J Radiat Oncol Biol Phys.* 2014;90:603–611. doi:10.1016/j.ijrobp.2014.05.055

57. Gauden S, Ramsay J, Tripcony L. The curative treatment by radiotherapy alone of stage I non-small cell carcinoma of the lung. *Chest.* 1995;108:1278–1282. doi:10.1378/chest.108.5.1278

58. Moore W, Talati R, Bhattacharji P, et al. Five-year survival after cryoablation of stage I non-small cell lung cancer in medically inoperable patients. *J Vasc Interv Radiol.* 2015;26:312–319. doi:10.1016/j.jvir.2014.12.006

59. Pereira PL, Salvatore M. Standards of practice: guidelines for thermal ablation of primary and secondary lung tumors. *Cardiovasc Interv Radiol.* 2012;35:247–254. doi:10.1007/s00270-012-0340-1

60. Ridge CA, Solomon SB. Percutaneous ablation of colorectal lung metastases. *J Gastrointest Oncol.* 2015;6:685–692. doi:10.3978/j.issn.2078-6891.2015.095

61. Carrafiello G, Mangini M, Fontana F, et al. Complications of microwave and radiofrequency lung ablation: personal experience and review of the literature. *La Radiologia Medica.* 2012;117:201–213. doi:10.1007/s11547-011-0741-2

62. Palussière J, Canella M, Cornelis F, et al. Retrospective review of thoracic neural damage during lung ablation — what the interventional radiologist needs to know about neural thoracic anatomy. *Cardiovasc Interv Radiol.* 2013;36:1602–1613. doi:10.1007/s00270-013-0597-z

63. Kashima M, Yamakado K, Takaki H, et al. Complications after 1000 lung radiofrequency ablation sessions in 420 patients: a single center's experiences. *Am J Roentgenol.* 2011;197:W576–W580. doi:10.2214/AJR.11.6408

64. de Baere T, Tselikas L, Woodrum D, et al. Evaluating cryoablation of metastatic lung tumors in patients — safety and efficacy: the ECLIPSE trial — interim analysis at 1-Year. *Cardiol Rev.* 2015;10(10):1468–1474. doi:10.1097/jto.0000000000000632

65. Wang H, Littrup PJ, Duan Y, et al. Thoracic masses treated with percutaneous cryotherapy: initial experience with more than 200 procedures. *Radiology.* 2005;235:289–298. doi:10.1148/radiol.2351030747

66. Deandreis D, Leboulleux S, Dromain C, et al. Role of FDG PET/CT and chest CT in the follow-up of lung lesions treated with radiofrequency ablation. *Radiology.* 2011;258:270–276. doi;10.1148/radiol.10092440

67. Sharma A, Lanuti M, He W, et al. Increase in fluorodeoxyglucose positron emission tomography activity following complete radiofrequency ablation of lung tumors. *J Comput Assist Tomogr.* 2013;37:9–14. doi:10.1097/RCT.0b013e3182732341

How I Treat Oligometastatic Colorectal Cancer With Adjuvant Chemotherapy

Andrea Cercek and Gustavo dos Santos Fernandes

INTRODUCTION

Metastatic colorectal cancer (CRC) is typically treatable and rarely curable. However, oligometastatic disease, in which only a small number of tumors form in one or two sites, is an outstanding exception. Multiple series have now confirmed that in this setting, cure is achieved in up to 50% of patients who undergo complete metastasectomy, especially if metastases are confined to a single organ and limited in number (<4) (1). Given these promising data and the lack of new systemic treatments for CRC, oligometastatic CRC is generally treated by surgery and other local therapies. For patients with more extensive disease involving multiple organs and/or numerous lesions, systemic cytotoxic chemotherapies are the first line of treatment (2).

Though neither the National Comprehensive Cancer Network (NCCN) nor the European Society for Medical Oncology (ESMO) has defined "oligometastatic disease," from a practical standpoint, it is defined by its amenability to local therapies. Thus, the criteria for local treatment of metastatic CRC vary considerably among institutions.

RATIONALE AND EVIDENCE FOR ADJUVANT CHEMOTHERAPY

While local therapy is the cornerstone treatment for oligometastatic disease, if that eliminates evidence of disease, systemic treatment is a rational option to reduce recurrence risk, as in early-stage disease. A limited number of trials have evaluated the benefit of systemic adjuvant chemotherapy, including single-agent fluoropyrimidine and its combination with oxaliplatin or irinotecan, but have not demonstrated improvements in survival over observation alone.

Single-Agent Fluoropyrimidines

Two randomized clinical trials (RCTs) of similar design evaluated systemic 5-fluorouracil (5-FU) and leucovorin (LV), one in France and one in Europe and Canada, but both were closed prematurely because of low accrual (3,4). The trials randomly assigned patients to either 6 months of postoperative FU and LV or observation alone following complete resection of metastases. A combined analysis of both trials, totaling 278 patients, found nonsignificant differences in median progression-free survival (PFS, 28 vs. 19 months, p = .058) and overall survival (OS, 62 vs. 47 months). More recently, a Japanese RCT with similar design but using uracil–tegafur (UFT)/LV, in 180 patients, found that at a median follow-up of 4.76 years, adjuvant UFT/LV was associated with a significant improvement in 3-year, relapse-free survival (39% vs. 32%; hazard ratio [HR] for relapse 0.56, 95% CI: 0.38–0.83) (5). However, as in the previous trials, there was no difference in OS (83% vs. 82% at 3 years).

Oxaliplatin-Based Regimens

Combination chemotherapy with a fluoropyrimidine and oxaliplatin was found to significantly reduce recurrence risk in patients with stage II or III CRC compared with fluoropyrimidine alone (6–8). To test whether this combination is also more effective in treating microscopic disease, an RCT from the European Organisation for Research and Treatment of Cancer (EORTC) evaluated perioperative FOLFOX chemotherapy (six cycles preoperatively and six postoperatively) versus

---

A Clinical Vignette ("How I Treat") is included at the end of the chapter.

surgery alone in patients with initially resectable liver metastases (9). FOLFOX was associated with an increase in 3-year PFS of 9.2% (from 33.2% to 42.4%; HR 0.73 [0.55–0.97]; *p* = .025) among patients who underwent resection (151 in the perioperative chemotherapy group, of whom 115 received a median of six postoperative cycles, and 152 in the surgery-alone group). In the latest update of this trial, 5-year OS was not significantly better in the chemotherapy group (52% vs. 48%, HR for death 0.88, 95% CI: 0.68–1.14) (10), though the trial was not powered to detect differences in OS. This combination is now considered the standard of care for nonpreviously treated patients with resected or resectable metastatic CRC.

Irinotecan-Based Regimens

Irinotecan is a very active drug in CRC and, in combination with infusional fluoropyrimidine, is one of the main treatments for metastatic CRC. Nonetheless, adding irinotecan to adjuvant regimens never proved to be beneficial in stage II and III CRC (11–13). This combination was evaluated in 321 patients undergoing resection of liver-limited metastases in a multicenter trial; patients were randomly assigned to short-term infusional 5-FU plus LV every other week for 24 weeks without or with irinotecan (180 mg/m² every other week) (14). At a median follow-up of 42 months, there was no significant disease-free survival advantage for adding irinotecan (median 25 vs. 22 months). Table 12.1 summarizes results of the major clinical trials of systemic adjuvant chemotherapy in oligometastatic CRC.

TARGETED THERAPY

Targeted therapy is widely used to treat metastatic CRC. Currently, six drugs of three different classes are approved to treat measurable metastatic disease: bevacizumab, ramucirumab, ziv-aflibercept, cetuximab, panitumumab, and regorafenib. Despite their activity in the metastatic setting, none have proven beneficial for treating micrometastatic disease. In large phase 3 trials, adding bevacizumab or cetuximab to standard adjuvant treatment for stage III disease failed to improve survival (16–18). Ramucirumab, ziv-aflibercept, regorafenib, and TAS-102 have yet to be studied in this setting.

In resected stage IV disease, only cetuximab has been assessed prospectively. In the New EPOC study, perioperative oxaliplatin plus a fluoropyrimidine chemotherapy with or without cetuximab (12 weeks preoperatively and 12 weeks postoperatively) was evaluated in patients with KRAS exon 2 wild-type resectable liver metastases, in which 128 patients were randomized to chemotherapy alone and 129 to chemotherapy with cetuximab (15). Surprisingly, PFS was significantly shorter in the chemotherapy plus cetuximab group than in the chemotherapy alone group (14.1 months vs. 20.5 months, HR 1.48, 95% CI: 1.04–2.12, *p* = .030), despite a higher response rate. Given these data and the lack of benefit

TABLE 12.1 Major Clinical Trials of Systemic Chemotherapy in Oligometastatic CRC

Trial	Treatment Arms	n	mOS (Months)	*p*	mPFS (Months)	*p*
FFCD 9002 and ENG (3)	5-FU	138	62.2	.095	27.9	.058
	Surgery	140	47.3		18.8	
ORTC 40983 (10)	FOLFOX	148*	51.2	.34	20.9	**.035**
	Surgery	152	47.8		12.5	
Ychou et al. (14)	FOLFIRI	153	NR	NA	24.7	.44
	5-FU/LV	153	NR		21.6	
New EPOC (15)	FOLFOX + cetuximab	129	NR	NA	14.1	**.03**
	FOLFOX	128	NR		20.5	

*Number of patients who received chemotherapy and underwent resection. Of these, 115 received postoperative chemotherapy.
5-FU, 5-fluorouracil; CRC, colorectal cancer; LV, leucovorin; m, median; NA, not applicable; NR, not reached; OS, overall survival; PFS, progression-free survival.

from cetuximab as adjuvant treatment for patients with stage II or III colon cancer, the use of cetuximab in this setting cannot be recommended.

HEPATIC ARTERIAL INFUSION (HAI) PLUS SYSTEMIC CHEMOTHERAPY

Despite the curative intent of surgery, in most patients who undergo liver resection for oligo-metastatic CRC, the metastases recur; in approximately half of those patients, the liver is the only site of initial recurrence. Therefore, adjuvant regional chemotherapy administered via the hepatic artery has been investigated. HAI of chemotherapy allows for the delivery of high dose of chemotherapy directly into the liver via a surgically implantable subcutaneous pump with a catheter in the gastroduodenal artery. Systemic chemotherapy has been administered in combination with HAI in most trials.

Two RCTs conducted in the 1990s, one at Memorial Sloan Kettering Cancer Center (MSKCC) and a multicenter study, found that adding HAI floxuridine (FUDR) to systemic flu-orouracil (FU) after resection of liver metastases was beneficial. The first demonstrated an increase in 2-year OS from 72% to 86% (p = .03) (19,20), and the second found a statisti-cally significant reduction in recurrence-free survival (RFS) and hepatic RFS (21). However, a third multicenter study that compared resection followed by HAI 5-FU with resection only was closed prematurely when no difference was found at interim analysis (22). As these trials were performed before the introduction of modern systemic chemotherapy such as oxaliplatin and irinotecan, a retrospective analysis of patients treated at MSKCC from 1992 to 2012 exam-ined the impact of adding HAI to perioperative systemic chemotherapy (23). With a median follow-up of 55 months, the median OS for patients treated with HAI (n = 785) was 67 months versus 44 months for those who did not receive HAI (n = 1,583; p = .001), despite more advanced disease in the HAI group; the difference was similar and equally significant when restricted to patients who received modern systemic chemotherapy. The HR adjusted for pro-pensity score (to control for prognostic factors) also demonstrated longer OS with HAI: 0.67 (95% CI: 0.59–0.76; p = .001).

In our view, HAI is a reasonable treatment option in the adjuvant setting for patients with a high risk of recurrence, especially those who have a limited response to standard neoadjuvant chemotherapy. A broader use of HAI as part of conversion strategies (where chemotherapy is given initially to reduce the size or number of metastases with the intent of rendering them resectable) or palliative treatment may be reasonable in certain situations, but is beyond the scope of this discussion.

ESMO AND NCCN GUIDELINES

The ESMO guidelines recommend proceeding with upfront resection in patients with clearly resectable disease (24). In patients with technically resectable disease where the prognosis is unclear or probably unfavorable, perioperative combination chemotherapy (FOLFOX or CAPOX) should be administered. Targeted agents should not be used in resectable patients where the indication for perioperative treatment is prognostic in nature.

In patients with favorable oncological and technical (surgical) criteria, who have not received perioperative chemotherapy, ESMO does not consider the evidence strong enough to support the use of adjuvant chemotherapy. In patients with unfavorable criteria who have not received any previous chemotherapy, adjuvant treatment with FOLFOX or CAPOX is recommended (unless patients were previously recently exposed to oxaliplatin-based adjuvant chemotherapy).

NCCN guidelines advise upfront surgery for resectable patients, and also suggest periop-erative FOLFOX/XELOX as an option (25). At experienced institutions, HAI with or without systemic chemotherapy is another option. For patients who have previously received chemo-therapy, the guidelines suggest observation rather than chemotherapy following resection.

PERSPECTIVES

Similar to other tumors, treatment of CRC is changing as our knowledge advances regarding its molecular underpinnings. The recent success of anti-PD-1 drugs in patients with mismatch repair deficient metastatic CRC generated overwhelming enthusiasm for immunotherapy

(26,27), but no data is yet available on their efficacy in the adjuvant setting for stage II, III, or resected stage IV disease. One clinical trial, Alliance A021502, is evaluating the addition of pembrolizumab to FOLFOX chemotherapy for patients with stage III microsatellite instability high (MSI-H) CRC. Despite not being directed to stage IV disease, this study will determine whether PD-L1 agents can treat micrometastatic disease.

Approximately 5% of CRCs carry the *BRAF V600* mutation (28), which is associated with a worse prognosis and reduced response to chemotherapy. Recently, clinical trials have shown that combining BRAF inhibitors with chemotherapy and anti-EGFR therapy can increase response rate and PFS in those patients (29,30), but the use of these agents to reduce recurrence following surgery is still investigational.

RECOMMENDATIONS AND CONCLUSIONS

- For patients with resected metastasis who have not previously been exposed to chemotherapy, we recommend 6 months of fluoropyrimidine and oxaliplatin.
- For patients with resected metastasis previously exposed to chemotherapy, we recommend observation.
- For patients whose treatment involves a conversion strategy, we suggest observation or complete chemotherapy for a total of 6 months.
- For patients with resectable metastatic disease limited to the liver, we consider utilization of liver-directed therapy via the HAI pump.

In conclusion, adjuvant therapy in the metastatic setting is dependent on the diagnosis and treatment history of the individual patient.

Clinical Vignette 12.1

Even this subpopulation of metastatic colorectal cancers can present in a variety of clinical scenarios, in which the goals of treatment may be distinct, as not all patients have the same probability of cure. For example, patients with a small burden of disease dispersed among multiple organs, despite having few metastases, are not good candidates for resection and instead may be better candidates for less invasive approaches aiming to extend survival. On the other hand, patients with ≤4 resectable liver or lung metastases have a higher cure rate and should be treated accordingly. Treatment for oligometastatic CRC should be tailored to fit patient characteristics and clinical aims. For discussion purposes, we consider two different cases of oligometastatic CRC:

- A 54-year-old female with a metachronous single liver metastasis from a KRAS-mutant, T3N0 adenocarcinoma of the ascending colon who has not received adjuvant therapy (Figure 12.1)
- A 70-year-old male with a recurrence of CRC involving the para-aortic lymph node and two lung nodules 1 year after finishing adjuvant FOLFOX following resection of a RAS/RAF wild-type T4N1(2/16) adenocarcinoma of the rectosigmoid (Figures 12.2 and 12.3)

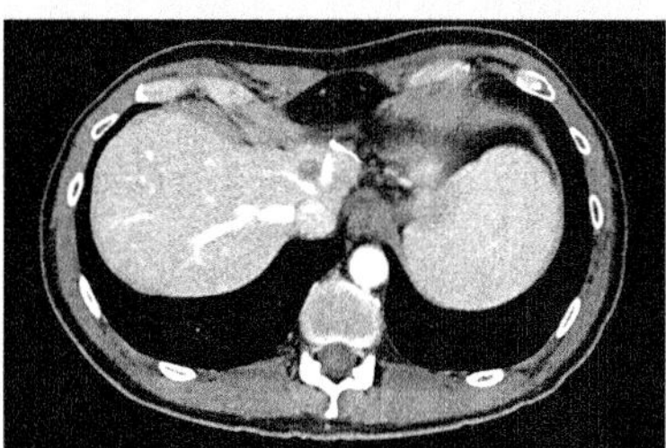

FIGURE 12.1 Single liver metastasis.

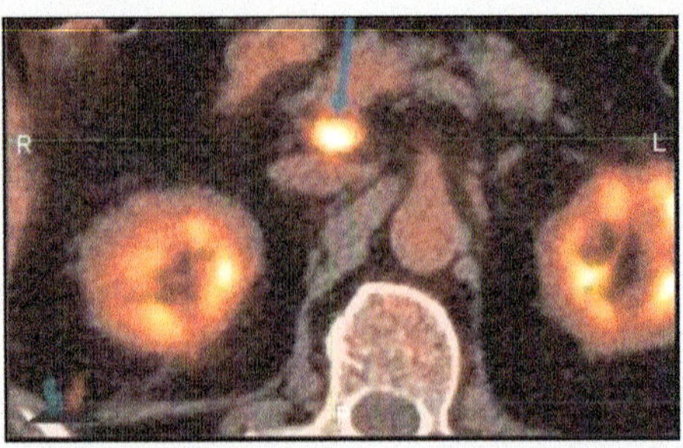

FIGURE 12.2   Para-aortic lymph node metastasis.

Both cases clearly represent oligometastatic disease, but the probability of cure differs greatly between the two, calling for distinct treatment strategies. In the first case, the patient is relatively young, presents initially with oligometastatic disease in only a single organ and a single metastasis, making her a perfect candidate for curative surgery. She would also be offered a combination of fluoropyrimidine and oxaliplatin, which reduces recurrence rates in this setting, though the ideal timing for chemotherapy is debatable. In general, preoperative chemotherapy provides a better understanding of an individual cancer's clinical behavior and sensitivity to chemotherapy, which can inform later treatment decisions, such as whether to continue chemo after resection. If the tumor recurs, this knowledge can also inform selection of the treatment regimen; for example, if the patient had no response to FOLFOX, it may be better to start with FOLFIRI. On the other hand, in rare cases the side effects of chemotherapy can seriously harm the patient and postpone a feasible and potentially curative surgery. Therefore, in patients with ≤3 clearly resectable lesions in the liver or lung, we recommend resecting the tumor first, followed by adjuvant chemotherapy.

The second case can be managed in several ways, all aiming to achieve the same treatment goals. While the cure rate for our first patient is around 50%, the chance of cure for the second is less than 10%; the intent of treatment would be palliative rather than curative. In this particular case, less invasive local treatments such as stereotactic body radiation therapy or radioablation would be better than surgery, as they provide a high rate of local control without the obvious inconvenience of a surgery and its recovery period. There are also two other reasonable approaches for this patient, the first of which is systemic chemotherapy. Chemotherapy would provide a better understanding of the clinical and biological behavior of the disease; if the cancer responds, it would be followed with local therapy. A less conventional but still defensible option is simply to monitor progression, as there are no data suggesting that starting chemo sooner rather than later is beneficial for asymptomatic patients for whom cure is unlikely. In this kind of case, it is important that management be planned in accordance with the patient's wishes and that the intensity of care be agreed upon by both the patient and the physician.

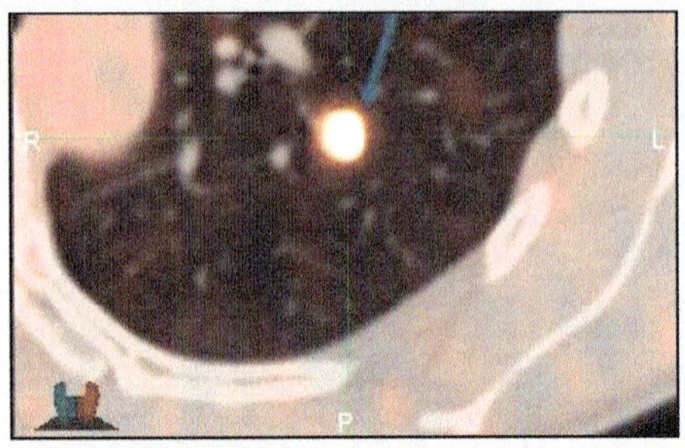

FIGURE 12.3   Low volume lung metastasis.

REFERENCES

1. House MG, Ito H, Gönen M, et al. Survival after hepatic resection for metastatic colorectal cancer: trends in outcomes for 1,600 patients during two decades at a single institution. *J Am Coll Surg.* 2010;210:744–752, 752–745. doi:10.1016/j.jamcollsurg.2009.12.040

2. Fakih MG. Metastatic colorectal cancer: current state and future directions. *J Clin Oncol.* 2015;33:1809–1824. doi:10.1200/jco.2014.59.7633

3. Mitry E, Fields ALA, Bleiberg H, et al. Adjuvant chemotherapy after potentially curative resection of metastases from colorectal cancer: a pooled analysis of two randomized trials. *J Clin Oncol.* 2008;26:4906–4911. doi:10.1200/jco.2008.17.3781

4. Portier G, Elias D, Bouche O, et al. Multicenter randomized trial of adjuvant fluorouracil and folinic acid compared with surgery alone after resection of colorectal liver metastases: FFCD ACHBTH AURC 9002 trial. *J Clin Oncol.* 2006;24:4976–4982. doi:10.1200/jco.2006.06.8353

5. Hasegawa K, Saiura A, Takayama T, et al. Adjuvant oral uracil-tegafur with leucovorin for colorectal cancer liver metastases: a randomized controlled trial. *PLoS One.* 2016;11:e0162400. doi:10.1371/journal.pone.0162400

6. Hong YS, Nam B-H, Kim K, et al. Oxaliplatin, fluorouracil, and leucovorin versus fluorouracil and leucovorin as adjuvant chemotherapy for locally advanced rectal cancer after preoperative chemoradiotherapy (ADORE): an open-label, multicentre, phase 2, randomised controlled trial. *Lancet Oncol.* 2014;15:1245–1253. doi:10.1016/s1470-2045(14)70377-8

7. Sobrero A, Lonardi S, Rosati G, et al. FOLFOX or CAPOX in stage II to III colon cancer: efficacy results of the Italian three or six colon adjuvant trial. *J Clin Oncol.* 2018;36:1478–1485. doi:10.1200/jco.2017.76.2187

8. Andre T, Boni C, Navarro M, et al. Improved overall survival with oxaliplatin, fluorouracil, and leucovorin as adjuvant treatment in stage II or III colon cancer in the MOSAIC trial. *J Clin Oncol.* 2009;27:3109–3116. doi:10.1200/jco.2008.20.6771

9. Nordlinger B, Sorbye H, Glimelius B, et al. Perioperative chemotherapy with FOLFOX4 and surgery versus surgery alone for resectable liver metastases from colorectal cancer (EORTC Intergroup trial 40983): a randomised controlled trial. *Lancet.* 2008;371:1007–1016. doi:10.1016/s0140-6736(08)60455-9

10. Nordlinger B, Sorbye H, Glimelius B, et al. Perioperative FOLFOX4 chemotherapy and surgery versus surgery alone for resectable liver metastases from colorectal cancer (EORTC 40983): long-term results of a randomised, controlled, phase 3 trial. *Lancet Oncol.* 2013;14:1208–1215. doi:10.1016/s1470-2045(13)70447-9

11. Saltz LB, Niedzwiecki D, Hollis D, et al. Irinotecan fluorouracil plus leucovorin is not superior to fluorouracil plus leucovorin alone as adjuvant treatment for stage III colon cancer: results of CALGB 89803. *J Clin Oncol.* 2007;25:3456–3461. doi:10.1200/jco.2007.11.2144

12. Van Cutsem E, Labianca R, Bodoky G, et al. Randomized phase III trial comparing biweekly infusional fluorouracil/leucovorin alone or with irinotecan in the adjuvant treatment of stage III colon cancer: PETACC-3. *J Clin Oncol.* 2009;27:3117–3125. doi:10.1200/jco.2008.21.6663

13. Ychou M, Raoul J-L, Douillard J-Y, et al. A phase III randomised trial of LV5FU2 + irinotecan versus LV5FU2 alone in adjuvant high-risk colon cancer (FNCLCC Accord02/FFCD9802). *Ann Oncol.* 2009;20:674–680. doi:10.1093/annonc/mdn680

14. Ychou M, Hohenberger W, Thezenas S, et al. A randomized phase III study comparing adjuvant 5-fluorouracil/folinic acid with FOLFIRI in patients following complete resection of liver metastases from colorectal cancer. *Ann Oncol.* 2009;20:1964–1970. doi:10.1093/annonc/mdp236

15. Primrose J, Falk S, Finch-Jones M, et al. Systemic chemotherapy with or without cetuximab in patients with resectable colorectal liver metastasis: the New EPOC randomised controlled trial. *Lancet Oncol.* 2014;15:601–611. doi:10.1016/s1470-2045(14)70105-6

16. Allegra CJ, Yothers G, O'Connell MJ, et al. Bevacizumab in stage II-III colon cancer: 5-year update of the National Surgical Adjuvant Breast and Bowel Project C-08 trial. *J Clin Oncol.* 2013;31:359–364. doi:10.1200/jco.2012.44.4711

17. de Gramont A, Cutsem EV, Schmoll H-J, et al. Bevacizumab plus oxaliplatin-based chemotherapy as adjuvant treatment for colon cancer (AVANT): a phase 3 randomised controlled trial. *Lancet Oncol.* 2012;13:1225–1233. doi:10.1016/s1470-2045(12)70509-0

18. Taieb J, Balogoun R, Le Malicot K, et al. Adjuvant FOLFOX +/− cetuximab in full RAS and BRAF wildtype stage III colon cancer patients. *Ann Oncol.* 2017;28:824–830. doi:10.1093/annonc/mdw687

19. Kemeny N, Huang Y, Cohen AM, et al. Hepatic arterial infusion of chemotherapy after resection of hepatic metastases from colorectal cancer. *N Engl J Med.* 1999;341:2039–2048. doi:10.1056/nejm199912303412702

20. Kemeny NE, Gonen M. Hepatic arterial infusion after liver resection. *N Engl J Med.* 2005;352:734–735. doi:10.1056/nejm200502173520723

21. Kemeny MM, Adak S, Gray B, et al. Combined-modality treatment for resectable metastatic colorectal carcinoma to the liver: surgical resection of hepatic metastases in combination with continuous infusion of chemotherapy--an intergroup study. *J Clin Oncol.* 2002;20:1499–1505. doi:10.1200/jco.2002.20.6.1499

22. Lorenz M, Müller H-H, Schramm H, et al. Randomized trial of surgery versus surgery followed by adjuvant hepatic arterial infusion with 5-fluorouracil and folinic acid for liver metastases of colorectal cancer. German Cooperative on Liver Metastases (Arbeitsgruppe Lebermetastasen). *Ann Surg.* 1998;228:756–762. doi:10.1097/00000658-199812000-00006

23. Groot Koerkamp B, Sadot E, Kemeny NE, et al. Perioperative hepatic arterial infusion pump chemotherapy is associated with longer survival after resection of colorectal liver metastases: a propensity score analysis. *J Clin Oncol.* 2017;35:1938–1944. doi:10.1200/jco.2016.71.8346

24. Van Cutsem E, Cervantes A, Adam R, et al. ESMO consensus guidelines for the management of patients with metastatic colorectal cancer. *Ann Oncol.* 2016;27:1386–1422. doi:10.1093/annonc/mdw235

25. Benson AB, Venook AP, Panel NG. *NCCN Clinical Practice Guidelines in Oncology: Colon Cancer.* https://www.nccn.org/professionals/physician_gls/pdf/colon.pdf; 2018.

26. Overman MJ, McDermott R, Leach JL, et al. Nivolumab in patients with metastatic DNA mismatch repair-deficient or microsatellite instability-high colorectal cancer (CheckMate 142): an open-label, multicentre, phase 2 study. *Lancet Oncol.* 2017;18:1182–1191. doi:10.1016/s1470-2045(17)30422-9

27. Le DT, Durham JN, Smith KN, et al. Mismatch repair deficiency predicts response of solid tumors to PD-1 blockade. *Science.* 2017;357:409–413. doi:10.1126/science.aan6733

28. Sclafani F, Gullo G, Sheahan K, et al. BRAF mutations in melanoma and colorectal cancer: a single oncogenic mutation with different tumour phenotypes and clinical implications. *Crit Rev Oncol Hematol.* 2013;87:55–68. doi:10.1016/j.critrevonc.2012.11.003

29. Hyman DM, Puzanov I, Subbiah V, et al. Vemurafenib in Multiple Nonmelanoma Cancers with BRAF V600 Mutations. *N Engl J Med.* 2015;373:726–736. doi:10.1056/NEJMoa1502309

30. Yaeger RD, Cercek A, O'Reilly EM, et al. Pilot study of vemurafenib and panitumumab combination therapy in patients with BRAF V600E mutated metastatic colorectal cancer. *J Clin Oncol.* 2015;33:611–611. doi:10.1200/jco.2015.33.3_suppl.611

How I Treat Oligometastatic Colorectal Cancer With Debulking/HIPEC in Limited Peritoneal Disease

Edward A. Levine

Key Points

1. Clinical factors such as age, comorbidities, smoking, and functional and nutritional status are important to minimize morbidity from cytoreductive surgery (CRS) and hyperthermic intraperitoneal chemotherapy (HIPEC).
2. Response to neoadjuvant chemotherapy and extent and volume of distribution of disease on imaging and or laparoscopy are important for selecting patients for CRS and HIPEC.
3. Peritoneal cancer index (PCI) ≤20 for colorectal cancer (CRC) for CRS and HIPEC.
4. PCI, experience, performance status, and completeness of resection are key outcome variables.
5. Long-term survival is possible with aggressive surgical therapy for peritoneal metastases from CRC.

INTRODUCTION

Colorectal cancer (CRC) is the third most common cancer worldwide (1) and up to 20% of the patients have distant metastases at the time of diagnosis (2). Approximately one-fifth of these will have isolated peritoneal spread (3) and peritoneal metastases are the third most common site of recurrence of CRC (after liver and lung) (4). Over the past two decades, the treatment of metastatic CRC has improved with new chemotherapeutic and biologic agents. These newer agents have improved the median overall survival (OS) for some stage IV CRC patients to 20+ months and beyond (5). However, when patients present with isolated colorectal hepatic metastases or pulmonary metastases, surgical resection has been shown in multiple large retrospective series to provide 5-year survival rates of 25% to 40% with a median OS of 30 to 40 months (6–8). Based on such data and the improved safety of hepatic resection using modern operative techniques and better critical care support, an aggressive surgical approach to isolated metastatic disease to the liver has become the standard of care accepted by oncologists of all disciplines. Resection of isolated pulmonary metastases has similar long-term outcomes. However, the resection and therapy of isolated peritoneal metastases has been more controversial.

Historically, peritoneal metastases were treated with therapeutic nihilism; patients typically received palliative chemotherapy and all too frequently permanent colostomy (9). Since there are no specific symptoms of peritoneal metastasis, it is often discovered in a very advanced stage with its attendant poor survival. However, the prognosis of patients with metastasis from CRC has significantly improved since the turn of the century. At the time of initial diagnosis of CRC, the peritoneal surface has metastatic disease in 10% to 15% of patients (10–14). After the liver, peritoneal surface disease (PSD) is the most common site for recurrence after curative primary tumor surgery, occurring in up to 50% of patients. In 10% to 35% of all patients with recurrent disease, PSD is the only site of cancer (11,12). Patients with isolated PSD from

---

A Clinical Vignette ("How I Treat") is included at the end of the chapter.

CRC have traditionally been treated with systemic therapy, which has clearly improved significantly since the turn of the century (5). The availability of newer agents such as oxaliplatin and irinotecan and biologic agents such as cetuximab, panitumumab, and bevacizumab has more than doubled the survival with systemic therapy alone (5,15). There are no randomized trials of modern systemic therapy limited to patients with PSD. However, there is a relevant retrospective study of the NCCTG 9741 and 9841 trials of systemic therapy for metastatic colon cancer stratified response by site of metastases (15). That study clearly showed inferior outcomes with "modern" systemic therapy for patients with peritoneal metastases compared with metastases to other sites (12.7 versus 17.6 months OS, $p < .001$, and 5.8 versus 7.2 months progression-free survival, $p < .001$). Despite this poorer outcome, it is noteworthy that with "modern" chemotherapy, there were a few 5-year survivors (4.1% with peritoneal metastases and 6% without peritoneal metastases), which represents a clear change from the era before newer agents for metastatic CRC became available when there were none reported (15).

The development of an aggressive regional therapeutic approach for peritoneal disease from CRC consisting of resection of peritoneal surface malignancy (PSM), also known as cytoreductive surgery (CRS), followed with intraperitoneal adjuvants such as hyperthermic intraperitoneal chemotherapy (HIPEC), has significantly improved outcomes. The use of CRS and HIPEC for PSD from CRC is a more recent development in oncologic surgery. Although originally described by Spratt in 1980 (16), the concept of aggressive cytoreduction and HIPEC was initially investigated by a handful of centers (9–11,17). The rationale for CRS for PSD is based on the premise that the peritoneum represents an organ site (such as liver or lung), which can be completely resected, with HIPEC or other intraperitoneal agents being used as an "adjuvant" to treat microscopic residual disease. The literature supporting such an approach is not as extensive as it is for hepatic resection; it mainly consists of many single institutional series, international multicenter retrospective reviews, and only three prospective randomized trials (18–20). Yet the reported outcomes are remarkably consistent, demonstrating 5-year OS rates of approximately 25% to 40% for patients undergoing a complete cytoreduction.

Despite the publication of consensus statements on the role of CS and HIPEC for PSD from CRC (21), the controversy continues regarding its efficacy, safety, and application in these patients. In contrast to hepatic resection, which is performed at virtually all major cancer centers worldwide, only a handful of high volume institutions have significant experience in this procedure. Due to the nature of this disease presentation, the surgical procedures required for complete cytoreduction of PSD have been associated with significant (but improving) (9,10,22) postoperative morbidity and mortality, which stresses patients, healthcare resources, and personnel.

PATIENT SELECTION FOR PERITONEAL CYTOREDUCTION FROM CRC

CRS and HIPEC is a major surgical undertaking that puts patients at risk for substantial postoperative morbidity and even mortality. According to an analysis of the National Surgical Quality Improvement Program (NSQIP) database, patients undergoing CRS and HIPEC have an average hospital stay of 13 days, an 11% readmission rate, an overall morbidity rate of >33%, and a mortality rate of 2% (23). In his presidential address to the Society of Surgical Oncology (SSO), Dr. Blake Cady stated that, "In the world of surgical oncology, biology is king; selection of cases is queen, and the technical details of surgical procedures are princes and princesses of the realm who frequently try to overthrow the powerful forces of the king and queen, usually to no long-term avail, although with some temporary apparent victories." This is particularly true for peritoneal metastases from CRC. Much of the long learning curve for the performance of CRS for peritoneal metastases from CRC lies in better patient selection.

It is imperative that appropriate candidates be selected for CRS and HIPEC for peritoneal dissemination from any site, but particularly for CRC. All colonic and proximal rectal primary tumors should be considered for HIPEC, although distal rectal cancers are rarely candidates (24). Although the appendix is anatomically part of the colon, the biology of low-grade appendiceal neoplasms is substantially different from most CRCs and is not addressed in this chapter. Major centers with significant experience and high case volumes have shorter hospital stays and lower morbidity and mortality rates, suggesting that experience is important in minimizing the adverse events attendant to these procedures. Both the individual and institutional learning curves are steep and long (25,26). Extensive prior surgery, recent smoking history, poor nutrition, diabetes, transfusion, poor functional status (Eastern Cooperative Oncology

Group [ECOG] >1), increasing number of visceral resections, higher peritoneal cancer index (PCI), longer operative times, transfusion, incomplete cytoreductions, and in some studies, advanced age (>70), correlated with higher risks of major morbidity (9–11,27–29). It is crucial to use the preoperative factors to guide patient selection, and all patients should be clearly informed of the substantial risks of morbidity, colostomy, and mortality prior to CRS and HIPEC.

Preoperative evaluation includes a complete history and thorough physical examination detailing comorbidities and functional status. Routine studies include review of biopsy material, contrast-enhanced CT or MRI, and laboratory examination including blood counts, carcinoembryonic antigen (CEA) levels renal and liver function panel. Endoscopy (if not done within the past 2 years) should be considered to seek additional primary lesions, and diagnostic laparoscopy (DL) has also been employed selectively to determine the resectability of PSD prior to CRS–HIPEC.

The social history should focus on patient support available to the patient, smoking, and use of alcohol and anxiolytics. Smoking cessation should be encouraged (30,31). A Cochrane review found that smoking cessation 4 to 8 weeks prior to surgery was associated with decreased postoperative complications and since many patients will be receiving chemotherapy for months prior to surgery there is ample time. Nutritional status must be assessed with body mass index, recent weight changes, body habitus, and albumin levels. Nutritional prehabilitation for malnourished patients has been shown in a systematic review to be associated with reductions in morbidity, length of stay, and infectious complications (32,33). Parenteral nutrition is occasionally necessary to replenish nutritional reserves in the perioperative period.

The volume of PSD is a key patient selection criterion. The PCI score is based on the amount of disease in each of the 13 abdominopelvic regions and does not stratify points based on the ease or difficulty of resecting the organs/structures within the abdominopelvic region (34). Also, preoperative imaging (via either CT or MRI) consistently underestimates the extent of disease. The PCI has been identified in several large cohort studies to be a major prognostic factor. Recently, Goere et al. even concluded that CRS and HIPEC does not offer any survival benefit in patients with a PCI score of 17 or higher (34). Others have demonstrated this as well reporting <10% 5-year OS for those with a PCI ≥17. I currently use a PCI cutoff >20 for CRC patients.

The following are selection criteria for consideration of CRS and HIPEC:

1. Stability or response of tumor to neoadjuvant systemic chemotherapy seen on imaging
2. The volume of disease on imaging must appear to be completely resectable
3. No evidence of extraperitoneal metastasis
4. No significant retroperitoneal or pericaval/periaortic lymphadenopathy
5. ECOG performance status ≤2
6. No evidence of extra-abdominal disease
7. Up to three small, resectable parenchymal hepatic metastases (resectable liver metastases are not a contraindication to CRS/HIPEC)
8. No evidence of biliary obstruction
9. No evidence of ureteral obstruction
10. No evidence of intestinal obstruction at more than one site
11. Small bowel involvement: no evidence of gross disease that would require >2 anastomoses and/or leave <100 cm of small bowel beyond the ligament of Treitz
12. No evidence of voluminous ascites

Diagnostic Laparoscopy

DL for staging is an excellent tool for assessing candidacy for CRS, which I employ selectively. The technique for DL I typically perform is a thorough evaluation of the abdominal cavity using a video port and one instrument port, gaining access with an Optiview cannula in the left upper quadrant. Adhesiolysis is performed only to the extent needed to provide adequate visualization. Particular attention is paid to the small bowel serosa as well as disease in the porta hepatis as these areas are particularly difficult to clear during cytoreduction. The PCI must be calculated at the time of DL, and I use a PCI >20 as a relatively strong contraindication for proceeding to cytoreduction for CRC. In addition, peritoneal biopsy and cytology can be obtained at the time of DL, which is particularly important for genetic studies in patients judged not to be candidates for CRS.

Patients considered amenable to CRS and HIPEC at laparoscopy are more likely to obtain complete cytoreduction (35–37). However, it must be kept in mind that even a favorable DL is not a guarantee of a compete cytoreduction. A multi-institutional study reported a successful completion of DL in 92.6% of patients with minimal morbidity and no port-site recurrence at short-term follow-up. Depending on the criteria utilized, DL can identify up to 31% of patients who have too extensive a disease burden for complete cytoreduction and thus spare them a nontherapeutic major laparotomy.

Additional adverse selection factors should include progression of disease through neo-adjuvant therapy and the presence of signet ring cells. However, long-term survival can be achieved in these patients with poor biology if complete cytoreduction can be achieved and therefore these are not *absolute* contraindications to CRS and HIPEC (34, 40). Patients with progression may be treated with additional chemotherapy or immunotherapy in an attempt to achieve response prior to reconsideration for CRS and HIPEC.

CRS AND HIPEC—CONDUCT OF THE OPERATION

Frank discussions with the patient regarding the magnitude of the resection's impact on life-style, including the possible need for colostomy or ileostomy formation, and the potential loss of mobility, fertility, and even mortality are required. Patients with preoperative imaging, which suggests the need for splenectomy, should undergo vaccinations for encapsulated organisms preoperatively. Preoperative consultations by anesthesia, enterostomal therapy nurses (if a stoma is anticipated), and potentially urology (for ureteral stent placement should complex pelvic anatomy from tumor or previous surgery require it) should be obtained. Mechanical bowel preparation, with oral antibiotics, is given the day prior to surgery. Preoperative antibiotics are given intravenously, and deep venous thrombosis prophylaxis using both chemical and mechanical approaches is appropriate. Patients are positioned in the supine position and cushioned as appropriate for the potentially lengthy operative intervention. If a rectal anastomosis is anticipated, lithotomy position is considered. General anesthesia may be supplemented with epidural catheters for postoperative analgesia. Arterial line monitoring is helpful for most patients. For patients with complex pelvic disease or extensive prior pelvic surgery, placement of externalized ureteral stents by urologic consultants is frequently a time-saving procedure. Patients are typically prepped from the mid chest (should tube thoracostomy be required) to the proximal thigh. Nasogastric and urinary catheters are routinely placed. Core temperature monitoring in the esophagus and/or bladder should be arranged with the anesthesia team.

SURGICAL TECHNIQUE

The goal of cytoreduction is the removal of all grossly apparent disease, while preserving organ function (38). I do not recommend peritonectomy procedures in the absence of visible disease. Although some patients with very low peritoneal disease burden may be approached laparoscopically, most cases are best approached with a generous midline incision. After making the incision, self-retaining retractors are deployed. The abdomen must be thoroughly and completely explored at this point, which requires lysis of *all* adhesions. The peritoneal carcinomatosis index is the most commonly utilized descriptor of tumor volume, and should be determined (range of 0–39) at this point (39). An assessment of the extent of visceral involvement must then be undertaken to direct planning for the remainder of the case. Close attention to the extent of small bowel disease is critical. Many cases have relative sparing of the small bowel, which facilitates complete resections. Resections that leave the patient with less than 100 cm small bowel (and attendant permanent short gut syndrome) should be avoided. The key assessment is whether the complete cytoreduction is feasible or if a palliative resection is all that can be achieved. The majority of patients (>90%), if properly assessed preoperatively, should be able to undergo a complete cytoreduction procedure.

Following evaluation of the peritoneal disease burden, an operative plan should then be formulated. Resecting the primary tumor (if not resected previously), as well as all gross disease, and determining which organs must be resected, should be thought out carefully. The necessity of peritoniectomy procedures should be decided upon so that the plan can be shared with the operative team.

The resection phase of the procedure begins with an omentectomy and is facilitated by entering the lesser sac just outside of the gastroepiploic arcades. If there is disease on the gastroepiploic arteries, they should be resected. However, resection preserving the gastroepiploic vessels can minimize delayed gastric emptying postoperatively. If the spleen has disease on its capsule, it should be resected, as stripping the splenic capsule is frequently associated with prohibitive loss. The spleen can be resected with the gastrosplenic ligament and omentum as a single unit. The left diaphragm can be stripped at this time, although it is not commonly needed for CRC.

The small bowel should be run from the ligament of Treitz to the ileocecal valve, removing disease from the mesentery as well as the serosa of the bowel. For predominantly mucinous lesions, an ultrasonic surgical aspirator can facilitate resection of small modules particularly on the mesentery. For more sclerotic lesions, an argon beam coagulator or plasma jet dissector can be helpful. Caution must be taken with the serosal implants; if the muscular wall must be resected to clear the implants, they should immediately be repaired with Lembert sutures. If small bowel resection is necessary, measurement *with a ruler* of residual small bowel, beyond the ligament of Treitz, after all resections are completed, should be performed prior to resecting. Rarely should more than two anastomoses be required.

The colon and mesocolon is then run in a similar fashion. The tenia epiploicae are a frequent site of peritoneal metastasis and these should be resected if diseased. When amputating tenia epiploica, it is important to be cautious not to open a colonic diverticulum. Should a colonic diverticulum be encountered, it should be closed with suture and oversewn with 3-0 Lembert sutures.

The pelvis is dealt with next, and follows clearance of the distal sigmoid colon. The pelvic cul-de-sac should be thoroughly inspected as it is a frequent site of "drop metastasis." This can usually be dissected off the rectum without the need for proctectomy. Should there be significant disease found on the anterior rectum which cannot be removed without resection, proctectomy should be undertaken to remove gross disease. A restorative anastomosis is usually feasible; however, proximal diversion is routinely performed to minimize the risk of a leak after perfusion with any rectal anastomosis. The internal inguinal rings should always be inspected for metastasis and cleared of any grossly apparent disease. This may require resection of the gonadal vessels in some cases. Pelvic peritoniectomy procedures may be required to clear gross disease. They are not required when no disease is apparent. If needed, the stripping of the peritoneum should begin at the superior portion of the bladder and proceed ever deeper into the pelvis. The bladder muscle can be thin at the dome, and care must be taken to avoid cystotomy. However, if the tumor is adherent to the bladder, a partial cystectomy can be performed and closed in two layers with 3-0 absorbable suture. The peritoniectomy can be taken around the cul-de-sac onto either the uterus or the rectum and laterally onto the pelvic sidewalls if needed.

In women, the ovary is a common site of metastasis and should be resected when any disease is apparent upon the ipsilateral tube or ovary. A hysterectomy is required only if there is disease that cannot be removed from the surface of the uterus. A supracervical hysterectomy is a reasonable choice if disease does not extend beyond the neck of the uterus. If there is disease encroaching upon the neck of the uterus or the cervix, a complete hysterectomy is then appropriate.

The upper quadrants of the abdomen are then addressed. Involvement of the right diaphragm is much more common than the left. The lesser omentum can be resected off the stomach while preserving the nerves of Latarjet when feasible if disease is present. If lesser omental disease requires division of both the nerves of Latarjet, a pyloromyotomy should be considered. The round ligament of the liver should be resected deep into the umbilical fissure of the liver, as it is a common site for metastasis and recurrence. The lesser sac is widely exposed at this point and disease should be cleared from it at this time. Should disease be found to be adherent to the stomach, partial gastrectomy is preferred. Total gastrectomy is rarely necessary, and should be undertaken *only* if it is the limiting site to complete cytoreduction, and in cases where substantial small bowel resection is not required, as a Roux-en-y reconstruction would be necessary.

The right upper quadrant is dealt with next. The porta hepatis should be carefully inspected. Bulk disease on the hepatoduodenal ligament which cannot be cleared is a contraindication to chemotherapy perfusion and should have been assessed in the initial evaluation. The peritoneum on the anterior surface of the hepatoduodenal ligament can be stripped while preserving the vasculature and bile duct. Should disease be found on the gallbladder, a cholecystectomy is indicated. If there is disease on the right diaphragm, mobilization of the right lobe of the liver is required, and must include division of the right triangular ligament. Frequently, peritoneal disease on the_right diaphragm can be stripped entirely as the tumor tends to thicken and stiffen the peritoneum. However, this is not feasible in all cases. Peritonectomy of the right diaphragm should begin just beneath the ribs to proceed progressively deeper into the abdomen. High-power cautery and good traction/countertraction facilitate this maneuver. A Cobb dissector can also be quite helpful in stripping the diaphragm. Should disease be apparent in the right gutter, the anterior lamina of Gerota's fascia can be resected with the right diaphragm stripping as a single unit. If disease is found on a portion of the diaphragm that cannot be stripped, full thickness resection of the diaphragm can be performed, with closure using a non-absorbable suture. A tube thoracostomy can then be placed with fresh gloves and instruments to try to avoid pleural contamination with cancer cells.

Disease on the liver capsule can be stripped as individual metastases if limited in number. If larger areas of disease or confluent disease are found, the entire liver capsule can be stripped off by incising the capsule and bluntly removing large areas of the capsule. Hemostasis is typically not difficult to obtain after parietal peritoneal stripping, and may be facilitated by high-power cautery or an argon beam coagulator.

Whether to perform restorative anastomoses at this time or after the perfusion is controversial. I have found it advantageous to perform the anastomosis, prior to perfusion, to allow them to be inspected after the perfusion is complete. While this has the theoretical risk of not perfusing tissue incorporated into the anastomoses, I have not found failure at these sites to be problematic with this approach.

HIPEC ADMINISTRATION

The delivery of intraperitoneal chemotherapy can be performed with either an open or closed technique. The open technique requires the abdomen to be open and filled with fluid during the time of perfusion. Since evaporation with chemotherapy vapor is attendant to this technique, it may violate occupational and health and safety administration rules, which vary state by state. I use exclusively a closed abdominal technique to avoid this issue (9). The closed technique requires placement of cannulas for inflow and outflow. I use two inflow and two outflow cannulas, which is a simple system that works well. Inflow cannulas, of 22 French, are placed via small incisions and carried through the subcutaneous tissue into the pelvis or lower quadrants. The outflow cannulas, of 34 French, are placed via separate incisions, through the subcutaneous tissue and positions in the upper quadrants. A device to diffuse suction is required on the outflow cannulas to avoid suction injuries to the bowel. The skin is then temporarily closed with a running suture. Each cannula is also sutured in position. The two inflow and two outflow cannulas are connected with Y-connectors. One-quarter inch tubing is connected to the inflow cannulas, and three-eighths inch tubing is connected to the outflow cannulas. The tubing is then connected to the pump to complete the circuit.

Thermistors are attached to the inflow and outflow to monitor temperature. A 3 L crystalloid solution is used to prime the circuit. The perfusion pump and heat exchanger manipulate the temperature of the perfusate. Gentle massage of the abdomen should remove all air from the peritoneal cavity. Toward the end of the extirpative portion of the procedure, communication with the anesthesia service should allow for discontinuation of warning devices to allow the patient to passively cool to approximately 35°C. The perfusate inflow is warmed to ~42°C and manipulated to maintain outflow temperatures of 40°C.

When the perfusion circuit is stabilized, the chemotherapy is then introduced. Mitomycin C is the most commonly used chemotherapeutic agent at most centers. Typically, 30 mg is given at the initiation of perfusion, with an additional 10 mg dose given into the circuit 1 hour into the perfusion, to maintain drug levels in the circuit. Oxaliplatin is an alternative agent, more commonly utilized in Europe. I use a dose of 200 mg/M^2 of oxaliplatin as a single dose into the HIPEC circuit. Most centers perfuse the peritoneum for 60 to 120 minutes (our protocol is for 120 minutes), at a flow rate of at least 1 L per minute. At the end of the perfusion, the circuit is drained, the abdomen reopened, the retractor repositioned, and the cannulas removed. I redose systemic antibiotics at this time as antibiotic levels are washed out with the perfusate.

RE-EXPLORATION AND DEFINITIVE CLOSURE

After completion of the perfusion, the self-retaining retractor is replaced, all cannulas are removed, and the abdomen is re-explored. Complete hemostasis is then confirmed.

Anastomoses are inspected, and if a colostomy or ileostomy is required it is created at this point. The nasogastric tube should be confirmed to be in good position. Typically, a naso-jejunal feeding tube is positioned in the proximal jejunum to facilitate early postoperative enteral alimentation.

Fascial closure is performed with absorbable number one suture. The subcutaneous tissue can be approximated if thick and the skin closed at the midline, as well as at the cannula sites. If a stoma is required, it is then matured and dressed with an appropriate appliance. The patients are typically extubated and taken to the recovery area. Intensive care unit monitoring is required for approximately half of the cases. Operative dictation should be completed immediately following the procedure to ensure that all relevant details are crisply recalled. Long-term follow-up is greatly facilitated by notes that include the areas where disease was encountered, the peritoneal carcinomatosis index, and the completeness of resection, as well as the volume of residual disease if any.

Patients undergoing substantial resection with HIPEC typically stay in the ICU overnight. Antibiotics are discontinued after the day of surgery. Patients are encouraged to be out of bed on the first postoperative day and on their feet the second day. Ureteral stents (if placed) are removed if there are no urinary clots, typically on the first postoperative day, with the urinary catheter removed on the second day. Patients with nasojejunal feeding tubes have nutrition initiated the day after the procedure. Venous thrombosis prophylaxis is continued with fractionated heparin *and* sequential compression stockings, with the fractionated heparin continued for a few weeks after discharge.

CLINICAL TRIALS

The first randomized trial with CRS and HIPEC was conducted in Holland, beginning in 1998, and randomized patients to CRS and HIPEC with systemic chemotherapy versus systemic chemotherapy alone (18). Despite the high perioperative mortality (8% in this study), the trial found nearly a doubling of survival compared to the control arm (22.3 months vs. 12.6 months median OS). Patients in whom a complete cytoreduction was unobtainable had survival that was similar to those treated with systemic chemotherapy alone and these patients clearly did not benefit from cytoreduction. Long-term follow-up demonstrates a median survival of 48 months and a 5-year survival of 45% for those patients for whom a complete cytoreduction could be achieved (18,40). This randomized trial was not only critical in establishing cytoreduction and HIPEC as a potential standard of care in patients with peritoneal metastasis from CRC, but it also demonstrated that in carefully selected patients, perioperative morbidity and mortality could be reduced and long-term survival obtained. A smaller, but similar randomized trial was performed in Sweden, reaching the same conclusions.

Despite difficulties in conducting prospective randomized trials for PSD from CRC, several centers have persevered, with European centers making significant progress. The French Prodige 7 trial randomized patients with peritoneal dissemination from colon cancer after *complete* cytoreduction to observation or HIPEC (with oxaliplatin 460 mg/M^2 for 30 minutes at 42°C). This trial of 280 patients was reported in abstract form at the American Society of Clinical Oncology meeting in Chicago in June, 2018 (19). The study was initially reported as a negative trial overall; however, the results of this study were positive for a benefit for intermediate levels of PCI. However, at the Paris 2018 Peritoneal Surface Oncology Group International (PSOGI) meeting, a reanalysis of the data using patients who crossed over to HIPEC in the analysis rather than intention to treat was positive for a benefit for HIPEC. The utility of this trial will be debated since both the high dose of oxaliplatin and short duration HIPEC are not commonly utilized outside of France. Further, this technique for HIPEC is associated with a 15% rate of late postoperative bleeding and will not become a standard regimen. A key conclusion of the Prodige 7 trial is the favorable impact of the CRS, the finding of a 5-year survival of 36.7% clearly establishing CRS in the treatment of peritoneal metastases.

Another French trial reported in June of 2018 is the PROPHYLOCHIP trial (41), which randomized 150 patients with CRC at very high risk for peritoneal metastases, after 6 months of adjuvant chemotherapy and no sign of disease to surveillance versus systematic second look surgery and HIPEC. During second look surgery, peritoneal disease was found in 52% with a PCI of 4. The surveillance group would find clinical peritoneal recurrence in 33%, of whom 64% underwent CRS and HIPEC. There was no difference in 3-year disease-free survival (44% vs. 51%) or OS (80% vs. 79%) with early intervention. This study confirms the importance of close follow-up of at-risk patients for peritoneal progression, but did not find an advantage to early intervention for CRS and HIPEC for CRC.

Another interesting trial from the French group is the Prodige 15 study, which plans for 130 patients, evaluating "high-risk" colorectal patients (those with perforation, ovarian metastasis, or a few peritoneal lesions completely resected with the primary lesion) and randomizing them, after 6 months of adjuvant systemic therapy to surveillance or second look surgery with HIPEC.

Despite substantial sustained efforts, randomized surgical trials have proven difficult to perform in the United States, and to date none have been completed for CRC in the Western hemisphere. Further, cooperative group trials are not currently on the horizon in North America. The ICARuS trial is currently accruing patients with CRC and appendiceal peritoneal metastases at several sites in the United States. The study randomizes patients achieving "optimal" cytoreduction to either HIPEC with mitomycin C or early postoperative intraperitoneal chemotherapy with floxuridine (FUDR). The study plan is for 212 patients with accrual likely to be completed in 2019.

CONCLUSIONS

The role of CRS for peritoneal disease from CRC is clearly established for appendiceal cancer, ovarian cancer, and peritoneal mesothelioma. The outcomes for CRS for colon cancer with complete resection of peritoneal metastases are not substantially different from that found with hepatic resection (42,43). Long-term disease-free survival is possible when complete cytoreduction can be achieved. Consequently, treating all patients with peritoneal metastasis with therapeutic nihilism is clearly no longer appropriate.

Although there are some who have suggested that CRS and intraperitoneal chemotherapy is an alternative to systemic chemotherapy, for peritoneal metastasis from colon cancer, it is best approached *with* systemic chemotherapy *and not* in lieu of it. Close collaboration between medical oncologists and surgical oncologists experienced in the evaluation of, and operative therapy for, peritoneal disease is important to optimize the survival of patients with metastases from colorectal carcinoma (44). Based upon currently available data, surgery with intraperitoneal chemotherapy should be considered for patients with isolated peritoneal disease who are otherwise fit.

Clinical Vignette 13.1

Case 1: An otherwise fit 53-year-old man is found to have peritoneal dissemination, with low volume ascites at the time of a sigmoid resection for a nearly obstructing adenocarcinoma. Imaging finds no extra-abdominal disease. The operative note describes only "multiple" peritoneal metastases on viscera. Pathology confirms a T3N2M1 adenocarcinoma with peritoneal metastases. He is referred to a medical oncologist, who treats the patient with FOLFOX and Avastin, and the CT scan after six cycles reveals "stable" disease. He is referred for consideration of CRS and HIPEC. To evaluate him for this, he undergoes diagnostic laparoscopy and is found to have moderate ascites and a PCI of 23. He is referred back to medical oncology for consideration of a second-line regimen, or clinical trial. Outcomes for patients with PCI scores over 15–20, particularly those who do not respond or progress, are poor candidates for CRS and HIPEC.

Case 2: An otherwise fit 53-year-old man is found to have low peritoneal dissemination to the omentum without ascites at the time of a staging CT obtained for a nonobstructing sigmoid adenocarcinoma. His medical oncologist refers the patient for evaluation for CRS and HIPEC. The surgical oncologist obtains a CEA determination (18.2) at the HIPEC center and suggests preoperative oxaliplatin-based chemotherapy. The patient receives six cycles of FOLFOX with bevacizumab. This regimen is well tolerated and the CEA level decreases from 18.2 to 7.1. The patient is taken to the operating room where CRS including a left colectomy, omentectomy, and left abdominal/pelvic peritoniectomy and complete resection of all gross disease is achieved (R1 or CC-0 resection) and HIPEC with mitomycin (40 mg at 40°C). Final pathology confirms a T3N1M1 with two nodes positive and an excellent response to chemotherapy. After recovery, he returns to the medical oncologist for completion of an additional six cycles and then moves into long-term follow-up.

REFERENCES

1. Parkin DM, Bray F, Ferlay J, et al. Global cancer statistics, 2002. *CA Cancer J Clin*. 2005;55(2):74–108. doi:10.3322/canjclin.55.2.74
2. Howlader N, Noone A, Krapcho M, et al. SEER Cancer Statistics Review, 1975-2014, National Cancer Institute. *Bethesda, MD, based on November 2016 SEER data submission, posted to the SEER web site*. April 2017. https://seer.cancer.gov/data
3. Segelman J, Granath F, Holm T, et al. Incidence, prevalence and risk factors for peritoneal carcinomatosis from colorectal cancer. *Br J Surg*. 2012;99(5):699–705. doi:10.1002/bjs.86794.
4. Goéré D, Sourrouille I, Gelli M, et al. Peritoneal metastases from colorectal cancer: treatment principles and perspectives. *Surg Oncol Clin N Am*. 2018;27:563–583. doi:10.1016/j.soc.2018.02.011
5. Kelly H, Goldberg RM. Systemic therapy for metastatic colorectal cancer: current options, current evidence. *J Clin Oncol*. 2005;23:4553–4560. doi:10.1200/JCO.2005.17.749
6. Rosen CB, Nagorney DM, Taswell HF, et al. Perioperative blood transfusion and determinants of survival after liver resection for metastatic colorectal carcinoma. *Ann Surg*. 1992;216:493–504. doi:10.1097/00000658-199210000-00012
7. Nordlinger B, Guiguet M, Vaillant JC, et al. Surgical resection of colorectal carcinoma metastases to the liver. A prognostic scoring system to improve case selection, based on 1568 patients. Association Française de Chirurgie. *Cancer*. 1996;77:1254–1262. doi:10.1002/(SICI)1097-0142(19960401)77:7<1254::AID-CNCR5>3.0.CO;2-I
8. Fong Y, Fortner J, Sun RL, et al. Clinical score for predicting recurrence after hepatic resection for metastatic colorectal cancer: analysis of 1001 consecutive cases. *Ann Surg*. 1999;230:309–318. doi:10.1097/00000658-199909000-00004
9. Levine EA, Stewart JH, Shen P, et al. Cytoreductive surgery and intraperitoneal hyperthermic chemotherapy for peritoneal surface malignancy: experience with 1,000 patients. *J Am Coll Surg*. 2014;518:573–587. doi:10.1016/j.jamcollsurg.2013.12.013
10. Goere D, Sourroville I, Gelli M, et al. Peritoneal metastases from colorectal cancer: treatment principles and perspectives. *Surg Oncol Clin N Am*. 2018;27:563–583. doi:10.1016/j.soc.2018.02.011
11. Glehen O, Kwiatkowski F, Sugarbaker PH, et al. Cytoreductive surgery combined with perioperative intraperitoneal chemotherapy for the management of peritoneal carcinomatosis from colorectal cancer: a multi-institutional study. *J Clin Oncol*. 2004;22:3284–3292. doi:10.1200/JCO.2004.10.01212.
12. Dawson LE, Russell AH, Tong D, et al. Adenocarcinoma of the sigmoid colon: sites of initial dissemination and clinical patterns of recurrence following surgery alone. *J Surg Oncol*. 1983;22:95–99. doi:10.1002/jso.2930220208
13. Benson AB, Venook AP, Bekaii-Saab T, et al. Rectal Cancer, Version 2.2015. J *Natl Compr Canc Netw*. 2015;13(6):719–728.
14. Chu DZ, Lang NP, Thompson C, et al. Peritoneal carcinomatosis in nongynecologic malignancy. A prospective study of prognostic factors. *Cancer*. 1989;63:364–367. doi:10.1002/1097-0142(19890115)63:2<364::AID-CNCR2820630228>3.0.CO;2-V
15. Franko J, Shi Q, Goldman CD, et al. Treatment of colorectal peritoneal carcinomatosis with systemic chemotherapy: a pooled analysis of North Central Cancer treatment group phase III trials N9741 and 9841. *J Clin Oncol*. 2012;30:263–267. doi:10.1200/JCO.2011.37.1039
16. Spratt JS, Adcock RA, Muskovin M, et al. Clinical delivery system for intraperitoneal hyperthermic chemotherapy. *Cancer Res*. 1980;40(2):260.
17. Lambert LA. Recent advances in understanding and treating peritoneal carcinomatosis. *Cancer J Clin*. 2014;65:283–298. doi:10.3322/caac.21277
18. Verwaal VJ, van Ruth S, de Bree E, et al. Randomized trial of cytoreduction and hyperthermic intraperitoneal chemotherapy versus systemic chemotherapy and palliative surgery in patients with peritoneal carcinomatosis of colorectal cancer. *J Clin Oncol*. 2003;21:3737–3743. doi:10.1200/JCO.2003.04.187

19. Quenet F, Elias D, Roca L, et al. A UNICANCER phase III trial of hyperthermic intraperitoneal chemotherapy (HIPEC) for colorectal peritoneal carcinomatosis: PRODIGE 7. *J Clin Oncol.* 2018;36(18_suppl):LBA5303. doi:10.1200/jco.2018.36.18_suppl.lba3503

20. Cashin PH, Mahteme H, Spang N, et al. Cytoreductive surgery and intraperitoneal chemotherapy versus systemic chemotherapy for colorectal peritoneal metastases: a randomized trial. *Eur J Cancer.* 2016:53:155–162. doi:10.1016/j.ejca.2015.09.017

21. Esquivel J, Sticca R, Sugarbaker P, et al. Cytoreductive surgery and hyperthermic intraperitoneal chemotherapy in the management of peritoneal surface malignancies of colonic origin: a consensus statement. *Ann Surg Oncol.* 2007;14:128–133. doi:10.1245/s10434-006-9185-7

22. Barratti D, Kusamura S, Lusco, D, et al. Postoperative complications after cytoreductive surgery and hyperthermic intraperitoneal chemotherapy affect long-term outcome of patients with peritoneal metastases from colorectal cancer: a two-center study of 101 patients. *Dis Colon Rectum.* 2014;57(7):858–868. doi:10.1097/DCR.0000000000000149

23. Jafari MD, Halabi WJ, Stamos MJ, et al. Surgical outcomes of hyperthermic intraperitoneal chemotherapy: analysis of the American College of Surgeons National Surgical Quality Improvement Program. *JAMA Surg.* 2014;149(2):170–175. doi:10.1001/jamasurg.2013.3640

24. Votanopoulos KI, Aaron Blackham A, Ihemelandu C, et al. Cytoreductive surgery with hyperthermic intraperitoneal chemotherapy in peritoneal carcinomatosis from rectal cancer. *Ann Surg Oncol.* 2013;20(4):1088–1092. doi:10.1245/s10434-012-2787-325.

25. Smeenk RM, Verwaal VJ, Zoetmulder FA. Learning curve of combined modality treatment in peritoneal surface disease. *Br J Surg.* 2007;94(11):1408–1414. doi:10.1002/bjs.5863

26. Polanco PM, Ding Y, Knox JM, et al. Institutional learning curve of cytoreductive surgery and hyperthermic intraperitoneal chemoperfusion for peritoneal malignancies. *Ann Surg Oncol.* 2015;22(5):1673–1679. doi:10.1245/s10434-014-4111-x

27. Ihemelandu CU, McQuellon R, Shen P, et al. Predicting postoperative morbidity following cytoreductive surgery with hyperthermic intraperitoneal chemotherapy (CS+HIPEC) with preoperative FACT-C (functional assessment of cancer therapy) and patient-rated performance status. *Ann Surg Oncol.* 2013;20:3519–3526. doi:10.1245/s10434-013-3049-8

28. Votanopoulos KI, Newman NA, Russell G, et al. Outcomes of cytoreductive surgery (CRS) with hyperthermic intraperitoneal chemotherapy (HIPEC) in patients older than 70 years; survival benefit at considerable morbidity and mortality. *Ann Surg Oncol.* 2013;20:3497–3503. doi:10.1245/s10434-013-3053-z29

29. Votanopoulos KI, Swords DS, Swett KR, et al. Obesity and peritoneal surface disease; outcomes following cytoreductive surgery (CRS) with hyperthermic intraperitoneal chemotherapy (HIPEC) for appendiceal and colon primaries. *Ann Surg Oncol.* 2013;20:3899–3904. doi:10.1245/s10434-013-3087-230

30. Tonnesen H, Nielsen PR, Lauritzen JB, et al. Smoking and alcohol intervention before surgery: evidence for best practice. *Br J Anaesth.* 2009;102(3):297–306. doi:10.1093/bja/aen401

31. Thomsen T, Villebro N, Moller AM. Interventions for preoperative smoking cessation. *Cochrane Database Syst Rev.* 2014;(3):CD002294. doi:10.1002/14651858.CD002294.pub4

32. Jie B, Jiang Z-M, Nolan MT, et al. Impact of preoperative nutritional support on clinical outcome in abdominal surgical patients at nutritional risk. *Nutrition.* 2012;28(10):1022–1027. doi:10.1016/j.nut.2012.01.017

33. Dineen SP, Robinson KA, Roland CL, et al. Feeding tube placement during cytoreductive surgery and heated intraperitoneal chemotherapy does not improve postoperative nutrition and is associated with longer length of stay and higher readmission rates. *J Surg Res.* 2016;200(1):158–163. doi:10.1016/j.jss.2015.08.003

34. Goere D, Souadka A, Faron M, et al. Extent of colorectal peritoneal carcinomatosis: attempt to define a threshold above which HIPEC does not offer survival benefit: a comparative study. *Ann Surg Oncol.* 2015;22(9):2958–2964. doi:10.1245/s10434-015-4387-5

35. Jayakrishnan TT, Zacharias AJ, Sharma A, et al. Role of laparoscopy in patients with peritoneal metastases considered for cytoreductive surgery and hyperthermic intraperitoneal chemotherapy (HIPEC). *World J Surg Oncol.* 2014;12:270. doi:10.1186/1477-7819-12-270

36. Tabrizian P, Jayakrishnan TT, Zacharias A, et al. Incorporation of diagnostic laparoscopy in the management algorithm for patients with peritoneal metastases: a multi-institutional analysis. *J Surg Oncol.* 2015;111(8):1035–1040. doi:10.1002/jso.23924

37. Marmor RA, Kelly KJ, Lowy AM, et al. Laparoscopy is safe and accurate to evaluate peritoneal surface metastasis prior to cytoreductive surgery. *Ann Surg Oncol.* 2016;23(5):1461–1467. doi:10.1245/s10434-015-4958-5

38. Levine, EA. Cytroreductive surgery and hyperthermic intraperitoneal chemotherapy for cancers of the appendix and colon in mastery of surgery, 7th edition. In: Fischer JE, ed. *Fischer's Mastery of Surgery.* Lippincott, Williams and Wilkins; 2018:1877-1882.

39. Jacquet P, Sugarbaker PH. Clinical research methodologies in diagnosis and staging of patients with peritoneal carcinomatosis. *Cancer Treat Res*. 1996;82:359–374. doi:10.1007/978-1-4613-1247-5_23

40. Verwaal VJ, Bruin S, Boot H, et al. 8-year follow-up of randomized trial: cytoreduction and hyperthermic intraperitoneal chemotherapy versus systemic chemotherapy in patients with peritoneal carcinomatosis of colorectal cancer. *Ann Surg Oncol*. 2008;15(9):2426–2432. doi:10.1245/s10434-008-9966-2

41. Goere, D, Quenet F, Ducreaux M, et al. Results of a randomized phase 3 study evaluating the potential benefit of a second-look surgery plus HIPEC in patients with high risk of developing colorectal peritoneal metastases (PROPHYLOCHIP-NTC01226384). *J Cin Oncol*. 2018;36(15_suppl):3531.

42. Varban O, Levine EA, Stewart JH, et al. Outcomes associated with cytoreductive surgery and intraperitoneal hyperthermic chemotherapy in colorectal cancer patients with peritoneal surface disease and hepatic metastases. *Cancer*. 2009;115(15):3427–3436. doi:10.1002/cncr.24385

43. Blackham AU, Russell GB, Stewart JH, et al. Metastatic colorectal cancer: survival comparison of hepatic resection versus cytoreductive surgery and hyperthermic chemotherapy. *Ann Surg Oncol*. 2014;21:2667–2674. doi:10.1245/s10434-014-3563-344.

44. Turaga K, Levine E, Barone R, et al. Consensus guidelines from The American Society of Peritoneal Surface Malignancies on Standardizing the Delivery of Hyperthermic Intraperitoneal Chemotherapy (HIPEC) in colorectal cancer patients in the United States. *Ann Surg Oncol*. 2013;21(5):1501-1505. doi:10.1245/s10434-013-3061-z

How I Treat Metastatic Colorectal Cancer With Chemotherapy and Choice of Biologics

Satya Das and Kristen K. Ciombor

INTRODUCTION AND HISTORICAL CONTEXT OF SURVIVAL IN METASTATIC COLORECTAL CANCER (mCRC)

Treatment for mCRC patients has dramatically improved over the past few decades. With the optimization of combinatorial chemotherapy, development of biologic agents, improved understanding of tumor biology, and better supportive care, patients are living longer. Median overall survival (OS) in mCRC patients increased from 14.2 months in 1990 to 29.3 months in 2006 (1). In the more recently reported FIRE-3 and CALGB-80405 studies, OS for stage IV colorectal cancer (CRC) patients was greater than 29 months (2,3). While improved surgical techniques and expertise have contributed to this improvement, much of the survival benefit has been driven by more effective systemic therapies.

COMBINATORIAL CHEMOTHERAPY FOR mCRC

Over the past two decades, much of the improvement in survival for mCRC patients has come from incremental improvement in combinatorial chemotherapy regimens. Until the year 2000, single agent 5-fluorouracil (5-FU) and leucovorin were the standard of care for mCRC patients. Various regimens were investigated, and the de Gramont regimen of bimonthly infusional 5-FU produced an OS of more than 10 months in patients with mCRC (4). IFL (irinotecan, leucovorin, and bolus 5-FU) was the first combination regimen to garner frontline approval in mCRC patients based on the trial published by Saltz et al. (5). In this study, IFL produced an OS of 14.8 months compared to 12.1 months with bolus 5-FU and leucovorin. These findings echoed results from an earlier trial published the same year by Douillard et al. (6). In this study, median OS in previously treatment-naïve mCRC patients treated with IFL was 17.4 months, compared to 14.1 months with infusional 5-FU and bolus calcium folinate. The N9741 trial established FOLFOX (infusional 5-FU, leucovorin, and oxaliplatin) as an optimal first-line regimen in mCRC patients compared to IFL. The median OS for patients on the trial with FOLFOX was 20 months compared to 14.1 months with IFL (7). Tournigand et al. established the equivalency of FOLFIRI (infusional 5-FU, leucovorin, and irinotecan) with FOLFOX in treatment-naïve mCRC patients (8). Median OS was 21.4 months with FOLFIRI compared to 20.6 months with FOLFOX (nonstatistically significant difference). More recently, the STEAM trial demonstrated a trend toward improved objective response rate (ORR) in mCRC patients treated in the first line with FOLFOXIRI (infusional 5-FU, oxaliplatin, leucovorin, and irinotecan) plus bevacizumab compared to FOLFOX plus bevacizumab (73% vs. 62%) (9). The TRIBE study compared FOLFOXIRI plus bevacizumab to FOLFIRI plus bevacizumab in the first-line setting and met its primary end point of improved progression-free survival (PFS) (10). Median PFS and OS in patients treated with triplet chemotherapy was 12.1 months and 29.8 months, respectively, compared to 7.5 months and 25.8 months, respectively, in patients treated with doublet chemotherapy. For most patients with widely metastatic CRC and ultimately incurable disease, the optimal choice of backbone chemotherapy regimen depends on the patient's performance status, treatment goals, and consideration of potential chemotherapy toxicities.

A Clinical Vignette ("How I Treat") is included at the end of the chapter.

ANTIANGIOGENIC THERAPIES IN mCRC

Bevacizumab, a monoclonal antibody against VEGF-A, was first added to single agent 5-FU in a trial reported by Kabbinavar et al. in 2003 (11). In this study, OS was reported as high as 21.5 months with the addition of the antiangiogenic agent. Hurwitz et al. first reported findings from a trial that added bevacizumab to a first-line chemotherapy doublet in 2005 (12). In this study, IFL plus bevacizumab increased OS from 15.6 months to 20.3 months compared to IFL alone. Shortly thereafter in 2007, the Eastern Cooperative Oncology Group (ECOG) 3200 trial touted the benefit of adding bevacizumab to FOLFOX in the second-line setting in patients who had progressed on IFL (13). In this trial, second-line mCRC patients who received FOLFOX plus bevacizumab had an OS of 12.9 versus 10.8 months in patients receiving FOLFOX alone. The BICC-C trial established FOLFIRI plus bevacizumab over IFL plus bevacizumab in first-line mCRC patients with a median OS of 28 months in the former group and 19.3 months in the latter group (14). The question of whether to continue bevacizumab beyond progression was answered in the ML18147 trial (15). In this study, 820 mCRC patients who had progressed on first-line chemotherapy plus bevacizumab within the prior 3 months were randomized to second-line chemotherapy plus bevacizumab versus chemotherapy alone. Median OS for the bevacizumab continuation arm was 11.1 months compared to 9.8 months for the chemotherapy alone arm, suggesting a benefit to the continued use of bevacizumab beyond progression.

The success of incorporating bevacizumab into the care of mCRC patients led to trials with other antiangiogenics such as aflibercept and ramucirumab in this patient population. The role of aflibercept, a decoy receptor that binds VEGF-A, VEGF-B, and placental growth factor, was assessed by Van Cutsem et al. in the AFFIRM study, which randomized second-line mCRC patients to aflibercept plus FOLFIRI or FOLFIRI alone (16). Patients who received FOLFIRI plus aflibercept demonstrated a median OS and PFS of 13.5 months and 6.9 months, respectively. Patients who received FOLFIRI alone demonstrated a median OS and PFS of 12.06 months and 4.67 months, respectively. Ramucirumab, a humanized IgG1 antibody targeting the VEGF receptor 2 extracellular domain, was evaluated by Tabernero et al. in the RAISE trial (17). In this study, mCRC patients who had progressed on FOLFOX plus bevacizumab were randomized to FOLFIRI plus ramucirumab or FOLFIRI. Median OS and PFS were 13.3 months and 5.7 months, respectively, in the ramucirumab arm versus 11.7 months and 4.5 months, respectively, in the FOLFIRI alone arm. Practically speaking, often due to costs or other toxicities, aflibercept and ramucirumab are far less commonly used in the mCRC setting than bevacizumab.

ANTI–EPIDERMAL GROWTH FACTOR RECEPTOR (EGFR) THERAPIES IN mCRC

EGFR inhibitors such as cetuximab and panitumumab were utilized in the first-line setting with chemotherapy prior to clinicians' understanding the predictive role of RAS mutations in mCRC patients. This finding was determined retrospectively through the CRYSTAL, PRIME, and FIRE-3 studies (18–20). The CRYSTAL study investigated cetuximab plus FOLFOX, while the PRIME study studied panitumumab plus FOLFOX in previously untreated mCRC patients. In the CRYSTAL trial, KRAS exon 2 wild-type (WT) patients demonstrated an OS survival with cetuximab plus FOLFOX of 23.5 months versus 20.0 months with FOLFOX alone. In the PRIME study, KRAS/NRAS exon 2,3,4 WT patients demonstrated an OS of 25.8 months with FOLFOX plus panitumumab versus 20.2 months with FOLFOX alone. The FIRE-3 study looked at FOLFIRI plus cetuximab versus FOLFIRI plus bevacizumab in first-line mCRC patients who were KRAS exon 2 WT. Retrospectively, the RAS WT definition was expanded to include KRAS/NRAS exon 2,3,4 WT patients. Cetuximab plus FOLFIRI, rather than bevacizumab plus FOLFIRI, created a pronounced survival benefit of 33.1 versus 25 months in these patients.

COMBINED ANTIANGIOGENIC AND ANTI-EGFR THERAPIES: MORE IS NOT ALWAYS BETTER

Approaches combining anti-EGFR therapies plus anti-VEGF agents in the first-line metastatic setting have been investigated but have not been found to confer benefit. The CAIRO-2 study randomized 736 mCRC patients to capecitabine, oxaliplatin, and bevacizumab, with or without cetuximab (21). PFS (9.4 months) was shorter in the combined biologic arm compared to the capecitabine, oxaliplatin, and bevacizumab arm (10.7 months), while OS was not statistically different between the two arms. Even when looking only at KRAS WT patients, PFS and OS were not statistically different between the two arms. More grade III/IV adverse events were observed in the combined biologic arm (81.7%) versus the chemotherapy plus bevacizumab arm (73.2%).

BRAF MUTANT mCRC

BRAF mutations are found in 8% to 12% of mCRC patients, with V600E representing the most common mutation (22). As a prognostic marker, *BRAF V600E* mutant patients fare worse than their WT counterparts. The predictive role for BRAF in predicting the absence of response to EGFR-directed antibody therapy is somewhat controversial, with some studies suggesting a lack of benefit to EGFR inhibitors in his population, while others suggest there is not enough evidence to make that determination (23). Treatment strategies targeting this group of patients remain a challenge given the absence of single-agent response to BRAF inhibitors as seen in other tumor types such as melanoma. A subgroup analysis from the TRIBE study suggested an OS and PFS benefit of FOLFOXIRI plus bevacizumab compared to FOLFIRI plus bevacizumab in *BRAF V600E* mutant mCRC patients. This benefit was not demonstrated in a subset analysis of *BRAF V600E* mutant patients from the STEAM trial comparing FOLFOXIRI plus bevacizumab versus FOLFOX plus bevacizumab, where no difference in PFS or OS was seen between the two regimens.

Strategies targeting multiple components in the RAS/RAF pathway are under way. Some of these approaches include utilizing BRAF inhibitors along with MEK and EGFR inhibitors and combining BRAF and MEK inhibitors with traditional chemotherapy. The SWOG 1406 study from Kopetz et al. randomized BRAF V600E mutant mCRC patients to irinotecan and cetuximab with or without vemurafenib (24). Median PFS in the vemurafenib-treated patients was 4.4 months and 2 months in patients who did not receive the agent. A nonstatistically significant trend toward improved ORR was seen in the patients who received vemurafenib compared to those who did not (16% vs. 4%). Hujberts et al. recently presented data from the safety lead-in portion of the BEACON CRC study (25). 30 *BRAF V600E* mutant mCRC patients were safely treated with the combination of encorafenib, binimetinib, and cetuximab with only 7% of patients experiencing grade III fatigue and 3% experiencing grade III diarrhea; no grade IV adverse events were reported. Given the safety of the therapy, patients are now being randomized to encorafenib and cetuximab with or without binimetinib versus investigator's choice therapy of FOLFIRI and cetuximab or irinotecan and cetuximab.

While *BRAF V600E* mutations often confer a poorer prognosis in this disease, mCRC patients with non-*V600E BRAF* mutations have better outcomes than their *BRAF V600E* mutant counterparts. From Jones et al., outcomes in 9,643 mCRC patients who had undergone next-generation sequencing were analyzed; 2.2% were found to have non-V600E BRAF mutations (26). Compared to patients with *BRAF V600E* mutations (11.3 months) and BRAF WT disease (40.3 months), non-*V600E BRAF* mutant patients had a median OS of 60.7 months (hazard ratio [HR] 0.18) (26).

HER2 AMPLIFICATION

HER2 amplification is found in 4% to 7% of RAS WT mCRC (27). In the open-label HERACLES trial, 27 heavily pretreated (74% with four lines or more of prior therapy) patients with HER2 amplification (IHC 3+ or IHC 2+ with FISH confirmation) received lapatinib and trastuzumab (28). A total of 30% of patients achieved an overall response to therapy, while 59% of patients achieved disease control (stable disease plus partial response plus complete response). Patients with an HER2 copy number greater than 9.45 (determined by a receiver operating characteristic [ROC] curve) had a median PFS of 29 weeks, compared to 16 weeks in those with an HER2 copy number <9.45. More updated results suggest disease control in patients on the study was 70% (29). Hurwitz et al. published interim data from the HER2 cohort of metastatic CRC patients from the phase II MyPathway trial (30). Thirty-four patients with an average of four lines of prior lines of therapy were treated with the combination of pertuzumab plus trastuzumab. Thirty-five percent of patients achieved an objective response to therapy, while 44% of patients achieved disease control; responses were durable with a median duration of 11.1 months.

PRIMARY TUMOR SIDEDNESS AND THE EFFECT OF ANTI-EGFR THERAPIES ON SURVIVAL IN mCRC

Early insights about the prognostic role of primary tumor sidedness were suggested by O'Dwyer et al. in the analysis of the E2290 study (31). Metastatic CRC patients in this study were treated with 5-FU alone and those with left-sided primaries had an OS of 15.8 months compared to 10.9 months in patients with right-sided primaries. This was formally reported by Venook et al. in an analysis from the CALGB/SWOG 80405 study (32). In this study, 1,137 patients with RAS WT tumors were randomized to first-line cetuximab or bevacizumab plus either FOLFOX or FOLFIRI. Patients with left-sided primary tumors had a median OS of 33.3 months compared to 19.4 months in patients with right-sided primary tumors. Furthermore, primary tumor sidedness seemed to play a predictive role in determining benefit from cetuximab as left-sided (from splenic flexure to descending colon) tumor patients who received the anti-EGFR antibody had a median OS of 36 months compared to 16.7 months in right-sided (from cecum to hepatic flexure) tumor patients. These findings were reaffirmed by an analysis from Tejpar et al. where the authors retrospectively analyzed outcomes from the CRYSTAL and FIRE-3 trial by tumor sidedness (33). In both studies, RAS WT mCRC patients with left-sided primary tumors had improved PFS and OS compared to patients with right-sided primary tumors. In the CRYSTAL study, left-sided primary tumor patients treated with cetuximab plus FOLFIRI had a median OS of 28.7 months compared to 18.5 months in right-sided primary tumor patients treated with the same combination. In the FIRE-3 study, left-sided primary tumor patients treated with FOLFIRI plus cetuximab had a median OS of 38.3 months compared to 18.3 months in right-sided primary tumor patients treated with the same agents. Distinct tumor biology and molecular drivers likely play a role in outcome differences between right-sided and left-sided primary tumors, with right-sided tumors having higher frequencies of RAS/BRAF V600E mutations and microsatellite instability compared to left-sided tumors. Other crucial elements, such as microbiome variation based on colonic location, contributing to the primary sidedness phenomenon have yet to be fully explained.

SYSTEMIC CHEMOTHERAPY OPTIONS FOR mCRC BEYOND FOLFOX, FOLFIRI, ANTI-VEGF, AND ANTI-EGFR THERAPIES

After progression on FOLFOX- and FOLFIRI-based chemotherapy, as well as anti-VEGF and anti-EGFR therapies, mCRC patients with the desire to receive further therapy and adequate performance status have both regorafenib and trifluridine/tipiracil (TAS-102) as Food and Drug Administration (FDA) approved options. Regorafenib, an oral VEGFR2 and TIE2 tyrosine kinase inhibitor, demonstrated an OS benefit compared to placebo in the CORRECT trial (34). In this study from Grothey et al., mCRC patients treated with regorafenib had a median OS of 6.4 months compared to 5 months with placebo. Given the toxicity seen in patients treated with regorafenib at 160 mg, a more optimal dosing schedule was explored in the recently presented ReDOS trial by Bekaii-Saab et al. (35). In this randomized study, mCRC patients were randomized to standard regorafenib dosing at 160 mg daily or a weekly dose escalation schedule of regorafenib at 80 mg, then 120 mg, and then 160 mg daily in the absence of toxicity. In the alternate dosing arm, 43% of patients completed two cycles of therapy and proceeded to a third cycle while only 25% in the routine treatment arm were able to do so. TAS-102, a combination of a thymidine-based analog and an agent that inhibits its degradation, improved OS compared to placebo in refractory mCRC patients in a study from Mayer et al. (36). In this study, mCRC patients who received TAS-102 had a median OS of 7.1 months compared to 5.3 months in patients who received placebo. Xu et al. published the experience of refractory Asian mCRC patients with TAS-102 (37). In this study, median OS in patients who received TAS-102 was 7.8 months, compared to 7.1 months in the placebo arm.

CONCLUSIONS

Overall, systemic chemotherapy for metastatic CRC has improved patient outcomes dramatically over the past two decades. The development of multiple cytotoxic chemotherapeutic agents and biologics such as antiangiogenics and anti-EGFR antibodies is in large part responsible for these improvements. Questions remain regarding ideal combinations and treatment sequences of these agents, but a sample treatment algorithm based on standard CRC classifications (genomic and primary tumor location) is included here in Figure 14.1. As

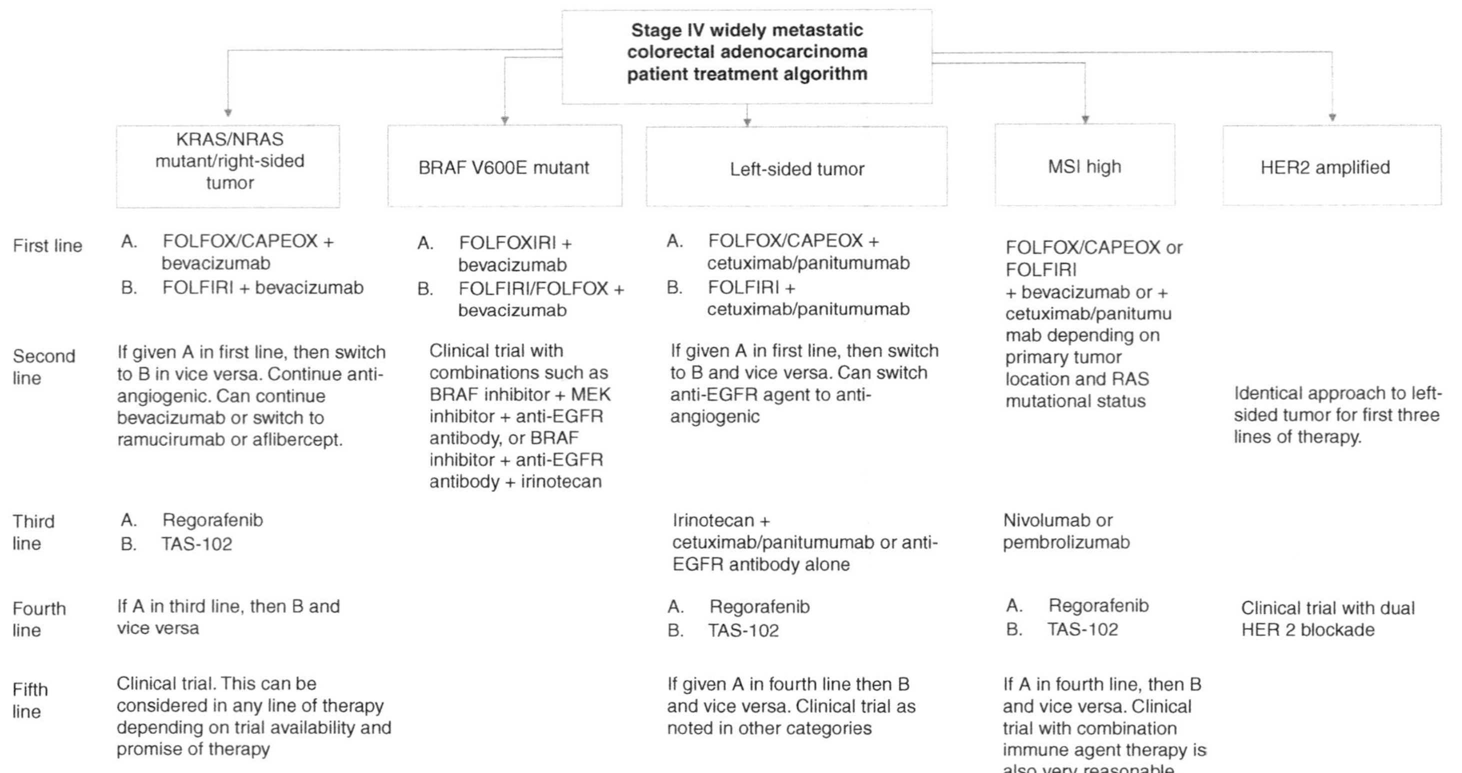

FIGURE 14.1   Sample treatment algorithm for an mCRC patient based on location of primary tumor and genomic characteristics.

Note: Clinical trials can also be considered with any line of therapy depending on patient interest, eligibility, and trial availability.

our understanding of the biologic underpinnings of this disease evolves, we will hopefully be able to maximize our treatment responses and patient survival and minimize toxicities for the patient. The following case discussion illustrates the required personalization of chemotherapy regimen strategy and sequencing employed by medical oncologists on a daily basis for patients with mCRC.

Clinical Vignette 14.1

A 53-year-old previously healthy gentleman presented with unremitting right upper quadrant pain in April 2015. A subsequent colonoscopy revealed a nonobstructive fungating mass in his cecum, which was biopsied and determined to be poorly differentiated adenocarcinoma, microsatellite stable (MSS) by immunohistochemistry (IHC), with signet ring features. He underwent staging contrasted CT scans of his chest and abdomen, which only revealed a 3.4 × 3.8 cm mass in the distal cecum with adjacent mildly prominent mesenteric lymph nodes (Figure 14.2). He was taken to the operating room in May 2015 for a right hemicolectomy; however, several peritoneal deposits were noted at the time of surgery. He underwent a right colon resection, along with biopsy of the most visible peritoneal deposit. His final pathologic staging was T3N1M1 with biopsy proven metastatic disease. Preoperative carcinoembryonic antigen (CEA) was 1.0. His case was discussed at our multidisciplinary tumor board conference and given his limited peritoneal disease, he was felt to be a potential future hyperthermic intraperitoneal chemotherapy (HIPEC) candidate if systemic control was able to be achieved with chemotherapy.

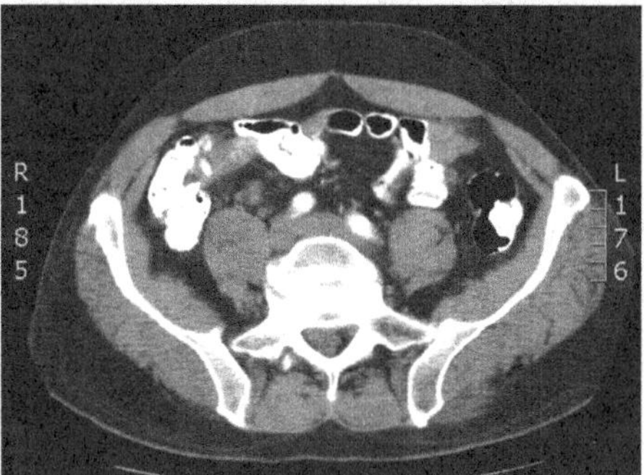

FIGURE 14.2   Initial abdominal CT scan of the patient demonstrating 3.4 cm area of irregularity at the cecum.

The patient initially received four cycles of FOLFOX and then was taken to the operating room for cytoreductive debulking and HIPEC in September 2015. The patient underwent nodule resection in his peritoneum, omentectomy, and removal of his pelvic peritoneum along with administration of intraperitoneal mitomycin. There were only a few tumor cells found in large mucinous pools in the pelvic peritoneum specimen with no other residual disease elsewhere. Postoperatively, he received 8 more cycles of FOLFOX to complete a total of 12 cycles. He remained free of disease until August 2016 when a CT scan revealed a new mesenteric nodule (Figure 14.3); his CEA was 1.2 at this time. The nodule was confirmed to be FDG-avid on PET, and the patient was taken for an exploratory laparotomy in September 2016. Multiple mesenteric nodules were found during the operation, with the largest one adjacent to the superior mesenteric vein (SMV). These were biopsied and recurrence was confirmed. Foundation One® next-generation sequencing (NGS) was obtained from this tissue and demonstrated the presence of SMAD4 and TP53 mutations but no alterations in KRAS, NRAS, HRAS, BRAF, or HER2. His performance status remained excellent.

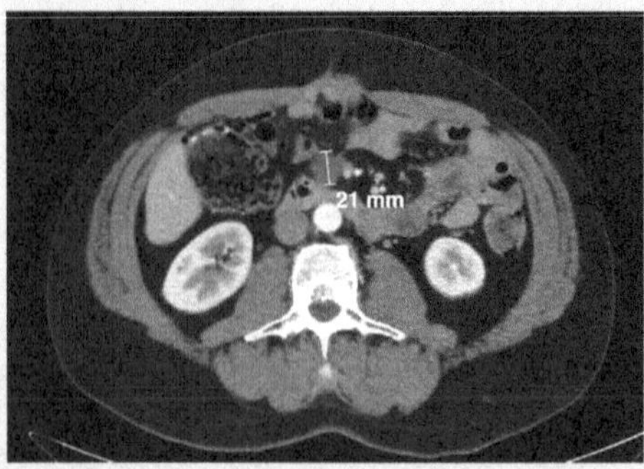

FIGURE 14.3 Abdominal CT scan of the patient at the time of disease recurrence, demonstrating a 2.1 cm mesenteric metastasis abutting the SMV.

SMV, superior mesenteric vein.

The patient was then started on FOLFOXIRI and bevacizumab because of an excellent performance status and the hope that the therapy would make him eligible for potential repeat debulking surgery and HIPEC. He was given bevacizumab despite RAS WT status of his tumor because of the right-sided location of his primary tumor and the reduced benefit of adding an anti-EGFR antibody to a chemotherapy backbone for primary tumors in this location. He received eight cycles of FOLFOXIRI plus bevacizumab from November 2016 to March 2017. Subsequent scans revealed the persistence of a central mesenteric lesion. Unfortunately, it was deemed unresectable due to proximity to the SMV. After another tumor board discussion, the patient received concurrent capecitabine and XRT to 54 Gy, directed toward the nodule, which was completed in May 2017. His subsequent scans in June 2017 revealed residual abutment of the nodule with the SMV, which continued to preclude surgical resection. At this point, the patient was completely asymptomatic and requested a therapy break with close surveillance. His surveillance scans revealed no progression until March 2018 when small new peritoneal lesions and left inguinal lymphadenopathy were noted (Figure 14.4). He has been scheduled for an excisional biopsy of his largest left inguinal lymph node. If the node is positive for colorectal adenocarcinoma as expected, systemic therapy will be restarted. Future chemotherapy options also include regorafenib, TAS-102, and consideration of a clinical trial. If the inguinal lymph node biopsy is negative for malignancy and all his disease remains confined to the peritoneum, surgical debulking and HIPEC may still be possible future options for him.

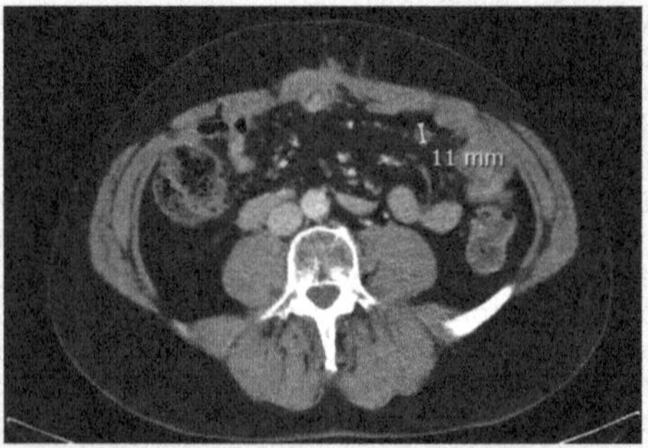

FIGURE 14.4 Most recent abdominal CT scan of the patient demonstrating peritoneal progression in the left lower mesenteric quadrant.

This patient initially received FOLFOX based on the N741 trial (7). Despite presenting with metastatic disease at diagnosis, given that all of his disease was resected, he was treated with 6 months of perioperative FOLFOX (38). The decision to move forward with cytoreductive surgery and HIPEC was made based on his poor risk signet ring cell tumor morphology and limited peritoneal disease, despite conflicting data about the effectiveness of the treatment modality (39,40). After he recurred in an unresectable mesenteric location, he was given FOLFOXIRI plus bevacizumab, based on response rates demonstrated by patients in the TRIBE-3 and STEAM studies, to try to make him eligible for surgical resection. He was given bevacizumab instead of an anti-EGFR monoclonal antibody in the metastatic setting due to the lack of benefit seen with anti-EGFR antibodies in right-sided primary colonic tumors, regardless of RAS status; this was illustrated by retrospective analyses from the CALGB 80405, FIRE-3, and CRYSTAL studies. Given his recent disease progression, he will likely be a candidate for further intravenous systemic chemotherapy, regorafenib, TAS-102, or a clinical trial.

REFERENCES

1. Kopetz S, Chang GJ, Overman MJ, et al. Improved survival in metastatic colorectal cancer is associated with adoption of hepatic resection and improved chemotherapy. *J Clin Oncol.* 2009;27(22):3677–3683. doi:10.1200/jco.2008.20.5278
2. Venook AP, Niedzwiecki D, Lenz H-J, et al. CALGB/SWOG 80405: Phase III Trial of Irinotecan/5-FU/Leucovorin (FOLFIRI) or Oxaliplatin/5-FU/Leucovorin (mFOLFOX6) with Bevacizumab (BV) or Cetuximab (CET) for Patients (Pts) with KRAS Wild-Type (Wt) Untreated Metastatic Adenocarcinoma of the Colon or Rectum (MCRC). *J Clin Oncol.* 2014;32(18_suppl):LBA3. doi:10.1200/jco.2014.32.18_suppl.lba3
3. Heinemann V, von Weikersthal LF, Decker T, et al. FOLFIRI plus cetuximab versus FOLFIRI plus bevacizumab as first-line treatment for patients with metastatic colorectal cancer (FIRE-3): a randomised, open-label, phase 3 trial. *Lancet Oncol.* 2014;15(10):1065–1075. doi:10.1016/s1470-2045(14)70330-4
4. De Gramont A, Bosset JF, Milan C, et al. Randomized trial comparing monthly low-dose leucovorin and fluorouracil bolus with bimonthly high-dose leucovorin and fluorouracil bolus plus continuous infusion for advanced colorectal cancer: a French Intergroup Study. *J Clin Oncol.* 1997;15(2):808–815. doi:10.1200/jco.1997.15.2.808
5. Saltz LB, Cox JV, Blanke C, et al. Irinotecan plus fluorouracil and leucovorin for metastatic colorectal cancer. *N Engl J Med.* 2000;343(13):905–914. doi:10.1056/nejm200009283431302
6. Douillard JY, Cunningham D, Roth AD, et al. Irinotecan combined with fluorouracil compared with fluorouracil alone as first-line treatment for metastatic colorectal cancer: a multicentre randomised trial. *Lancet.* 2000;355(9209):1041–1047. doi:10.1016/s0140-6736(00)02034-1
7. Goldberg RM, Sargent DJ, Morton RF, et al. Randomized controlled trial of reduced-dose bolus fluorouracil plus leucovorin and irinotecan or infused fluorouracil plus leucovorin and oxaliplatin in patients with previously untreated metastatic colorectal cancer: a North American Intergroup Trial. *J Clin Oncol.* 2006;24(21):3347–3353. doi:10.1200/jco.2006.06.1317
8. Tournigand C, André T, Achille E, et al. FOLFIRI followed by FOLFOX6 or the reverse sequence in advanced colorectal cancer: a randomized GERCOR study. *J Clin Oncol.* 2004;22(2):229–237. doi:10.1200/jco.2004.05.113
9. Hurwitz H, Tan BH, Reeves JA, et al. Updated efficacy, safety, and biomarker analyses of STEAM, a randomized, open-label, phase II trial of sequential (s) and concurrent (c) FOLFOXIRI-bevacizumab (BV) vs FOLFOX-BV for first-line (1L) treatment (Tx) of patients with metastatic colorectal cancer (MCRC). *J Clin Oncol.* 2017;35(4_suppl):657–657. doi:10.1200/jco.2017.35.4_suppl.657
10. Cremolini C, Loupakis F, Antoniotti C, et al. FOLFOXIRI plus bevacizumab versus FOLFIRI plus bevacizumab as first-line treatment of patients with metastatic colorectal cancer: updated overall survival and molecular subgroup analyses of the open-label, phase 3 TRIBE study. *Lancet Oncol.* 2015;16(13):1306–1315. doi:10.1016/s1470-2045(15)00122-9
11. Kabbinavar F, Hurwitz HI, Fehrenbacher L, et al. Phase II, randomized trial comparing bevacizumab plus fluorouracil (FU)/leucovorin (LV) with FU/LV alone in patients with metastatic colorectal cancer. *J Clin Oncol.* 2003;21(1):60–65. doi:10.1200/jco.2003.10.066

12. Hurwitz H, Fehrenbacher L, Novotny W, et al. Bevacizumab plus irinotecan, fluorouracil, and leucovorin for metastatic colorectal cancer. *N Engl J Med*. 2004;350(23):2335–2342. doi:10.1056/nejmoa032691

13. Giantonio BJ, Catalano PJ, Meropol NJ, et al. Bevacizumab in combination with oxaliplatin, fluorouracil, and leucovorin (FOLFOX4) for previously treated metastatic colorectal cancer: results from the Eastern Cooperative Oncology Group Study E3200. *J Clin Oncol*. 2007;25(12):1539–1544. doi:10.1200/jco.2006.09.6305

14. Fuchs CS, Marshall J, Mitchell E, et al. Randomized, controlled trial of irinotecan plus infusional, bolus, or oral fluoropyrimidines in first-line treatment of metastatic colorectal cancer: results from the BICC-C study. *J Clin Oncol*. 2007;25(30):4779–4786. doi:10.1200/jco.2007.11.3357

15. Bennouna J, Sastre J, Arnold D, et al. Continuation of bevacizumab after first progression in metastatic colorectal cancer (ML18147): a randomised phase 3 trial. *Lancet Oncol*. 2013;14(1):29–37. doi:10.1016/s1470-2045(12)70477-1

16. Van Cutsem E, Tabernero J, Lakomy R, et al. Addition of aflibercept to fluorouracil, leucovorin, and irinotecan improves survival in a phase III randomized trial in patients with metastatic colorectal cancer previously treated with an oxaliplatin-based regimen. *J Clin Oncol*. 2012;30(28):3499–3506. doi:10.1200/JCO.2012.42.8201

17. Tabernero J, Yoshino T, Cohn AL, et al. Ramucirumab versus placebo in combination with second-line FOLFIRI in patients with metastatic colorectal carcinoma that progressed during or after first-line therapy with bevacizumab, oxaliplatin, and a fluoropyrimidine (RAISE): a randomised, double-blind, multicentre, phase 3 study. *Lancet Oncol*. 2015;6(5):499–508. doi:10.1016/S1470-2045(15)70127-0

18. Van Cutsem E, Lenz H-J, Köhne C-H, et al. Fluorouracil, leucovorin, and irinotecan plus cetuximab treatment and RAS mutations in colorectal cancer. *J Clin Oncol*. 2015;33(7):692–700. doi:10.1200/jco.2014.59.4812

19. Douillard J-Y, Siena S, Cassidy J, et al. Randomized, phase III trial of panitumumab with infusional Fluorouracil, Leucovorin, and Oxaliplatin (FOLFOX4) versus FOLFOX4 alone as first-line treatment in patients with previously untreated metastatic colorectal cancer: the PRIME study. *J Clin Oncol*. 2010;28(31):4697–4705. doi:10.1200/jco.2009.27.4860

20. Stintzing S, Modest DP, Rossius L, et al. FOLFIRI plus Cetuximab versus FOLFIRI plus bevacizumab for metastatic colorectal cancer (FIRE-3): a post-hoc analysis of tumour dynamics in the final RAS wild-type subgroup of this randomised open-label phase 3 trial. *Lancet Oncol*. 2016;17(10):1426–1434. doi:10.1016/s1470-2045(16)30269-8

21. Tol J, Koopman M, Cats A, et al. Chemotherapy, bevacizumab, and cetuximab in metastatic colorectal cancer. *N Engl J Med*. 2009;360:563–572. doi:10.1056/NEJMoa0808268

22. Barras D. BRAF mutation in colorectal cancer: an update. *Biomark Cancer*. 2015;7s1:BIC. S25248. doi:10.4137/bic.s25248

23. Rowland A, Dias MM, Wiese MD, et al. Meta-analysis of BRAF mutation as a predictive biomarker of benefit from anti-EGFR monoclonal antibody therapy for RAS wild-type metastatic colorectal cancer. *Br J Cancer*. 2015;112(12):1888–1894. doi:10.1038/bjc.2015.173

24. Kopetz S, McDonough SL, Lenz H-J, et al. Randomized trial of irinotecan and cetuximab with or without vemurafenib in BRAF-mutant metastatic colorectal cancer (SWOG S1406). *J Clin Oncol*. 2017;35(suppl_15):3505–3505. doi:10.1200/JCO.2017.35.15_suppl.3505

25. Huijberts S, Schellens JHM, Elez E, et al. 517P BEACON CRC: Safety lead-in (SLI) for the combination of binimetinib (BINI), encorafenib (ENCO), and cetuximab (CTX) in patients (Pts) with BRAF-V600E metastatic colorectal cancer (MCRC). *Ann Oncol*. 2017;28(suppl_5). doi:10.1093/annonc/mdx393.043

26. Jones JC, Renfro LA, Al-Shamsi HO, et al. Non-V600BRAF mutations define a clinically distinct molecular subtype of metastatic colorectal cancer. *J Clin Oncol*. 2017;35(23):2624–2630. doi:10.1200/jco.2016.71.4394

27. Kavuri SM, Jain N, Galimi F, et al. HER2 activating mutations are targets for colorectal cancer treatment. *Cancer Discov*. 2015;5(8):832–841. doi:10.1158/2159-8290.cd-14-1211

28. Sartore-Bianchi A, Trusolino L, Martino C, et al. Dual-targeted therapy with trastuzumab and lapatinib in treatment-refractory, KRAS codon 12/13 wild-type, HER2-Positive Metastatic Colorectal Cancer (HERACLES): a proof-of-concept, multicentre, open-label, phase 2 trial. *Lancet Oncol*. 2016;17(6):738–746. doi:10.1016/s1470-2045(16)00150-9

29. Siena S, Sartore-Bianchi A, Trusolino L, et al. Abstract CT005: final results of the HERACLES Trial in HER2-amplified colorectal cancer. *Cancer Res*. 2017;77(suppl_13):CT005. doi:10.1158/1538-7445.am2017-ct005

30. Hurwitz H, Raghav KPS, Burris HA, et al. Pertuzumab trastuzumab for HER2-amplified/overexpressed metastatic colorectal cancer (MCRC): interim data from MyPathway. *J Clin Oncol*. 2017;35(4_suppl);676–676. doi:10.1200/jco.2017.35.4_suppl.676

31. O'Dwyer PJ, Manola J, Valone FH, et al. Fluorouracil modulation in colorectal cancer: lack of improvement with N -Phosphonoacetyl- l -aspartic acid or oral leucovorin or interferon, but enhanced therapeutic index with weekly 24-hour infusion schedule. An Eastern Cooperative Oncology Group/Cancer and Leukemia Group B study. *J Clin Oncol*. 2001;19(9):2413–2421. doi:10.1200/jco.2001.19.9.2413

32. Venook A, Ou F-S, Lenz H-J, et al. Primary (1°) tumor location as an independent prognostic marker from molecular features for overall survival (OS) in patients (pts) with metastatic colorectal cancer (mCRC): analysis of CALGB / SWOG 80405 (Alliance). *J Clin Oncol*. 2017;35(15_suppl):3503. doi:10.1200/JCO.2017.35.15_suppl.3503

33. Tejpar S, Stintzing S, Ciardiello F, et al. Prognostic and predictive relevance of primary tumor location in patients with RAS wild-type metastatic colorectal cancer. *JAMA Oncology*. 2017;3(2):194. doi:10.1001/jamaoncol.2016.3797

34. Grothey A, Van Cutsem E, Sobrero A, et al. Regorafenib monotherapy for previously treated metastatic colorectal cancer (CORRECT): an international, multicentre, randomised, placebo-controlled, phase 3 trial. *Lancet*. 2013;381(9863):303–312. doi:10.1016/S0140-6736(12)61900-X

35. Bekai-Saab T, Ou F-S, Anderson DM, et al. Regorafenib dose optimization study (ReDOS): randomized phase II trial to evaluate dosing strategies for regorafenib in refractory metastatic colorectal cancer (mCRC)—An ACCRU Network study. *J Clin Oncol*. 2018;36(4_suppl):611–611. doi:10.1200/JCO.2018.36.4_suppl.611

36. Mayer R, Van Cutsem E, Falcone A, et al. Randomized trial of TAS-102 for refractory metastatic colorectal cancer. *N Engl J Med*. 2015;372(20):1909–1919. doi:10.1056/NEJMoa1414325

37. Xu J, Kim TW, Shen L, et al. Results of a randomized, double-blind, placebo-controlled, phase III trial of Trifluridine/Tipiracil (TAS-102) monotherapy in Asian patients with previously treated metastatic colorectal cancer: the TERRA study. *J Clin Oncol*. 2018;36(4):350–358. doi:10.1200/JCO.2017.74.3245

38. Andre T, Boni C, Navarro M, et al. Improved overall survival with oxaliplatin, fluorouracil, and leucovorin as adjuvant treatment in stage II or III colon cancer in the MOSAIC trial. *J Clin Oncol*. 2009;27(19);3109–3116. doi:10.1200/JCO.2008.20.6771

39. Elias D, Gilly F, Boutitie F, et al. Peritoneal colorectal carcinomatosis treated with surgery and perioperative intraperitoneal chemotherapy: retrospective analysis of 523 patients from a multicentric French study. *J Clin Oncol*. 2010;28(1):63–68. doi:10.1200/JCO.2009.23.9285

40. Quenet F, Elias D, Roca L, et al. Perioperative outcomes of cytoreductive surgery and hyperthermic intra-peritoneal chemotherapy versus cytoreductive surgery alone for colorectal peritoneal carcinomatosis: PRODIGE 7 randomized trial. *Eur J Surg Oncol*. 2016;42(9):S107. doi:10.1016/j.ejso.2016.06.105

15

How I Treat Metastatic Colorectal Cancer With Maintenance Therapies

Sakti Chakrabarti and Joleen M. Hubbard

INTRODUCTION

The first-line treatment of metastatic colorectal cancer (mCRC) generally consists of a cytotoxic doublet, commonly oxaliplatin plus 5-fluorouracil and leucovorin (5-FU/LV), commonly referred to as FOLFOX regimen or capecitabine plus oxaliplatin (CAPOX), along with a biologic, commonly bevacizumab. However, after 4 to 5 months of oxaliplatin-containing regimens, approximately 18% of patients develop grade 3 or higher neurotoxicity. As a result, more patients come off therapy because of toxic effects than because of progressive disease (1,2). Two strategies have been developed to address this issue:

1. *Chemotherapy-free interval (treatment holiday)*: complete discontinuation of treatment after initial response and reintroduction of therapy at progression
2. *Maintenance therapy*: omission of more toxic oxaliplatin/irinotecan and continuation of a fluoropyrimidine with or without a biologic

Chemotherapy-Free Interval
The COIN trial was a noninferiority study investigating overall survival (OS) with chemotherapy holidays versus continuous therapy (3). 1,630 patients were randomly assigned to six cycles of FOLFOX followed by a chemotherapy-free interval until disease progression or continuous therapy until disease progression, unacceptable toxicity, or the patient's decision to stop. The median OS was similar in the continuous versus intermittent arm, 19.6 months versus 18 months, hazard ratio (HR) 1.084 (confidence interval [CI]: 1.008–1.165) in the intention-to-treat population and 1.087 (0.986–1.198) in the per-protocol population. Since the upper limit of the CI exceeded the predefined noninferiority boundary interval for survival, the noninferiority of the intermittent treatment strategy could not be established.

Maintenance Therapy
The primary goal of maintenance therapy is prolongation of disease control with minimal or manageable toxicities. Table 15.1 lists clinical trials investigating maintenance therapy regimens. The OPTIMOX trials set the stage for the intermittent oxaliplatin administration strategy utilizing fluoropyrimidines as maintenance therapy. After bevacizumab was approved, subsequent trials investigated fluoropyrimidines and/or bevacizumab as maintenance therapy.

MAINTENANCE THERAPY WITH A FLUOROPYRIMIDINE ALONE

The OPTIMOX1 trial (4) randomized previously untreated patients with mCRC to FOLFOX4 continuously until disease progression, or FOLFOX7 for six cycles, followed by maintenance therapy with biweekly infusional 5-FU and reintroduction of oxaliplatin at the time of disease progression. Median OS was similar between the continuous treatment and maintenance therapy arms (19.3 vs. 21.2 months respectively, *p* = .49). Individuals in the maintenance therapy arm had a significantly lower risk of developing grade 3 or 4 toxicity during cycles 6 to 18.

A Clinical Vignette ("How I Treat") is included at the end of the chapter.

TABLE 15.1 Maintenance Strategies Evaluated in Major Clinical Trials

Clinical Trial	Number of Patients	Control Arm	Maintenance Arm	End Point (Months)	OS (Months)
OPTIMOX1 (4)	620	**FOLFOX4** until progression	**FOLFOX7** for 6 cycles followed by **5-FU/LV** until progression	Duration of disease control: 9 vs. 10.6	19.3 vs. 21.3
OPTIMOX2 (5)	202	**mFOLFOX7** for 6 cycles followed by observation until progression	**mFOLFOX7** x 6 cycles followed by 5-**FU/LV** until progression	Duration of disease control: 9.2 vs. 13.1	19.5 vs. 23.8
CAIRO3 (6)	558	**CAPOX+ Bev** x 6 cycles followed by observation → reintroduction of **CAPOX+Bev** on progression	**CAPOX+Bev** x 6 cycles followed by **Cape+Bev** until progression▢ reintroduction of **CAPOX+Bev** on progression	PFS2: 8.5 vs. 11.7	18.2 vs. 21.7
PRODIGE 9 (7)	491	**FOLFIRI+Bev** x 12 cycles followed by observation until progression	**FOLFIRI+Bev** x 12 cycles followed by maintenance with **Bev** until progression	Tumor control duration: 15 (both groups)	21.7 vs. 22 months
CONcePT (8)	139	**FOLFOX7+Bev** until progression	**FOLFOX7+Bev** x 8 cycles followed by **5-FU/LV+Bev** x 8 cycles	Time to treatment failure: 4.2 vs. 5.7	Not reported
AIO KRK 0207 (9)	473	**FOLFOX7+Bev** followed by observation (arm A)	**FOLFOX7+Bev** followed by **Bev** (arm B) or **FOLFOX7+Bev** followed by **5-FU/LV+ Bev**(arm C)	Time to failure of strategy: C better than A	23.4 (equivalent in all groups)
STOP and GO (10)	123	**CAPOX+Bev** until progression	**CAPOX+Bev** x 6 cycles followed by **Cape+Bev** until progression	PFS 8.3 vs. 11	20.2 vs. 23.8

Bev, bevacizumab; Cape, capecitabine; CAPOX, capecitabine plus oxaliplatin; FOLFOX, 5-fluorouracil, leucovorin, and oxaliplatin; LV, leucovorin; OS, overall survival; PFS, progression-free survival.

In the OPTIMOX2 trial, patients with untreated mCRC were randomly assigned to receive six cycles of mFOLFOX7 followed by biweekly 5-FU/LV until progression or six cycles of mFOLFOX7 before a complete stop of chemotherapy (5). Reintroduction of mFOLFOX7 was planned after tumor progression in both arms. The median duration of disease control was 13.1 months in patients assigned to the maintenance arm and 9.2 months in patients assigned to the chemotherapy-free interval arm, which was statistically significant (p = .046). The conclusion of the trial was that complete discontinuation of therapy had an adverse impact on prognosis.

Capecitabine as maintenance therapy for mCRC patients has also been shown to improve progression-free survival (PFS) compared to observation after induction chemotherapy with an oxaliplatin-based regimen (11). Based on the data discussed earlier, 5-FU/LV or capecitabine is currently recommended as maintenance therapy for those patients who are not candidates for treatment with bevacizumab.

MAINTENANCE THERAPY WITH THE COMBINATION OF A FLUOROPYRIMIDINE AND BEVACIZUMAB

The CAIRO3 trial (6) randomized patients who had achieved at least stable disease after six cycles of induction therapy with capecitabine, oxaliplatin, and bevacizumab (CAPOX-B) to observation versus maintenance therapy with capecitabine and bevacizumab. CAPOX-B was to be reintroduced upon first progression. The primary end point of CAIRO3 was PFS from the time of randomization until disease progression after the reintroduction of CAPOX-B (PFS2). The primary end point of the study was reached: median PFS2 was 8.5 months in the observation group and 11.7 months in the maintenance group (HR 0.67, 95% CI: 0.56–0.81; $p < .0001$), in spite of the imbalance of reinduction treatment (60% patients in the observation group vs. 47% in the maintenance group). The time to tumor progression on maintenance treatment versus observation was more than doubled with the use of maintenance therapy (4.1 months in the observation group vs. 8.5 months in the maintenance group, $p < .0001$). There was a trend toward improved median OS in the maintenance group (21.6 months) versus the observation group (was 18.1 months), which was not statistically significant ($p = .22$).

As listed in Table 15.1, several other trials (8–10) have also confirmed improved disease control (exact end points differ among the trials) with the use of a fluoropyrimidine plus bevacizumab as a maintenance therapy strategy. Based on the consistent improvement of disease control with a fluoropyrimidine plus bevacizumab as a maintenance therapy across multiple clinical trials, it has become a standard of care for patients with mCRC who have achieved at least stable disease after 4 months of first-line treatment with a bevacizumab-containing regimen.

MAINTENANCE THERAPY WITH BEVACIZUMAB ALONE

Two trials made a comparison between bevacizumab alone as maintenance therapy and no maintenance therapy (7,12). Both trials failed to demonstrate a benefit in disease control with single agent bevacizumab compared to observation. Based on these results, bevacizumab alone is not recommended as maintenance therapy.

MAINTENANCE THERAPY WITH ERLOTINIB PLUS BEVACIZUMAB

The OPTIMOX3 (13) and Nordic ACT trial (14) have compared erlotinib plus bevacizumab versus bevacizumab alone as maintenance therapy in mCRC patients after induction therapy with a bevacizumab-containing regimen. Neither trial showed a PFS benefit with the combination. In the OPTIMOX3 trial, there was a statistically significant improvement of OS in the bevacizumab plus erlotinib group compared with the bevacizumab alone group (24.9 months vs. 22.1 months, $p = .035$), but the Nordic ACT trial did not confirm the same finding. At the current time, erlotinib plus bevacizumab is not recommended as a maintenance therapy approach.

CONCLUSIONS ON MAINTENANCE THERAPY

Based on the results of multiple clinical trials discussed earlier, several conclusions can be drawn:

1. The intermittent use of oxaliplatin reduces the symptoms of sensory neuropathy.
2. Compared to the continuous administration of oxaliplatin-containing regimens until disease progression, utilizing a maintenance therapy approach does not compromise survival.
3. The use of a fluoropyrimidine with or without bevacizumab as maintenance therapy leads to improved PFS compared to complete chemotherapy holidays.
4. Bevacizumab alone or combined with erlotinib is not recommended as maintenance therapy.

Figure 15.1 depicts our approach regarding maintenance therapy in unresectable mCRC.

One argument against the use of maintenance therapy compared to complete chemotherapy-free intervals is that the maintenance therapy trials have not demonstrated an OS benefit.

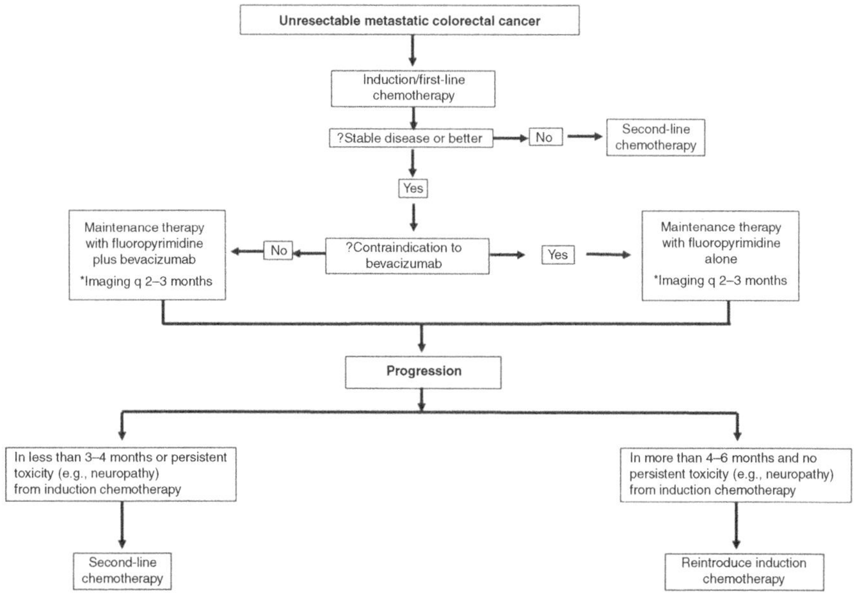

FIGURE 15.1 Suggested algorithm for maintenance chemotherapy in unresectable metastatic colorectal cancer.

It is important to recognize that these trials were not powered to demonstrate an OS benefit. There are a number of subsequent treatment options and varying practice patterns after first-line therapy that can influence OS outcomes. A recent meta-analysis of eight randomized trials of continuous versus intermittent strategies did not demonstrate inferior OS with an intermittent as compared with continuous treatment strategy (15). In the same meta-analysis, however, one subgroup analysis of the three trials (CAIRO3, OPTIMOX2, COIN, n = 2,403), which included an arm of an induction phase followed by no maintenance until progression, revealed a small but statistically significant benefit in favor of continuous treatment (HR = 1.10, 95% CI: 1.00–1.20, p = .049).

BACK TO OUR CASE

For our patient AB mentioned in Clinical Vignette 15.1, we recommended maintenance chemotherapy with bevacizumab and infusional 5-FU/LV for 2 days every 2 weeks with the omission of bolus 5-FU (he completed eight cycles of induction chemotherapy). Imaging studies as well as carcinoembryonic antigen (CEA) were obtained every 2 months. AB stayed on maintenance therapy for 6 months and progressed thereafter. At that time, he was restarted on mFOLFOX7 plus bevacizumab.

Clinical Vignette 15.1

AB is a 56-year-old man in good general health, with an Eastern Cooperative Oncology Group (ECOG) performance status of 1, who presented with a 2-month history of fatigue and intermittent rectal bleeding. A colonoscopy revealed a partially obstructing sigmoid colon mass and biopsy confirmed a moderately differentiated adenocarcinoma. Molecular analysis of the tumor revealed a KRAS mutation. Staging CT scans revealed multiple liver metastases, numerous bilateral lung nodules, and an elevated carcinoembryonic antigen (CEA) level of 97 ng/ml. The patient was initiated on modified FOLFOX7 (mFOLFOX7, 5-fluorouracil, leucovorin, and oxaliplatin) plus bevacizumab. After four cycles, a CT scan showed partial response and CEA decreased to 12 ng/ml. He received four more cycles of the same regimen. At this time, he started to experience more fatigue and neuropathic symptoms limiting his ability to perform fine motor movements thereby leading to a significant decline of his quality of life. CT scans were repeated, which showed further shrinkage of the metastatic lesions, most prominently in his lungs (Figure 15.2). His CEA dropped to 4 ng/ml. AB has returned for follow-up after eight cycles of treatment to discuss further plan of care.

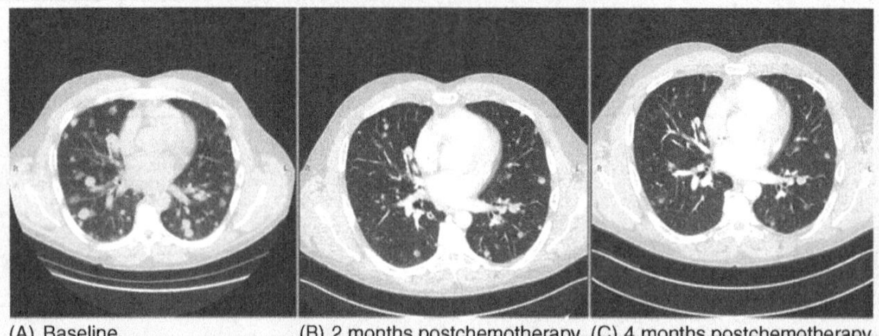

FIGURE 15.2 Serial CT scans show extensive bilateral pulmonary metastatic disease in a patient of metastatic colon cancer at baseline (A), partial response after 2 months of therapy (B), and further regression after 4 months of therapy (C).

REFERENCES

1. Goldberg RM, Sargent DJ, Morton RF, et al. A randomized controlled trial of fluorouracil plus leucovorin, irinotecan, and oxaliplatin combinations in patients with previously untreated metastatic colorectal cancer. *J Clin Oncol*. 2004;22(1):23–30. doi:10.1200/JCO.2004.09.046
2. Saltz LB, Clarke S, Díaz-Rubio E, et al. Bevacizumab in combination with oxaliplatin-based chemotherapy as first-line therapy in metastatic colorectal cancer: a randomized phase III study. *J Clin Oncol*. 2008;26(12):2013–2019. doi:10.1200/JCO.2007.14.9930
3. Adams RA, Meade AM, Seymour MT, et al. Intermittent versus continuous oxaliplatin and fluoropyrimidine combination chemotherapy for first-line treatment of advanced colorectal cancer: results of the randomised phase 3 MRC COIN trial. *Lancet Oncol*. 2011;12(7):642–653. doi:10.1016/S1470-2045(11)70102-4
4. Tournigand C, Cervantes A, Figer A, et al. OPTIMOX1: a randomized study of FOLFOX4 or FOLFOX7 with oxaliplatin in a stop-and-go fashion in advanced colorectal cancer--a GERCOR study. *J Clin Oncol*. 2006;24(3):394–400. doi:10.1200/JCO.2005.03.0106
5. Chibaudel B, Maindrault-Goebel F, Lledo G, et al. Can chemotherapy be discontinued in unresectable metastatic colorectal cancer? The GERCOR OPTIMOX2 Study. *J Clin Oncol*. 2009;27(34):5727–5733. doi:10.1200/JCO.2009.23.4344
6. Simkens LH, van Tinteren H, May A, et al. Maintenance treatment with capecitabine and bevacizumab in metastatic colorectal cancer (CAIRO3): a phase 3 randomised controlled trial of the Dutch Colorectal Cancer Group. *Lancet*. 2015;385(9980):1843–1852. doi:10.1016/S0140-6736(14)62004-3
7. Aparicio T, Bennouna J, Le Malicot K, et al. Final results of PRODIGE 9, a randomized phase III comparing no treatment to bevacizumab maintenance during chemotherapy-free intervals in metastatic colorectal cancer. *J Clin Oncol*. 2016;34(15_suppl):3531–3531. doi:10.1200/jco.2016.34.15_suppl.3531
8. Hochster HS, Grothey A, Hart L, et al. Improved time to treatment failure with an intermittent oxaliplatin strategy: results of CONcePT. *Ann Oncol*. 2014;25(6):1172–1178. doi:10.1093/annonc/mdu107

9. Hegewisch-Becker S, Graeven U, Lerchenmüller CA, et al. Maintenance strategies after first-line oxaliplatin plus fluoropyrimidine plus bevacizumab for patients with metastatic colorectal cancer (AIO 0207): a randomised, non-inferiority, open-label, phase 3 trial. *Lancet Oncol.* 2015;16(13):1355–1369. doi:10.1016/S1470-2045(15)00042-X

10. Yalcin S, Uslu R, Dane F, et al. Bevacizumab + capecitabine as maintenance therapy after initial bevacizumab + XELOX treatment in previously untreated patients with metastatic colorectal cancer: phase III 'stop and go' study results--a Turkish Oncology Group Trial. *Oncology.* 2013;85(6):328–335. doi:10.1159/000355914

11. Luo HY, Li YH, Wang W, et al. Single-agent capecitabine as maintenance therapy after induction of XELOX (or FOLFOX) in first-line treatment of metastatic colorectal cancer: randomized clinical trial of efficacy and safety. *Ann Oncol.* 2016;27(6):1074–1081. doi:10.1093/annonc/mdw101

12. Koeberle D, Betticher DC, von Moos R, et al. Bevacizumab continuation versus no continuation after first-line chemotherapy plus bevacizumab in patients with metastatic colorectal cancer: a randomized phase III non-inferiority trial (SAKK 41/06). *Ann Oncol.* 2015;26(4):709–714. doi:10.1093/annonc/mdv011

13. Tournigand C, Chibaudel B, Samson B, et al. Bevacizumab with or without erlotinib as maintenance therapy in patients with metastatic colorectal cancer (GERCOR DREAM; OPTIMOX3): a randomised, open-label, phase 3 trial. *Lancet Oncol.* 2015;16(15):1493–1505. doi:10.1016/S1470-2045(15)00216-8

14. Johnsson A, Hagman H, Frödin J-E, et al. A randomized phase III trial on maintenance treatment with bevacizumab alone or in combination with erlotinib after chemotherapy and bevacizumab in metastatic colorectal cancer: the Nordic ACT Trial. *Ann Oncol.* 2013;24(9):2335–2341. doi:10.1093/annonc/mdt236

15. Berry SR, Cosby R, Asmis T, et al. Continuous versus intermittent chemotherapy strategies in metastatic colorectal cancer: a systematic review and meta-analysis. *Ann Oncol.* 2015;26(3):477–485. doi:10.1093/annonc/mdu272

How I Treat Metastatic Colorectal Cancer With Emerging Therapeutic Strategies

Niharika B. Mettu and John H. Strickler

INTRODUCTION

Recent advances in the genomic characterization of colorectal cancer (CRC) have led to the identification of genes and pathways that are responsible for malignant transformation, progression, and metastasis (1). Several of these genomic alterations and molecular pathways are recurrent in metastatic colorectal cancer (mCRC) (2,3). CRC tumors are genetically heterogeneous, and this heterogeneity has complicated efforts to target molecular drivers. Despite this heterogeneity, some CRC tumors have aberrations that are critical to their growth and development, and these aberrations are potentially susceptible to therapeutic interventions. In some patients, these alterations are potentially actionable with therapies that are already approved by the Food and Drug Administration (FDA) for other tumor types; in other patients, these alterations are promising targets for novel therapeutic strategies. This chapter focuses on many of these molecularly targeted strategies, including those designed to target alterations in *KRAS* and *NRAS (RAS), MET, HER2, BRAF, EGFR,* and others in mCRC.

KRAS

The Kirsten Ras (*KRAS*) oncogene encodes a guanosine triphosphate (GTP)- guanosine diphosphate (GDP) binding protein downstream of the epidermal growth factor receptor (EGFR) in the MAP kinase (MAPK) cell signaling pathway. *KRAS* mutations occur in approximately 40% to 50% of patients with mCRC; these driver mutations are responsible for initiation, proliferation, and progression of the disease (3–5). Mutations in *KRAS* occur in exons 2 (codons 12 and 13), 3 (codons 59 and 61), and 4 (codons 117 and 146), with the most common mutation being a glycine to aspartic acid amino acid substitution in codon 12 (G12D). Other *KRAS* mutations outside of exons 2–4 have been reported, though the function and pathogenicity of these rare variants are less established (6). Mutations in *NRAS*, which confer similar pathogenicity and predict negative response to anti-EGFR antibodies, are found at an incidence of approximately 5% in mCRC (4,7).

Despite the importance of *KRAS* and *NRAS* mutations in mCRC, the development of therapeutic strategies targeting the RAS signaling pathway has presented many clinical challenges and limited success. Ras proteins require membrane association for their activity, and essential to this process is lipid modification by a farnesyl isoprenoid (8). A phase II trial of the farnesyl transferase inhibitor (FTI) SCH 66336 resulted in no objective responses (9). The failure of FTIs is likely due to membrane association of KRAS and NRAS via other mechanisms (8). Besides membrane association of Ras proteins, there may be a role for drugs that are involved in processing of Ras proteins; efforts to target Ras chaperone proteins—such as PDE-delta—have been shown to impair oncogenic KRAS signaling, and these strategies could be explored further in mCRC (10). Another area of therapeutic potential is targeting KRAS with siRNAs in synthetic nanoparticles, which has been shown to prevent the growth of KRAS-driven lung tumors in vivo (11). The prospect of suppressing KRAS activity and preventing drug resistance to anti-EGFR therapies by specifically targeting KRAS with siRNAs warrants further studies.

A Clinical Vignette ("How I Treat") is included at the end of the chapter.

MEK is downstream of RAS and RAF in the MAPK signaling pathway and has been the focus of several drug development efforts. In a phase II, multicenter, open-label study, 67 patients with breast, colon, non–small cell lung, and pancreatic cancers were treated with the first-generation MEK inhibitor CI-1040 (PD-184352). Stable disease (SD) lasting a median of 4.4 months was confirmed in eight patients, only two of whom had colon cancer. Given the limited antitumor activity of this molecule, further development of CI-1040 in colon cancer was not pursued (12). PD-0325901 is a second-generation MEK inhibitor, further developed to target the MAPK signaling pathway. PD-0325901 is a derivative of CI-1040 with 50-fold greater potency and longer duration of target suppression. The first-in-human trial of PD-0325901 in 35 evaluable patients showed only two partial responses (PRs) in melanoma patients, and 8 patients with SD, 1 of whom had CRC. PD-0325901 was subsequently evaluated in a phase II study in 34 patients with advanced non–small cell lung cancer (NSCLC), but the study was terminated due to a lack of objective responses and concerns about ocular toxicity and neurotoxicity (13). Another second-generation MEK inhibitor selumetinib (AZD6244) was compared with capecitabine monotherapy in 69 patients with mCRC (14). There was no difference in objective response rate (ORR) between the treatment groups, and progression-free survival (PFS) was 81 days and 88 days in the selumetinib and capecitabine groups, respectively. Given the failure of selumetinib and other MEK inhibitors to provide meaningful clinical benefit for patients with mCRC, further development of MEK inhibitors as a single agent has not been pursued.

Despite the failure of single-agent MEK inhibition in mCRC, combinatorial approaches to target *KRAS*- or *NRAS*-mutated mCRC are ongoing. Gene expression profiling of 55 *KRAS*-mutated mCRC tumors identified functional enrichment in cell cycle and mitosis processes, including the mitotic transcription factor FOXM1 (15). CDK 4/6 is an upstream regulator of FOXM1, and dual inhibition of CDK 4/6 and MEK markedly attenuated cell growth and colony formation in *KRAS*-mutant CRC cell lines and inhibited tumor growth in *KRAS*-mutant patient derived xenografts (16,17). Further studies of the CDK 4/6 inhibitor palbociclib in combination with cetuximab in mCRC (NCT03446157) and in combination with cisplatin or carboplatin in advanced solid tumors (NCT02897375) are ongoing.

Given the importance of *KRAS* in multiple advanced solid tumors, it has been the focus of extensive drug development. Early efforts to block RAS activity have been hampered by either primary or acquired resistance. Resistance often develops as a result of second-site mutations, and these mutations limit the effectiveness of targeted strategies. Additionally, RAS inhibitors may paradoxically stimulate oncogenic pathways by preventing feedback inhibition of upstream signaling proteins (18). Further characterizing mechanisms of resistance may identify novel combinatorial strategies that could be employed—either initially or at the development of resistance—to improve the effectiveness of RAS-targeting therapies.

MET

The receptor tyrosine kinase cMET (mesenchymal–epithelial transition factor) is associated with tumor cell invasiveness, metastasis, and proliferation (19). Binding of its only known ligand, hepatocyte growth factor (HGF), leads to receptor homodimerization, and downstream activation of the PI3K-AKT, RAS-MAPK, RAP1-FAK, and RAC1-CDC42-cadherin pathways (20). Overexpression of cMET is relatively common in CRC tumors, occurring in nearly half of tumors (21). On the other hand, *MET* gene amplification is rare, occurring in less than 3% of treatment-naïve mCRC tumors (22). Because *MET* amplification drives resistance to anti-EGFR therapies, the frequency of *MET* amplification tends to increase after exposure to anti-EGFR therapies (23–25).

In patients with various *MET* amplified advanced solid tumors, MET inhibitors have demonstrated single-agent activity. A case series of two patients with metastatic NSCLC and high level *MET* gene amplification (*MET/CEP7* ratio >5) demonstrated substantial clinical activity for the MET inhibitor crizotinib (26). In addition, several phase I studies of selective MET inhibitors have noted single-agent activity in patients with *MET* amplified advanced solid tumors, including ABT-700 (27), AMG337 (28), and SAR125844 (29). Despite these signals of activity in gastric, lung, and ovarian cancers, the activity of MET inhibitors against *MET* amplified mCRC is unknown. A study of cabozantinib, an orally bioavailable inhibitor of VEGFR2, TIE-2, RET, AXL, and cMET, is ongoing in patients with *MET* amplified mCRC (NCT02008383).

Dual inhibition of the MET and EGFR receptors may also result in enhanced therapeutic activity, though results have been inconclusive thus far. In a randomized phase II study testing the combination of panitumumab with the anti-HGF monoclonal antibody rilotumumab (AMG102), patients receiving panitumumab/rilotumumab had greater response rate (RR) and PFS than those receiving panitumumab/placebo (RR 31% vs. 21%; PFS 5.2 months vs. 3.7 months) (30). It is unknown if the clinical benefits of panitumumab/ rilotumumab were even greater in patients with cMET overexpressing or *MET* amplified tumors. A study evaluating the clinical activity of cabozantinib and panitumumab in patients with *RAS*-wild-type mCRC is ongoing (NCT02008383). In addition, a study evaluating the combination of the MEK inhibitor binimetinib combined with the cMET inhibitor crizotinib is under way in patients with *RAS*-mutated and *RAS*-wild-type mCRC (NCT02510001). This study will further evaluate the combination in patients with cMET overexpressing, *MET* mutated, and *MET* amplified mCRC.

HER2

HER2 is a member of a family of four related receptor tyrosine kinases, including HER1 (EGFR), HER2, HER3, and HER4. HER2 is encoded by the *ERBB2* gene. Amplification of *ERBB2* leads to HER2 receptor overexpression and HER2 pathway addiction. In other cancers that have *ERBB2* amplification or HER2 protein overexpression, targeted therapies that block HER2 have become important therapeutic interventions (31,32).

In patients with mCRC, the prevalence of *ERBB2* amplification is approximately 3% (1,33). However, among patients with *RAS*- and *BRAF*-wild-type mCRC, the prevalence of ERBB2 amplification is approximately 5–10% (34,35). *ERBB2* amplification is a likely driver of EGFR antibody resistance (34,36,37). Anti-HER2 therapies are active in patients with *ERBB2* amplified mCRC. In a single-arm, phase II trial conducted in 27 patients with refractory HER2-positive mCRC (HER2 3+ by immunohistochemistry or amplified by in situ hybridization), dual HER2 blockade with lapatinib and trastuzumab resulted in a 30% RR, and a nearly 5-month median time to progression (35). In addition, the multicenter, open-label, phase IIA MyPathway multibasket study (NCT02091141) evaluated pertuzumab and trastuzumab in 37 patients with treatment-refractory HER2+ mCRC. This dual HER2 targeting strategy demonstrated an RR of 38% (95% CI: 23%–55%), and an additional four patients had SD lasting longer than 120 days. The median duration of response was 11 months (38,39). Further study of trastuzumab and pertuzumab in patients with HER2-positive mCRC is ongoing in the SWOG 1613 trial. This study will compare the PFS of trastuzumab/pertuzumab versus cetuximab/irinotecan (NCT03365882). In addition, novel anti-HER2 targeting strategies are currently under investigation for HER2+ mCRC. Tucatinib is an oral, potent, tyrosine kinase inhibitor that is highly specific for HER2. A phase II, open-label study of tucatinib combined with trastuzumab in patients with HER2+ mCRC is currently underway (NCT03043313). HER2 testing is advised to support clinical trial enrollment and maximize therapeutic options.

BRAF

B-type Raf kinase V600E (BRAF^{V600E}) mutations are present in 7% to 10% of patients with mCRC and are associated with aggressive biology, short overall survival (OS), and poor response to standard chemotherapy (1,40–43). BRAF^{V600E} results in constitutive activation of MEK1 and MEK2, leading to activation of the MAPK signaling cascade (44,45). *BRAF* mutations are usually mutually exclusive with *KRAS* or *NRAS* mutations (46). Due to the limited therapeutic options for patients with *BRAF*-mutated mCRC, a number of therapeutic options have been evaluated (47).

BRAF inhibitors have limited single-agent activity against BRAF-mutated mCRC. EGFR-mediated reactivation of the RAS-MAPK pathway prevents sustained MAPK pathway inhibition and leads to therapeutic escape (48). In a phase II study of vemurafenib in patients with BRAF-mutated mCRC, only 1 of 21 patients treated with vemurafenib had a confirmed PR, 7 other patients had SD, and the median PFS was only 2.1 months (48–51). In addition to EGFR-mediated activation of the RAS-MAPK pathway, other mechanisms of resistance to BRAF inhibitors include activation of the phosphoinositide 3-kinase (PI3K) and Wnt-β-catenin pathways (43,48,50–54).

Understanding mechanisms of resistance to BRAF inhibitors has helped to identify possible combinatorial strategies. Dual inhibition of BRAF and EGFR produces sustained suppression of MAPK signaling and resensitization to BRAF inhibitors in preclinical models (55–60). In the randomized phase 2 SWOG S1406 study, patients with BRAF^{V600E} mutated mCRC who had received one or two prior regimens of systemic chemotherapy were randomized to either cetuximab/irinotecan versus cetuximab/irinotecan/vemurafenib. The study met its primary end point, with the combination of cetuximab/irinotecan/vemurafenib improving PFS (4.3 months vs. 2 months, HR: 0.42, $p < .0001$), RR (16% vs. 4%, $p = .09$), and disease control rate (67% vs. 22%, $p < .001$) (61). Despite high rates of cross-over, survival also favored the combination of cetuximab/irinotecan/vemurafenib, though this difference was not statistically significant (9.6 months vs. 5.9 months, HR: 0.73, $p = .19$). Based on these results, the combination of cetuximab/irinotecan/vemurafenib has been added to the NCCN guidelines for BRAF-mutated mCRC.

Other anti-BRAF therapeutic strategies may be active against BRAF-mutated mCRC. In vitro and preclinical studies suggested improved antitumor activity with the addition of MEK inhibition to BRAF and EGFR inhibitors. In a phase Ib/II study, 102 patients with advanced BRAF-mutated mCRC were randomized 1:1 to encorafenib/cetuximab versus encorafenib/cetuximab/alpelisib (PI3Kα inhibitor) (58). The triplet combination compared to the doublet had superior PFS (5.4 vs. 4.2 months; HR = 0.69) and RR (27% vs. 22%). Although the combination of encorafenib/cetuximab/alpelisib shows promising clinical activity, the addition of a PI3Kα inhibitor adds additional toxicity. The BEACON CRC (NCT02928224) study is currently evaluating the combination of the selective BRAF inhibitor encorafenib, the MEK inhibitor binimetinib, and cetuximab in patients with BRAF^{V600E} mutated mCRC. Six-hundred fifteen patients will be randomized 1:1:1 to encorafenib/binimetinib/cetuximab, encorafenib/cetuximab, or control (investigator's choice of irinotecan/cetuximab or FOLFIRI/cetuximab). The primary end point of this study is OS of the triplet combination versus the control (62). Results from the safety lead-in among the first 30 patients demonstrated a median PFS of 8 months, a confirmed overall RR (ORR) of 48%, and 3 patients who achieved complete response (CR) (63). Furthermore, the ORR was 62% in 16 patients who had only received one prior line of therapy. These results demonstrate the potential benefit of the triplet combination for patients with BRAF^{V600E} mutated mCRC, for whom treatment options have been historically limited.

EGFR

EGFR mutations are rare in primary CRC tumor tissue, but somatic mutations in the EGFR ectodomain (ECD) are implicated in acquired resistance to anti-EGFR antibodies. Genomic profiling of cell-free DNA (cfDNA) has identified acquired EGFR ECD mutations in approximately 10% of patients who develop resistance to anti-EGFR therapy (64,65). EGFR ECD mutations are the target of novel anti-EGFR antibody therapies, including MM-151 and Sym004. MM-151 is a combination of three antibodies that simultaneously engage distinct, nonoverlapping epitopes on the EGFR ECD with subnanomolar affinities (66). Treatment with MM-151 reduces the mutant allele frequency of EGFR ECD mutations in the peripheral blood of patients with mCRC who had previously developed EGFR antibody resistance (67). In the phase I study of MM-151 in 57 patients with refractory solid tumors, PRs were observed in 2 patients with mCRC and SD greater than 4 months was observed in 8 patients (68). Various combination studies of MM-151, however, were either terminated or withdrawn, and further development of this drug has not been pursued. Sym004 is a mixture of two monoclonal antibodies, futuximab and modotuximab, that bind to nonoverlapping epitopes in EGFR ECD III, leading to highly efficient receptor internalization and degradation (69,70). Despite promising preliminary data, in a randomized phase II study Sym004 failed to improve survival compared to investigator choice therapy (71). Therapeutic strategies that target EGFR ECD mutations may be limited by tumor heterogeneity. In an analysis of 42 patients with mCRC who had EGFR ECD mutations, 91% of patients had at least one additional co-occurring resistance alteration, including *KRAS* mutations, *NRAS* mutations, *MET* amplification, and *ERBB2* amplification (72). Tumor heterogeneity remains a significant challenge for the design of molecularly targeted therapies, particularly in the setting of acquired EGFR antibody resistance (73).

NEW AND EMERGING TARGETS

Other therapeutic targets have been explored in mCRC. The fibroblast growth factor receptor (FGFR) is a receptor tyrosine kinase that stimulates tumor growth, metastasis, and resistance to apoptosis. Though preclinical studies have pointed to a putative role of FGFR in mCRC, results have thus far been mixed (74–77). Regorafenib is an inhibitor of multiple kinases, including FGFR, with a survival benefit in patients with mCRC (76). Nintedanib is an oral tyrosine kinase inhibitor that targets multiple cell surface receptors including VEGFR, platelet-derived growth factor (PDGFR) and FGFR1-4. In the LUME-Colon 1 phase III trial, nintedanib improved the disease control rate compared to placebo, but survival was not improved (78). FGFR inhibitors have significant activity in patients with tumors that have FGFR fusions (e.g., FGFR-BICC2), though these fusions are rare in patients with mCRC. Additionally, FGF9 amplification has been observed in approximately 5% of mCRC patients, and is associated with resistance to anti-EGFR therapies, suggesting that in some cases FGFR-targeted therapy may help overcome resistance to anti-EGFR therapy (79).

ALK, ROS1, and *NTRK* fusions are rare chromosomal aberrations present in 0.2% to 2.4% of CRC tumors (80). Chromosomal rearrangements in *NTRK1* gene (encoding the TRKA protein) result in constitutive activation of the kinase domain of TRKA. Screening for rearrangements involving *NTRK* may identify patients who could benefit from TRK inhibitors, including entrectinib and larotrectinib (81). One of these TRK inhibitors—larotrectinib—demonstrated dramatic and durable antitumor responses in patients with TRK fusion-positive cancers, 7% of whom had CRC (82).

Though *PIK3CA* mutations are relatively common in patients with mCRC, therapeutic strategies targeting PIK3CA and the PI3K pathway have thus far been unsuccessful. A randomized, phase II study of cetuximab with or without PX-866, an irreversible oral PI3K inhibitor, did not improve PFS, ORR, or OS (83). Additionally, the combination of another PI3K inhibitor, BKM120, with mFOLFOX in patients with refractory solid tumors resulted in limited clinical benefit (84). Though there is scientific rationale and preclinical data for the combination of PI3K/AKT/mTOR inhibition with RAS/RAF/MEK inhibition, a biomarker-driven phase 2 study of the AKT 1/2/3 inhibitor MK-2206 with selumetinib did not result in clinical benefit (85). Given the limited activity of PI3K inhibitors thus far, novel therapeutic strategies will require a rational biomarker-driven approach or a novel combination strategy.

Wnt-β-catenin pathway activation is ubiquitous in CRC tumors, making it a particularly attractive drug development target. Tankyrase inhibitors prevent degradation of axin, leading to destabilization of β-catenin and disrupting cell proliferation and survival. Tankyrase inhibitors reduce the growth of *APC*-mutant CRC tumors in xenograft models, but can also block tumor development in mice lacking *Apc* (86,87). Furthermore, tankyrase inhibitors have shown activity in combination with targeted agents—including AKT and PI3K inhibitors—in preclinical models (88,89). Wnt-β-catenin signaling is also disrupted by inhibitors of porcupine O-acyltransferase (PORCN), an enzyme that is critical to secretion of Wnt proteins. Inhibition of PORCN may be particularly effective in Wnt-driven cancers that do not have downstream Wnt-β-catenin pathway-activating mutations. Fusions involving *RSPO2* and *RSPO3* are examples of genetic alterations that result in Wnt-β-catenin pathway activation, independent of *APC* or *CTNNB1* mutations. The PORCN inhibitor ETC-1922159 has shown efficacy in xenografts derived from CRC patients bearing the *RSPO*-translocation. PORCN inhibitors may also be active in tumors with Rnf43 and Znrf3 mutations, which encode negative regulators of Wnt signaling (89,90). Further development of Wnt-β-catenin pathway targeting strategies is ongoing.

CONCLUSIONS

In recent years, novel technologies—including next-generation sequencing (NGS) of tumor tissue and identification of cfDNA in the blood—have improved the understanding of the genomic landscape of mCRC (72,91). With the improved understanding of genomic drivers in mCRC, therapeutic strategies have emerged to target specific alterations. The possibility of identifying actionable alterations, treating those alterations, and tracking in real time the clonal evolution of tumors offers the potential to fulfill the promise of personalized medicine. Currently, the number of patients with therapeutically actionable molecular targets is low; however, emerging targeted strategies may ultimately offer improved outcomes and better quality of life for select subsets of patients with mCRC.

Clinical Vignette 16.1

A 62-year-old female presented with abdominal pain. CT revealed thickening of the sigmoid colon with involvement of the right adnexa. The patient underwent a segmental resection of the sigmoid colon and proximal rectum with involvement of the right fallopian tube and ovary. The pathologic stage was pT4bN0M1. The patient was initially treated with FOLFOX–bevacizumab. Initial testing revealed no mutations in *KRAS* or *NRAS*, so at the time of clinical progression, she was treated with FOLFIRI–cetuximab. Upon further progression, she received trifluridine–tipiracil, panitumumab, and regorafenib. Her performance status remained Eastern Cooperative Oncology Group (ECOG) 1, even 5 years out from her initial diagnosis. She was evaluated at a tertiary care center and underwent a liver biopsy, upon which next-generation sequencing was performed and revealed wild-type *KRAS*, *NRAS*, and *BRAF* genes; no mismatch repair enzyme deficiency; *APC* mutation; *TP53* mutation; and *HER2* amplification.

REFERENCES

1. Cancer Genome Atlas Network. Comprehensive molecular characterization of human colon and rectal cancer. *Nature*. 2012;487(7407):330–337. doi:10.1038/nature11252
2. Fearon ER. Molecular genetics of colorectal cancer. *Annu Rev Pathol*. 2011;6:479–507. doi:10.1146/annurev-pathol-011110-130235
3. Mody K, Bekaii-Saab T. Clinical trials and progress in metastatic colon cancer. *Surg Oncol Clin N Am*. 2018;27(2):349–365. doi:10.1016/j.soc.2017.11.008
4. Douillard JY, Oliner KS, Siena S, et al. Panitumumab-FOLFOX4 treatment and RAS mutations in colorectal cancer. *N Engl J Med*. 2013;369(11):1023–1034. doi:10.1056/NEJMoa1305275
5. Van Cutsem E, Kohne CH, Lang I, et al. Cetuximab plus irinotecan, fluorouracil, and leucovorin as first-line treatment for metastatic colorectal cancer: updated analysis of overall survival according to tumor KRAS and BRAF mutation status. *J Clin Oncol*. 2011;29(15):2011–2019. doi:10.1200/JCO.2010.33.5091
6. Zehir A, Benayed R, Shah RH, et al. Mutational landscape of metastatic cancer revealed from prospective clinical sequencing of 10,000 patients. *Nat Med*. 2017;23(6):703–713. doi:10.1038/nm.4333
7. Cercek A, Braghiroli MI, Chou JF, et al. Clinical features and outcomes of patients with colorectal cancers harboring NRAS mutations. *Clin Cancer Res*. 2017;23(16):4753–4760. doi:10.1158/1078-0432.CCR-17-0400
8. Cox AD, Der CJ, Philips MR. Targeting RAS membrane association: back to the future for anti-RAS drug discovery? *Clin Cancer Res*. 2015;21(8):1819–1827. doi:10.1158/1078-0432.CCR-14-3214
9. Sharma S, Kemeny N, Kelsen DP, et al. A phase II trial of farnesyl protein transferase inhibitor SCH 66336, given by twice-daily oral administration, in patients with metastatic colorectal cancer refractory to 5-fluorouracil and irinotecan. *Ann Oncol*. 2002;13(7):1067–1071.
10. Zimmermann G, Papke B, Ismail S, et al. Small molecule inhibition of the KRAS-PDEdelta interaction impairs oncogenic KRAS signalling. *Nature*. 2013;497(7451):638–642. doi:10.1038/nature12205
11. Xue W, Dahlman JE, Tammela T, et al. Small RNA combination therapy for lung cancer. *Proc Natl Acad Sci U S A*. 2014;111(34):E3553–E3561. doi:10.1073/pnas.1412686111
12. Rinehart J, Adjei AA, Lorusso PM, et al. Multicenter phase II study of the oral MEK inhibitor, CI-1040, in patients with advanced non-small-cell lung, breast, colon, and pancreatic cancer. *J Clin Oncol*. 2004;22(22):4456–4462. doi:10.1200/JCO.2004.01.185
13. Haura EB, Ricart AD, Larson TG, et al. A phase II study of PD-0325901, an oral MEK inhibitor, in previously treated patients with advanced non-small cell lung cancer. *Clin Cancer Res*. 2010;16(8):2450–2457. doi:10.1158/1078-0432.CCR-09-1920
14. Bennouna J, Lang I, Valladares-Ayerbes M, et al. A Ppase II, open-label, randomised study to assess the efficacy and safety of the MEK1/2 inhibitor AZD6244 (ARRY-142886) versus capecitabine monotherapy in patients with colorectal cancer who have failed one or two prior chemotherapeutic regimens. *Invest New Drugs*. 2011;29(5):1021–1028. doi:10.1007/s10637-010-9392-8
15. Pek M, Yatim S, Chen Y, et al. Oncogenic KRAS-associated gene signature defines co-targeting of CDK4/6 and MEK as a viable therapeutic strategy in colorectal cancer. *Oncogene*. 2017;36(35):4975–4986. doi:10.1038/onc.2017.120

16. Lee MS, Helms TL, Feng N, et al. Efficacy of the combination of MEK and CDK4/6 inhibitors in vitro and in vivo in KRAS mutant colorectal cancer models. *Oncotarget*. 2016;7(26):39595–39608. doi:10.18632/oncotarget.9153

17. Ziemke EK, Dosch JS, Maust JD, et al. Sensitivity of KRAS-mutant colorectal cancers to combination therapy that cotargets MEK and CDK4/6. *Clin Cancer Res*. 2016;22(2):405–414. doi:10.1158/1078-0432.CCR-15-0829

18. McCormick F. KRAS as a therapeutic target. *Clin Cancer Res*. 2015;21(8):1797–1801. doi:10.1158/1078-0432.CCR-14-2662

19. Gherardi E, Sandin S, Petoukhov MV, et al. Structural basis of hepatocyte growth factor/scatter factor and MET signalling. *Proc Natl Acad Sci U S A*. 2006;103(11):4046–4051. doi:10.1073/pnas.0509040103

20. Gherardi E, Birchmeier W, Birchmeier C, Vande Woude G. (2012). Targeting MET in cancer: rationale and progress. *Nature Rev. Cancer*. 2012;12(2):89–103. doi:10.1038/nrc3205

21. Gatalica Z, Millis S, Chen S, et al. Integrating molecular profiling into cancer treatment decision making: Experience with over 35,000 cases. *J Clin Oncol*. 2013;31(suppl).

22. Palma NA, Palmer GA, Ali SM, et al. Frequency of MET amplification determined by comprehensive next-generation sequencing (NGS) in multiple solid tumors and implications for use of MET inhibitors. *J Clin Oncol*. 2013;31(suppl).

23. Bardelli A, Corso S, Bertotti A, et al. Amplification of the MET receptor drives resistance to anti-EGFR therapies in colorectal cancer. *Cancer Disc*. 2013;3(6):658–673. doi:10.1158/2159-8290.CD-12-0558

24. Engelman JA, Zejnullahu K, Mitsudomi T, et al. MET amplification leads to gefitinib resistance in lung cancer by activating ERBB3 signaling. *Science*. 2007;316(5827):1039–1043. doi:10.1126/science.1141478

25. Turke AB, Zejnullahu K, Wu YL, et al. Preexistence and clonal selection of MET amplification in EGFR mutant NSCLC. *Cancer Cell*. 2010;17(1):77–88. doi:10.1016/j.ccr.2009.11.022

26. Caparica R, Yen CT, Coudry R, et al. Responses to Crizotinib Can Occur in High-Level MET-Amplified Non-Small Cell Lung Cancer Independent of MET Exon 14 Alterations. *J Thorac Oncol*. 2017;12(1):141–144. doi:10.1016/j.jtho.2016.09.116

27. Strickler JH, LoRusso P, Yen C-J, et al. Phase 1, open-label, dose-escalation, and expansion study of ABT-700, an anti-C-met antibody, in patients (pts) with advanced solid tumors. *J Clin Oncol*. 2014;32(15_suppl):2507. doi:10.1200/jco.2014.32.15_suppl.2507

28. Hong DS, LoRusso P, Hamid O, et al. First-in-human study of AMG 337, a highly selective oral inhibitor of MET, in adult patients (pts) with advanced solid tumors. *J Clin Oncol*. 2014;32(15 suppl):2508. doi:10.1200/jco.2014.32.15_suppl.2508

29. Angevin E, Spitaleri G, Hollebecque A, et al. A first-in-human (FIH) phase I study of SAR125844, a novel selective MET kinase inhibitor, in patients (pts) with advanced solid tumors: Dose escalation results. *J Clin Oncol*. 2014;32(15_suppl):2506. doi:10.1200/jco.2014.32.15_suppl.2506

30. Cutsem EV, Eng C, Tabernero J, et al. A randomized, phase I/II trial of AMG 102 or AMG 479 in combination with panitumumab (pmab) compared with pmab alone in patients (pts) with wild-type (WT) KRAS metastatic colorectal cancer (mCRC): safety and efficacy results. *J Clin Oncol*. 2011;29(4_suppl):366. doi:10.1200/jco.2011.29.4_suppl.366

31. Blackwell KL, Burstein HJ, Storniolo AM, et al. Randomized study of Lapatinib alone or in combination with trastuzumab in women with ErbB2-positive, trastuzumab-refractory metastatic breast cancer. *J Clin Oncol*. 2010;28(7):1124–1130. doi:10.1200/JCO.2008.21.4437

32. Blackwell KL, Burstein HJ, Storniolo AM, et al. Overall survival benefit with lapatinib in combination with trastuzumab for patients with human epidermal growth factor receptor 2-positive metastatic breast cancer: final results from the EGF104900 Study. *J Clin Oncol*. 2012;30(21):2585–2592. doi:10.1200/JCO.2011.35.6725

33. Ross JS, Fakih M, Ali SM, et al. Targeting HER2 in colorectal cancer: The landscape of amplification and short variant mutations in ERBB2 and ERBB3. *Cancer*. 2018;124(7):1358–1373. doi:10.1002/cncr.31125

34. Raghav KP, Overman MJ, Yu R, et al. HER2 amplification as a negative predictive biomarker for anti-epidermal growth factor receptor antibody therapy in metastatic colorectal cancer. *J Clin Oncol*. 2016;34(15_suppl):3517.doi:10.1200/jco.2016.34.15_suppl.3517.

35. Sartore-Bianchi A, Trusolino L, Martino C, et al. Dual-targeted therapy with trastuzumab and lapatinib in treatment-refractory, KRAS codon 12/13 wild-type, HER2-positive metastatic colorectal cancer (HERACLES): a proof-of-concept, multicentre, open-label, phase 2 trial. *Lancet Oncol*. 2016;17(6):738–746. doi:10.1016/S1470-2045(16)00150-9

36. Bertotti A, Migliardi G, Galimi F, et al. A molecularly annotated platform of patient-derived xenografts ("xenopatients") identifies HER2 as an effective therapeutic target in cetuximab-resistant colorectal cancer. *Cancer Disc*. 2011;1(6):508–523. doi:10.1158/2159-8290.CD-11-0109

37. Martin V, Landi L, Molinari F, et al. HER2 gene copy number status may influence clinical efficacy to anti-EGFR monoclonal antibodies in metastatic colorectal cancer patients. *Br J Cancer.* 2013;108(3):668–675. doi:10.1038/bjc.2013.4
38. Hainsworth JD, Meric-Bernstam F, Swanton C, et al. Targeted therapy for advanced solid tumors on the basis of molecular profiles: results from mypathway, an open-label, phase IIa multiple basket study. *J Clin Oncol.* 2018;36(6):536–542. doi:10.1200/JCO.2017.75.3780
39. Hurwitz H, Raghav K, Burris HA, et al. Pertuzumab + trastuzumab for HER2-amplified/overexpressed metastatic colorectal cancer (mCRC): Interim data from MyPathway. *J Clin Oncol.* 2017;35(4_suppl):676.
40. Bokemeyer C, Van Cutsem E, Rougier P, et al. Addition of cetuximab to chemotherapy as first-line treatment for KRAS wild-type metastatic colorectal cancer: pooled analysis of the CRYSTAL and OPUS randomised clinical trials. *Eur J Cancer.* 2012;48(10):1466–1475. doi:10.1016/j.ejca.2012.02.057
41. Morris V, Overman MJ, Jiang ZQ, et al. Progression-free survival remains poor over sequential lines of systemic therapy in patients with BRAF-mutated colorectal cancer. *Clin Colorectal Cancer.* 2014;13(3):164–171. doi:10.1016/j.clcc.2014.06.001
42. Scartozzi M, Giampieri R, Aprile G, et al. The distinctive molecular, pathological and clinical characteristics of BRAF-mutant colorectal tumors. *Expert Rev Mol Diagn.* 2015;15(8):979–987. doi:10.1586/14737159.2015.1047346
43. Strickler JH, Wu C, Bekaii-Saab T. Targeting BRAF in metastatic colorectal cancer: Maximizing molecular approaches. *Cancer Treat Rev.* 2017;60:109–119. doi:10.1016/j.ctrv.2017.08.006
44. Davies H, Bignell GR, Cox C, et al. Mutations of the BRAF gene in human cancer. *Nature.* 2002;417(6892):949–954. doi:10.1038/nature00766
45. Dhillon AS, Hagan S, Rath O, et al. MAP kinase signalling pathways in cancer. *Oncogene.* 2007;26(22):3279–3290. doi:10.1038/sj.onc.1210421
46. Tie J, Gibbs P, Lipton L, et al. Optimizing targeted therapeutic development: analysis of a colorectal cancer patient population with the BRAF(V600E) mutation. *Int J Cancer.* 2011;128(9):2075–2084. doi:10.1002/ijc.25555
47. Clarke CN, Kopetz ES. BRAF mutant colorectal cancer as a distinct subset of colorectal cancer: clinical characteristics, clinical behavior, and response to targeted therapies. *J Gastrointest Oncol.* 2015;6(6):660–667. doi:10.3978/j.issn.2078-6891.2015.077
48. Corcoran RB, Ebi H, Turke AB, et al. EGFR-mediated re-activation of MAPK signaling contributes to insensitivity of BRAF mutant colorectal cancers to RAF inhibition with vemurafenib. *Cancer Disc.* 2012;2(3):227–235. doi:10.1158/2159-8290.CD-11-0341
49. Kopetz S, Desai J, Chan E, et al. Phase II pilot study of vemurafenib in patients with metastatic BRAF-mutated colorectal cancer. *J Clin Oncol.* 2015;33(34):4032–4038. doi:10.1200/JCO.2015.63.2497
50. Poulikakos PI, Zhang C, Bollag G, et al. RAF inhibitors transactivate RAF dimers and ERK signalling in cells with wild-type BRAF. *Nature.* 2010;464(7287):427–430. doi:10.1038/nature08902
51. Prahallad A, Sun C, Huang S, et al. Unresponsiveness of colon cancer to BRAF(V600E) inhibition through feedback activation of EGFR. *Nature.* 2012;483(7387):100–103. doi:10.1038/nature10868
52. Ahmed D, Eide PW, Eilertsen IA, et al. Epigenetic and genetic features of 24 colon cancer cell lines. *Oncogenesis.* 2013;2:e71. doi:10.1038/oncsis.2013.35
53. Anastas JN, Kulikauskas RM, Tamir T, et al. WNT5A enhances resistance of melanoma cells to targeted BRAF inhibitors. *J Clin Invest.* 2014;124(7):2877–2890. doi:10.1172/JCI70156
54. Suraweera N, Robinson J, Volikos E, et al. Mutations within Wnt pathway genes in sporadic colorectal cancers and cell lines. *Int J Cancer.* 2006;119(8):1837–1842. doi:10.1002/ijc.22046
55. Corcoran RB, Andre T, Atreya CE, et al. Combined BRAF, EGFR, and MEK Inhibition in Patients with BRAF(V600E)-Mutant Colorectal Cancer. *Cancer Discov.* 2018;8(4):428–443. doi:10.1158/2159-8290.CD-17-1226
56. Desai J, Markman B, Ananda S, et al. A phase I/II trial of combined BRAF and EGFR inhibition in patients (pts) with BRAF V600E mutated (BRAFm) metastatic colorectal (mCRC): the EViCT (Erlotinib and Vemurafenib in Combination Trial) study. *J Clin Oncol.* 2017;35(15_suppl):3557.
57. Hyman DM, Puzanov I, Subbiah V, et al. Vemurafenib in Multiple Nonmelanoma Cancers with BRAF V600 Mutations. *N Engl J Med.* 2015;373(8):726–736. doi:10.1056/NEJMoa1502309
58. Tabernero J, Van Geel R, Guren TK, et al. Phase 2 results: Encorafenib (ENCO) and cetuximab (CETUX) with or without alpelisib (ALP) in patients with advanced BRAF-mutant colorectal cancer (BRAFm CRC). *J Clin Oncol.* 2016;34(15_suppl):3544. doi:10.1200/jco.2016.34.15_suppl.3544
59. van Geel R, Tabernero J, Elez E, et al. A Phase Ib Dose-Escalation Study of Encorafenib and Cetuximab with or without Alpelisib in Metastatic BRAF Mutant Colorectal Cancer. *Cancer Discov.* 2017;7(6):610–619. doi:10.1158/2159-8290.CD-16-0795

60. Yaeger R, Cercek A, O'Reilly EM, et al. Pilot trial of combined BRAF and EGFR inhibition in BRAF-mutant metastatic colorectal cancer patients. *Clin Cancer Res.* 2015;21(6):1313–1320. doi:10.1158/1078-0432.CCR-14-2779

61. Kopetz S, McDonough SL, Lenz HJ, et al. Randomized trial of irinotecan and cetuximab with or without vemurafenib in BRAF-mutant metastatic colorectal cancer (SWOG S1406). *J Clin Oncol.* 2017;35(15):3505.

62. Huijberts S, Schellens JH, Fakih MG, et al. BEACON CRC (binimetinib [BINI], encorafenib [ENCO], and cetuximab [CTX] combined to treat BRAF-mutant metastatic colorectal cancer [mCRC]): A multicenter, randomized, open-label, three-arm phase III study of ENCO plus CTX plus or minus BINI vs irinotecan (IRI)/CTX or infusional 5-fluorouracil/folinic acid/IRI (FOLFIRI)/ CTX with a safety lead-in of ENCO + BINI + CTX in patients (Pts) with BRAFV600E mCRC. *J Clin Oncol.* 2017;35(15_suppl):TPS3622. doi:10.1200/jco.2017.35.15 suppl.tps3622

63. Van Cutsem E, Cuyle P-J, Huijberts S, et al. BEACON CRC study safety lead-in (SLI) in patients with BRAFV600E metastatic colorectal cancer (mCRC): Efficacy and tumor markers. *J Clin Oncol.* 2018;36(4):627.

64. Arena S, Bellosillo B, Siravegna G, et al. Emergence of Multiple EGFR Extracellular Mutations during Cetuximab Treatment in Colorectal Cancer. *Clin Cancer Res.* 2015;21(9):2157–2166. doi:10.1158/1078-0432.CCR-14-2821

65. Morelli MP, Overman MJ, Dasari A, et al. Characterizing the patterns of clonal selection in circulating tumor DNA from patients with colorectal cancer refractory to anti-EGFR treatment. *Ann Oncol.* 2015;26(4):731–736. doi:10.1093/annonc/mdv005

66. Kearns JD, Bukhalid R, Sevecka M, et al. Enhanced Targeting of the EGFR Network with MM-151, an Oligoclonal Anti-EGFR Antibody Therapeutic. *Mol Cancer Ther.* 2015;14(7):1625–1636. doi:10.1158/1535-7163.MCT-14-0772

67. Arena S, Siravegna G, Mussolin B, et al. MM-151 overcomes acquired resistance to cetuximab and panitumumab in colorectal cancers harboring EGFR extracellular domain mutations. *Sci Transl Med.* 2016;8(324):324ra314. doi:10.1126/scitranslmed.aad5640

68. Lieu CH, Harb WA, Beeram M, et al. Phase 1 trial of MM-151, a novel oligoclonal anti-EGFR antibody combination in patients with refractory solid tumors. *J Clin Oncol.* 2014;32(15_suppl):2518. doi:10.1200/jco.2014.32.15_suppl.2518

69. Dienstmann R, Patnaik A, Garcia-Carbonero R, et al. Safety and Activity of the First-in-Class Sym004 Anti-EGFR Antibody Mixture in Patients with Refractory Colorectal Cancer. *Cancer Discov.* 2015;5(6):598–609. doi:10.1158/2159-8290.CD-14-1432

70. Sanchez-Martin FJ, Bellosillo B, Gelabert M, et al. The first-in-class anti-EGFR antibody mixture Sym004 overcomes cetuximab-resistance mediated by EGFR extracellular domain mutations in colorectal cancer. *Clin Cancer Res.* 2016;22(13):3260–3267. doi:10.1158/1078-0432.CCR-15-2400

71. Montagut C, Argiles G, Ciardiello F, et al. Efficacy of Sym004 in patients with metastatic colorectal cancer with acquired resistance to anti-EGFR therapy and molecularly selected by circulating tumor DNA analyses: a phase 2 randomized clinical trial. *JAMA Oncol.* 2018;4(4):e175245. doi:10.1001/jamaoncol.2017.5245

72. Strickler JH, Loree JM, Ahronian LG, et al. Genomic Landscape of Cell-Free DNA in Patients with Colorectal Cancer. *Cancer Disc.* 2018;8(2):164–173. doi:10.1158/2159-8290.CD-17-1009

73. McGranahan N, Swanton C. Clonal heterogeneity and tumor evolution: past, present, and the future. *Cell.* 2017;168(4):613–628. doi:10.1016/j.cell.2017.01.018

74. Knuchel S, Anderle P, Werfelli P, et al. Fibroblast surface-associated FGF-2 promotes contact-dependent colorectal cancer cell migration and invasion through FGFR-SRC signaling and integrin alphavbeta5-mediated adhesion. *Oncotarget.* 2015;6(16):14300–14317. doi:10.18632/ oncotarget.3883

75. Lee CK, Lee ME, Lee WS, et al. Dovitinib (TKI258), a multi-target angiokinase inhibitor, is effective regardless of KRAS or BRAF mutation status in colorectal cancer. *Am J Cancer Res.* 2015;5(1):72–86.

76. Grothey A, Van Cutsem E, Sobrero A, et al. Regorafenib monotherapy for previously treated metastatic colorectal cancer (CORRECT): an international, multicentre, randomised, placebo-controlled, phase 3 trial. *Lancet.* 2013;381(9863):303–312. doi:10.1016/S0140-6736(12)61900-X

77. Yao TJ, Zhu JH, Peng DF, et al. AZD-4547 exerts potent cytostatic and cytotoxic activities against fibroblast growth factor receptor (FGFR)-expressing colorectal cancer cells. *Tumour Biol.* 2015;36(7):5641–5648. doi:10.1007/s13277-015-3237-1

78. Lenz HJ, Tabernero J, Yoshino T, et al. LUME-Colon 1: A double-blind, randomized phase III study of nintedanib plus best supportive care (BSC) versus placebo plus BSC in patients with colorectal cancer (CRC) refractory to standard therapies. *J Clin Oncol.* 2015;33(3_suppl):TPS794. doi:10.1200/jco.2015.33.3_suppl.tps794

79. Mizukami T, Togashi Y, Naruki S, et al. Significance of FGF9 gene in resistance to anti-EGFR therapies targeting colorectal cancer: a subset of colorectal cancer patients with FGF9 upregulation may be resistant to anti-EGFR therapies. *Mol Carcinog*. 2017;56(1):106–117. doi:10.1002/mc.22476

80. Pietrantonio F, Di Nicolantonio F, Schrock AB, et al. ALK, ROS1, and NTRK Rearrangements in Metastatic Colorectal Cancer. *J Natl Cancer Inst*. 2017;109(12). doi:10.1093/jnci/djx089

81. Milione M, Ardini E, Christiansen J, et al. Identification and characterization of a novel SCYL3-NTRK1 rearrangement in a colorectal cancer patient. *Oncotarget*. 2017;8(33):55353–55360. doi:10.18632/oncotarget.19512

82. Drilon A, Laetsch TW, Kummar S, et al. Efficacy of larotrectinib in TRK fusion-positive cancers in adults and children. *N Engl J Med*. 2018;378(8):731–739. doi:10.1056/NEJMoa1714448

83. Bowles DW, Kochenderfer M, Cohn A, et al. A randomized, phase II trial of cetuximab with or without PX-866, an irreversible oral phosphatidylinositol 3-kinase inhibitor, in patients with metastatic colorectal carcinoma. *Clin Colorectal Cancer*. 2016;15(4):337–344.e332. doi:10.1016/j.clcc.2016.03.004

84. McRee AJ, Sanoff HK, Carlson C, et al. A phase I trial of mFOLFOX6 combined with the oral PI3K inhibitor BKM120 in patients with advanced refractory solid tumors. *Invest New Drugs*. 2015;33(6):1225–1231. doi:10.1007/s10637-015-0298-3

85. Do K, Speranza G, Bishop R, et al. Biomarker-driven phase 2 study of MK-2206 and selumetinib (AZD6244, ARRY-142886) in patients with colorectal cancer. *Invest New Drugs*. 2015;33(3):720–728. doi:10.1007/s10637-015-0212-z

86. Lau T, Chan E, Callow M, et al. A novel tankyrase small-molecule inhibitor suppresses APC mutation-driven colorectal tumor growth. *Cancer Res*. 2013;73(10):3132–3144. doi:10.1158/0008-5472.CAN-12-4562

87. Waaler J, Machon O, Tumova L, et al. A novel tankyrase inhibitor decreases canonical Wnt signaling in colon carcinoma cells and reduces tumor growth in conditional APC mutant mice. *Cancer Res*. 2012;72(11):2822–2832. doi:10.1158/0008-5472.CAN-11-3336

88. Arques O, Chicote I, Puig I, et al. Tankyrase inhibition blocks Wnt/beta-catenin pathway and reverts resistance to PI3K and AKT inhibitors in the treatment of colorectal cancer. *Clin Cancer Res*. 2016;22(3):644–656. doi:10.1158/1078-0432.CCR-14-3081

89. Punt CJ, Koopman M, Vermeulen L. From tumour heterogeneity to advances in precision treatment of colorectal cancer. *Nature Rev. Clin Oncol*. 2017;14(4):235–246. doi:10.1038/nrclinonc.2016.171

90. Koo BK, van Es JH, van den Born M, et al. Porcupine inhibitor suppresses paracrine Wnt-driven growth of Rnf43;Znrf3-mutant neoplasia. *Proc Natl Acad Sci U S A*. 2015;112(24):7548–7550. doi:10.1073/pnas.1508113112

91. Bertotti A, Papp E, Jones S, et al. The genomic landscape of response to EGFR blockade in colorectal cancer. *Nature*. 2015;526(7572):263–267. doi:10.1038/nature14969

How I Treat Metastatic Colorectal Cancer With Immunotherapy

Michael Lam and Shubham Pant

NIVOLUMAB OR PEMBROLIZUMAB SHOULD BE OFFERED TO MSI/dMMR METASTATIC COLORECTAL CANCER

Patients with metastatic colorectal cancers (mCRCs) that display defective mismatch repair (dMMR) protein expression or microsatellite instability (MSI) should be offered inhibitors to immune checkpoint programmed cell death-1 (PD-1) after progression on first-line therapy. Impressive response rates were demonstrated in mCRC that was selected by dMMR or MSI status in a number of early phase KEYNOTE studies and the CHECKMATE-142 trial. These responses also led to durable progression-free survival (PFS) and overall survival (OS), which continue with longer follow-up from these trials.

Immunotherapy has traditionally displayed little efficacy when tested in unselected mCRC (1,2). However, dMMR/MSI mCRC has been associated with increased cytotoxic lymphocyte infiltration, which is associated with elevated levels of multiple immune checkpoints (3–5). MSI typing is expensive and not widely available. MSI type may be predicted by tumor-infiltrating lymphocytes (TILs). The risk of dMMR is elevated in individuals who inherit a defective allele in associated genes such as in Lynch syndrome or can occur through epigenetic mechanisms such as methylation of MutL homolog 1 (MLH1). The resultant dMMR leads to a hypermutator state with the rise in neoantigens theoretically increasing the likelihood of tumor recognition by the immune system. Cancers that typically respond to immunotherapy strategies such as melanoma and lung cancer have high somatic mutational burden from external exposures like tobacco and ultraviolet radiation. Responses to immune checkpoint therapy in mCRC were postulated by appropriate selection for hypermutators within mCRC. This was proposed through either immunohistochemistry (IHC) via loss of protein expression of mismatch repair (MMR) proteins compared to normal or by measuring the contraction or expansion of repetitive nucleotide regions prone to changes as a result of dMMR (microsatellites).

In a proof of concept phase 2 study, investigators assessed the efficacy of pembrolizumab in three cohorts. Two of these arms included treatment refractory mCRC that was divided into dMMR and proficient MMR (pMMR) groups (6), an anti-programmed death 1 immune checkpoint inhibitor, in 41 patients with progressive metastatic carcinoma with or without MMR deficiency. Pembrolizumab was administered intravenously at a dose of 10 mg per kilogram of body weight every 14 days in patients with MMR-deficient colorectal cancers, patients with pMMR colorectal cancers, and patients with MMR-deficient cancers that were not colorectal. The coprimary end points were the immune-related objective response rate and the 20-week immune-related PFS rate.

RESULTS

The immune-related objective response rate (ORR) and immune-related PFS rate were 40% (4 of 10 patients). The coprimary end points were ORR and 20-week immune-related PFS. The ORR was 40% in the dMMR group and 0% in the pMMR group at a median follow-up of 20 and 36 weeks, respectively. Twenty-week immune-related PFS was 78% and 11% in dMMR and pMMR CRC. Coprimary end points were similar in the dMMR CRC and dMMR across other tumor types. These findings demonstrated that mCRC is responsive to immune

---

A Clinical Vignette ("How I Treat") is included at the end of the chapter.

checkpoint therapy with appropriate selection. The lack of efficacy in the pMMR group also illustrated that dMMR/MSI status was a predictive biomarker for response. Results from an expanded trial were in agreement with these results (7). At a median follow-up time of 8.7 months, the response rate was 50% versus 16% in the dMMR compared to the pMMR group. Median progression-free survival (mPFS) was not reached in the dMMR group and 2.4 months in the pMMR cohort. Similarly, median OS was not reached in the dMMR group and 6 months in the pMMR group (hazard ratio [HR]: 0.247, 95% confidence interval [CI]: 0.043–0.191, *p* < .0001). This effect was durable in the dMMR group with 24-month PFS and OS rates of 66% and 61% with longer follow-up. When considered against the expected mPFS of 8 to 10 months in the first-line mCRC setting with standard-of-care (SOC) chemotherapy and biological agents, these results at 2 years are clinically remarkable in a predominantly treatment refractory group.

In 2017, the Food and Drug Administration (FDA) approved pembrolizumab for the treatment of MSI/dMMR mCRC for patients who have progressed after fluoropyrimidine, oxaliplatin, and irinotecan after consideration of this data in addition to other results from similar patients in pembrolizumab studies (8). The ORR for this combined population was 36%.

It is important to note that MSI/dMMR constitutes approximately 5% of the mCRC population. Defective MMR occurs more frequently in earlier stage disease where the reported rates of MSI are 21%, 14%, and 5% in stage II, III, and IV disease, respectively (9,10). Despite this, presence of MSI or dMMR should be tested in all mCRC given the high response rates and potential for long-term disease control with pembrolizumab. This is currently the recommendation of the National Comprehensive Cancer Network (NCCN) to select appropriate patients for immunotherapy (11,12).

The data for nivolumab, a PD-1 inhibitor, is similar to that of pembrolizumab. Patients with dMMR CRC who had progressed on prior fluoropyrimidine, oxaliplatin, or irinotecan were treated with either nivolumab or nivolumab and ipilumumab (CTLA-4 inhibitor) in a nonrandomized manner to assess ORR. Early reports demonstrated an ORR with pembrolizumab of 27% in MSI CRC. In a small number of non-MSI patients treated with nivolumab and ipilumumab combinations, the mPFS was 1.4 months (1.2–1.9 months) and there were no objective responses, recapitulating the role of dMMR/MSI status as a predictive marker of response to PD-1 blockade (13).

More mature data has reaffirmed results seen with pembrolizumab. At a median follow-up of 12 months, nivolumab monotherapy resulted in an ORR of 31% with 23 confirmed responders from 74 patients. Disease control rate (DCR) was 69% defined as stable disease or better with a duration over 12 weeks. Responses were seen irrespective of Lynch syndrome status, PD-L1 expression (dichotomized as high or low at a cutoff of 1%), and RAS or BRAF mutation status (14). The most recent report of the nivolumab monotherapy arm at a median of 21 months follow-up demonstrates a 34% ORR and more complete responders with longer follow-up (9%) (15). Median PFS was 6.6 months and median OS was still not reached. More impressively, both PFS and OS estimations displayed stability with time with the 12- and 18-month rates of PFS (44% and 44%) and OS (72% and 67%), respectively (15). Nivolumab appeared safe with a serious adverse event rate of 20% with 7% of patients discontinuing therapy due to treatment induced toxicity. These findings led to the approval of nivolumab by the FDA for MSI mCRC after progression on prior therapy with a fluoropyrimidine, oxaliplatin, or irinotecan (16). Although efficacy and toxicity appear similar between pembrolizumab and nivolumab, no definitive head-to-head trial exists to conclude superiority of either.

All patients with mCRCs that display features suggestive of MSI/dMMR should be offered pembrolizumab or nivolumab after progression or intolerance on fluoropyrimidine, oxaliplatin, or irinotecan (Figure 17.1).

NEW ISSUES ARISING FROM IMMUNOTHERAPY

Improved ORR and duration of response have led to new management issues. Imaging may need to be supplemented with other forms of assessment for adequate measures of disease activity. In the case of mixed responses, consideration of a biopsy may be required. Pseudoprogression has been described whereby patients who progress on immunotherapy by RECIST criteria subsequently have response confirmed on later scans. The true incidence of this may be as low as 4% and the majority of data about pseudoprogression exists in melanoma and lung cancer for which the mechanisms remain unclear (17) stimulating host

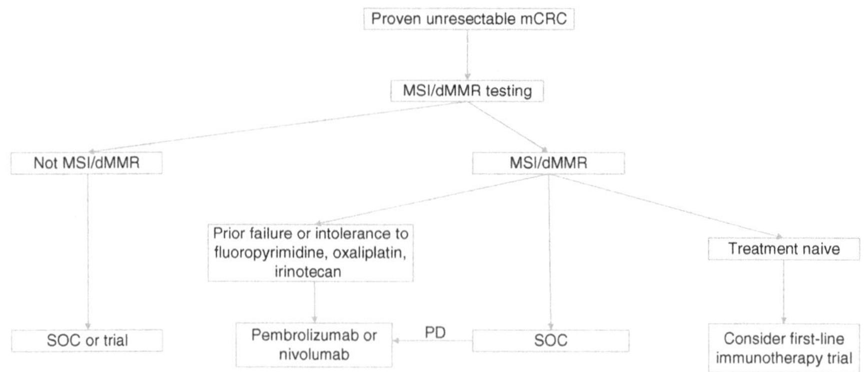

FIGURE 17.1 Algorithm for immunotherapy in mCRC.

dMMR, defective mismatch repair; mCRC, metastatic colorectal cancer; MSI, microsatellite instability; SOC, standard of care.

antitumor response. Tumor cells generate an immunosuppressive milieu with multiple mechanisms to evade immune destruction, including disruption of effective antigen presentation, reduction of effector T-cell function, and upregulation of pathways that promote tolerance and T-cell energy. 1 The programmed death (PD). In mCRC, 20 patients from the previously described MOI pembrolizumab study who had evidence of radiological disease were biopsied, after starting treatment in a time period from 1 to 5 months (18). Twelve of the biopsies contained no viable tumor with only inflammation or fibrosis evident. In this case presented, surgery was undertaken to resect stable residual disease. Pathology revealed no viable tumor. The size of an individual lesion or its presence may not always correlate to active disease on immune checkpoint therapy. Although case numbers are small, a biopsy to supplement imaging as a measure for response should be considered. This would be particularly pertinent to discontinuation decisions in the event of long-term disease control or borderline serious immune adverse events where treatment continuation entails ongoing risk.

The optimal duration of treatment is also uncertain. Studies to date have stopped therapy after 2 years if patients have continued to benefit without toxicity. In one of the pembrolizumab studies, 11 patients with complete response stopped therapy at 2 years and 7 patients with residual disease stopped prior to 2 years due to intolerance or toxicity. None of these patients have had recurrence since stopping (18). Based on these small numbers, stopping therapy in responders does not appear to impact on long-term response although this requires more investigation with long-term follow-up.

ON THE HORIZON

The successes of immunotherapy approaches in MSI/dMMR mCRC have led to strategies to enhance efficacy further. One of the arms of the CHECKMATE-142 study is testing combination immune checkpoint therapy with ipilumumab (a CTLA-4 inhibitor) and nivolumab. The ORR was 55% (65 of 119 patients) and the DCR of over 12 weeks was 80% at a median of 13.4 months follow-up (19). PFS rates at 9 and 12 months were 76% and 71%, respectively. Adverse events of grade 3 or higher were 32% with the most common being transaminitis (8%). While ORR, DCR, and PFS of the combination therapy appear to be higher than nivolumab monotherapy, this comes at the expense of increased but manageable adverse events. A direct comparison between the combination versus monotherapy is not generalizable given the nonrandomized nature of the study.

The success of immune checkpoint therapy in refractory MSI mCRC has led to questions of benefit in the first-line setting. First-line metastatic trials are now evaluating FOLFOX/bevacizumab versus the addition of nivolumab or atezolimab (PD-ligand-1 inhibitor) in separate studies (20,21). Given the impressive responses and potential for long-term disease control previously described, newly diagnosed MSI mCRC patients should be strongly encouraged to consider such trials.

New approaches for eliciting immune responses in the microsatellite stable (MSS) population, which forms the majority of mCRC, are being investigated. These may target necessary elements of an effective antitumoral response such as increasing immunogenicity of tumor cells or overcoming an immunosuppressive tumor microenvironment. For example, preclinical evidence suggested enhanced priming of cytotoxic T-cell recognition, localization and engagement in tumors with mitogen-activated protein kinase (MEK) inhibition and synergistic activity when combined with a PD-L1 inhibitor (22). In a phase 1 setting, atezolizumab and cobimetinib (MEK inhibitor) reported a response rate of 17% in an MSS, predominantly KRAS mutated mCRC population (23). However, updated results from the atezolizumab and cobimetinib study reported a drop in response rate to 8% (24), promotes intratumoral T-cell accumulation and improves anti?PD-L1 responses (Ebert, Immunity. 2016 and early reports suggest that there is no difference in OS in the phase 3 setting with this combination versus atezolizumab monotherapy or regorafenib monotherapy (25,26).

An alternative to enhancing immune responses is better selection of patients for immunomodulatory approaches by novel CRC classification systems. The consensus molecular subtypes (CMSs) represent CRC heterogeneity by gene expression into four distinct biologically relevant categories (27). we formed an international consortium dedicated to large-scale data sharing and analytics across expert groups. We show marked interconnectivity between six independent classification systems coalescing into four consensus molecular subtypes (CMSs). Two of the four subtypes (CMS1 and CMS4) are immunologically active but are skewed toward upregulation of cytotoxic lymphocytic pathways versus an inflammatory, predominantly stromal, immunosuppressive pathway (28). CMS1 mainly represents MSI CRC. Stromal-based approaches directing therapies toward immunosuppressive cells and their molecules are being tested. Although investigational at present, CMS1 and, in particular, CMS4, may represent a rational mCRC population to target for novel targeted agents directed at overcoming an immunosuppressive tumor microenvironment. For example, the bispecific antibody that targets PD-1 and transforming growth factor (TGF)-β simultaneously is an illustration of a potential approach toward CMS4, which overexpresses TGFb pathways as a hallmark feature (29). Selection based on CRC subtypes may, in the future, extend immune modulating approaches beyond MSI mCRC.

SUMMARY

Improved response rates and durable clinical outcomes for pembrolizumab and nivolumab in MSI mCRC have led to approval for use after progression or intolerance to first-line therapy. Patients can have durable responses with many median PFS and OS end points not yet reached in clinical studies assessing their use. These issues have led to questions about when to stop therapy and how best to evaluate disease in the case of mixed responses or long term radiologically evident, but stable disease. Functional imaging or biopsies may be required as

Clinical Vignette 17.1

A previously well 70-year-old female with a history of osteoarthritis, osteoporosis, and hyperlipidemia presents with a 30 pound unintentional weight loss over 4 months associated with progressive worsening of postprandial bloating, pain, and anorexia (Figure 17.2). A CT of the abdomen reveals a cecal mass and surrounding lymphadenopathy effacing the psoas and ureter (Figures 17.3 and 17.4). A colonoscopy confirms a nonobstructing adenocarcinoma that demonstrates loss of MLH1 and postmeiotic segregation2 (PMS2) protein expression. Her baseline carcinoembryonic antigen (CEA) is on the upper limit of normal (5.1 ng/mL). Due to the locally advanced nature of the disease, a diverting procedure and neoadjuvant chemotherapy is discussed prior to definitive surgery, conditional to response. The patient completes 4 cycles of FOLFOX after her loop ileostomy with minimal improvement in her abdominal symptoms. A restaging scan demonstrates progression of the nodal disease and a questionable new liver metastasis. Her CEA is elevated (21.7 ng/mL). Molecular testing reveals a BRAFV600E mutation and MLH1 methylation consistent with sporadic MSI/dMMR status.

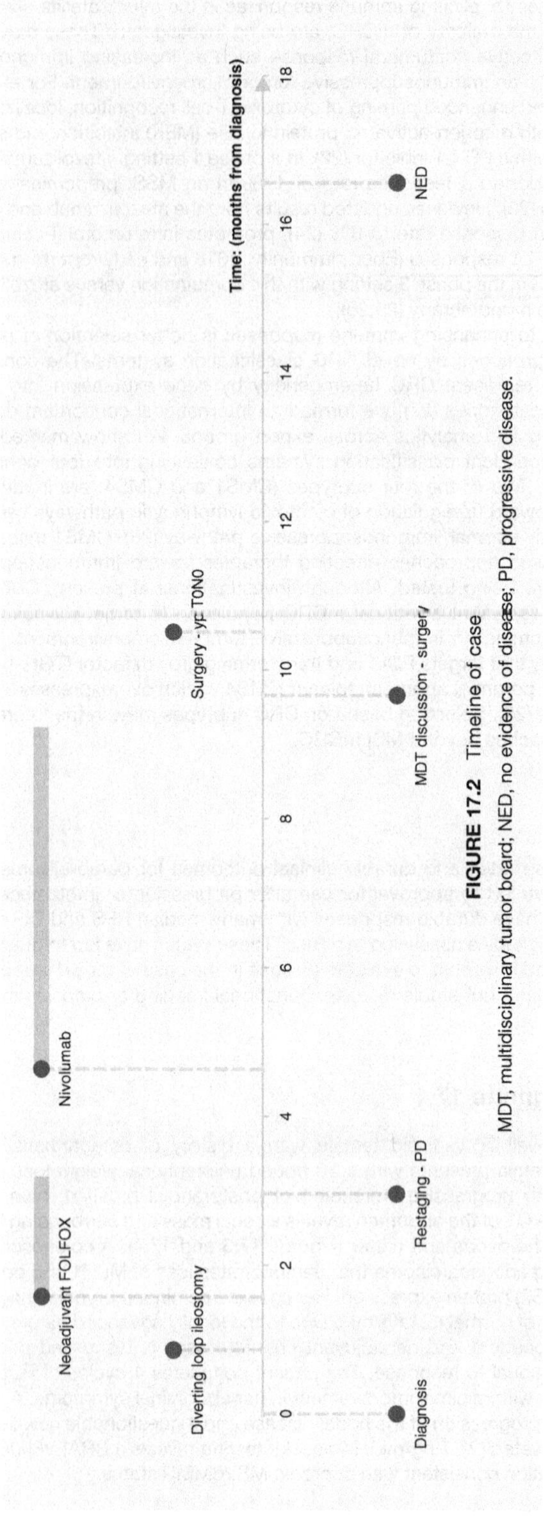

FIGURE 17.2   Timeline of case

MDT, multidisciplinary tumor board; NED, no evidence of disease; PD, progressive disease.

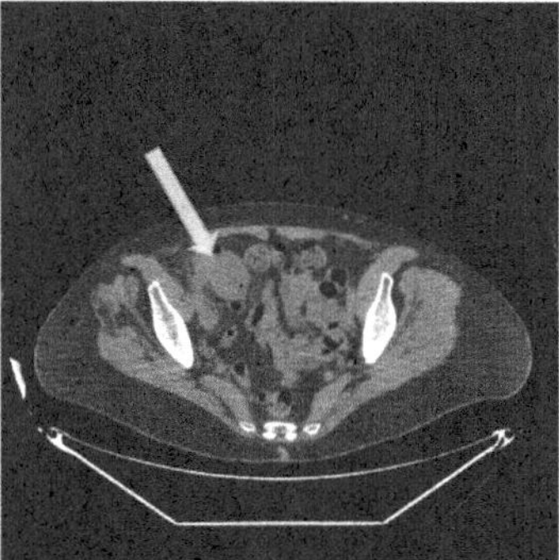

Diagnosis

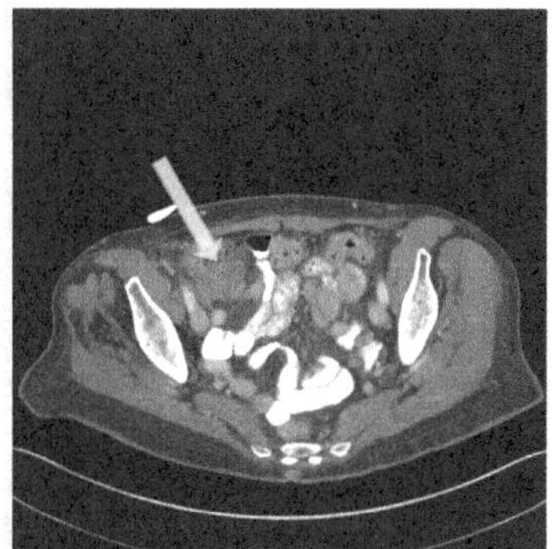

Post 5 doses of nivolumab

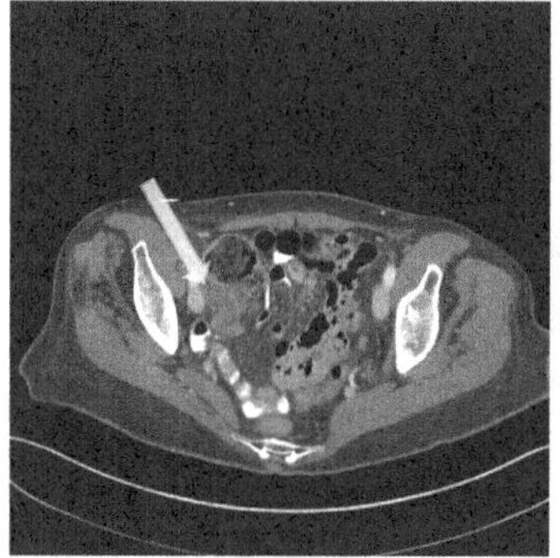

Post 10 doses of nivolumab

FIGURE 17.3 Primary lesion.

Note: Primary post FOLFOX is not included because of incomplete imaging.

The patient starts nivolumab at a performance status of Eastern Cooperative Oncology Group (ECOG) 2. After five doses, her abdominal symptoms are mildly improved. Reimaging reveals an improved appearance of the primary, and the associated lymphadenopathy shows less enhancement (Figures 17.3 and 17.4). Her CEA has also declined to 9.8 ng/mL. After an additional five doses, her CEA has declined to 5.4 ng/mL and she is feeling stronger with improved appetite and weight gain. Repeat imaging shows stable disease (Figures 17.3 and 17.4). Because of the improvement in her radiological findings and clinical state, her case is discussed at a tumor board. The liver metastasis is felt to be fatty infiltration rather than a true metastasis. She proceeds to surgery after 1 month post her last dose of nivolumab. Pathology from her partial colectomy, closure of enterostomy, and takedown of her diverting ileostomy reveals no viable tumor in the primary or in the associated lymph nodes (ypT0N0) with evidence of treatment effect. She remains disease free at 8 months post her last dose of nivolumab with clinical improvement illustrated by steady weight gain, increased physical activity, and normal CEA (Figure 17.2).

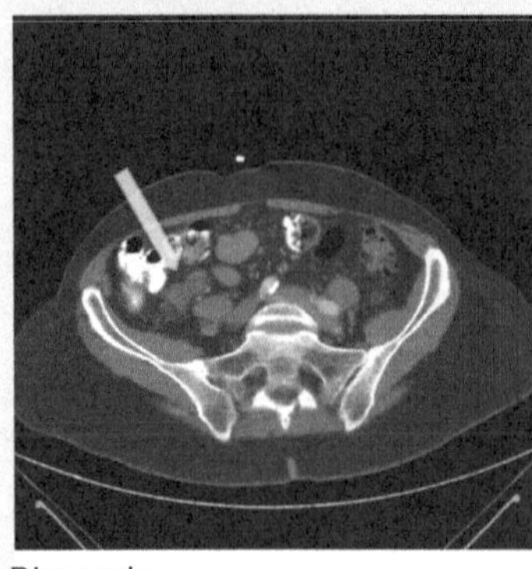

Diagnosis

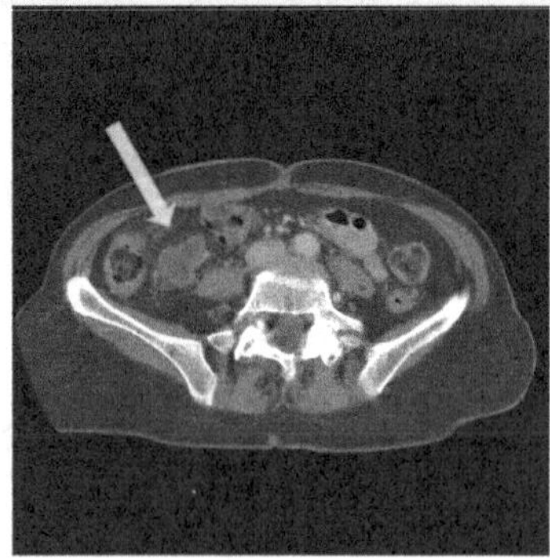

Post 4 cycles of FOLFOX

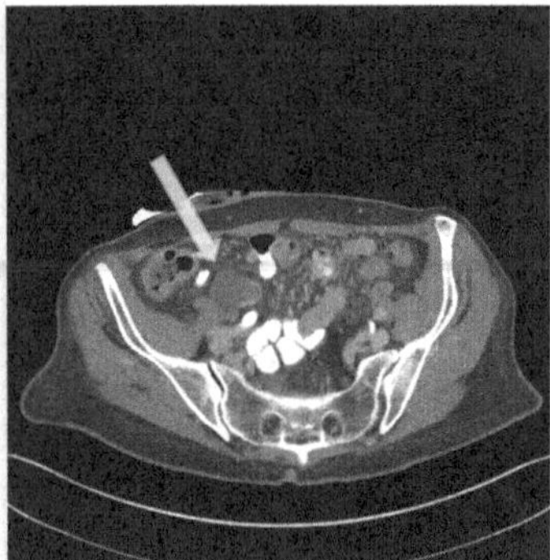

Post 5 doses of nivolumab

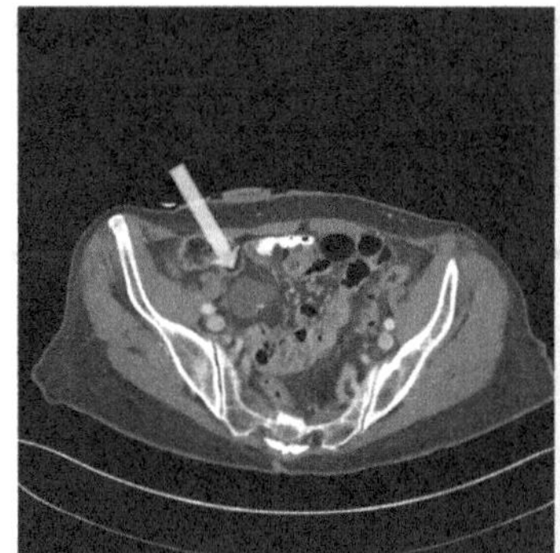

Post 10 doses of nivolumab

FIGURE 17.4 Mesenteric nodules.

an assessment of disease. Impressive outcomes have resulted in ongoing clinical evaluation in the first-line setting for PD-1/PD-L1 directed therapy. For the majority of MSS mCRC, strategies that involve increasing immunogenicity of tumors by targeting pathways or mediators of immunosuppression are being evaluated.

REFERENCES

1. Brahmer JR, Tykodi SS, Chow LQM, et al. Safety and activity of anti–PD-L1 antibody in patients with advanced cancer. *N Engl J Med*. 2012;366(26):2455–2465. doi:10.1056/NEJMoa1200694
2. Brahmer JR, Drake CG, Wollner I, et al. Phase I study of single-agent anti-programmed death-1 (MDX-1106) in refractory solid tumors: safety, clinical activity, pharmacodynamics, and immunologic correlates. *J Clin Oncol*. 2010;28(19):3167–3175. doi:10.1200/JCO.2009.26.7609
3. Smyrk TC, Watson P, Kaul K,et al. Tumor-infiltrating lymphocytes are a marker for microsatellite instability in colorectal carcinoma. *Cancer*. 2001;91(12):2417–2422. doi:10.1002/1097-0142 (20010615)91
4. Llosa NJ, Cruise M, Tam A, et al. The vigorous immune microenvironment of microsatellite instable colon cancer is balanced by multiple counter-inhibitory checkpoints. *Cancer Discov*. 2015;5(1):43–51. doi:10.1158/2159-8290.CD-14-0863
5. Dolcetti R, Viel A, Doglioni C, et al. High prevalence of activated intraepithelial cytotoxic T lymphocytes and increased neoplastic cell apoptosis in colorectal carcinomas with microsatellite instability. *Am J Pathol*. 1999;154(6):1805–1813. doi:10.1016/S0002-9440(10)65436-3

6. Le DT, Uram JN, Wang H, et al. PD-1 blockade in tumors with mismatch-repair deficiency. *N Engl J Med*. 2015;372(26):2509–2520. doi:10.1056/NEJMoa1500596

7. Le DT, Uram JN, Wang H, et al. Programmed death-1 blockade in mismatch repair deficient colorectal cancer. *J Clin Oncol*. 2016;34(15_suppl):103. doi:10.1200/JCO.2016.34.15_suppl.103

8. Accelerated approval of pembrolizumab for mCRC. https://www.accessdata.fda.gov/drug-satfda_docs/appletter/2017/125554Orig1s034ltr.pdf; 2017.

9. Bertagnolli MM, Redston M, Compton CC, et al. Microsatellite instability and loss of heterozygosity at chromosomal location 18q: prospective evaluation of biomarkers for stages II and III colon cancer--a study of CALGB 9581 and 89803. *J Clin Oncol*. 2011;29(23):3153–3162. doi:10.1200/JCO.2010.33.0092

10. Venderbosch S, Nagtegaal ID, Maughan TS, et al. Mismatch repair status and BRAF mutation status in metastatic colorectal cancer patients: a pooled analysis of the CAIRO, CAIRO2, COIN, and FOCUS studies. *Clin Cancer Res*. 2014;20(20):5322–5330. doi:10.1158/1078-0432.CCR-14-0332

11. National Comprehensive Cancer Network. Colon Cancer — Version 2.2018. https://www.nccn.org/professionals/physician_gls/pdf/colon.pdf; 2018.

12. National Comprehensive Cancer Network. Rectal Cancer — Version 1.2018. https://www.nccn.org/professionals/physician_gls/pdf/rectal.pdf; 2018.

13. Overman MJ, Kopetz S, McDermott RS, et al. Nivolumab ± ipilimumab in treatment (tx) of patients (pts) with metastatic colorectal cancer (mCRC) with and without high microsatellite instability (MSI-H): checkMate-142 interim results. *J Clin Oncol*. 2016;34(15_suppl):3501. doi:10.1200/JCO.2016.34.15_suppl.3501

14. Overman MJ, Lonardi S, Leone F, et al. Nivolumab in patients with DNA mismatch repair deficient/microsatellite instability high metastatic colorectal cancer: update from CheckMate 142. *J Clin Oncol*. 2017;35(4_suppl):519–519. doi:10.1200/JCO.2017.35.4_suppl.519

15. Overman MJ, Bergamo F, McDermott RS, et al. Nivolumab in patients with DNA mismatch repair-deficient/microsatellite instability-high (dMMR/MSI-H) metastatic colorectal cancer (mCRC): long-term survival according to prior line of treatment from CheckMate-142. *J Clin Oncol*. 2018;36(4_suppl):554. doi:10.1200/JCO.2018.36.4_suppl.554

16. U.S. Food and Drug Administration. Approved Drugs - FDA grants nivolumab accelerated approval for MSI-H or dMMR colorectal cancer. https://www.fda.gov/Drugs/InformationOnDrugs/ApprovedDrugs/ucm569366.htm; 2018.

17. Chiou VL, Burotto M. Pseudoprogression and immune-related response in solid tumors. *J Clin Oncol*. 2015;33(31):3541–3543. doi:10.1200/JCO.2015.61.6870

18. Le DT, Durham JN, Smith KN, et al. Mismatch-repair deficiency predicts response of solid tumors to PD-1 blockade. *Science*. 2017;6733(June):1–11. doi:10.1126/science.aan6733

19. Overman MJ, Lonardi S, Wong KYM, et al. Durable clinical benefit with nivolumab plus ipilimumab in DNA mismatch repair–deficient/microsatellite instability–high metastatic colorectal cancer. *J Clin Oncol*. 2018;36(8):JCO.2017.76.990. doi:10.1200/JCO.2017.76.9901

20. ClinicalTrials.gov Identifier: NCT03414983. An investigational immunotherapy study of nivolumab with standard of care therapy vs standard of care therapy for first-line treatment of colorectal cancer that has spread. https://clinicaltrials.gov/ct2/show/NCT03414983?term=nivolumab&cond=colorectal&rank=4; 2018.

21. ClinicalTrials.gov Identifier: NCT02997228. Combination chemotherapy, bevacizumab, and/or atezolizumab in treating patients with deficient DNA mismatch repair metastatic colorectal cancer. https://clinicaltrials.gov/ct2/show/NCT02997228?term=NCT02997228&rank=1; 2018.

22. Ebert PJR, Cheung J, Yang Y, et al. MAP kinase inhibition promotes T cell and anti-tumor activity in combination with PD-L1 checkpoint blockade. *Immunity*. 2016;44(3):609–621. doi:10.1016/j.immuni.2016.01.024

23. Bendell JC, Kim TW, Goh BC, et al. Clinical activity and safety of cobimetinib (cobi) and atezolizumab in colorectal cancer (CRC). *J Clin Oncol*. 2016;34(15_suppl):3502. doi:10.1200/JCO.2016.34.15_suppl.3502

24. Bendell JC, Bang Y-J, Chee CE, et al. A phase Ib study of safety and clinical activity of atezolizumab (A) and cobimetinib (C) in patients (pts) with metastatic colorectal cancer (mCRC). *J Clin Oncol*. 2018;36(4_suppl):560. doi:10.1200/JCO.2018.36.4_suppl.560

25. ClinicalTrials.gov Identifier: NCT02788279. A study to investigate efficacy and safety of cobimetinib plus atezolizumab and atezolizumab monotherapy versus regorafenib in participants with metastatic colorectal adenocarcinoma (COTEZO IMblaze370). https://clinicaltrials.gov/ct2/show/NCT02788279?term=NCT02788279&rank=1; 2018.

26. Atezolizumab, cobimetinib combo falls short in phase III mCRC trial. https://www.onclive.com/web-exclusives/atezolizumab-cobimetinib-combo-falls-short-in-phase-iii-mcrc-trial; 2018.

27. Guinney J, Dienstmann R, Wang X, et al. The consensus molecular subtypes of colorectal cancer. *Nat Med*. 2015;21(11):1350–1356. doi:10.1038/nm.3967

28. Becht E, de Reyniès A, Giraldo NA, et al. Immune and stromal classification of colorectal cancer is associated with molecular subtypes and relevant for precision immunotherapy. *Clin Cancer Res*. 2016;22(16):4057–4066. doi:10.1158/1078-0432.CCR-15-2879

29. ClinicalTrials.gov Identifier: NCT03436563. M7824 in Consensus Molecular Subtype 4, Treatment-Refractory Metastatic Colorectal Cancer. https://clinicaltrials.gov/ct2/show/NCT03436563?term=CMS4&rank=3; 2018.

II

Pancreatic Cancer

Epidemiology of Pancreatic Cancer

*Mehmet Akce, Alexandra G. Lopez-Aguiar, David A. Kooby, Field F. Willingham,
Gregory B. Lesinski, and Shishir K. Maithel*

INTRODUCTION

Pancreatic cancer (ductal adenocarcinoma and its subtypes) is the fourth most common
cause of cancer-related mortality in the United States, and it is projected to cause more than
44,000 deaths in 2018 (1). Death rates due to pancreatic cancer for men and women were
12.6/100,000 and 9.5/100,000 between 2011 and 2015 in the United States (1). It is estimated
to become the second most common cause of cancer-related mortality by 2030 and the most
common cause of cancer-related mortality by 2050 in the United States (2,3). Worldwide, it
causes 331,000 deaths annually, and it is the seventh most common cause of cancer-related mortality (4). The age estimated incidence of pancreatic cancer is 4.9/100,000 in men
and 3.6/100,000 in women globally (4). The age estimated incidence of pancreatic cancer in
men is 8.6/100,000 in more developed countries and 3.3/100,000 in less developed countries, whereas in women it is 5.9/100,000 in more developed countries and 2.4/100,000 in less
developed countries. Striking differences exist in the pancreatic cancer incidence and mortality between more developed and less developed regions globally, which could be due to differences in quality of registries, availability of diagnostic tools, or imperfect reporting. Pancreatic
ductal adenocarcinoma (PDAC) is the most common type and comprises more than 90% of all
pancreatic cancers (5). Pancreatic neuroendocrine tumors are the second most common solid
neoplasm of the pancreas and comprise <5% of all pancreas cancers (6). The median age of
diagnosis of PDAC is 71; about 90% of cases are diagnosed after the age of 55, less than 3%
of cases are diagnosed prior to the age of 44, and the incidence is 30% more common in men
(5–8). The incidence of PDAC is higher in African American men and women compared to other
racial and ethnic groups in the United States, 17.1/100,000 and 14.4/100,000, respectively
(5,8). According to Surveillance, Epidemiology, and End Results (SEER) data analysis between
1974 and 2013, pancreatic cancer incidence in the United States has increased in Caucasian
non-Hispanic and Hispanic men and remained stable in African American and Asian/Pacific
Islander men for the majority of histologic subtypes including PDAC during the 1992–2013
period (5). The rates increased in women in all racial and ethnic categories except African
American women for the same period. PDAC has the lowest survival rate for all stages combined among all cancers between 2007 and 2013 in the United States; 5-year overall survival
(OS) rate is 8% (1). Despite significant survival improvements in many cancer types, the PDAC
death rate has increased by 0.3% per year in men in recent years (1).

MODIFIABLE AND GENETIC RISK FACTORS

Multiple modifiable and genetic risk factors play a role in the development of PDAC. Modifiable
risk factors include smoking, diabetes, obesity, high fat diet, history of chronic pancreatitis,
certain infections and abdominal surgeries, occupational exposures, and environment factors;
nonmodifiable risk factors include African American ethnic origin, non–O blood group, male
sex, and genetic factors (9,10); see Table 18.1. Among all risk factors, smoking is the most
preventable risk factor for pancreatic cancer.

Smoking
Smoking is considered the most important risk factor for pancreatic cancer, and about 25% of
cases are attributable to smoking (11). There is 71% increased risk of PDAC in current smokers

TABLE 18.1 Risk Factors Associated With Pancreatic Cancer

Occupational Risk Factors	Environmental/ Lifestyle Risk Factors	Race/Ethnic Risk Factors	Medical Conditions
Methylene chloride (chlorinated hydrocarbons) Paint/paint thinners Varnish Solvents	Cigarettes or tobacco smoke exposure	African American men and women	Cirrhosis
Pesticides/herbicides/ fertilizers	Heavy alcohol	Ashkenazi Jews	Diabetes mellitus
Asbestos and lead exposure	High fat/ cholesterol diet	Non–O blood type	Chronic pancreatitis
Cement manufacturing	Processed meats	Above average height (+ 2.54 cm)	Obesity

Source: From Jarnagin WR, Belghiti J, Blumgart LH. *Blumgart's surgery of the liver, biliary tract, and pancreas.* 5th ed. Philadelphia, PA: Elsevier Saunders; 2012. https://www.clinicalkey.com/dura/browse/bookChapter/3-s2.0-C20111001236

and 19% increased risk in former smokers according to a large prospective European cohort study (12). Additionally, the risk increases with the current intensity of smoking and pack-years of smoking. Environmental tobacco smoke is also associated with increased risk of PDAC compared to no smoking (12). In a recent meta-analysis based on more than 2 million individuals from the general population, the risks of PDAC in current and former smokers compared to nonsmokers were reported to be 66% and 40%, respectively (3). The risk of pancreatic cancer persists up to 10 years after smoking cessation (13). Furthermore smoking is associated with poorer survival in patients with pancreatic cancer (14). The population attributable risk factor was estimated to be 20%, and smoking cessation has a significant impact on decreasing pancreatic cancer related deaths, should be encouraged by all physicians (13). Smoking cessation is of paramount significance in patients with existing risk factors such as hereditary pancreatitis.

Alcohol

The association between alcohol intake and pancreatic cancer development is less certain, as results of many studies may be confounded by concurrent smoking history (15,16). It is possible that alcohol consumption increases the risk of PDAC by causing chronic pancreatitis due to repeated episodes of acute pancreatitis although other mechanisms may exist. Heavy alcohol consumption and >30 grams daily alcohol intake is associated with moderately increased risk of pancreatic cancer (3,16). In a pooled nested case control study which analyzed 12 prospective cohort studies no significant association was observed in moderate alcohol consumption and PDAC development. However, high levels of alcohol (>45 g/day liquor) were associated with an increased risk of PDAC. Heavy alcohol consumption seems to increase risk of PDAC.

Pancreatitis

Pancreatitis is a known risk factor for development of PDAC. Different types of pancreatitis are associated with different risks, and hereditary pancreatitis is associated with the highest risk for PDAC, 50 to 70 times compared to general population (17). According to a pooled analysis in the international pancreatic cancer case–control consortium, strong association between pancreatitis and PDAC development was reported. The odds ratio (OR) was very high (OR: 13.56, 95% confidence interval [CI]: 8.72–21.90) in patients who had history of pancreatitis and were diagnosed with PDAC in less than 2 years (18). Population attributable risk was reported to be 1.3% in the same study indicating a small proportion of pancreatic cancer could be avoided with the prevention of pancreatitis. Similarly, a high risk for the development of PDAC was reported in a meta-analysis indicating a relative risk of 13.3 (6.1–28.9) for PDAC development in patients with chronic pancreatitis (19). While conflicting results were reported between acute pancreatitis and association with PDAC in certain cases acute pancreatitis can be the first sign of pancreatic cancer and can be developed because of ductal obstruction due to tumor.

Obesity

Obesity is associated with increased risk of PDAC, disease onset at a younger age, and worse survival in patients who are diagnosed with PDAC (20). Chronic inflammation and peripheral insulin resistance may be related to an associated risk for PDAC development although the exact pathophysiology remains unknown (21). A higher body mass index (BMI) at baseline has been shown to be associated with more advanced PDAC stage at diagnosis and decreased survival; this association was stronger in patients with longer duration of obesity in analysis of patients with large prospective cohort studies (21). In another analysis of a prospectively studied population, BMI ≥30 was associated with an increased risk of death from PDAC in both men and women, with a relative risk of 1.41. For BMI >40, the relative risks are 1.49 and 2.76, respectively (22). These results emphasize the importance of maintaining a healthy BMI.

Diabetes

Diabetes is one of the risk factors for PDAC; however, new onset diabetes could also be the first sign of pancreatic cancer (11). Diabetes is associated with a 1.8-fold increased risk of pancreatic cancer according to a pooled analysis of large case–control studies (23). Even though the risk of pancreatic cancer decreases with the increased duration of diabetes, it remains elevated at 1.4-fold even after 15 years of diabetes history. When there is a short time period between the diabetes development and a new diagnosis of pancreatic cancer, this could suggest the diabetes could be a consequence of the PDAC.

Pancreatic Cystic Lesions

Pancreatic cystic neoplasms may increase the risk of PDAC. Intraductal papillary mucinous neoplasm (IMPN), cystic islet cell tumors, solid pseudopapillary neoplasms, mucinous cystic neoplasms, and serous cystic tumors are some of the epithelial neoplastic cystic lesions of the pancreas (24). IPMN is considered premalignant and characterized by papillary growth of ductal epithelium and significant mucin production. It could involve the main pancreatic duct (MPD) or a branch duct, and the risk of pancreatic cancer development is higher for main duct IPMN (25). It is usually located in the head of the pancreas and mostly seen after the age of 50 with similar frequencies in both sexes. Worrisome features of IMPN on imaging include cyst size ≥3 cm, thickened enhanced cyst walls, enhanced mural nodule <5 mm, MPD size 5 to 9 mm, adjacent lymphadenopathy, distal pancreatic atrophy with abrupt change in the size of MPD, and rapid CA 19-9 rise with cyst growth >5 mm/2 years (26). High-risk stigmata on imaging include enhanced mural nodule ≥5 mm, MPD size ≥10 mm, and clinical obstructive jaundice in a patient with cystic lesion in the head of the pancreas. These are managed by surgical resection in clinically appropriate cases. Patients with cysts <3 cm in size without worrisome features are followed with close surveillance (26).

Genetic Factors

PDAC could also present as part of a genetic syndrome and about 5% to 10% of the patients have a family history of pancreatic cancer (27). The hereditary disorders associated with increased risk of PDAC are listed in Table 18.2, and the risk of PDAC in these hereditary disorders is substantial, up to 132-fold increased risk compared to the general population (7). There is a ninefold increase in the risk of PDAC in first-degree relatives of patients with familial PDAC and a twofold increase in first-degree relatives of patients with sporadic PDAC (28). Furthermore, the patients with family history of pancreatic cancer have increased risk of dying from other types of cancers including colon, liver, bile ducts, prostate, ovarian, and breast cancers (29). Consensus guidelines for management of patients with increased risk for familial pancreatic cancer recommend screening by magnetic resonance cholangiopancreatography and/or endoscopic ultrasonography for individuals who are first-degree relatives of patients with pancreatic cancer from familial pancreatic cancer kindred with at least two affected first-degree relatives; patients with Peutz–Jeghers syndrome; *BRCA2, p16,* or hereditary nonpolyposis colorectal cancer mutation carriers with one or more affected first-degree relatives (30). There is no recommendation for the screening interval or appropriate age to start or end the screening.

The common genetic abnormalities encountered in PDAC include *CDKN2A, SMAD4,* and *TP53* tumor suppressor genes and *KRAS* oncogene (31). Somatic mutations in *KRAS* oncogene are encountered in more than 90% of PDAC, and alterations in *CDKN2A* tumor suppressor gene are seen in about more than 90% of PDAC (7). The mutation status of the PDAC has implications in targeted therapy approaches.

TABLE 18.2 Inherited Disorders With Increased Risk of Pancreatic Ductal Adenocarcinoma

	Gene*	Chromosome	Risk Ratio
Familial breast and ovarian cancer	*BRCA2*	13	3.5–10
Familial atypical multiple mole melanoma syndrome	*CDKN2A (P16)*	9	9–47
Peutz–Jeghers syndrome	*STK11 (LKB1)*	19	132
Hereditary pancreatitis	*PRSS1; SPINK1*	7;5	50–80
Hereditary nonpolyposis colorectal cancer (Lynch syndrome)	Multiple	Multiple	9
Familial pancreatic cancer	*PALB2*	16	6
Familial pancreatic cancer (monoallelic); ataxia–telangiectasia (biallelic)	*ATM*	11	Unknown

*Gene synonyms are shown in parentheses.

Source: From Kamisawa T, Wood LD, Itoi T, Takaori K. Pancreatic cancer. *Lancet.* 2016;388(10039): 73–85. doi:10.1016/s0140-6736(16)00141-0

SIGNS AND SYMPTOMS

Presenting signs or symptoms of PDAC depend on the location of the pancreatic mass; however, the disease often presents in advanced stages with no prior signs or symptoms. About 60% to 70% of PDAC are located in the head of the pancreas; jaundice due to biliary obstruction, abdominal pain radiating to back, and pruritus are the typical presenting symptoms in these cases (32,33). Approximately 25% of PDAC are located in the body or tail of the pancreas (33). Abdominal pain is usually the most common symptom in pancreatic body and tail tumors, and these tumors often present at advanced stages (32). The common symptoms of early-stage PDAC include weight loss, nausea, vomiting, bloating, dyspepsia, abdominal pain, lethargy, changes in bowel habits, shoulder pain, jaundice, pruritus, and new onset diabetes (34). Keane et al. identified lethargy, back pain, and new onset diabetes as unique features of PDAC in their case–control study. Of the presenting symptoms of advanced PDAC, abdominal pain and diabetes are most frequently reported as the presenting symptoms (35). In certain cases, acute pancreatitis due to pancreatic duct obstruction could be the initial symptom of PDAC. Less common signs and symptoms of the disease include thrombophlebitis, panniculitis, depression, and gastric outlet obstruction (9).

OUTCOMES

Surgical resection remains the only potentially curative treatment option for PDAC; however, only about 20% of patients present with resectable disease (9). Relation of the primary pancreatic mass to the surrounding blood vessels is paramount in determining the resectability. Following surgical resection, the 5-year OS rate ranges between 20% and 25% (9). Adjuvant therapy is the standard for resected PDAC. Approximately 35% of patients present with locally advanced unresectable disease and 50% present with metastatic disease (36). Median OS ranges between 8.5 months and 11.1 months with the current standard systemic treatments in the metastatic setting (37,38). Distant recurrence is more common than local recurrence following curative surgical resection of PDAC, >70% versus >20%, respectively (9). The number of different therapeutic options is limited in patients who fail standard first-line systemic chemotherapy. Although early diagnosis impacts prognosis dramatically, there are no effective screening tests for pancreas cancer. Primary prevention by improving potentially modifiable risk factors such as smoking, diabetes, and obesity is crucial for the prevention of pancreatic cancer. Individuals with a high risk for pancreatic cancer could benefit from screening strategies as outlined by consensus-based guidelines.

REFERENCES

1. Siegel RL, Miller KD, Jemal A. Cancer statistics, 2018. *CA Cancer J Clin*. 2018;68(1):7–30. doi:10.3322/caac.21442
2. Rahib L, Smith BD, Aizenberg R, et al. Projecting cancer incidence and deaths to 2030: the unexpected burden of thyroid, liver, and pancreas cancers in the United States. *Cancer Res*. 2014;74(11):2913–2921. doi:10.1158/0008-5472.CAN-14-0155
3. Korc M, Jeon CJ, Edderkaoui M, et al. Tobacco and alcohol as risk factors for pancreatic cancer. *Best Pract Res Clin Gastroenterol*. 2017;31(5):529–536. doi:10.1016/j.bpg.2017.09.001
4. Ferlay J, Soerjomataram I, Dikshit R, et al. Cancer incidence and mortality worldwide: sources, methods and major patterns in GLOBOCAN 2012. *Int J Cancer*. 2015;136(5):E359–E386. doi:10.1002/ijc.29210
5. Gordon-Dseagu VL, Devesa SS, Goggins M, et al. Pancreatic cancer incidence trends: evidence from the Surveillance, Epidemiology and End Results (SEER) population-based data. *Int J Epidemiol*. 2017;47(2):427–439. doi:10.1093/ije/dyx232
6. Ilic M, Ilic I. Epidemiology of pancreatic cancer. *World J Gastroenterol*. 2016;22(44):9694–9705. doi:10.3748/wjg.v22.i44.9694
7. Kamisawa T, Wood LD, Itoi T, et al. Pancreatic cancer. *Lancet*. 2016;388(10039):73–85. doi:10.1016/s0140-6736(16)00141-0
8. Yeo TP. Demographics, epidemiology, and inheritance of pancreatic ductal adenocarcinoma. *Semin Oncol*. 2015;42(1):8–18. doi:10.1053/j.seminoncol.2014.12.002
9. Vincent A, Herman J, Schulick R, et al. Pancreatic cancer. *Lancet*. 2011;378(9791):607–620. doi:10.1016/S0140-6736(10)62307-0
10. Becker AE, Hernandez YG, Frucht H, et al. Pancreatic ductal adenocarcinoma: risk factors, screening, and early detection. *World J Gastroenterol*. 2014;20(32):11182–11198. doi:10.3748/wjg.v20.i32.11182
11. Wolfgang CL, Herman JM, Laheru DA, et al. Recent progress in pancreatic cancer. *CA Cancer J Clin*. 2013;63(5):318–348. doi:10.3322/caac.21190
12. Vrieling A, Bueno-de-Mesquita HB, Boshuizen HC, et al. Cigarette smoking, environmental tobacco smoke exposure and pancreatic cancer risk in the European Prospective Investigation into Cancer and Nutrition. *Int J Cancer*. 2010;126(10):2394–2403. doi:10.1002/ijc.24907
13. Iodice S, Gandini S, Maisonneuve P, et al. Tobacco and the risk of pancreatic cancer: a review and meta-analysis. *Langenbecks Arch Surg*. 2008;393(4):535–545. doi:10.1007/s00423-007-0266-2
14. Yuan C, Morales-Oyarvide V, Babic A, et al. Cigarette smoking and pancreatic cancer survival. *J Clin Oncol*. 2017;35(16):1822–1828. doi:10.1200/JCO.2016.71.2026
15. Michaud DS, Vrieling A, Jiao L, et al. Alcohol intake and pancreatic cancer: a pooled analysis from the pancreatic cancer cohort consortium (PanScan). *Cancer Causes Control*. 2010;21(8):1213–1225. doi:10.1007/s10552-010-9548-z
16. Genkinger JM, Spiegelman D, Anderson KE, et al. Alcohol intake and pancreatic cancer risk: a pooled analysis of fourteen cohort studies. *Cancer Epidemiol Biomarkers Prev*. 2009;18(3):765–776. doi:10.1158/1055-9965.EPI-08-0880
17. Carrera S, Sancho A, Azkona E, et al. Hereditary pancreatic cancer: related syndromes and clinical perspective. *Hered Cancer Clin Pract*. 2017;15:9. doi:10.1186/s13053-017-0069-6
18. Duell EJ, Lucenteforte E, Olson SH, et al. Pancreatitis and pancreatic cancer risk: a pooled analysis in the International Pancreatic Cancer Case-Control Consortium (PanC4). *Ann Oncol*. 2012;23(11):2964–2970. doi:10.1093/annonc/mds140
19. Raimondi S, Lowenfels AB, Morselli-Labate AM, et al. Pancreatic cancer in chronic pancreatitis; aetiology, incidence, and early detection. *Best Pract Res Clin Gastroenterol*. 2010;24(3):349–358. doi:10.1016/j.bpg.2010.02.007
20. Li D, Morris JS, Liu J, et al. Body mass index and risk, age of onset, and survival in patients with pancreatic cancer. *JAMA*. 2009;301(24):2553–2562. doi:10.1001/jama.2009.886
21. Yuan C, Bao Y, Wu C, et al. Prediagnostic body mass index and pancreatic cancer survival. *J Clin Oncol*. 2013;31(33):4229–4234. doi:10.1200/JCO.2013.51.7532
22. Calle EE, Rodriguez C, Walker-Thurmond K, et al. Overweight, obesity, and mortality from cancer in a prospectively studied cohort of U.S. adults. *N Engl J Med*. 2003;348(17):1625–1638. doi:10.1056/NEJMoa021423
23. Li D, Tang H, Hassan MM, et al. Diabetes and risk of pancreatic cancer: a pooled analysis of three large case-control studies. *Cancer Causes Control*. 2011;22(2):189–197. doi:10.1007/s10552-010-9686-3
24. The European Study Group on Cystic Tumours of the Pancreas. European evidence-based guidelines on pancreatic cystic neoplasms. *Gut*. 2018;67(5):789–804. doi:10.1136/gutjnl-2018-316027

25. Pagliari D, Saviano A, Serrichio ML, et al. Uptodate in the assessment and management of intraductal papillary mucinous neoplasms of the pancreas. *Eur Rev Med Pharmacol Sci.* 2017;21(12):2858–2874.
26. Tanaka M, Fernández-del Castillo C, Kamisawa T, et al. Revisions of international consensus Fukuoka guidelines for the management of IPMN of the pancreas. *Pancreatology.* 2017;17(5):738–753. doi:10.1016/j.pan.2017.07.007
27. Chen F, Roberts NJ, Klein AP. Inherited pancreatic cancer. *Chin Clin Oncol.* 2017;6(6):58. doi:10.21037/cco.2017.12.04
28. Klein AP, Brune KA, Petersen GM, et al. Prospective risk of pancreatic cancer in familial pancreatic cancer kindreds. *Cancer Res.* 2004;64(7):2634–2638. doi:10.1158/0008-5472.CAN-03-3823
29. Wang L, Brune KA, Visvanathan K, et al. Elevated cancer mortality in the relatives of patients with pancreatic cancer. *Cancer Epidemiol Biomarkers Prev.* 2009;18(11):2829–2834. doi:10.1158/1055-9965.EPI-09-0557
30. Canto MI, Harinck F, Hruban RH, et al. International Cancer of the Pancreas Screening (CAPS) Consortium summit on the management of patients with increased risk for familial pancreatic cancer. *Gut.* 2013;62(3):339–347. doi:10.1136/gutjnl-2012-303108
31. Sausen M, Phallen J, Adleff V. Clinical implications of genomic alterations in the tumour and circulation of pancreatic cancer patients. *Nat Commun.* 2015;6:7686. doi:10.1038/ncomms8686
32. Modolell I, Guarner L, Malagelada JR. Vagaries of clinical presentation of pancreatic and biliary tract cancer. *Ann Oncol.* 1999;10 Suppl 4:82–84. doi:10.1093/annonc/10.suppl_4.S82
33. Ryan DP, Hong TS, Bardeesy N. Pancreatic adenocarcinoma. *N Engl J Med.* 2014;371(11):1039–1049. doi:10.1056/NEJMra1404198
34. Keane MG, Horsfall L, Rait G, et al. A case-control study comparing the incidence of early symptoms in pancreatic and biliary tract cancer. *BMJ Open;*2014:4(11):e005720. doi:10.1136/bmjopen-2014-005720
35. Sharma C, Eltawil KM, Renfrew PD, et al. Advances in diagnosis, treatment and palliation of pancreatic carcinoma: 1990-2010. *World J Gastroenterol.* 2011;17(7):867–897. doi:10.3748/wjg.v17.i7.867
36. Weledji EP, Enoworock G, Mokake M, et al. How grim is pancreatic cancer? *Oncol Rev.* 2016;10(1):294. doi:10.4081/oncol.2016.294
37. Von Hoff DD, Ervin T, Arena FP, et al. Increased survival in pancreatic cancer with nab-paclitaxel plus gemcitabine. *N Engl J Med.* 2013;369(18):1691–1703. doi:10.1056/NEJMoa1304369
38. Conroy T, Desseigne F, Ychou M, et al. FOLFIRINOX versus gemcitabine for metastatic pancreatic cancer. *N Engl J Med.* 2011;364(19):1817–1825. doi:10.1056/NEJMoa1011923

19

Biological Basis for Pancreatic Cancer

Michael Brandon Ware, Mehmet Akce, Alexandra G. Lopez-Aguiar, David A. Kooby, Field F. Willingham, Shishir K. Maithel, and Gregory B. Lesinski

INTRODUCTION

Pancreatic ductal adenocarcinoma (PDAC) is a devastating disease with limited treatment options. This malignancy has a 5-year overall survival rate of less than 9% (1). Perhaps even more alarming are published models predicting that PDAC will surpass breast and colon cancer to become the second leading cause of cancer-related deaths by the year 2030 (2). One of the key factors accounting for poor outcomes in PDAC is its clinical silence. Typically, the disease only becomes apparent after the tumor becomes invasive into surrounding tissues or metastasizes to distant organs (3). For a number of years, the standard of care for advanced PDAC patients was gemcitabine-based regimens. More recently, combined administration of gemcitabine with nab-paclitaxel (Abraxane) has been widely used, while in patients with good performance status, more aggressive chemotherapy regimens (e.g., FOLFIRINOX) have emerged in practice (4). These treatments are often being used as a strategy to debulk the tumor and improve candidacy for surgery. The overall poor outcomes for patients with PDAC underscore the need for significant advances in both early diagnosis of the disease, particularly in high-risk individuals, and improving therapeutic options for patients. This chapter focuses on the biologic properties of PDAC, highlighting several tumor-cell intrinsic features including key mutation patterns that drive the disease process. In addition, we emphasize the controversial role of the stroma associated with pancreatic tumors in influencing the disease process and response to treatment. Finally, the unique immunologic features of the tumor microenvironment are described with an appreciation for pathways that facilitate cross-talk between these multiple cellular compartments.

KEY BIOLOGIC PROPERTIES AND MUTATIONS OF RELEVANCE TO PANCREATIC CANCER

PDAC is characterized by several dominant genetic features, although the exact nature of its pathogenesis remains quite complicated. A recent integrated genomic, transcriptomic, and proteomic analysis of 150 PDAC samples revealed recurrent somatic mutations in *KRAS*, *TP53*, *CDKN2A*, *SMAD4*, *RNF43*, *ARID1A*, *TGFβR2*, *GNAS*, *RREB1*, and *PBRM1* (5). In tumors with wild-type *KRAS*, other oncogenic drivers were altered including *GNAS*, *BRAF*, and *CTNNB1* along with additional RAS pathway genes. These observations highlight the complex molecular landscape of PDAC and suggest that it will be challenging to identify broad pharmacologic options to target driver oncogenes that are mutated across a wide range of tumors. Unfortunately, due to a concurrent lack of neoantigens, immunotherapy approaches may also be at a disadvantage. The lack of efficacy for both targeted small molecule and immunotherapy agents in PDAC certainly supports this premise. However, the *G12D* mutation within the *KRAS* gene represents a characteristic hallmark of PDAC. In fact, this mutation is found in over 90% of PDAC cases and regulates downstream growth of transformed cells through a variety of downstream signal transduction pathways including the MAPK, PI3K, RAL-GEF, PLC pathways, inflammatory STAT signaling, and NF-κB mediated cytokine production. More recently, other mutations in *KRAS* have been shown to afford a survival advantage to malignant cells, demonstrating the redundancy in this gene and its downstream pathways in PDAC (6). The majority of the *KRAS* mutations in PDAC are limited to codon 12 (G12D, G12V, and G12R) with a subset of tumors exhibiting *KRAS* mutations in codon 61 (7). While the high prevalence of this mutation may signify an obvious node for therapeutic intervention, the biochemical nature of the mutated KRAS protein renders it a particularly challenging therapeutic target. Efforts are ongoing to interfere with this key mutation; however, attention has turned to alternative targets as potential strategies to interfere with the oncogenic circuits within transformed cells. More recently, differing oncogenic gains in *KRAS*[G12D] have been shown to alternatively drive early aggressiveness and metastasis in PDAC (8). The early occurrence of point mutations in *KRAS* creates selective pressure for amplifications in alleles bearing these mutations as well as loss of wild-type *KRAS*. In cases lacking these oncogenic gains in *KRAS*[G12D], transcriptional increases are present and MYC, YAP1, and NFKB2 amplification have been found to drive progression of PDAC tumors (7). Separate studies utilized murine tumors derived from Kras[G12D] mice failing to express this mutated transgene (9). Investigation of transcriptional changes in these tumors lacking Kras[G12D] expression found amplification of chromosomal arms containing *Yap1* and the antiapoptotic genes *Birc2* and *Birc3* (9). Further research revealed redundancy in YAP1 and KRAS, as *Yap1* knockdown in these tumors led to expression of the *Kras*[G12D] transgene. YAP1 was found to allow oncogenic bypass upon loss of *Kras*[G12D], working through the transcription factors TEAD2 and E2F1 to drive tumor growth and proliferation (9). YAP1 has also been found to have increased transcriptional profiles in early development of PanIN lesions with *Kras*[G12D] mutations and has been demonstrated to drive JAK-STAT activation (10–12). These data concerning YAP1 are highly relevant in the tumors harboring *Kras*[G12D] mutations as well as in the relapse setting, where PDAC cases falling into the quasimesenchymal subset exhibit KRAS independence.

Mutated *KRAS* is often accompanied by passenger mutations in genes encoding proteins such as p53, p16, BRCA, various receptor tyrosine kinases, and others (13–15). Evidence from studies involving genetically engineered mouse models (GEMMs) of PDAC indicates that mutations in *Kras* are not sufficient for driving development of PDAC in preclinical models (16,17). Interestingly, *Kras* mutations are found in premalignant lesions known as pancreatic intraepithelial neoplasias (PanINs), supporting the notion that these mutations occur quite early in the malignant process. Emerging evidence has demonstrated a role for *KRAS* mutations in altering the tumor microenvironment (TME), inducing cytokine production, and leading to increased infiltration of immune suppressive T-regulatory cells and myeloid-derived suppressor cells (MDSCs) (18–20). This proinflammatory environment induced by mutated *KRAS* assists in the progression of PanIN lesions into PDAC. In most instances, the transition from a premalignant lesion to a PDAC is likely due to the acquisition of additional mutations in tumor suppressor genes such as *PTEN, INK4a, SMAD4,* or *TP53* in cells previously harboring mutant *KRAS* (21,22). The data from experiments utilizing GEMMs suggest that *Kras* mutations confer selective pressure on preneoplastic cells to develop mutations in these other tumor suppressor genes. These studies also showed that mutations in *Ink4ra* or *Tp53* alone are not sufficient to drive a malignant phenotype. However, once these additional mutations in tumor suppressors occur in cells with *Kras* mutations, the onset of aggressive PDAC happens in a remarkably rapid manner (16,17).

The genetic instability leading to these mutations in pancreatic tumors is variable, and currently four dominant subtypes of PDAC are described based on genetic instability alone (15). Studies characterizing these subtypes found the majority of PDAC cases to exhibit little genomic rearrangement events outside of local chromosomal rearrangements. Some genomic instability can be attributed to mutations in genes encoding proteins like BRCA that are involved in DNA repair pathways; there is even a percentage of pancreatic cancer cases (13%–17%) that have a mismatch repair deficient phenotype due to mutations in the mismatch repair pathway (15,23–26). Cases of PDAC exhibiting high microsatellite instability (~1% of cases) have demonstrated robust responses to therapy with immune checkpoint blockade, while the majority of PDAC cases are refractory to chemotherapy, radiation, and currently available targeted agents (27,28). While *KRAS*[G12D] mutations are highly prevalent in cases of PDAC, these investigations unveil a complex genetic heterogeneity that must be considered in the clinical treatment of this deadly disease.

The underlying causes of pancreatic cancer are still unclear; however, pancreatitis has been correlated with increased risk for pancreatic cancer and many of the underlying mechanisms are common between the two. Pancreatitis results from acute or chronic inflammation of the pancreas, specifically involving the acinar cells of the pancreas. Inflammation or injury due to pancreatitis or other factors can lead to the differentiation of these acinar cells, accompanied by the acquisition of cancer-related mutations or gene signatures and a ductal epithelial identity (29). This differentiation has become a recognized transformation termed "acinar-to-ductal metaplasia" (ADM), and has most recently been linked to increased expression of Kruppel-like factor 5 (KLF5) (30,31). Induction of KLF5 expression precedes PanIN formation and, due to its activity downstream of KRAS and the MAPK pathway, can be found upregulated in over 70% of PDAC cases (1). In the process of ADM and PanIN progression, KLF5 has demonstrated the ability to induce STAT3 phosphorylation and expression of ductal markers, while reducing expression of the tumor suppressor N-myc downregulated gene 2 (NDRG2) (30). In vivo evaluation of KLF5 in murine models has highlighted an essential role for KLF5 in ADM and a requirement for this transcription factor in the progression of *KRAS*[G12D]-induced PanINs to PDAC (30,31).

THE STROMA IS A UNIQUE FEATURE OF THE MICROENVIRONMENT IN PANCREATIC CANCER

One prominent histopathological feature of PDAC is a dense fibrotic stroma that surrounds tumors and intercalates throughout the tumor microenvironment. This pattern of fibrosis is prominent within pancreatic cancer and has emerged as a major player in regulating the metastatic propensity of these tumors and their ability to enforce an immune suppressive phenotype. The microenvironment of these tumors is quite heterogeneous and encompasses cell types from several lineages. It is quite intriguing that the actual transformed cells often only comprise a fraction of the cellular content within a pancreatic tumor. Other components including extracellular matrix (ECM) factors such as collagen, immune cells, and fibroblasts are estimated to make up to 90% of the volume within a pancreatic tumor (32). Of particular abundance within this space are activated myofibroblast-like cells termed pancreatic stellate cells (PSCs) that surround each tumor (32–37). These supporting stromal cells are themselves quite heterogeneous in their phenotypic properties, but can have a great deal of plasticity that influences their complicated biology. This concept and our emerging understanding of their role in PDAC are discussed in detail in the following.

The fibroblast components within the PDAC tumor microenvironment have recently gained a great deal of attention. In particular, PSCs are cells that reside in the pancreas that are equipped to respond to an inflammatory or injurious stimulus within the organ to facilitate wound repair. The PSCs are normally quiescent, where they accumulate vitamin A and retinyl palmitate storing lipid droplets and contribute to tissue homeostasis (38). PSCs localize mainly to the exocrine compartment of the pancreas, sitting directly adjacent to enzyme secreting acinar cells, exterior to the lumen of acini (39). Upon exposure to an appropriate inflammatory stimulus, these cells become activated whereby they release their vitamin A and lipid stores, alter their phenotype, and secrete large amounts of ECM to facilitate in wound healing and repair. Concurrently, activated PSCs elicit a sustained burst in cytokine and chemokine secretion, presumably to attract immune cells to the site of pancreatic inflammation. Soluble factors such as platelet-derived growth factor β (PDGFβ), transforming growth factor β (TGF-β), and fibroblast growth factor 2 (FGF2) produced by the PSCs stimulate the production of the ECM components that lead to the classical fibrosis observed in PDAC (40). There is also evidence that PSCs produce some of these factors that may signal through feedforward autocrine loops to maintain activation of the PSCs (41–43). Consistent with these functional roles, PSCs usually display an activated phenotype in the setting of acute or chronic pancreatitis, as well as in PDAC. These disease states are accompanied by remarkably high levels of fibrosis in the organ, and both local and systemic increases in inflammatory cytokine mediators that exacerbate the disease process. Traditionally, PSCs have been identified using distinct phenotypic markers including alpha-smooth muscle actin (αSMA) or interleukin-6 (IL-6), while subsets express surface markers consistent with a fibroblast phenotype including fibroblast activation protein alpha (FAPα), fibroblast specific protein 1 (FSP-1), and PDGFR-β (44).

The phenotypic and functional classification of PSCs in the setting of PDAC has recently come under careful scrutiny. In fact, recent studies have appreciated the heterogeneous nature of PSCs in this disease, and suggest there may be individual classifications or subtypes of stroma. These classifications were based on both stromal characterization (normal vs. inflammatory genotypes) as well as tumoral subtypes (classical vs. basal genotypes) and demonstrated the complex heterogeneity of stromal and tumoral subtypes across PDAC tumors (45). A more recent publication has further delineated PSC into at least two distinct functional and phenotypically defined subsets based on histological analysis of tumors and a series of eloquent organoid-based studies (46). In this manuscript, differential expression of αSMA and IL-6 were used as distinct markers to define separate "myofibroblastic" and "inflammatory" PSC subsets (46). Certainly other subtypes of cancer-associated fibroblasts (CAFs) beyond these two phenotypes exist in the literature and have been studied in other cancers. Hence there remains some controversy on the defined subtypes of fibroblast cell populations within PDAC due to this heterogeneity. Nonetheless, the functional difference between these two very well-characterized PSC subsets is quite interesting and warrants further discussion in what follows.

The first myofibroblastic subset, termed myCAFs, is responsible for creating the periglandular border of fibroblasts that surrounds and physically supports cancerous cells within the pancreas (46). This thin border of myofibroblasts is surmised to provide a layer of protection and support for the glandular clusters of cancer cells in PDAC. The myCAF populations are typically located directly adjacent to cancer cells and are marked by expression of FAP, with significantly elevated levels of αSMA (46). An established matrix of collagen and other ECM components deposited by myCAFs separates malignant cells from a thin border of the myofibroblastic stellate cells. This physical cellular barrier is postulated to limit access of treatments such as chemotherapy due to the physical blockage of drugs moving into the area and prevent vascular growth and function (47), leading to a hypoxic tumor microenvironment (48–50). This hypoxic environment also contributes to therapy resistance, making radiation a seemingly ineffective treatment (50).

The second inflammatory subset, which has been termed iCAFs, composes the larger proportion of PSC within a pancreatic tumor (46). The iCAF subset has lower overall expression of αSMA but more elevated levels of IL-6 and leukemia inhibitory factor (Lif), which both play a tumor supportive and immunomodulatory role (46). This elevated propensity to produce modulatory cytokines supports a dynamic, three-way interaction, affecting the inflammatory cells in the microenvironment, sustaining PSC activation, and altering the characteristics of the tumor itself. Interestingly, this elevated IL-6 production is associated with PSC only in the presence of cancer cells or conditioned media from cancer cells, indicating a tumor supportive role for IL-6. These data also suggest that iCAFs can be induced by signaling from pancreatic cancer cells themselves (51). Notably, PSCs derived from PDAC patient biopsies have been shown to express abundant levels of IL-6 at both the transcript and protein levels, thereby maintaining an inflammatory activated state in the absence of cancer cells (52).

These two phenotypically defined PSC subsets also display plasticity that depends on exposure to tumor cells or tumor-derived soluble factors. Evidence for this reciprocal relationship is derived from studies using tumor organoids. For instance, in the absence of pancreatic cancer cells, the cocultured PSCs lost their high αSMA expression and exhibited a phenotype more characteristic of the inflammatory subset (46,53). Currently, it is unknown whether this plasticity is due only to direct interaction between the cancer cells and PSC, or if there exists communication to maintain a homeostatic balance between the various subtypes. myCAFs and iCAFs represent two well-characterized subsets of PSCs; however, further research is needed to fully elucidate the distinct populations and their effect on tumor growth and development.

CONTROVERSIAL ROLE OF THE STROMA IN THE PANCREATIC DISEASE PROCESS

The topic of stromal components as promoting or inhibiting PDAC growth and progression has become somewhat controversial (32,54,55). Data from multiple studies support a role for PSCs and the reactive microenvironment they reside in as key contributors to both the aggressiveness of PDAC and its resistance to therapy. Historically, chemotherapy and other treatments for PDAC are thought to be limited by this stromal reaction, which may inhibit drug delivery and promote resistance to therapy (47). Increasing evidence supports the concept that the PDAC stroma contributes to tumor growth indirectly, via secretion of growth factors to adjacent tumor cells or even through direct, physical interaction with cancer cells. Certainly the PSCs in the stroma produce collagen, growth factors, and soluble factors such as cytokines that modulate the immune reaction to cancer as well as inhibiting therapeutic response. Direct interaction between the PSCs and cancer occurs through growth factor signaling to pancreatic cancer cells and contact mediated promotion of growth and metastasis.

Despite this prevailing view, more recent evidence indicates the abundant stromal reaction in PDAC can have a paradoxical role in protecting the host from metastasis. A provocative study highlighted this possibility, showing genetic ablation of αSMA+ stromal cells accelerated metastasis and disease progression in a mutant *KRAS*-driven model of PDAC (56). These data suggest that stromal fibroblasts were actually protective to the host by limiting the spread of the tumor cells beyond the local microenvironment allowed for greater access to systemic spread. Despite these data, another key observation was made. Immunotherapy with anti-CTLA4 Ab was more effective in these animals harboring aggressive PDAC tumors but lacking αSMA+ cells. These observations suggest that while the presence of activated fibroblasts can limit tumor metastasis, they also inhibit immune recognition of the tumors. Likewise, other studies demonstrated that targeting FAP+ cells maintain the stroma and suppress antitumor immunity, although these data did not demonstrate a role for FAP+ cells in regulating tumor metastasis (57–59). Other publications demonstrate that PSCs derived from PDAC stroma secrete a variety of cytokines or other soluble factors that can shape the fibrosis and immune cellular composition within the TME (52,60). Together, these results suggest that immunity against tumors is restrained by the stroma and that targeting key pathways may augment the efficacy of immunotherapy.

TARGETING DOMINANT PATHWAYS IN THE TUMOR MICROENVIRONMENT

Rather than targeting entire populations of cells in the tumor microenvironment, great insight has been gained from attempts at targeting key pathways relevant in the development of the PDAC associated stroma. One key example is derived from studies targeting the Sonic hedgehog pathway in PDAC. Hedgehog pathway inhibitors were applied in mouse models of PDAC with the hypothesis that disrupting the activation of the fibrotic stromal barrier may allow for better drug delivery to the site of disease, enhancing the effect of chemotherapy (47). Sonic hedgehog ligand is produced by cancer cells, and possibly other stromal members, and signals to myofibroblasts that express Gli-1 (61). This leads to activation of myofibroblasts as previously described and initiates the excretion of collagen I, formation of fibrosis, and development of the desmoplastic stroma (61). One of the early studies applying this concept of hedgehog inhibition enhancing chemotherapy found that the hedgehog inhibitor IPI-926 was able to partially restore vascular density and led to an increase in the intratumoral concentration of gemcitabine (47). This study also showed that while tumor cells from these mice were sensitive to gemcitabine in vitro, the gemcitabine had little effect on tumor cell viability in vivo as a single agent (47). This supports prior hypotheses that the cancer cells themselves are not resistant to these therapies and that devising therapies to increase drug delivery would have a significant impact on tumor burden and overall survival. While these preclinical trials showed promise, a clinical trial (NCT01130142) combining the hedgehog inhibitor saridegib and gemcitabine was halted early due to accelerated disease progression in the combination arm. Research into the hedgehog pathway in PDAC has revealed a complex interplay between the stroma and tumor and the role of the hedgehog pathway in mediating cross-talk between these compartments (62,63).

Contrary to these findings are positive data whereby interfering with hyaluronidase represents a stroma-targeted approach with encouraging early results in clinical trials. Hyaluronic acid (HA), an upregulated ECM component in PDAC, can be secreted by fibroblasts and cancer cells in PDAC (64). This polysaccharide has been found to localize to desmoplastic regions of PDAC and is thought to contribute to the fibrosis mediated drug resistance associated with the PDAC stroma (65). Clinical trials have utilized therapeutics blocking HA, one of which is a PEGylated form of recombinant hyaluronidase (66). Hyaluronidases are enzymes that depolymerize HA, and are thought to relieve the rigid fibrosis associated with PDAC to improve delivery and effectiveness of chemotherapy or other drugs (67). Indeed, a phase III clinical trial utilized PEGPH20 (a PEGylated recombinant hyaluronidase) and found a clinical benefit for patients expressing high levels of HA (68). For this subset of patients, PEGPH20 in combination with chemotherapy improved survival by 4 months (9.2 months vs. 5.2 months) compared to chemotherapy alone (58). Without considering HA expression in patients, survival only increased by a margin of a few weeks, indicating a drastic heterogeneous role for HA between patients (49).

Taken together, the aforementioned studies demonstrate a heterogeneous response among patients and mouse experiments to stromal modulation, emphasizing the importance of understanding the cancer in the context of the stroma, the body, and the immune system.

Further research is needed to elicit the mechanisms responsible for differential modulation of the stroma by the cancer and vice versa. Studies should also consider how the immune system might play a role in mediating this interaction, as differences in immune modulation between patients and in vivo studies may provide some insight into why responses to therapy are so variable.

Other pathways with shared functional roles between the cancerous and stromal cells may also represent key mediators of PDAC development and progression. For example, the IL-6/JAK-STAT signaling axis can orchestrate carcinogenesis, metastasis, and the complex immunologic changes that accompany PDAC (69,70). IL-6 is a pleiotropic cytokine that binds membrane receptor complexes containing the common signal transducing receptor chain gp130 (glycoprotein 130) (71), thereby initiating a complex series of signaling events that include the JAK-STAT, MAPK, and PI3K pathways (65,68). In particular, STAT3 is activated via phosphorylation at Tyr[705] in most human PDAC specimens and cooperates with activated *Kras* to drive initiation and progression of PDAC in murine models (8,72). The IL-6/STAT3 axis can simultaneously promote the expansion of immunosuppressive cells. Among the most notable of these subsets are MDSCs and T-regulatory cells (T regs). Several groups have shown that these cells are expanded, and are poor prognostic indicators in patients with advanced gastrointestinal cancer (73–75). In this manner, IL-6 can cooperate with other cytokines either systemically or in the tumor microenvironment to further amplify immune changes in patients. Recent studies using an inducible *KRAS*-mediated PDAC mouse model also showed that IL-6 was instrumental for PDAC progression (69,76). In fact, lack of IL-6 completely ablated cancer progression even in the presence of oncogenic *KRAS* (69). In agreement with these data are recent results that emphasize the importance of systemic IL-6 in PDAC patients (77). For example, analysis of plasma from n = 73 untreated patients with metastatic or nonresectable PDAC revealed IL-6, IL-10, and MCP-1 were associated with overall survival, with IL-6 having a strong inverse relationship. Further studies confirm a majority of IL-6 is in stromal regions of human PDAC tumors (46,78). Published data further show that PSCs from PDAC patients are an abundant source of cytokines that act via STAT3 to expand MDSCs, a key mediator of immune suppression in advanced cancers (60). Consistent with these observations were a series of in vivo studies indicating that antibody-mediated targeting of IL-6 increased tumoral infiltration of effector T cells, and enhanced the efficacy of immune checkpoint blockade in four separate preclinical models of PDAC (52). Together, these data suggest stromal IL-6 orchestrates PDAC development and immune suppression and progression via signaling through the JAK-STAT pathway.

FUTURE ADVANCES THAT WILL IMPROVE OUR UNDERSTANDING OF PANCREATIC CANCER BIOLOGY

The field of pancreatic cancer research is moving quite rapidly, with innovative technology driving discoveries in the field. In particular, more sophisticated animal models have been developed that incorporate inducible systems to regulate expression of oncogenes including mutant *KRAS* at specified time points (79). Other studies have demonstrated the feasibility of developing patient-derived organoid systems to better recapitulate three-dimensional interactions occurring between tumor and stroma and do so in a high throughput fashion for advanced drug screening (80–82). Finally, an improved understanding of tumor immune interactions has led to clinical trials targeting key immunologic factors including CSF1-R, CCR2, and CD40 that are founded upon preclinical data and are demonstrating early signs of clinical activity (83–86). Overall, continued appreciation for the complexity of the PDAC tumor microenvironment will likely uncover additional therapeutic targets and better inform our use of existing therapies in combination.

REFERENCES

1. Siegel RL, Miller KD, Jemal A. Cancer statistics, 2018. *CA Cancer J Clin*. 2018;68(1):7–30. doi:10.3322/caac.21442
2. Rahib L, Smith BD, Aizenberg R, et al. Projecting cancer incidence and deaths to 2030: the unexpected burden of thyroid, liver, and pancreas cancers in the United States. *Cancer Res*. 2014;74(11):2913–2921. doi:10.1158/0008-5472.CAN-14-0155

3. Vincent A, Herman J, Schulick R, et al. Pancreatic cancer. *Lancet*. 2011;378(9791):607–620. doi:10.1016/S0140-6736(10)62307-0

4. Al-Hajeili M, Azmi AS, Choi M. Nab-paclitaxel: potential for the treatment of advanced pancreatic cancer. *Onco Targets Ther*. 2014;7:187–192. doi:10.2147/ott.s40705

5. Cancer Genome Atlas Research Network. Electronic address: andrew_aguirre@dfci.harvard.edu; Cancer Genome Atlas Research Network. Integrated Genomic Characterization of Pancreatic Ductal Adenocarcinoma. *Cancer Cell*. 2017;32(2):185–203.e13. doi:10.1016/j.ccell.2017.07.007

6. Zhu Z, Golay HG, Barbie DA. Targeting pathways downstream of KRAS in lung adenocarcinoma. *Pharmacogenomics*. 2014;15(11):1507–1518. doi:10.2217/pgs.14.108

7. Mueller S, Engleitner T, Maresch R, et al. Evolutionary routes and KRAS dosage define pancreatic cancer phenotypes. *Nature*. 2018;554(7690):62–68. doi:10.1038/nature25459

8. Corcoran RB, Contino G, Deshpande V, et al. STAT3 plays a critical role in KRAS-induced pancreatic tumorigenesis. *Cancer Res*. 2011;71(14):5020–5029. doi:10.1158/0008-5472.CAN-11-0908

9. Kapoor A, Yao W, Ying H, et al. Yap1 activation enables bypass of oncogenic Kras addiction in pancreatic cancer. *Cell*. 2014;158(1):185–197. doi:10.1016/j.cell.2014.06.003

10. Gruber R, Panayiotou R, Nye E, et al. YAP1 and TAZ control pancreatic cancer initiation in mice by direct up-regulation of JAK-STAT3 signaling. *Gastroenterology*. 2016;151(3):526–539. doi:10.1053/j.gastro.2016.05.006

11. Taniguchi K, Moroishi T, de Jong PR, et al. YAP-IL-6ST autoregulatory loop activated on APC loss controls colonic tumorigenesis. *Proc Natl Acad Sci U S A*. 2017;114(7):1643–1648. doi:10.1073/pnas.1620290114

12. Zhang W, Nandakumar N, Shi Y, et al. Downstream of mutant KRAS, the transcription regulator YAP is essential for neoplastic progression to pancreatic ductal adenocarcinoma. *Sci Signal*. 2014;7(324):ra42. doi:10.1126/scisignal.2005049

13. Rozenblum E, Schutte M, Goggins M, et al. Tumor-suppressive pathways in pancreatic carcinoma. *Cancer Res*. 1997;57(9):1731–1734.

14. Almoguera C, Shibata D, Forrester K, et al. Most human carcinomas of the exocrine pancreas contain mutant c-K-ras genes. *Cell*. 1988;53(4):549–554. doi:10.1016/0092-8674(88)90571-5

15. Waddell N, Australian Pancreatic Cancer Genome Initiative, Pajic M, et al. Whole genomes redefine the mutational landscape of pancreatic cancer. *Nature*. 2015;518(7540):495–501. doi:10.1038/nature14169

16. Aguirre AJ, Bardeesy N, Sinha M, et al. Activated Kras and Ink4a/Arf deficiency cooperate to produce metastatic pancreatic ductal adenocarcinoma. *Genes Dev*. 2003;17(24):3112–3126. doi:10.1101/gad.1158703

17. Bardeesy N, Cheng K, Berger JH, et al. Smad4 is dispensable for normal pancreas development yet critical in progression and tumor biology of pancreas cancer. *Genes Dev*. 2006;20(22):3130–3146. doi:10.1101/gad.1478706

18. Dias Carvalho P, Guimarães CF, Cardoso AP, et al. KRAS oncogenic signaling extends beyond cancer cells to orchestrate the microenvironment. *Cancer Res*. 2018;78(1):7–14. doi:10.1158/0008-5472.CAN-17-2084

19. Zdanov S, Mandapathil M, Eid RA, et al. Mutant KRAS conversion of conventional T cells into regulatory T cells. *Cancer Immunol Res*. 2016;4(4):354–365. doi:10.1158/2326-6066.CIR-15-0241

20. Busch SE, Hanke ML, Kargl J, et al. Lung cancer subtypes generate unique immune responses. *J Immunol*. 2016;197(11):4493–4503. doi:10.4049/jimmunol.1600576

21. Khan MA, Azim S, Zubair H, et al. Molecular drivers of pancreatic cancer pathogenesis: looking inward to move forward. *Int J Mol Sci*. 2017;18(4):779. doi:10.3390/ijms18040779

22. Ying H, Elpek KG, Vinjamoori A, et al. PTEN is a major tumor suppressor in pancreatic ductal adenocarcinoma and regulates an NF-kappaβ-cytokine network. *Cancer Discov*. 2011;1(2):158–169. doi:10.1158/2159-8290.CD-11-0031

23. Riazy M, Kalloger SE, Sheffield BS, et al. Mismatch repair status may predict response to adjuvant chemotherapy in resectable pancreatic ductal adenocarcinoma. *Mod Pathol*. 2015;28(10):1383–1389. doi:10.1038/modpathol.2015.89

24. Nakata B, Wang YQ, Yashiro M, et al. Prognostic value of microsatellite instability in resectable pancreatic cancer. *Clin Cancer Res*. 2002;8(8):2536–2540.

25. Ottenhof NA, Morsink FHM, ten Kate F, et al. Multivariate analysis of immunohistochemical evaluation of protein expression in pancreatic ductal adenocarcinoma reveals prognostic significance for persistent Smad4 expression only. *Cell Oncol (Dordr)*. 2012;35(2):119–126. doi:10.1007/s13402-012-0072-x

26. Yamamoto H, Itoh F, Nakamura H, et al. Genetic and clinical features of human pancreatic ductal adenocarcinomas with widespread microsatellite instability. *Cancer Res*. 2001;61(7):3139–3144.

27. Humphris JL, Patch A-M, Nones K, et al. Hypermutation in pancreatic cancer. *Gastroenterology*. 2017;152(1):68–74.e2. doi:10.1053/j.gastro.2016.09.060

28. Laghi L, Beghelli S, Spinelli A, et al. Irrelevance of microsatellite instability in the epidemiology of sporadic pancreatic ductal adenocarcinoma. *PLoS One*. 2012;7(9):e46002. doi:10.1371/journal.pone.0046002

29. Strobel O, Dor Y, Alsina J, et al. In vivo lineage tracing defines the role of acinar-to-ductal trans-differentiation in inflammatory ductal metaplasia. *Gastroenterology*. 2007;133(6):1999–2009. doi:10.1053/j.gastro.2007.09.009

30. He P, Yang JW, Yang VW, et al. Kruppel-like factor 5, increased in pancreatic ductal adeno-carcinoma, promotes proliferation, acinar-to-ductal metaplasia, pancreatic intraepithelial neo-plasia, and tumor growth in mice. *Gastroenterology*. 2018;154(5):1494–1508.e13. doi:10.1053/j.gastro.2017.12.005

31. David CJ, Huang Y-H, Chen M, et al. TGF-beta tumor suppression through a lethal EMT. *Cell*. 2016;164(5):1015–1030. doi:10.1016/j.cell.2016.01.009

32. Neesse A, Michl P, Frese KK, et al. Stromal biology and therapy in pancreatic cancer. *Gut*. 2011;60(6):861–868. doi:10.1136/gut.2010.226092

33. Apte MV, Haber PS, Applegate TL, et al. Periacinar stellate shaped cells in rat pancreas: identifi-cation, isolation, and culture. *Gut*. 1998;43(1):128–133. doi:10.1136/gut.43.1.128

34. Krizhanovsky V, Yon M, Dickins RA, et al. Senescence of activated stellate cells limits liver fibro-sis. *Cell*. 2008;134(4):657–667. doi:10.1016/j.cell.2008.06.049

35. Lonardo E, Frias-Aldeguer J, Hermann PC, et al. Pancreatic stellate cells form a niche for cancer stem cells and promote their self-renewal and invasiveness. *Cell Cycle*. 2012;11(7):1282–1290. doi:10.4161/cc.19679

36. Waghray M, Yalamanchili M, di Magliano MP, et al. Deciphering the role of stroma in pancreatic cancer. *Curr Opin Gastroenterol*. 2013;29(5):537–543. doi:10.1097/MOG.0b013e328363affe

37. Moffitt RA, Marayati R, Flate EL, et al. Virtual microdissection identifies distinct tumor- and stroma-specific subtypes of pancreatic ductal adenocarcinoma. *Nat Genet*. 2015;47(10):1168–1178. doi:10.1038/ng.3398

38. McCarroll JA, Phillips PA, Santucci N, et al. Vitamin A inhibits pancreatic stellate cell activa-tion: implications for treatment of pancreatic fibrosis. *Gut*. 2006;55(1):79–89. doi:10.1136/gut.2005.064543

39. Omary MB, Lugea A, Lowe AW, et al. The pancreatic stellate cell: a star on the rise in pancreatic diseases. *J Clin Invest*. 2007;117(1):50–59. doi:10.1172/JCI30082

40. Bachem MG, Schünemann M, Ramadani M, et al. Pancreatic carcinoma cells induce fibrosis by stimulating proliferation and matrix synthesis of stellate cells. *Gastroenterology*. 2005;128(4):907–921. doi:10.1053/j.gastro.2004.12.036

41. Ohnishi N, Miyata T, Ohnishi H, et al. Activin A is an autocrine activator of rat pancreatic stellate cells: potential therapeutic role of follistatin for pancreatic fibrosis. *Gut*. 2003;52(10):1487–1493. doi:10.1136/gut.52.10.1487

42. Aoki H, Ohnishi H, Hama K, et al. Existence of autocrine loop between interleukin-6 and transforming growth factor-beta1 in activated rat pancreatic stellate cells. *J Cell Biochem*. 2006;99(1):221–228. doi:10.1002/jcb.20906

43. Shek FW, Benyon RC, Walker FM, et al. Expression of transforming growth factor-beta 1 by pan-creatic stellate cells and its implications for matrix secretion and turnover in chronic pancreatitis. *Am J Pathol*. 2002;160(5):1787–1798. doi:10.1016/S0002-9440(10)61125-X

44. Ohlund D, Elyada E, Tuveson D. Fibroblast heterogeneity in the cancer wound. *J Exp Med*. 2014;211(8):1503–1523. doi:10.1084/jem.20140692

45. Moffitt RA, Marayati R, Flate EL, et al. Virtual microdissection identifies distinct tumor- and stro-ma-specific subtypes of pancreatic ductal adenocarcinoma. *Nat Genet*. 2015;47(10):1168–1178. doi:10.1038/ng.3398

46. Ohlund D, Handly-Santana A, Biffi G, et al. Distinct populations of inflammatory fibroblasts and myofibroblasts in pancreatic cancer. *J Exp Med*. 2017;214(3):579–596. doi:10.1084/jem.20162024

47. Olive KP, Jacobetz MA, Davidson CJ, et al. Inhibition of hedgehog signaling enhances delivery of chemotherapy in a mouse model of pancreatic cancer. *Science*. 2009;324(5933):1457–1461. doi:10.1126/science.1171362

48. Buchler P, Reber HA, Büchler M, et al. Hypoxia-inducible factor 1 regulates vascular endo-thelial growth factor expression in human pancreatic cancer. *Pancreas*. 2003;26(1):56–64. doi:10.1097/00006676-200301000-00010

49. Shibaji T, Nagao M, Ikeda N, et al. Prognostic significance of HIF-1 alpha overexpression in human pancreatic cancer. *Anticancer Res*. 2003;23(6C):4721–4727.

50. Koong AC, Mehta VK, Le QT, et al. Pancreatic tumors show high levels of hypoxia. *Int J Radiat Oncol Biol Phys*. 2000;48(4):919–922. doi:10.1016/S0360-3016(00)00803-8

51. Zhang Y, Yan W, Collins MA, et al. Interleukin-6 is required for pancreatic cancer progression by promoting MAPK signaling activation and oxidative stress resistance. *Cancer Res.* 2013;73(20):6359–6374. doi:10.1158/0008-5472.CAN-13-1558-T

52. Mace TA, Shakya R, Pitaressi JR, et al. IL-6 and PD-L1 antibody blockade combination therapy reduces tumour progression in murine models of pancreatic cancer. *Gut.* 2016;67(2):320-332. doi: 10.1136/gutjnl-2016-311585

53. Habisch H, Zhou S, Siech M, et al. Interaction of stellate cells with pancreatic carcinoma cells. *Cancers (Basel).* 2010;2(3):1661–1682. doi:10.3390/cancers2031661

54. Rhim AD, Oberstein PE, Thomas DH, et al. Stromal elements act to restrain, rather than support, pancreatic ductal adenocarcinoma. *Cancer Cell.* 2014;25(6):735–747. doi:10.1016/j.ccr.2014.04.021

55. Lee JJ, Perera RM, Wang H, et al. Stromal response to hedgehog signaling restrains pancreatic cancer progression. *Proc Natl Acad Sci U S A.* 2014;111(30):E3091–E3100. doi:10.1073/pnas.1411679111

56. Ozdemir BC, Pentcheva-Hoang T, Carstens JL, et al. Depletion of carcinoma-associated fibroblasts and fibrosis induces immunosuppression and accelerates pancreas cancer with reduced survival. *Cancer Cell.* 2014;25(6):719–734. doi:10.1016/j.ccr.2014.04.005

57. Fearon DT. The carcinoma-associated fibroblast expressing fibroblast activation protein and escape from immune surveillance. *Cancer Immunol Res.* 2014;2(3):187–193. doi:10.1158/2326-6066.CIR-14-0002

58. Feig C, Jones JO, Kraman M, et al. Targeting CXCL12 from FAP-expressing carcinoma-associated fibroblasts synergizes with anti-PD-L1 immunotherapy in pancreatic cancer. *Proc Natl Acad Sci U S A.* 2013;110(50):20212–20217. doi:10.1073/pnas.1320318110

59. Lo A, Wang L-CS, Scholler J, et al. Tumor-promoting desmoplasia is disrupted by depleting FAP-expressing stromal cells. *Cancer Res.* 2015;75(14):2800–2810. doi:10.1158/0008-5472.CAN-14-3041

60. Mace TA, Ameen Z, Collins A, et al. Pancreatic cancer-associated stellate cells promote differentiation of myeloid-derived suppressor cells in a STAT3-dependent manner. *Cancer Res.* 2013;73(10):3007–3018. doi:10.1158/0008-5472.CAN-12-4601

61. Bailey JM, Swanson BJ, Hamada T, et al. Sonic hedgehog promotes desmoplasia in pancreatic cancer. *Clin Cancer Res.* 2008;14(19):5995–6004. doi:10.1158/1078-0432.CCR-08-0291

62. Ozdemir BC, Pentcheva-Hoang T, Carstens JL, et al. Depletion of carcinoma-associated fibroblasts and fibrosis induces immunosuppression and accelerates pancreas cancer with reduced survival. *Cancer Cell.* 2014;25(6):719–734. doi:10.1016/j.ccr.2014.04.005

63. Rhim AD, Oberstein PE, Thomas DH, et al. Stromal elements act to restrain, rather than support, pancreatic ductal adenocarcinoma. *Cancer Cell.* 2014;25(6):735–747. doi:10.1016/j.ccr.2014.04.021

64. Sato N, Cheng X-B, Kohi S, et al. Targeting hyaluronan for the treatment of pancreatic ductal adenocarcinoma. *Acta Pharm Sin B.* 2016;6(2):101–105. doi:10.1016/j.apsb.2016.01.002

65. Scheller J, Chalaris A, Schmidt-Arras D, et al. The pro- and anti-inflammatory properties of the cytokine interleukin-6. *Biochim Biophys Acta.* 2011;1813(5):878–888. doi:10.1016/j.bbamcr.2011.01.034

66. Hingorani SR, Zheng L, Bullock AJ, et al. HALO 202: randomized phase II study of PEGPH20 plus nab-paclitaxel/gemcitabine versus nab-paclitaxel/gemcitabine in patients with untreated, metastatic pancreatic ductal adenocarcinoma. *J Clin Oncol.* 2018;36(4):359–366. doi:10.1200/JCO.2017.74.9564

67. Infante JR, Korn RL, Rosen LS, et al. Phase 1 trials of PEGylated recombinant human hyaluronidase PH20 in patients with advanced solid tumours. *Br J Cancer.* 2018;118(2):e3. doi:10.1038/bjc.2017.438

68. Fisher DT, Appenheimer MM, Evans SS. The two faces of IL-6 in the tumor microenvironment. *Semin Immunol.* 2014;26(1):38–47. doi:10.1016/j.smim.2014.01.008

69. Zhang Y, Yan W, Collins MA, et al. Interleukin-6 is required for pancreatic cancer progression by promoting MAPK signaling activation and oxidative stress resistance. *Cancer Res.* 2013;73(20):6359–6374. doi:10.1158/0008-5472.CAN-13-1558-T

70. Lesina M, Kurkowski MU, Ludes K, et al. Stat3/Socs3 activation by IL-6 transsignaling promotes progression of pancreatic intraepithelial neoplasia and development of pancreatic cancer. *Cancer Cell.* 2011;19(4):456–469. doi:10.1016/j.ccr.2011.03.009

71. Rose-John S, Scheller J, Elson G, et al. Interleukin-6 biology is coordinated by membrane-bound and soluble receptors: role in inflammation and cancer. *J Leukoc Biol.* 2006;80(2):227–236. doi:10.1189/jlb.1105674

72. Scholz A, Heinze S, Detjen KM, et al. Activated signal transducer and activator of transcription 3 (STAT3) supports the malignant phenotype of human pancreatic cancer. *Gastroenterology.* 2003;125(3):891–905. doi:10.1016/S0016-5085(03)01064-3

73. Gabitass RF, Annels NE, Stocken DD, et al. Elevated myeloid-derived suppressor cells in pancreatic, esophageal and gastric cancer are an independent prognostic factor and are associated with significant elevation of the Th2 cytokine interleukin-13. *Cancer Immunol Immunother.* 2011;60(10):1419–1430. doi:10.1007/s00262-011-1028-0

74. Markowitz J, Brooks TR, Duggan MC, et al. Patients with pancreatic adenocarcinoma exhibit elevated levels of myeloid-derived suppressor cells upon progression of disease. *Cancer Immunol Immunother.* 2015;64(2):149–159. doi:10.1007/s00262-014-1618-8

75. Mundy-Bosse BL, Young GS, Bauer T, et al. Distinct myeloid suppressor cell subsets correlate with plasma IL-6 and IL-10 and reduced interferon-alpha signaling in CD4(+) T cells from patients with GI malignancy. *Cancer Immunol Immunother.* 2011;60(9):1269–1279. doi:10.1007/s00262-011-1029-z

76. Goumas FA, Holmer R, Egberts J-H, et al. Inhibition of IL-6 signaling significantly reduces primary tumor growth and recurrencies in orthotopic xenograft models of pancreatic cancer. *Int J Cancer.* 2015;137(5):1035–1046. doi:10.1002/ijc.29445

77. Farren MR, Mace TA, Geyer S, et al. Systemic immune activity predicts overall survival in treatment-naive patients with metastatic pancreatic cancer. *Clin Cancer Res.* 2016;22(10):2565–2574. doi:10.1158/1078-0432.CCR-15-1732

78. Mace TA, Shakya R, Pitarresi JR, et al. IL-6 and PD-L1 antibody blockade combination therapy reduces tumour progression in murine models of pancreatic cancer. *Gut.* 2018;67(2):320–332. doi:10.1136/gutjnl-2016-311585

79. Collins MA, Bednar F, Zhang Y, et al. Oncogenic Kras is required for both the initiation and maintenance of pancreatic cancer in mice. *J Clin Invest.* 2012;122(2):639–653. doi:10.1172/JCI59227

80. Baker LA, Tiriac H, Clevers H, et al. Modeling pancreatic cancer with organoids. *Trends Cancer.* 2016;2(4):176–190. doi:10.1016/j.trecan.2016.03.004

81. Hou S, Tiriac H, Sridharan BP, et al. Advanced development of primary pancreatic organoid tumor models for high-throughput phenotypic drug screening. *SLAS Discov.* 2018;23(6):574–584. doi:10.1177/2472555218766842

82. Tiriac H, Bucobo JC, Tzimas D, et al. Successful creation of pancreatic cancer organoids by means of EUS-guided fine-needle biopsy sampling for personalized cancer treatment. *Gastrointest Endosc.* 2018;87(6):1474–1480. doi:10.1016/j.gie.2017.12.032

83. Beatty GL, Torigian DA, Chiorean EG, et al. A phase I study of an agonist CD40 monoclonal antibody (CP-870,893) in combination with gemcitabine in patients with advanced pancreatic ductal adenocarcinoma. *Clin Cancer Res.* 2013;19(22):6286–6295. doi:10.1158/1078-0432.CCR-13-1320

84. Cannarile MA, Weisser M, Jacob W, et al. Colony-stimulating factor 1 receptor (CSF1R) inhibitors in cancer therapy. *J Immunother Cancer.* 2017;5(1):53. doi:10.1186/s40425-017-0257-y

85. Nywening TM, Belt BA, Cullinan DR, et al. Targeting both tumour-associated CXCR2(+) neutrophils and CCR2(+) macrophages disrupts myeloid recruitment and improves chemotherapeutic responses in pancreatic ductal adenocarcinoma. *Gut.* 2017;67(6):1112–1123. doi:10.1136/gutjnl-2017-313738

86. Nywening TM, Wang-Gillam A, Sanford DE, et al. Targeting tumour-associated macrophages with CCR2 inhibition in combination with FOLFIRINOX in patients with borderline resectable and locally advanced pancreatic cancer: a single-centre, open-label, dose-finding, non-randomised, phase 1b trial. *Lancet Oncol.* 2016;17(5):651–662. doi:10.1016/S1470-2045(16)00078-4

Diagnosis and Staging of Pancreatic Cancer

Ramzi Mulki, Parit Mekaroonkamol, Alexandra G. Lopez-Aguiar,
Gregory B. Lesinski, David A. Kooby, Mehmet Akce, Shishir K. Maithel, and
Field F. Willingham

INTRODUCTION

The management of pancreatic adenocarcinoma is multifaceted, requiring a multidisciplinary team including medical oncologists, radiation oncologists, pancreatobiliary surgeons, interventional endoscopists, diagnostic radiologists, and pathologists. This chapter describes the modalities available for the diagnosis and staging of pancreatic adenocarcinoma.

CLINICAL PRESENTATION

The presenting symptoms and signs of pancreatic cancer are often vague and are dependent on the location of disease. Tumors tend to present late when the stage is advanced. Tumors in the head and uncinate process of the pancreas account for 60% to 70% of cases (1). These typically present with features of cholestasis such as jaundice, pruritus, and dark urine. In advanced disease, some patients may present with symptoms and signs of gastric outlet obstruction due to extrinsic compression or invasion into the duodenum (2). Tumors in the body and tail of the pancreas frequently present late, with pain being the most common symptom (1). Other symptoms include weight loss, steatorrhea, acute pancreatitis, and new onset diabetes. Recent studies highlight an association between new onset diabetes mellitus (DM) and pancreatic adenocarcinoma, and this possibility should be considered in patients with new onset DM without other risk factors (3,4).

DIAGNOSIS

It is not possible to diagnose pancreatic cancer based on these symptoms. Awareness of the symptoms and signs in a patient with risk factors for the development of pancreatic cancer may prompt earlier evaluation. Laboratory testing and imaging are typically indicated in the initial workup. This chapter reviews the diagnostic modalities for pancreatic carcinoma, some of which are involved in the staging process as well.

Biomarker and Laboratory Data

Serum carbohydrate antigen 19-9 (CA 19-9) is currently the best tumor marker for pancreatic cancer with a sensitivity and specificity of 79% to 81% and 80% to 90%, respectively (5). Several considerations exist: (a) its low positive predictive value diminishes its applicability in screening (6); (b) it can be falsely elevated in common benign conditions such as acute cholangitis, cirrhosis, and cholestatic diseases; (c) it is not specific to pancreatic cancer and may be elevated in other malignant conditions such as hepatobiliary, gastric, ovarian, and colorectal cancers (7); and (d) it requires the presence of the Lewis blood group antigen (a glycosyl transferase) to be expressed, which is absent in 5% to 10% of the population, and is therefore not useful as a tumor marker in this particular population (8,9). It is most useful as a marker of disease activity and in monitoring patients in the setting of a confirmed pancreatic cancer (10). The 2017 National Comprehensive Cancer Network (NCCN) practice guidelines recommended measuring CA 19-9 levels before surgery, immediately after, before adjuvant therapy, and for surveillance (11). Though nonspecific, other laboratory abnormalities that may be seen in those with pancreatic cancer include an elevated bilirubin, alkaline phosphatase, and transaminases.

Imaging

Initial diagnostic studies may be performed to evaluate symptoms and to work up abnormal laboratory results. Abdominal ultrasound is of little value in the evaluation of pancreatic cancer due to its low sensitivity for tumors less than 3 cm and due to the sonographic interference of bowel gas, which frequently overlies and obscures the pancreas. Abdominal ultrasound has a high sensitivity for detecting biliary ductal dilation and gallbladder abnormalities. When tumors can be visualized with transabdominal ultrasound, they most frequently appear as hypoechoic hypovascular solid mass lesions with irregular margins (12).

Axial imaging is required for staging and to determine resectability. Staging requires imaging of the chest, abdomen, and pelvis. Resectability determinations require high-resolution imaging with axial sections through the pancreas, which allows precise characterization of nodal, arterial, and venous involvement. CT and MRI may both be employed and are discussed in the following.

CT with pancreatic protocol involves triple-phase contrast-enhanced subcentimeter slices with images obtained in the portal venous and pancreatic phases of contrast enhancement (13,14). The difference in contrast enhancement between the normal tissue and adenocarcinoma is greatest during the pancreatic phase, providing a distinction between a hypodense lesion (cancer) and the remainder of the gland (Figure 20.1). The sensitivity and specificity of triple-phase contrast-enhanced pancreatic protocol CT is 89% to 97% and 95%, respectively for the detection of pancreatic cancer (12,15) comparable to the sensitivity and specificity of MRI (81%–99% and 70%–93%, respectively) (16). One advantage of MRI over CT is the ability to detect subtle liver metastasis. MRI is therefore frequently used as an adjunct to CT in patients with indeterminate liver lesions, or for those with contrast allergy (17,18). The utility and quality of MRI continue to evolve and the choice between CT and MRI is dependent on availability, expertise, and the clinician's comfort with one modality over another. MRI findings suggestive of pancreatic cancer include a hypointense lesion within an enhancing pancreatic

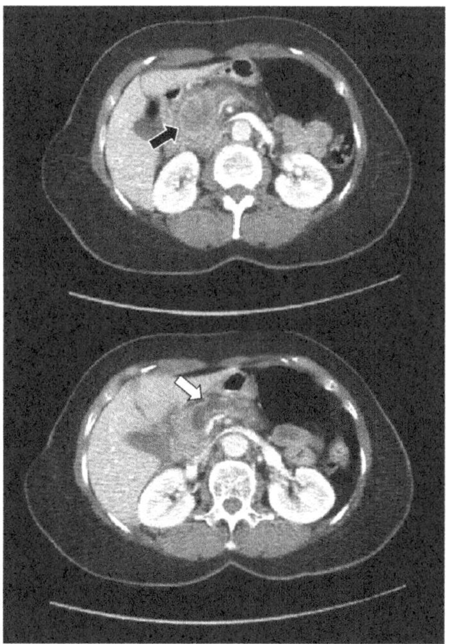

FIGURE 20.1   Abdominal CT with IV contrast demonstrating pancreatic adenocarcinoma in the head region (black arrow) with upstream pancreatic ductal dilation (white arrow).

IV, intravenous.

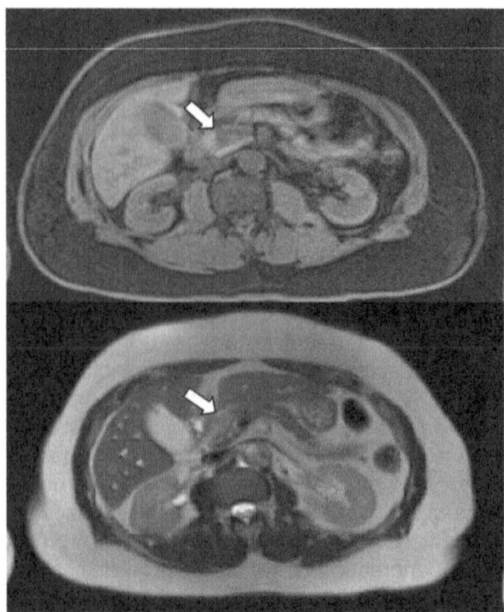

FIGURE 20.2   Pancreatic adenocarcinoma demonstrated as a 2-cm T1 hypointense, mildly T2 hyperintense, hypoenhancing mass within the head of the pancreas.

gland (Figure 20.2). Though the CT pancreatic protocol is favored in some guidelines for staging (11), institutional strengths are impactful and a multidisciplinary discussion on the preferred radiologic modality is encouraged. A recent consensus statement endorsed by the Society of Abdominal Radiology and the American Pancreatic Association puts forward a standardized imaging reporting template using universally accepted terms, with a goal of providing optimal characterization of the stage (19). Briefly, reporting a case of pancreatic cancer involves the detailed description of the morphological aspects of the tumor, its relationship with nearby arteries, veins, and extrapancreatic spread or metastasis (11,19).

PET is a technique based on a differential metabolic activity between neoplastic and non-neoplastic tissue, commonly using [18]fluorodeoxyglucose ([18]FDG) as a tracer of glucose metabolism (Figure 20.3). PET integrated with CT (PET/CT) has enhanced the diagnostic capabilities, particularly for masses <2 cm in size (20,21). The sensitivity of PET/CT reached 90.1%, which was significantly higher than PET alone (22). Currently, PET has not been formally endorsed by the NCCN or European Society for Medical Oncology (ESMO); however, the study continues to evolve and can be considered when additional staging is deemed necessary or for postoperative surveillance (11,23).

Diagnostic Procedures and Biopsy

Several diagnostic, endoscopic, and surgical options are available for tissue diagnosis (24). These include endoscopic ultrasound (EUS) with fine-needle aspiration (FNA), endoscopic retrograde cholangiopancreatography (ERCP), CT-guided FNA, and diagnostic laparoscopy. Obtaining a conclusive tissue diagnosis in a subtle pancreatic lesion can be challenging depending on the location and size of the mass and repeat sampling may be required in some cases (11). In some instances where there is a high suspicion of pancreatic adenocarcinoma in a patient with resectable disease who is fit for surgery, sampling or repeat sampling may not be required as a negative biopsy might not change the surgical management (11).

EUS uses a linear echoendoscope, an endoscope with an ultrasound probe and a biopsy channel at its tip, enabling it to obtain sonographic images and tissue sampling in real time. Sonographically, pancreatic cancer typically appears as an irregular hypoechoic mass in the pancreas and commonly presents with upstream pancreatic ductal dilation (Figure 20.4). EUS is considered to be the most sensitive test for pancreatic cancer with a high sensitivity ranging from 91% to 100%. EUS is also sensitive for tumors <2 cm; however, it may not image some distant metastatic lesions, and characterization of vascular involvement may be more in line

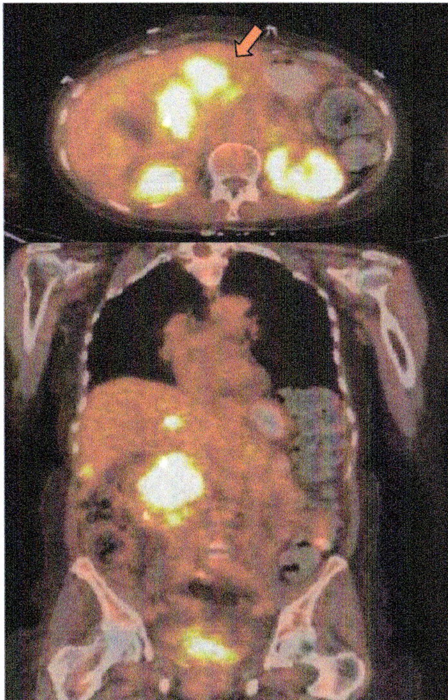

FIGURE 20.3 Pancreatic adenocarcinoma showing increased FDG uptake in the pancreatic head region on PET scan.

FDG, fluorodeoxyglucose.

with MRI or CT (25). Though endorsed by the American Society for Gastrointestinal Endoscopy (ASGE) for diagnosis and staging, the NCCN considers EUS in a complementary role to a pancreatic protocol CT (11,24). One major advantage of EUS lies in its ability to image the pancreas and obtain a tissue diagnosis in the same procedure (Figure 20.5). The presence of a cytopathologist during the procedure to offer an on-site evaluation and confirm adequate tissue procurement has been repeatedly shown to improve conclusive tissue diagnosis. Potential risks associated with EUS-guided sampling include bleeding, pancreatitis, and the potential for tumor seeding (24). A potential benefit of EUS as opposed to percutaneous sampling is that the areas traversed by EUS for tissue diagnosis are typically in the resection field at a subsequent surgery. When compared to CT-guided tissue sampling, EUS-FNA is the preferred method, endorsed in recent NCCN guidelines due to its higher diagnostic yield, safety, and lower risk of tumor seeding (11).

Findings on ERCP suggestive of pancreatic head malignancy include biliary and pancreatic duct strictures with upstream ductal dilation. Dilation of both ducts is referred to as the "double duct sign." Patients presenting with double ductal dilation should be carefully evaluated for tumors in the head of the pancreas. ERCP is primarily utilized for pancreaticobiliary stent placement to relieve obstructions caused by the tumor either for palliation or as a bridge to surgery (Figure 20.5). Brush cytology from intraductal biliary strictures can be obtained during ERCP. These brushings have a much lower diagnostic yield compared to EUS but when positive may spare patients additional procedures. The specificity of ERCP with brush cytology and biopsy approaches 100%; however, their sensitivity is low to moderate reaching 15% to 50% for brush cytology and 33% to 50% for biopsy (26). ERCP may be less frequently needed for tumors in the uncinate process, body, and tail as they have a lower propensity for biliary obstruction.

Small peritoneal and liver metastases can be missed on pancreatic protocol CT. Given the importance of accurate staging prior to potential surgical resection, laparoscopy may be

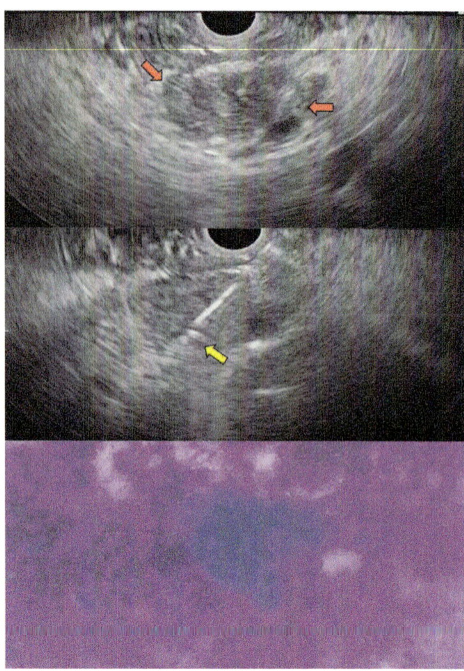

FIGURE 20.4   Endosonographic images show hypoechoic mass involving the head of the pancreas. Fine-needle aspiration (yellow arrow) confirmed pancreatic adenocarcinoma.

indicated as an additional diagnostic tool in certain situations (27). A recent Cochrane review was performed to determine the diagnostic accuracy of laparoscopy as an adjunctive test to CT scanning and found that diagnostic laparoscopy may decrease the rate of unnecessary laparotomy for pancreatic and periampullary cancers (28). This is due to the fact that small subtle peritoneal or liver metastasis may have been missed on CT imaging. However, it is important to note that approximately half of the studies included in the review were performed in the 1990s and so it is unlikely that modern CT techniques and equipment were used. Diagnostic laparoscopy is used in some institutions, and it is typically employed for patients with potentially resectable disease, but with higher risk features such as a very high CA19-9 level prior to surgery or chemoradiation.

STAGING AND RESECTABILITY

According to the eighth edition of the tumor, node, and metastasis (TNM) system of the combined American Joint Committee on Cancer (AJCC) and Union for International Cancer Control (UICC), patients are categorized as potentially resectable (stage I and II), locally advanced unresectable (stage III), and metastatic (stage IV); see Table 20.1 (29). Changes from the prior staging guidelines include changes to the T stage definitions with clear size cutoffs. T stages now focus on size rather than the depth of invasion. Metastasis to 1–3 regional lymph nodes is now classified as stage II if there is no arterial involvement. Any involvement of the celiac axis (CA), superior mesenteric artery (SMA), and/or common hepatic artery (CHA; T4) is classified as stage III disease, regardless of nodal metastasis. The staging is considered locally advanced (stage III) when any T size tumor is accompanied by N2 (metastasis to ≥4 regional lymph nodes) as described in Table 20.1 (29,30). These changes have been based on data demonstrating differences in the overall survival according to the size of the tumor and the number of lymph nodes involved (31–33).

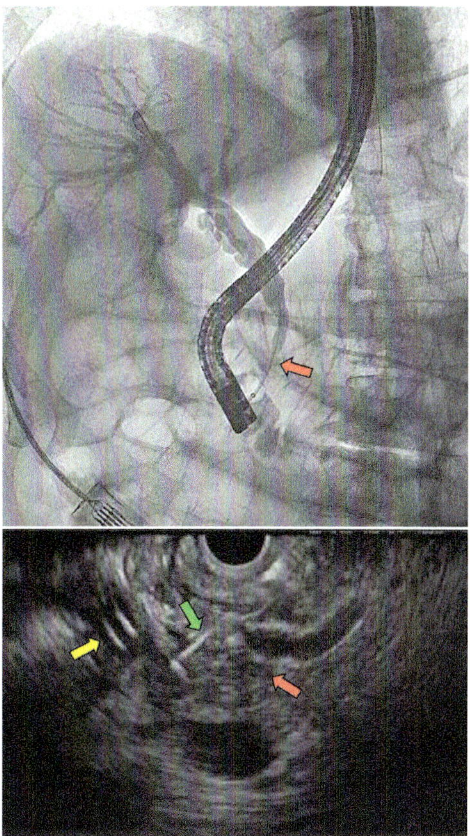

FIGURE 20.5 Cholangiogram performed during ERCP shows distal CBD stricture from pancreatic head mass (red arrow) as subsequently confirmed by endoscopic ultrasound (yellow arrow: stent in common bile duct, green arrow: endosonographic-guided needle biopsy).

CBD, common bile duct; ERCP, endoscopic retrograde cholangiopancreatography.

TABLE 20.1 TNM Staging for Pancreatic Cancer Based on the AJCC Criteria (Eighth Edition)

Anatomic Stage/Prognostic Groups			
Stage	**Primary Tumor[1] (T)**	**Regional Lymph Nodes[2] (N)**	**Distant Metastasis[3] (M)**
Stage 0	Tis	N0	M0
Stage IA	T1	N0	M0
Stage IB	T2	N0	M0
Stage IIA	T3	N0	M0
Stage IIB	T1	N1	M0
	T2	N1	M0
	T3	N1	M0

(continued)

TABLE 20.1 TNM Staging for Pancreatic Cancer Based on the AJCC Criteria (Eighth Edition) (*continued*)

Anatomic Stage/Prognostic Groups			
Stage	**Primary Tumor[1] (T)**	**Regional Lymph Nodes[2] (N)**	**Distant Metastasis[3] (M)**
Stage III	T1	N2	M0
	T2	N2	M0
	T3	N2	M0
	T4	Any N	M0
Stage IV	Any T	Any N	M1

[1]Primary Tumor (T)
TX   Primary tumor cannot be assessed
T0   No evidence of primary tumor
Tis   Carcinoma **in situ**
T1   Tumor $\leq$2 cm or less in greatest dimension
T1a   Tumor $\leq$0.5 cm in greatest dimension
T1b   Tumor >0.5 cm and <1 cm in greatest dimension
T1c   Tumor 1–2 cm in greatest dimension
T2   Tumor >2 cm and $\leq$4 cm in greatest dimension
T3   Tumor >4 cm in greatest dimension
T4   Tumor of any size that involves celiac axis, superior mesenteric artery, and/or common hepatic artery

[2]Regional Lymph Nodes (N)
NX   Regional lymph nodes cannot be assessed
N0   No regional lymph node metastasis
N1   Metastasis in one to three regional lymph nodes
N2   Metastasis in four or more regional lymph nodes

[3]Distant Metastasis (M)
M0   No distant metastasis
M1   Distant metastasis

AJCC, American Joint Committee on Cancer; TNM, tumor, node, and metastasis.

Source: From Kamarajah SK, Burns WR, Frankel TL, et al. Validation of the American Joint Commission on Cancer (AJCC) 8th edition staging system for patients with pancreatic adenocarcinoma: a Surveillance, Epidemiology and End Results (SEER) analysis. *Ann Surg Oncol.* 2017;24(7):2023–2030. doi:10.1245/s10434-017-5810-x

Complete surgical resection of pancreatic cancer is in most cases the only potentially curative option, and even following resection, recurrence is still seen in the majority of patients. Many patients and particularly those with borderline resectable tumors may benefit from neoadjuvant chemotherapy prior to surgery. The criteria for determining the potential for surgical resectability have been included in the 2017 NCCN practice guidelines, which are based on the consensus statement from the Society of Abdominal Radiology/American Pancreatic Association (11,19). The details of the criteria defining resectability are outlined in Table 20.2. Patients with distant metastasis are considered unresectable regardless of location. "Resectable" and "borderline resectable" characterizations are primarily dependent on tumor involvement of the surrounding arteries (SMA, CA, and CHA) and veins (superior mesenteric vein, inferior vena cava, and portal vein). The detailed diagnostic and staging algorithm is outlined in Figure 20.6.

TABLE 20.2 Criteria Defining Resectability Status

Criteria Defining Resectability		
Vascular Category	**Arterial**	**Venous**
Resectable	No arterial tumor contact (CA, SMA, CHA)	No tumor contact with SMV or PV or ≤180° contact without vein contour irregularity
Borderline resectable	Pancreatic head/uncinate process: • Solid tumor contact with CHA without extension to CA or hepatic artery bifurcation allowing for safe and complete resection and reconstruction. • Solid tumor contact with SMA of ≤180° • Solid tumor contact with variant arterial anatomy (e.g., accessary right hepatic artery, replaced right hepatic artery, replaced CHA, and the origin of replaced or accessory artery) and the presence and degree of tumor contact should be noted if present as it may affect surgical planning. Pancreatic body/tail: • Solid tumor contact with CA of ≤180° • Solid tumor contact with CA of >180° without involvement of the aorta and with intact and uninvolved GDA, thereby permitting a modified Appleby procedure.	• Solid tumor contact with the SMV or PV of >180°, contact of ≤180° with contour irregularity of the vein or thrombosis of the vein but with suitable vessel proximal and distal to the site of involvement allowing for safe and complete resection and vein reconstruction. • Solid tumor contact with the IVC
Unresectable	Distant metastasis (including nonregional LN metastasis) Head/uncinate process: • Solid tumor contact with SMA >180° solid tumor contact with CA >180° • Solid tumor contact with first jejunal SMA branch Body and tail: • Solid tumor contact of >180° with SMA or CA • Solid tumor contact with the CA and aortic involvement	Head/uncinate process: • Unreconstructable SMV/PV due to tumor involvement or occlusion (can be due to tumor or bland thrombus) • Contact with most proximal draining jejunal branch into SMV Body and tail: • Unreconstructable SMV/PV due to tumor involvement or occlusion (can be due to tumor or bland thrombus).

CA, celiac axis; CHA, common hepatic artery; GDA, gastroduodenal artery; IVC, inferior vena cava; LN, lymph node; PV, portal vein; SMA, superior mesenteric artery; SMV, superior mesenteric vein.

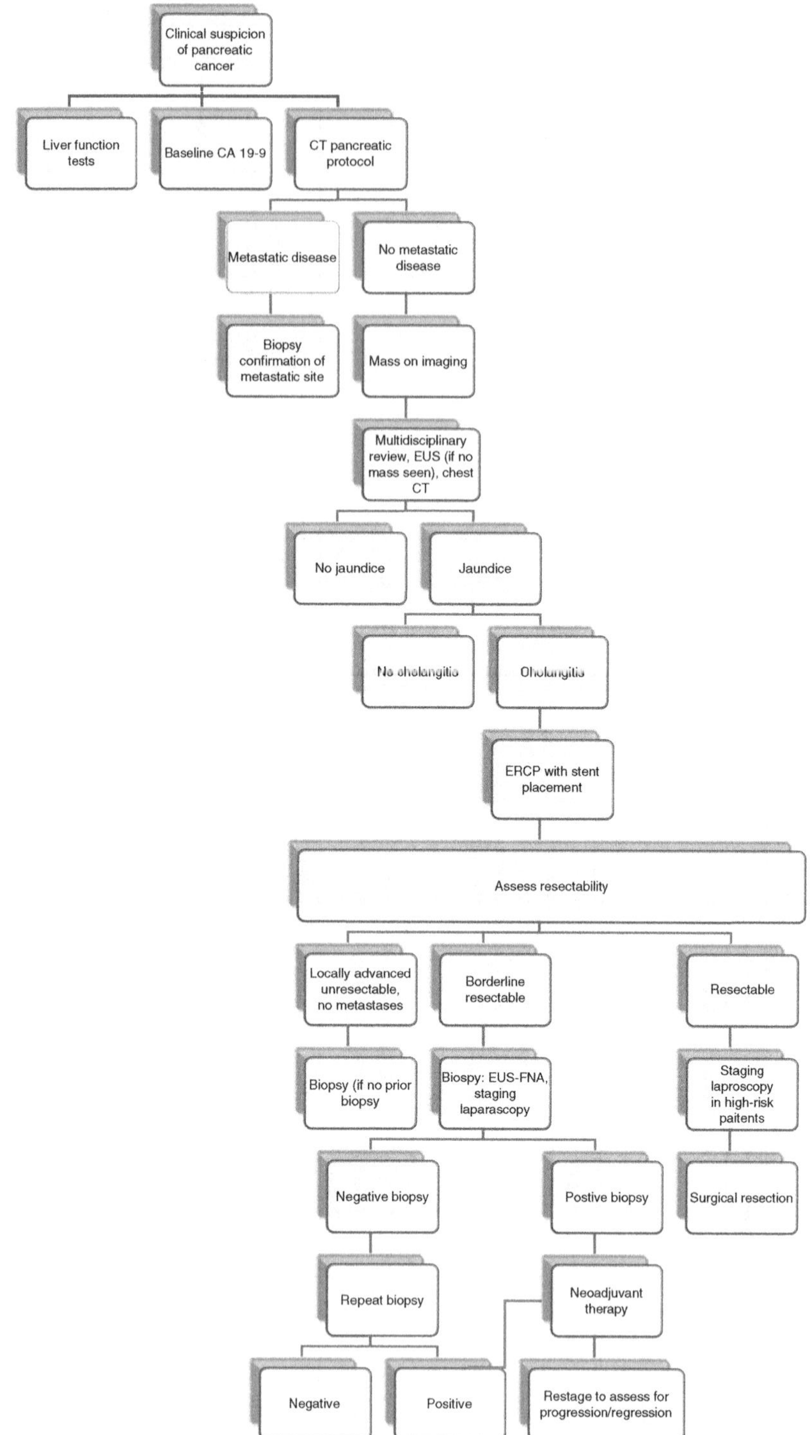

FIGURE 20.6 Diagnostic/staging algorithm.

ERCP, endoscopic retrograde cholangiopancreatography; EUS, endoscopic ultrasound; FNA, fine-needle aspiration.

REFERENCES

1. Modolell I, Guarner L, Malagelada JR. Vagaries of clinical presentation of pancreatic and biliary tract cancer. *Ann Oncol*. 1999;10 Suppl 4:82–84. doi:10.1093/annonc/10.suppl_4.S82
2. Watanapa P, Williamson RC. Surgical palliation for pancreatic cancer: developments during the past two decades. *Br J Surg*. 1992;79(1):8–20. doi:10.1002/bjs.1800790105
3. Gupta S, Vittinghoff E, Bertenthal D, et al. New-onset diabetes and pancreatic cancer. *Clin Gastroenterol Hepatol*. 2006;4(11):1366–1372; quiz 01. doi:10.1016/j.cgh.2006.06.024
4. Chari ST, Leibson CL, Rabe KG, et al. Probability of pancreatic cancer following diabetes: a population-based study. *Gastroenterology*. 2005;129(2):504–511. doi:10.1016/j.gastro.2005.05.007
5. Huang Z, Liu F. Diagnostic value of serum carbohydrate antigen 19-9 in pancreatic cancer: a meta-analysis. *Tumour Biol*. 2014;35(8):7459–7465. doi:10.1007/s13277-014-1995-9
6. Ballehaninna UK, Chamberlain RS. The clinical utility of serum CA 19-9 in the diagnosis, prognosis and management of pancreatic adenocarcinoma: an evidence based appraisal. *J Gastrointest Oncol*. 2012;3(2):105–119. doi:10.3978/j.issn.2078-6891.2011.021
7. Mann DV, Edwards R, Ho S, et al. Elevated tumour marker CA19-9: clinical interpretation and influence of obstructive jaundice. *Eur J Surg Oncol*. 2000;26(5):474–479. doi:10.1053/ejso.1999.0925
8. Lamerz R. Role of tumour markers, cytogenetics. *Ann Oncol*. 1999;10 Suppl 4:145–149. doi:10.1093/annonc/10.suppl_4.S145
9. Tempero MA, Uchida E, Takasaki H, et al. Relationship of carbohydrate antigen 19-9 and Lewis antigens in pancreatic cancer. *Cancer Res*. 1987;47(20):5501–5503.
10. Berger AC, Garcia M Jr, Hoffman JP, et al. Postresection CA 19-9 predicts overall survival in patients with pancreatic cancer treated with adjuvant chemoradiation: a prospective validation by RTOG 9704. *J Clin Oncol*. 2008;26(36):5918–5922. doi:10.1200/JCO.2008.18.6288
11. Tempero MA, Malafa MP, Al-Hawary M, et al. Pancreatic adenocarcinoma, version 2.2017, NCCN clinical practice guidelines in oncology. *J Natl Compr Canc Netw*. 2017;15(8):1028–1061. doi:10.6004/jnccn.2017.0131
12. Miura F, Takada T, Amano H, et al. Diagnosis of pancreatic cancer. *HPB (Oxford)*. 2006;8(5):337–342. doi:10.1080/13651820500540949
13. Horton KM, Fishman EK. Multidetector row CT with dual-phase CT angiography in the preoperative evaluation of pancreatic cancer. *Crit Rev Comput Tomogr*. 2002;43(5):323–360. doi:10.3109/20024091059189
14. Wong JC, Raman S. Surgical resectability of pancreatic adenocarcinoma: CTA. *Abdom Imaging*. 2010;35(4):471–480. doi:10.1007/s00261-009-9539-2
15. Kanji ZS, Gallinger S. Diagnosis and management of pancreatic cancer. *CMAJ*. 2013;185(14):1219–1226. doi:10.1503/cmaj.121368
16. Birchard KR, Semelka RC, Hyslop WB, et al. Suspected pancreatic cancer: evaluation by dynamic gadolinium-enhanced 3D gradient-echo MRI. *AJR Am J Roentgenol*. 2005;185(3):700–703. doi:10.2214/ajr.185.3.01850700
17. Holzapfel K, Reiser-Erkan C, Fingerle AA, et al. Comparison of diffusion-weighted MR imaging and multidetector-row CT in the detection of liver metastases in patients operated for pancreatic cancer. *Abdom Imaging*. 2011;36(2):179–184. doi:10.1007/s00261-010-9633-5
18. Motosugi U, Ichikawa T, Morisaka H, et al. Detection of pancreatic carcinoma and liver metastases with gadoxetic acid-enhanced MR imaging: comparison with contrast-enhanced multi-detector row CT. *Radiology*. 2011;260(2):446–453. doi:10.1148/radiol.11103548
19. Al-Hawary MM, Francis IR, Chari ST, et al. Pancreatic ductal adenocarcinoma radiology reporting template: consensus statement of the society of abdominal radiology and the American pancreatic association. *Gastroenterology*. 2014;146(1):291–304.e1. doi:10.1053/j.gastro.2013.11.004
20. Delbeke D, Martin WH. Update of PET and PET/CT for hepatobiliary and pancreatic malignancies. *HPB (Oxford)*. 2005;7(3):166–179. doi:10.1080/13651820510028909
21. Sahani DV, Bonaffini PA, Catalano OA, et al. State-of-the-art PET/CT of the pancreas: current role and emerging indications. *Radiographics*. 2012;32(4):1133–1158; discussion 58–60. doi:10.1148/rg.324115143
22. Tang S, Huang G, Liu J, et al. Usefulness of 18F-FDG PET, combined FDG-PET/CT and EUS in diagnosing primary pancreatic carcinoma: a meta-analysis. *Eur J Radiol*. 2011;78(1):142–150. doi:10.1016/j.ejrad.2009.09.026
23. Ducreux M, Cuhna AS, Caramella C, et al. Cancer of the pancreas: ESMO Clinical Practice Guidelines for diagnosis, treatment and follow-up. *Ann Oncol*. 2015;26 Suppl 5:v56–v68. doi:10.1093/annonc/mdv295
24. ASGE Standards of Practice Committee, Eloubeidi MA, Decker GA, et al. The role of endoscopy in the evaluation and management of patients with solid pancreatic neoplasia. *Gastrointest Endosc*. 2016;83(1):17–28. doi:10.1016/j.gie.2015.09.009

25. Dewitt J, Devereaux BM, Lehman GA, et al. Comparison of endoscopic ultrasound and computed tomography for the preoperative evaluation of pancreatic cancer: a systematic review. *Clin Gastroenterol Hepatol*. 2006;4(6):717–725; quiz 664. doi:10.1016/j.cgh.2006.02.020

26. De Bellis M, Sherman S, Fogel EL, et al. Tissue sampling at ERCP in suspected malignant biliary strictures (Part 1). *Gastrointest Endosc*. 2002;56(4):552–561. doi:10.1067/mge.2002.128132

27. Ahmed SI, Bochkarev V, Oleynikov D, et al. Patients with pancreatic adenocarcinoma benefit from staging laparoscopy. *J Laparoendosc Adv Surg Tech*. 2006;16(5):458–463. doi:10.1089/lap.2006.16.458

28. Allen VB, Gurusamy KS, Takwoingi Y, et al. Diagnostic accuracy of laparoscopy following computed tomography (CT) scanning for assessing the resectability with curative intent in pancreatic and periampullary cancer. *Cochrane Database of Syst Rev*. 2013;(11). doi:10.1002/14651858. CD009323.pub2

29. *Amin MB, Edge S, Greene F, et al. AJCC Cancer Staging Manual*. 8th ed. New York, NY; Springer International Publishing; 2017.

30. Amin MB, Edge S, Greene F, et al. The eighth edition AJCC cancer staging manual: continuing to build a bridge from a population-based to a more "personalized" approach to cancer staging. *CA Cancer J Clin*. 2017;67(2):93–99. doi:10.3322/caac.21388

31. Allen PJ, Kuk D, Castillo CF, et al. Multi-institutional validation study of the American joint commission on cancer (8th Edition) changes for T and N staging in patients with pancreatic adenocarcinoma. *Ann Surg*. 2017;265(1):185–191. doi:10.1097/SLA.0000000000001763

32. Kamarajah SK, Burns WR, Frankel TL, et al. Validation of the American Joint Commission on Cancer (AJCC) 8th edition staging system for patients with pancreatic adenocarcinoma: a Surveillance, Epidemiology and End Results (SEER) analysis. *Ann Surg Oncol*. 2017;24(7):2023–2030. doi:10.1245/s10434-017-5810-x

33. Chun YS, Pawlik TM, Vauthey J-N. 8th edition of the AJCC cancer staging manual: pancreas and hepatobiliary cancers. *Ann Surg Oncol*. 2017;25(4):845–847. doi:10.1245/s10434-017-6025-x

The Role and Timing of Surgery in Pancreatic Cancer

Mark J. Truty

PANCREAS CANCER: THE ROLE AND TIMING OF SURGERY

Specific treatment recommendations for pancreatic ductal adenocarcinoma (PDAC) have been largely determined according to initial radiologic staging and, as the majority of patients present with distant metastatic disease, palliative chemotherapy alone is recommended for most cases. Despite the high prevalence of systemic dissemination, approximately 50% of patients with PDAC will have radiologic nonmetastatic disease on initial diagnostic imaging (1). Of these nonmetastatic tumors, approximately two-thirds have been historically classified as surgically unresectable due to extrapancreatic tumor extension involving critical vasculature, and these patients typically receive a combination of systemic chemotherapy and/or locoregional chemoradiation alone. In the remaining minority of patients with localized tumors that are considered "resectable," recommendations are to proceed with curative-intent upfront resection as the initial presumed optimal treatment strategy, as surgery is the only known curative treatment modality. Although this approach has been the standard of care for decades, this paradigm has resulted in standard outcomes, which are suboptimal from a patient perspective, and the realization that alternative treatment sequencing is required if we intend to change historical outcomes.

Surgical treatment of localized pancreatic cancer has a long and storied history with the initial reports of resection dating back to the late 1800s with the first distal pancreatectomy, and this continued until the mid-20th century with various iterations until the development of the one-stage pancreatoduodenectomy, described by Dr. Allen Whipple, that became synonymous with pancreatic cancer surgery (2,3). Despite initial technical success, major perioperative complications with associated mortality combined with the poor long-term survival outcomes tempered the enthusiasm of surgery for this disease during this era. Beginning in the 1980s with more surgical specialization and focus on perioperative safety, multiple reports from high-volume centers resulted in significant improvement in surgical outcomes with operative mortality less than 5% and surgery was reintroduced and popularized as the treatment of choice for PDAC (4–7). Since then surgical resection has demonstrated significantly improved survival outcomes for resectable PDAC when compared to chemotherapy and/or radiation therapy alone, and is the only treatment modality to offer potential cure and long-term survival for these patients (8,9). Further refinements in techniques have continued and, currently, minimally invasive resections for PDAC include both laparoscopic and robotic approaches (10–13). During this evolution in surgical technique, the critical importance of obtaining negative surgical margins was established as one of the primary surgical contributions to a patient's outcome from an oncologic perspective (14,15). As a result, significant efforts to define "resectability" in the context of margin risk using standardized radiologic criteria were established over time. This has resulted in multiple radiologic classification systems, all of which include varied degrees of venous and/or arterial involvement. Concurrent with these surgical advances, numerous trials in resectable PDAC have solidified the importance of postoperative adjuvant systemic chemotherapy in order to improve the particularly limited long-term survival outcomes after resection alone (16–20). Despite our best efforts over time, the majority of patients succumb to distant recurrence postoperatively even with curative-intent operations. We have reached a surgical plateau in terms of outcomes with a surgery-first approach for PDAC and this is exemplified with the Hopkins four decade experience (Figure 21.1). In this seminal paper, there was marked improvement in perioperative complications and operative mortality over time. However, there was also decreasing incremental improvement in survival during that same time period suggesting that technical refinements do not significantly affect biology and more than an operation alone is needed to optimize patient survival (21).

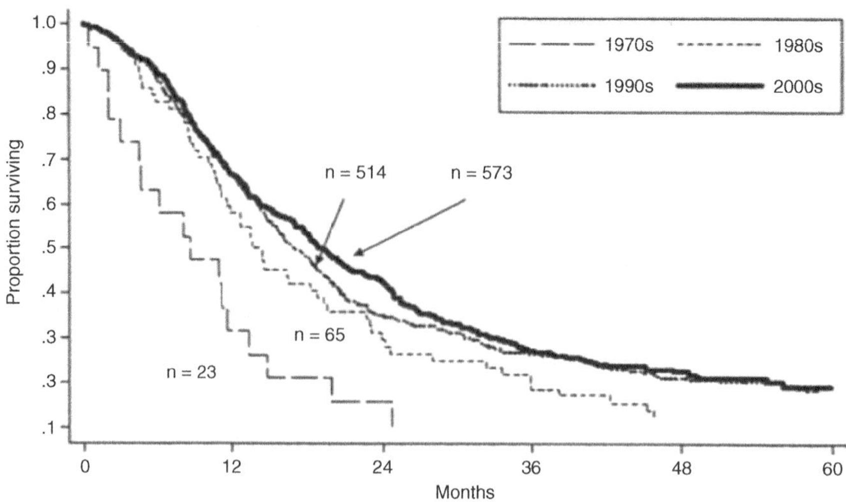

FIGURE 21.1   Kaplan–Meier survival curves for patients undergoing pancreatoduodenectomy for ductal adenocarcinoma of the pancreas at Johns Hopkins, by decade.

Source: From Winter JM, Cameron JL, Campbell KA, et al. 1423 pancreaticoduodenectomies for pancreatic cancer: a single-institution experience. *J Gastrointest Surg.* 2006;10(9):1199–1210. doi:10.1016/j.gassur.2006.08.018

The classic standard strategy that has been practiced focuses on a small proportion of patients with "resectable" disease using upfront resection with the hopes of attaining a negative margin followed by adjuvant therapy if feasible. This approach has been recently challenged. Much of our understanding of the biology of PDAC metastatic progression stems from quantitative analysis of genomic and mutational sequencing in this disease, and this has revealed novel insights into the genetic features underlying pancreatic cancer progression suggesting that most patients, regardless of initial radiologic staging, likely harbor occult systemic metastases at initial presentation (22). This has also been supported with recent computational modeling based on validated patient datasets using mutational analyses and cancer cell growth metrics of localized PDAC that appears to be directly correlated with primary tumor size (Figure 21.2). Furthermore, such modeling has also suggested that there may be an actual biological detriment with a surgery-first approach whereby complete locoregional tumor resection, although removing 99.9% of disease burden, may leave behind a fraction of occult metastatic cells leading to exponential expansion while the patient is recovering from surgery, a clinical observation that has been observed in most patients (23). The problem with the traditional approach of upfront surgical resection in seemingly resectable tumors is that this leads to little understanding of patient or tumor biology, has led to disappointing survival outcomes that have had minimal improvements over time despite improved surgical care, and does not account for several critically important resectability variables that have significant influence on postoperative outcomes. Thus, a new strategy is required if we intend to improve upon historical results of surgical resection for PDAC, a strategy that determines the suitability and the order of treatment sequencing for a safe and potentially curative operation in the greatest number of patients. In order to address this, we must risk-stratify patients using various preoperative factors in order to determine the optimal sequencing of therapy.

Risk Stratification and Clinical Resectability Classification

There is a significant difference between removability and resectability. Removability is the ability to surgically separate a tumor from a patient, whereas resectability is surgical removability with various anatomical, biological, and conditional constraints. It is these three factors that are used for risk stratification in order to assign a clinical resectability classification for patients to guide sequencing of therapy based on the answers to three critically important

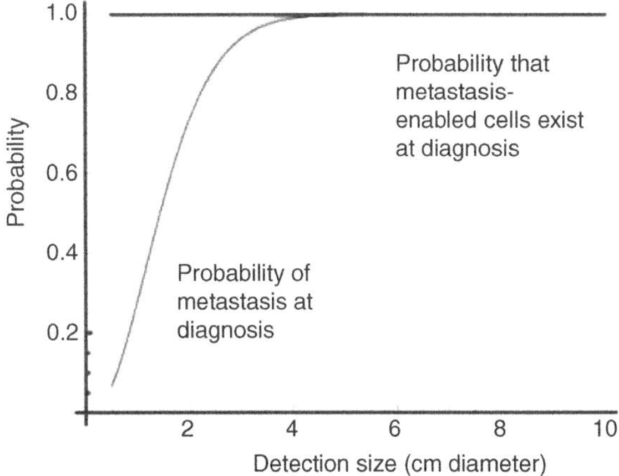

FIGURE 21.2   Probability of metastasis at diagnosis (gray curve) and the probability of the existence of cells in the primary tumor that have evolved the potential to metastasize (black curve) correlated with tumor size (cm).

Source: From Haeno H, Gonen M, Davis MB, et al. Computational modeling of pancreatic cancer reveals kinetics of metastasis suggesting optimum treatment strategies. *Cell.* 2012;148(1–2):362–375. doi:10.1016/j.cell.2011.11.060

questions: (a) Can the tumor be successfully surgically removed with a high likelihood of a negative margin?, (b) Will the cancer recur soon after surgery due to occult metastases?, and (c) What is the patient's risk of surgical complications and ultimate failure to receive any chemotherapy? Patients are then stratified according to these questions as clinically resectable, borderline resectable, or unresectable. Borderline resectable, a term coined by Katz et al., describes those patients with localized disease who have, however, tumor or patient characteristics that may preclude immediate surgery with good outcomes (24) Borderline simply implies higher risk with an upfront resection, and it is an indication to consider neoadjuvant treatment sequencing. Although much of the literature has focused on borderline anatomy (high risk of positive margin resection with a surgery-first approach), there is also borderline biology (high risk of occult metastases and early postoperative recurrence) and borderline condition (high risk of perioperative complications and failure to receive chemotherapy). Most patients have a combination of these factors at initial presentation.

Borderline Anatomy
The rationale for standardized anatomical classification is driven by the established known detriment that a positive surgical margin has on postoperative patient survival. Margins are classified as R0—microscopically negative, R1—microscopically positive, and R2—grossly positive. There has been much debate as to what is the optimal assessment of margin positivity from a histologic examination perspective (25–27). Regardless of the pathologic assessment technique, positive margins have been demonstrably shown to not only significantly mitigate the survival benefit of surgical resection but also negatively affect any potential derived added benefit of adjuvant therapy (28,29). Based on meta-analysis of data obtained from randomized controlled trials in PDAC, there were widely variable margin positive rates ranging from 0% to 80% despite higher levels of standardization of anatomic resectability inclusion criteria in these controlled studies (30). Remarkably consistent in all, however, was the fact that a positive margin resulted in up to a 50% reduction in postoperative survival. Notwithstanding poor surgical technique, positive margins cannot be predicted with certainty by preoperative imaging alone. PDAC can be microscopically infiltrative far distant from the primary tumor, and previous work has shown that radiologic distance poorly predicts microscopic margins even when an optimal oncologic operation is performed. It is this histologic finding that explains why at least 20% of pancreatic cancer operations with "resectable" anatomy result in R1 resections despite high-quality preoperative anatomical imaging (31). As surgeons, we traditionally

accepted the fact that a fraction of patients, despite good oncologic surgical techniques, would end up with a positive margin, with resultant worse survival outcomes. These suboptimal survival outcomes were superior, however, when compared to those patients undergoing palliative procedures; thus we accepted a certain proportion of R1 resections as there were no better treatment alternatives, with some centers even suggesting the benefit of R2 resections over palliative procedures (32,33). However, we are in a new era and there is a new survival comparator due to the advances in nonoperative treatment modalities. Gemcitabine was the first approved agent for advanced PDAC disease; however, with response rates of less than 10%, it rarely led to any meaningful benefit as a single agent for nearly 20 years (34). In the modern era, however, with the advent of more efficacious combinatorial systemic regimens including FOLFIRINOX and gemcitabine plus nab-paclitaxel combined with improvements in locoregional control with various chemoradiation strategies, the outcomes for nonoperative therapy, even in patients with anatomically inoperable tumors, have improved significantly over time. Currently median survivals in unresectable cancers are approaching those typically seen in previous surgery-first series with clearly resectable tumors (35–38). Thus our modern day comparator is no longer the palliative operation, and if we intend to continue to assert that surgical resection offers significant survival benefit for patients with localized disease, we must demonstrate superior outcomes to modern nonoperative modalities.

Despite the various proposed classifications systems, the Alliance (Intergroup) criteria are likely the current and future standard in radiologic anatomical resectability assessment based on its simple classification system, increased utilization of similar radiologic templated reporting at most centers, and its subsequent validation in current and ongoing surgical trials (39). Regardless of which anatomic resectability classification is utilized, we need to consider that all of them are based on two primary assumptions: an upfront surgery-first approach, and traditional anatomical plane based pancreatic resection techniques without en bloc vascular and/ or multivisceral resection. Patients without significant radiologic involvement and clear tissue planes between tumor and venous (portal/superior mesenteric vein) or arterial structures (superior mesenteric artery, celiac axis, hepatic artery) are currently considered anatomically resectable, and in these patients an R0 is likely, but not certain (Figure 21.3A). In these anatomically resectable patients, a surgery-first approach followed by adjuvant therapy will lead to standard survival outcomes. In contrast, those with more extensive venous involvement or limited abutment of arterial structures are considered anatomically borderline and a surgery-first approach will lead to a higher likelihood of a positive margin resection in the absence of preoperative therapy or en bloc vascular resection (Figure 21.3B). Finally, in those patients who have locally advanced anatomy, an R2 resection is likely, or often, tumors are strictly inoperable due to extensive anatomical restrictive limitations, or only performed with extensive en bloc resection at specialized centers with experience (Figure 21.3C). However, although patients may have anatomical features that place them into the borderline or locally advanced category, this does not imply inoperability, only that margin risk is higher if these patients undergo upfront standard resectional surgery as the initial treatment. Thus margin risk can be potentially modified with either the use of neoadjuvant therapy (chemotherapy and/or chemoradiation) or the judicious use of en bloc vascular resection as indicated by anatomical limitations and surgeon technical skillset and experience. Both modern induction systemic combinatorial chemotherapy and/or locoregional chemoradiation have been suggested to anatomically downstage tumors prior to resection in order to increase the probability of a negative margin. Both modalities, used either as sole therapy or in combination, have demonstrated improved margin negative operations often in conjunction with en bloc vascular resection. Thus for any patient with borderline or locally advanced anatomy, treatment sequencing should include some form of neoadjuvant therapy prior to reassessment for surgical resectability in the absence of development of metastatic disease. The optimal sequencing of this therapy is currently the topic of significant debate and will likely be the focus of all future studies in this disease. However, regardless of these anatomic factors, anatomy alone still poorly predicts long-term outcome as many patients with early-stage and clearly resectable tumors still succumb to distant metastatic disease with high frequency. Thus we need to consider other relevant factors that allow us to optimally triage and determine the appropriate sequencing strategy for patients with PDAC.

Borderline Biology

One of the most remarkably consistent findings in all surgical studies in PDAC is the associated overall survival curves. Within the confines of these survival outcomes, there are two specific groups with divergently different outcomes—approximately 25% of patients who develop early

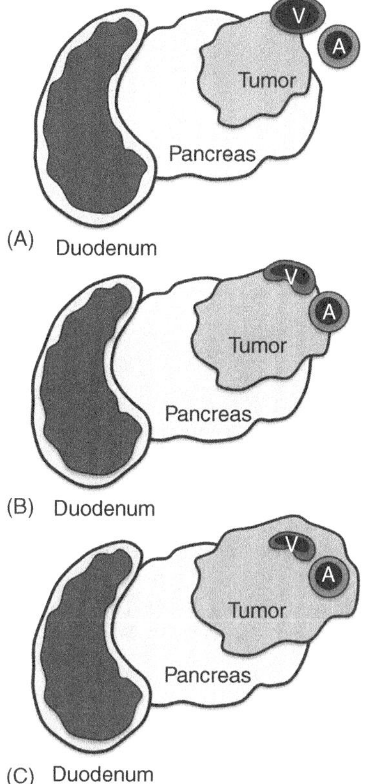

FIGURE 21.3 Radiologic assessment of anatomic resectability based on extent of venous and/or arterial involvement: (A) anatomically resectable; (B) borderline resectable; (C) locally advanced.

recurrence and death within 12 months of operation, and a similar proportion of long-term survivors beyond 5 years (Figure 21.4) (40). Thus there is a subgroup of patients who derived no benefit whatsoever from an operative intervention and another group that was seemingly cured or at least enjoyed long-term survival. It is this clinical reality that highlights how anatomic resectability alone cannot accurately predict tumor biology using a surgery-first approach strategy. Given the high rate of systemic recurrence following an upfront resection approach with PDAC, there are patients who are at higher risk for distant failure. This has been clearly demonstrated in an often-cited National Cancer Database (NCDB) study looking at the utilization of surgery as a curative-intent modality in early-stage PDAC (41). In this study, authors found that only 27% of early-stage pancreatic cancer (preclinical stage I) underwent resection with an associated median survival of 19.1 months in contrast to the remaining 73% without operation with a survival of only 8.4 months from diagnosis. The conclusion of this study was that there was a national failure to offer potentially curative-intent resection to the majority of patients with seemingly early-stage disease. However, another interpretation is that if those 73% were truly "early stage" why was the survival so poor? The data would highly suggest that those patients likely harbored unmeasured biological factors other than just lack of operative intervention that could explain such dismal outcomes in otherwise early-stage anatomically resectable tumors. There are several primary factors readily available at diagnosis that can assist in defining these patients that include: radiographic findings suggestive of possible metastatic disease such as small indeterminate hepatic, pulmonary, or peritoneal lesions (including small-volume ascites), suspicious or obviously involved regional nodal metastases, and elevation of circulating tumor markers (CA 19-9). The rationales for this are that many of these indeterminate radiologic lesions have a probability of being metastatic when followed over time, nodal metastases are surrogate

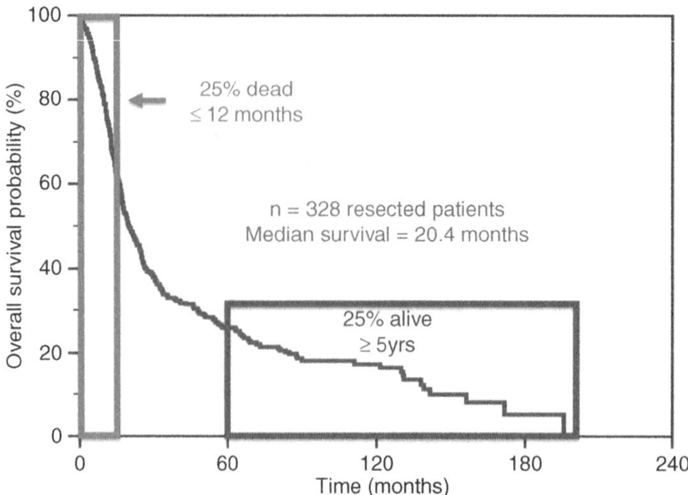

FIGURE 21.4   Typical overall survival curve after curative-intent resection for PDAC reveals recurrence in 25% of patients and death within 12 months of operation and long-term survival in another 25% of patients.

Source: Adapted from Katz MH, Wang H, Fleming JB, et al. Long-term survival after multidisciplinary management of resected pancreatic adenocarcinoma. *Ann Surg Oncol.* 2009;16(4):836–847. doi:10.1245/ s10434-008-0295-2

for more advanced disease and higher stage (IIB) with detriment to survival with a surgery-first approach similar in magnitude to those with a positive margin (<12 months), and patients with markedly elevated carbohydrate antigen 19-9 (CA 19-9) at diagnosis have worse outcomes after upfront resection (42–44). Patients with any of these biologically borderline factors have a nearly 50% likelihood of developing early metastatic disease compared to 15% of patients without (45). Of these factors, CA 19-9 elevation likely has the greatest prognostic influence and is the simplest measure of biological aggressiveness. CA 19-9 is a Lewis blood group antigen that is found in a variety of gastrointestinal (GI) malignancies including pancreas, biliary tract, and gastric cancer among others. It has a specific mechanism as it is the ligand for endothelial cell selectin; thus, patients with elevated levels have a higher risk of developing hematogenous metastases (46). This tumor marker has not been found significantly effective as a screening or diagnostic biomarker as up to 10% of the population does not express the fucosyltransferase required for production. Thus, it is unmeasurable in these patients, and CA 19-9 can be falsely elevated in patients with biliary tract obstruction, cholangitis, or inflammation. Numerous single-center studies have confirmed that CA 19-9 elevation leads to worse prognosis after resection but no specific cutoff had been universally established that would preclude operation in otherwise anatomically resectable tumors. In a simple but profound German study, all patients were stratified by CA 19-9 levels at diagnosis, regardless of the level of jaundice, and survival remarkably correlated with the level of CA 19-9 elevation, with the greatest survival in those patients with normal preoperative levels with significantly worse outcomes for each increased strata of CA 19-9 elevation (Figure 21.5) (47). A recent, larger scale NCDB study revealed that any elevation of CA 19-9 above normal, regardless of extent, resulted in a worse stage-for-stage survival compared to patients with either normal levels or CA 19-9 nonsecretors with the largest survival detriment seen in otherwise resectable stage I/II tumors (48). Furthermore, when treatment sequencing was considered and other significant factors were adjusted for (margins, node status, etc.), the most optimal treatment sequence that mitigated the negative affect of CA 19-9 elevation was neoadjuvant systemic therapy followed by surgery, even when analyses were done on an intent-to-treat basis and were still superior to surgery-first followed by systemic adjuvant chemotherapy (Figure 21.6). Although most currently consider baseline CA 19-9 levels >1,000 u/mL to be of major significance, there is still debate for those patients whose CA 19-9 is elevated but <1,000 u/mL, specifically in those with larger tumors or patients

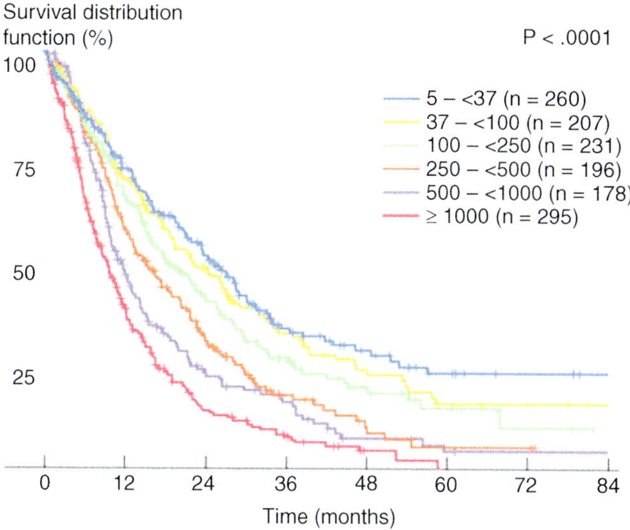

FIGURE 21.5   Preoperative CA 19-9 serum levels and survival.

CA 19-9, carbohydrate antigen 19-9.

Source: From Hartwig W, Strobel O, Hinz U, et al. CA 19-9 in potentially resectable pancreatic cancer: perspective to adjust surgical and perioperative therapy. *Ann Surg Oncol.* 2013;20(7):2188–2196. doi:10.1245/s10434-012-2809-1

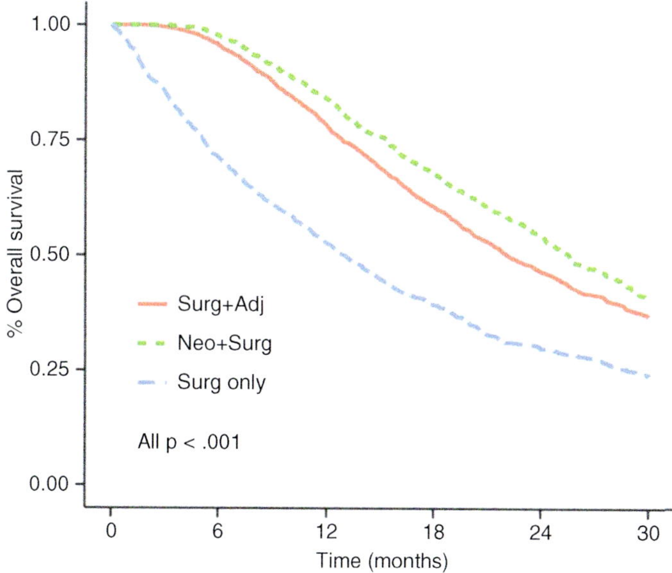

FIGURE 21.6   Survival outcomes in all patients with any CA 19-9 elevation by treatment sequencing.

CA 19-9, carbohydrate antigen 19-9.

Source: From Bergquist JR, Puig CA, Shubert CR, et al. Carbohydrate antigen 19-9 elevation in anatomically resectable, early stage pancreatic cancer is independently associated with decreased overall survival and an indication for neoadjuvant therapy: a national cancer database study. *J Am Coll Surg.* 2016;223(1):52–65. doi:10.1016/j.jamcollsurg.2016.02.009

who are jaundiced at the time of biomarker measurement. In jaundiced patients, some authors have suggested adjusting the tumor marker levels by dividing CA 19-9 by the serum bilirubin level although no scientific basis for this calculated adjustment was provided (49). Our group has reviewed our own institutional data (unpublished) looking at the correlation of CA 19-9 with tumor size and/or bilirubin levels at diagnosis in those patients with intermediate levels of CA 19-9 elevation (>37 but <1,000 u/mL), and we found little to no correlation of CA 19-9 with bilirubin level or tumor size even when adjusting for bilirubin elevation (Figure 21.7A,B). The only factor that CA 19-9 elevation correlated with was worse postoperative survival, even in the earliest stages of disease (stage 1) undergoing a surgery-first approach (Figure 21.7C). Thus in the absence of more modern biomarkers of occult systemic disease, CA 19-9 elevation is a major predictor of systemic metastases in otherwise anatomically resectable tumors regardless of the extent of marker elevation, tumor size, or level of jaundice, and so upfront surgical resection in these patients should proceed with caution. Despite the significant ability of CA 19-9 to predict postoperative survival, CA 19-9 is still markedly underutilized as an indication for neoadjuvant therapy and is actually not even measured in nearly three-fourths of patients at diagnosis, suggesting that the historical perception of the survival benefits of an operation alone continues to guide treatment decisions despite significant evidence to the contrary, a bias that needs to be corrected if we aim to improve survival outcomes in the future. Notwithstanding these biological borderline features, there is still a small fraction of patients, up to 15%, who will develop

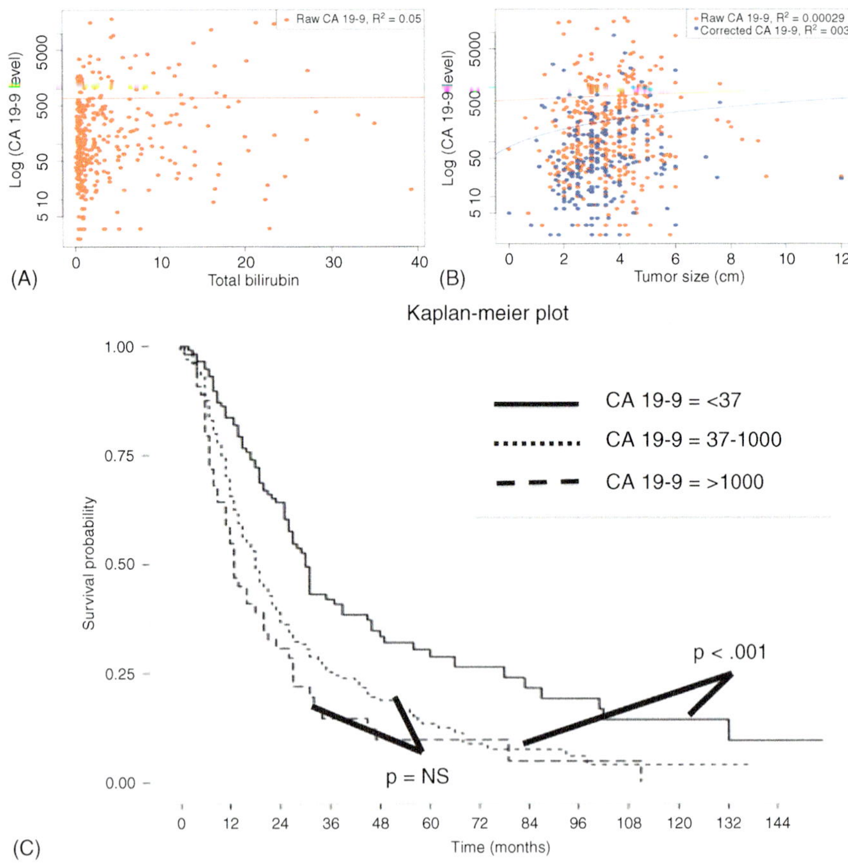

FIGURE 21.7   Correlation of CA 19-9 levels in patients undergoing resection for early stage 1 tumors with: (A) bilirubin levels; (B) tumor size with bilirubin correction; (C) and overall survival. (unpublished data)

CA 19-9, carbohydrate antigen 19-9.

rapid postoperative recurrence without any of these borderline features with an upfront surgery approach and patients need to be counseled about this realistic probability despite curative-intent upfront resection. Further work into the identification of predictive biomarkers in this subset of aggressive cancers is needed.

Borderline Condition

The final criteria utilized for risk stratification include both patient and operative factors to determine the optimal sequencing of therapy. Pancreatectomy, although having marked improvements in perioperative morbidity and mortality over time, continues to result in significant debilitation postoperatively. There are, however, factors that can be used to assist in identifying these higher risk conditional patients prior to resection. These include patient age and fitness, associated comorbidities, weight loss and nutritional status, presence of cancer symptoms (pain, depression, etc.), and complexity of operation. The rationale for this is based on historical outcomes in patients with these factors.

There has been a significant amount of work related to risks of pancreatectomy in older PDAC patients, although age alone has not traditionally been a contraindication to potential curative-intent resection in otherwise resectable patients in most centers. Although having proven feasible in several high-volume center reports, the associated morbidity, mortality, and survival outcomes of pancreatectomy in older adults (>80) are likely underestimated in these single-institution reports as large population-based studies have demonstrated increased risks with advanced age (50,51). Furthermore, over one-third of patients above 80 years of age require nursing home discharge after pancreatectomy compared to 10% for those <70 years of age (52). Stage-for-stage, elderly patients (>80 years of age) do worse oncologically than similarly staged younger patients with 5-year survivals of less than 10% for elderly patients with seemingly "early-stage" disease (stage I/II) (53). These poor outcomes are more than just age bias as those patients with noncancer indications for surgery enjoy significantly improved survival over those undergoing pancreatectomy for PDAC, hence likely a biological reality. Complications after pancreatectomy occur at much higher rates than other GI cancer operations, with at least 25% of patients having serious complications, prolonged hospital stay, or readmission, and this significantly reduces the likelihood of receipt of multimodality adjuvant therapy (54,55). Furthermore, any major morbidity alone can contribute to worse outcomes by some yet to be identified physiological mechanisms independent of adjuvant therapy receipt (56–59). Finally, many cancer-associated symptoms found in a significant proportion of PDAC patients at presentation, such as pain, depression, weight loss, and cachexia, are often markers of more advanced occult systemic disease. Using data from ACS-NSQIP assessing risk factors for morbidity and mortality in patients undergoing pancreatectomy, the authors found that the single most predictive factor for worse perioperative outcomes was age >80, followed by comorbidities, complexity of resection, and nutritional status (54). One of the drivers of morbidity after pancreatic resection is the development of postoperative pancreatic fistula (POPF) or pancreatic leak. Recent multicenter evaluations have validated the finding that there are several nonmodifiable patient factors that can predict the incidence and severity of clinically relevant POPF that include histologic diagnosis, texture of pancreas pancreatic duct diameter, and operative blood loss (60). Other than blood loss, many of these factors can be inferred preoperatively to predict the likelihood of this specific complication. Regardless of the complication type, one-third of patients undergoing pancreatectomy are conditionally borderline and not only at higher risk for, but also less able to be rescued from, major complications postoperatively (61). Although we know that receipt of systemic adjuvant chemotherapy leads to improvement in long-term survival, a large proportion of patients still do not receive this recommended care. As there are marked differences in recovery from certain types of operations (Whipple vs. distal) and approaches (laparoscopic vs. open), perhaps the extent of operation is the primary driver of the national failure of patients receiving adjuvant therapy? We recently specifically evaluated this question and found that one-third of patients undergoing a surgery-first approach did not receive adjuvant chemotherapy and this was no different for patients undergoing distal versus proximal (Whipple) resections despite a larger proportion of distal pancreatectomies performed via a minimally invasive approach, with lower hospital stays and more rapid recovery (62). Surprisingly, the primary reason identified for the failure of adjuvant chemotherapy receipt was that it was not recommended by their treating oncologists. Thus there is a perceived benefit of upfront surgery that pervades the oncologic community and appears to drive treatment sequencing recommendations for better or worse.

Although necessary for long-term survival, surgery alone is not sufficient in the majority of patients. As discussed, there are three critical survival factors required in order to maximize surgical benefit: negative margin resection, absence of occult metastatic disease, and receipt of adjuvant chemotherapy. All of these are independent factors and not mutually inclusive. We recently reviewed (unpublished data) the NCDB to assess the perceived benefit of an upfront surgery approach with early-stage resectable tumors (stage I/II) looking at these specific factors. Patients were given a point for each successful factor: (a) negative margin operation, (b) nonelevated preoperative CA 19-9 (surrogate for occult metastases), and (c) receipt of adjuvant chemotherapy. We categorically scored these patients according to the various combinations of factors with a total score of 0 to 3, and evaluated the proportion of patients with these factors and associated survival outcomes compared to similarly staged patients undergoing neoadjuvant chemotherapy on an intent-to-treat basis, regardless of whether they ultimately underwent curative resection. Despite our perception of optimal outcomes with surgery, only 1 in 5 patients had all three factors with the resultant best survival, with worse outcomes for each failing factor (Figure 21.8). However, there was an actual higher probability of patients

Treatment strategy	Score category	% of Pts.			HR, [95% CI], p-value	Median overall survival (months)		
Surgery-first	ABC, score = 3	20.2%		79.8%	Reference	31.2		19.6
	AC only, score = 2	32.6%			1.28, [1.18, 1.39], <0.001	23.9	23.4	
	AB only, score = 2	8.5%			1.42, [1.26, 1.60], <0.001	23.3		
	BC only, score = 2	5.9%			1.48, [1.30, 1.69], <0.001	21.3		
	C only, score = 1	11.4%	32.8%		1.74, [1.57, 1.93], <0.001	17.5	14.7	
	A only, score = 1	13.9%			2.08, [1.88, 2.30], <0.001	15.2		
	B only, score = 1	2.4%			2.20, [1.83, 2.65], <0.001	10.4		
	None, score = 0	5.1%			3.32, [2.92, 3.78], <0.001	7.9		
Neoadjuvant (ITT)	-	100%			1.37, [1.25, 1.49]	24.9		
A = Negative research margin, B = Normal Pre-Op CA 19-9, C = Receipt of adjuvant chemotherapy								

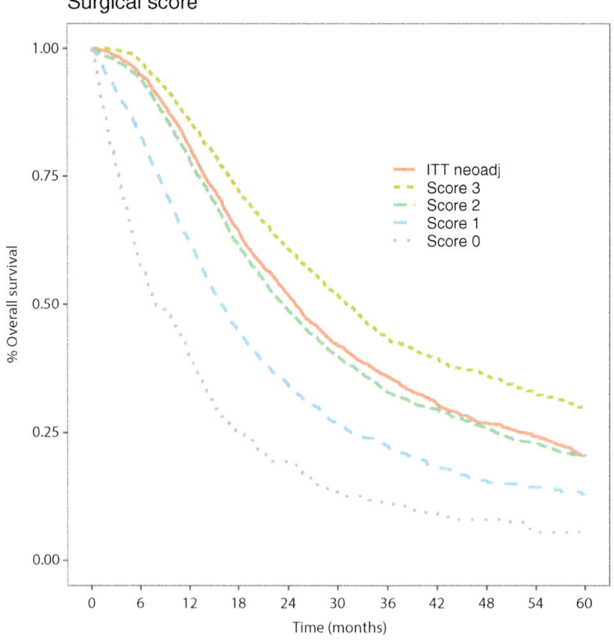

FIGURE 21.8   Actual proportion of patients and associated survival outcomes of patients undergoing upfront resection based on critical survival factors compared to ITT neoadjuvant therapy (unpublished data).

CI, confidence interval; ITT, intention to treat.

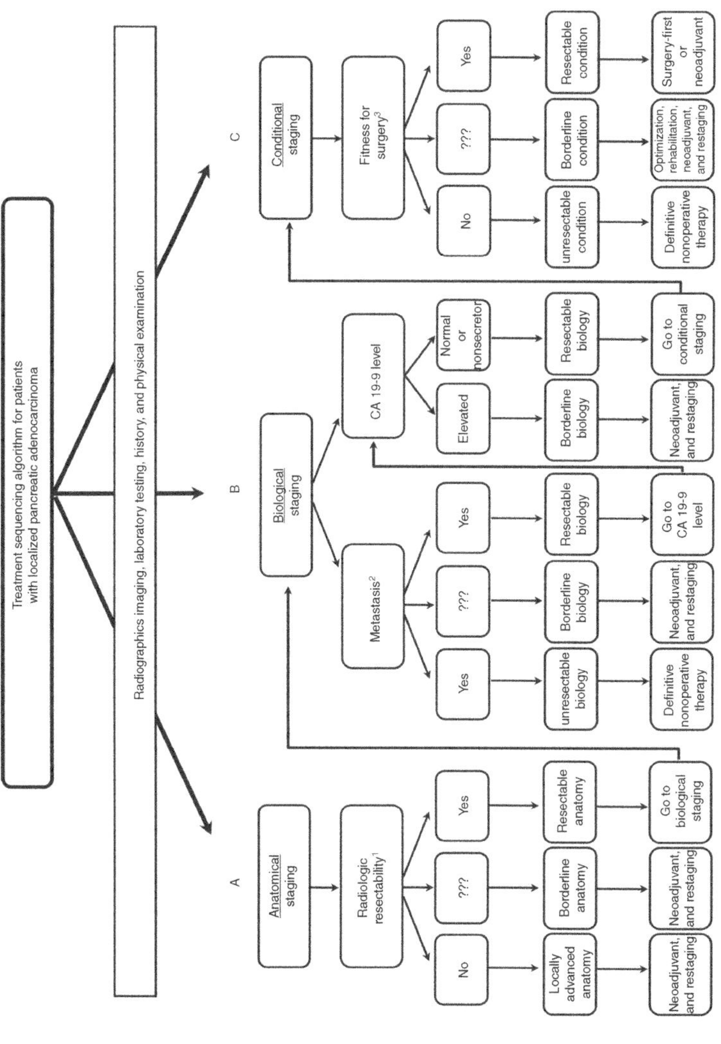

FIGURE 21.9 Treatment sequencing algorithm based on clinical resectability risk stratification.

¹Based on Alliance criteria (or other classification systems).

²Indeterminate radiologic lesions or regional nodal metastases.

³Age, comorbidities, performance status, nutrition/weight loss, and cancer symptoms.

CA 19-9, carbohydrate antigen 19-9.

only having 1 or none of these factors and these patients unsurprisingly had the worse survival. In contrast, outcomes for patients undergoing neoadjuvant chemotherapy on an intent-to-treat analysis were superior to nearly 80% of patients undergoing a surgery-first strategy. Thus statistically, patients are more likely to do the worst than the best with an upfront surgery approach when taking into account these repeatedly demonstrated survival factors.

To summarize, patients with any borderline anatomical, biological, or conditional factors should be considered high risk and thus neoadjuvant treatment sequencing should be highly considered over a surgery-first approach (Figure 21.9). In patients without any of these borderline features, we currently do not have enough high level data to suggest a neoadjuvant approach is superior to upfront surgery. However, we must keep in mind that at least 20% of anatomically resectable tumors will result in a positive (R1) margin that cannot be predicted with preoperative imaging. Up to 15% of patients will have rapid recurrent disease that we cannot currently identify via any available predictive markers, and one-third of patients will likely not receive any systemic adjuvant chemotherapy regardless of the extent of operation either due to postoperative complications and/or delayed recovery or the perception that surgery alone is sufficient. Thus patients should have full disclosure as to the actual probability of maximal survival benefit with a surgery-first approach based on actual outcomes and not simply historical perceptions of benefit.

REFERENCES

1. Cancer Stat Facts: Pancreatic Cancer 2018. www.seer.cancer.gov
2. Griffin JF, Poruk KE, Wolfgang CL. Pancreatic cancer surgery: past, present, and future. *Chin J Cancer Res*. 2015;27(4):332–348.
3. Whipple AO. A reminiscence: pancreaticduodenectomy. *Rev Surg*. 1963;20:221–225.
4. Trede M, Schwall G, Saeger HD. Survival after pancreatoduodenectomy. 118 consecutive resections without an operative mortality. *Ann Surg*. 1990;211(4):447–458. doi:10.1097/00000658-199004000-00011
5. Miedema BW, Sarr MG, van Heerden JA, et al. Complications following pancreaticoduodenectomy. Current management. *Arch Surg*. 1992;127(8):945–949; discussion 949–950. doi:10.1001/archsurg.1992.01420080079012
6. Fernandez-del Castillo C, Rattner DW, Warshaw AL. Standards for pancreatic resection in the 1990s. *Arch Surg*. 1995;130(3):295–299; discussion 299–300. doi:10.1001/archsurg.1995.01430030065013
7. Yeo CJ, Cameron JL, Sohn TA, et al. Six hundred fifty consecutive pancreaticoduodenectomies in the 1990s: pathology, complications, and outcomes. *Ann Surg*. 1997;226(3):248–257; discussion 57–60. doi:10.1097/00000658-199709000-00004
8. Imamura M, Doi R, Imaizumi T, et al. A randomized multicenter trial comparing resection and radiochemotherapy for resectable locally invasive pancreatic cancer. *Surgery*. 2004;136(5):1003–1011. doi:10.1016/j.surg.2004.04.030
9. Doi R, Imamura M, Hosotani R, et al. Surgery versus radiochemotherapy for resectable locally invasive pancreatic cancer: final results of a randomized multi-institutional trial. *Surg Today*. 2008;38(11):1021–1028. doi:10.1007/s00595-007-3745-8
10. Gagner M, Pomp A. Laparoscopic pylorus-preserving pancreatoduodenectomy. *Surg Endosc*. 1994;8(5):408–410. doi:10.1007/BF00642443
11. Giulianotti PC, Sbrana F, Bianco FM, et al. Robot-assisted laparoscopic pancreatic surgery: single-surgeon experience. *Surg Endosc*. 2010;24(7):1646–1657. doi:10.1007/s00464-009-0825-4
12. Croome KP, Farnell MB, Que FG, et al. Total laparoscopic pancreaticoduodenectomy for pancreatic ductal adenocarcinoma: oncologic advantages over open approaches? *Ann Surg*. 2014;260(4):633–638; discussion 638–640. doi:10.1097/SLA.0000000000000937
13. Croome KP, Farnell MB, Que FG, et al. Pancreaticoduodenectomy with major vascular resection: a comparison of laparoscopic versus open approaches. *J Gastrointest Surg*. 2015;19(1):189–194; discussion 194. doi:10.1007/s11605-014-2644-8
14. Allema JH, Reinders ME, van Gulik TM, et al. Prognostic factors for survival after pancreaticoduodenectomy for patients with carcinoma of the pancreatic head region. *Cancer*. 1995;75(8):2069–2076. doi:10.1002/1097-0142(19950415)75:8<2069::AID-CNCR2820750807>3.0.CO;2-7
15. Willett CG, Lewandrowski K, Warshaw AL, et al. Resection margins in carcinoma of the head of the pancreas. Implications for radiation therapy. *Ann Surg*. 1993;217(2):144–148. doi:10.1097/00000658-199302000-00008
16. Kalser MH, Ellenberg SS. Pancreatic cancer. Adjuvant combined radiation and chemotherapy following curative resection. *Arch Surg*. 1985;120(8):899–903. doi:10.1001/archsurg.1985.01390320023003

17. Klinkenbijl JH, Jeekel J, Sahmoud T, et al. Adjuvant radiotherapy and 5-fluorouracil after curative resection of cancer of the pancreas and periampullary region: phase III trial of the EORTC gastrointestinal tract cancer cooperative group. *Ann Surg*. 1999;230(6):776–782; discussion 782–784. doi:10.1097/00000658-199912000-00006

18. Neoptolemos JP, Dunn JA, Stocken DD, et al. Adjuvant chemoradiotherapy and chemotherapy in resectable pancreatic cancer: a randomised controlled trial. *Lancet*. 2001;358(9293):1576–1585. doi:10.1016/S0140-6736(01)06651-X

19. Neoptolemos JP, Stocken DD, Tudur Smith C, et al. Adjuvant 5-fluorouracil and folinic acid vs observation for pancreatic cancer: composite data from the ESPAC-1 and -3(v1) trials. *Br J Cancer*. 2009;100(2):246–250. doi:10.1038/sj.bjc.6604838

20. Oettle H, Post S, Neuhaus P, et al. Adjuvant chemotherapy with gemcitabine vs observation in patients undergoing curative-intent resection of pancreatic cancer: a randomized controlled trial. *JAMA*. 2007;297(3):267–277. doi:10.1001/jama.297.3.267

21. Winter JM, Cameron JL, Campbell KA, et al. 1423 pancreaticoduodenectomies for pancreatic cancer: a single-institution experience. *J Gastrointest Surg*. 2006;10(9):1199–1210; discussion 1210–1211. doi:10.1016/j.gassur.2006.08.018

22. Yachida S, Jones S, Bozic I, et al. Distant metastasis occurs late during the genetic evolution of pancreatic cancer. *Nature*. 2010;467(7319):1114–1117. doi:10.1038/nature09515

23. Haeno H, Gonen M, Davis MB, et al. Computational modeling of pancreatic cancer reveals kinetics of metastasis suggesting optimum treatment strategies. *Cell*. 2012;148(1–2):362–375. doi:10.1016/j.cell.2011.11.060

24. Katz MH, Pisters PW, Evans DB, et al. Borderline resectable pancreatic cancer: the importance of this emerging stage of disease. *J Am Coll Surg*. 2008;206(5):833–846; discussion 846–848. doi:10.1016/j.jamcollsurg.2007.12.020

25. Verbeke CS, Leitch D, Menon KV, et al. Redefining the R1 resection in pancreatic cancer. *Br J Surg*. 2006;93(10):1232–1237. doi:10.1002/bjs.5397

26. Esposito I, Kleeff J, Bergmann F, et al. Most pancreatic cancer resections are R1 resections. *Ann Surg Oncol*. 2008;15(6):1651–1660. doi:10.1245/s10434-008-9839-8

27. Menon KV, Gomez D, Smith AM, et al. Impact of margin status on survival following pancreatoduodenectomy for cancer: the Leeds Pathology Protocol (LEEPP). *HPB (Oxford)*. 2009;11(1):18–24. doi:10.1111/j.1477-2574.2008.00013.x

28. Neoptolemos JP, Stocken DD, Dunn JA, et al. Influence of resection margins on survival for patients with pancreatic cancer treated by adjuvant chemoradiation and/or chemotherapy in the ESPAC-1 randomized controlled trial. *Ann Surg*. 2001;234(6):758–768. doi:10.1097/00000658-200112000-00007

29. Neoptolemos JP, Palmer DH, Ghaneh P, et al. Comparison of adjuvant gemcitabine and capecitabine with gemcitabine monotherapy in patients with resected pancreatic cancer (ESPAC-4): a multicentre, open-label, randomised, phase 3 trial. *Lancet*. 2017;389(10073):1011–1024. doi:10.1016/S0140-6736(16)32409-6

30. Butturini G, Stocken DD, Wente MN, et al. Influence of resection margins and treatment on survival in patients with pancreatic cancer: meta-analysis of randomized controlled trials. *Arch Surg*. 2008;143(1):75–83. doi:10.1001/archsurg.2007.17

31. Katz MH, Wang H, Balachandran A, et al. Effect of neoadjuvant chemoradiation and surgical technique on recurrence of localized pancreatic cancer. *J Gastrointest Surg*. 2012;16(1):68–78.

32. Koninger J, Wente MN, Muller-Stich BP, et al. R2 resection in pancreatic cancer—does it make sense? *Langenbecks Arch Surg*. 2008;393(6):929–934. doi:10.1007/s00423-008-0308-4

33. Wellner UF, Makowiec F, Bausch D, et al. Locally advanced pancreatic head cancer: margin-positive resection or bypass? *ISRN Surg*. 2012;2012:513241. doi: 10.5402/2012/513241

34. Burris HA 3rd, Moore MJ, Andersen J, et al. Improvements in survival and clinical benefit with gemcitabine as first-line therapy for patients with advanced pancreas cancer: a randomized trial. *J Clin Oncol*. 1997;15(6):2403–2413. doi:10.1200/JCO.1997.15.6.2403

35. Conroy T, Desseigne F, Ychou M, et al. FOLFIRINOX versus gemcitabine for metastatic pancreatic cancer. *N Engl J Med*. 2011;364(19):1817–1825. doi:10.1056/NEJMoa1011923

36. Von Hoff DD, Ervin T, Arena FP, et al. Increased survival in pancreatic cancer with nab-paclitaxel plus gemcitabine. *N Engl J Med*. 2013;369(18):1691–1703. doi:10.1056/NEJMoa1304369

37. Kharofa J, Tsai S, Kelly T, et al. Neoadjuvant chemoradiation with IMRT in resectable and borderline resectable pancreatic cancer. *Radiother Oncol*. 2014;113(1):41–46. doi:10.1016/j.radonc.2014.09.010

38. Torgeson A, Lloyd S, Boothe D, et al. Multiagent induction chemotherapy followed by chemoradiation is associated with improved survival in locally advanced pancreatic cancer. *Cancer*. 2017;123(19):3816–3824. doi:10.1002/cncr.30780

39. Katz MH, Shi Q, Ahmad SA, et al. Preoperative modified FOLFIRINOX treatment followed by capecitabine-based chemoradiation for borderline resectable pancreatic cancer: alliance for clinical trials in oncology trial A021101. *JAMA Surg.* 2016;151(8):e161137. doi:10.1001/jamasurg.2016.1137

40. Katz MH, Wang H, Fleming JB, et al. Long-term survival after multidisciplinary management of resected pancreatic adenocarcinoma. *Ann Surg Oncol.* 2009;16(4):836–847. doi:10.1245/s10434-008-0295-2

41. Bilimoria KY, Bentrem DJ, Ko CY, et al. National failure to operate on early stage pancreatic cancer. *Ann Surg.* 2007;246(2):173–180. doi:10.1097/SLA.0b013e3180691579

42. Ferrone CR, Finkelstein DM, Thayer SP, et al. Perioperative CA 19-9 levels can predict stage and survival in patients with resectable pancreatic adenocarcinoma. *J Clin Oncol.* 2006;24(18):2897–2902. doi:10.1200/JCO.2005.05.3934

43. Cameron JL, Crist DW, Sitzmann JV, et al. Factors influencing survival after pancreaticoduodenectomy for pancreatic cancer. *Am J Surg.* 1991;161(1):120–124; discussion 124–125. doi:10.1016/0002-9610(91)90371-J

44. Bhalla M, Aldakkak M, Kulkarni NM, et al. Characterizing indeterminate liver lesions in patients with localized pancreatic cancer at the time of diagnosis. *Abdom Radiol (NY).* 2018;43(2):351–363. doi:10.1007/s00261-017-1404-0

45. Tzeng CW, Fleming JB, Lee JE, et al. Defined clinical classifications are associated with outcome of patients with anatomically resectable pancreatic adenocarcinoma treated with neoadjuvant therapy. *Ann Surg Oncol.* 2012;19(6):2045–2053. doi:10.1245/s10434-011-2211-4

46. Kannagi R. Carbohydrate antigen sialyl Lewis a—its pathophysiological significance and induction mechanism in cancer progression. *Chang Gung Med J.* 2007;30(3):189–209.

47. Hartwig W, Strobel O, Hinz U, et al. CA 19-9 in potentially resectable pancreatic cancer: perspective to adjust surgical and perioperative therapy. *Ann Surg Oncol.* 2013;20(7):2188–2196. doi:10.1245/s10434-012-2809-1

48. Bergquist JR, Puig CA, Shubert CR, et al. Carbohydrate antigen 19-9 elevation in anatomically resectable, early stage pancreatic cancer is independently associated with decreased overall survival and an indication for neoadjuvant therapy: a national cancer database study. *J Am Coll Surg.* 2016;223(1):52–65. doi:10.1016/j.jamcollsurg.2016.02.009

49. La Greca G, Sofia M, Lombardo R, et al. Adjusting CA 19-9 values to predict malignancy in obstructive jaundice: influence of bilirubin and C-reactive protein. *World J Gastroenterol.* 2012;18(31):4150–4155. doi:10.3748/wjg.v18.i31.4150

50. Riall TS. What is the effect of age on pancreatic resection? *Adv Surg.* 2009;43:233–249. doi:10.1016/j.yasu.2009.02.004

51. Hardacre JM, Simo K, McGee MF, et al. Pancreatic resection in octogenarians. *J Surg Res.* 2009;156(1):129–132. doi:10.1016/j.jss.2009.03.047

52. Finlayson E, Fan Z, Birkmeyer JD. Outcomes in octogenarians undergoing high-risk cancer operation: a national study. *J Am Coll Surg.* 2007;205(6):729–734. doi:10.1016/j.jamcollsurg.2007.06.307

53. Sener SF, Fremgen A, Menck HR, et al. Pancreatic cancer: a report of treatment and survival trends for 100,313 patients diagnosed from 1985-1995, using the National Cancer Database. *J Am Coll Surg.* 1999;189(1):1–7. doi:10.1016/S1072-7515(99)00075-7

54. Wu W, He J, Cameron JL, et al. The impact of postoperative complications on the administration of adjuvant therapy following pancreaticoduodenectomy for adenocarcinoma. *Ann Surg Oncol.* 2014;21(9):2873–2881. doi:10.1245/s10434-014-3722-6

55. Merkow RP, Bilimoria KY, Tomlinson JS, et al. Postoperative complications reduce adjuvant chemotherapy use in resectable pancreatic cancer. *Ann Surg.* 2014;260(2):372–377. doi:10.1097/SLA.0000000000000378

56. Reddy DM, Townsend CM Jr, Kuo YF, et al. Readmission after pancreatectomy for pancreatic cancer in Medicare patients. *J Gastrointest Surg.* 2009;13(11):1963–1974; discussion 1974–1975.

57. Ahmad SA, Edwards MJ, Sutton JM, et al. Factors influencing readmission after pancreaticoduodenectomy: a multi-institutional study of 1302 patients. *Ann Surg.* 2012;256(3):529–537. doi:10.1097/SLA.0b013e318265ef0b

58. Yermilov I, Bentrem D, Sekeris E, et al. Readmissions following pancreaticoduodenectomy for pancreas cancer: a population-based appraisal. *Ann Surg Oncol.* 2009;16(3):554–561. doi:10.1245/s10434-008-0178-6

59. Le AT, Huang B, Hnoosh D, et al. Effect of complications on oncologic outcomes after pancreaticoduodenectomy for pancreatic cancer. *J Surg Res.* 2017;214:1–8. doi:10.1016/j.jss.2017.02.036

60. Miller BC, Christein JD, Behrman SW, et al. A multi-institutional external validation of the fistula risk score for pancreatoduodenectomy. *J Gastrointest Surg*. 2014;18(1):172–179; discussion 179–180. doi:10.1007/s11605-013-2337-8
61. Tzeng CW, Katz MH, Fleming JB, et al. Morbidity and mortality after pancreaticoduodenectomy in patients with borderline resectable type C clinical classification. *J Gastrointest Surg*. 2014;18(1):146–155; discussion 155–156. doi:10.1007/s11605-013-2371-6
62. Bergquist JR, Ivanics T, Shubert CR, et al. Type of resection (Whipple vs. istal) does not affect the national failure to provide post-resection adjuvant chemotherapy in localized pancreatic cancer. *Ann Surg Oncol*. 2017;24(6):1731–1738. doi:10.1245/s10434-016-5762-6

How I Treat Resectable Pancreatic Cancer With Adjuvant Therapy

Philip A. Philip and Mandana Kamgar

INTRODUCTION

Pancreatic cancer is a systemic disease with a high potential for early dissemination even in patients who are clinically and radiologically deemed to have disease localized to the pancreas. Following surgical resection of localized and resectable pancreatic cancer, observation alone would lead to 5-year survival of approximately 10% (1,2). However, the addition of adjuvant chemotherapy will improve disease-free and overall survival of patients undergoing pancreatic resection. The role of radiation therapy in the adjuvant setting remains not clearly defined.

ADJUVANT SYSTEMIC CHEMOTHERAPY

Choice of Chemotherapy
Clinical Trial Participation
Even with the utilization of combination adjuvant chemotherapy, 5-year survival rate only modestly increased to not more than ~30% (3). We therefore strongly encourage all patients with resected localized or locally advanced pancreatic cancer and good performance status to participate in adjuvant therapy trials using newer agents. Table 22.1 shows examples of ongoing or recently completed adjuvant clinical trials.

Combination Versus Single-Agent Adjuvant Chemotherapy
Combination of FOLFIRINOX is our first choice for adjuvant chemotherapy in patients with good performance status who are either not eligible or not interested in clinical trials. Gemcitabine combined with capecitabine is another acceptable first-line chemotherapy for patients not eligible for FOLFIRINOX, especially those who have preexisting significant neuropathy. Gemcitabine/nab-paclitaxel regimen is no consideration at this time, pending the outcome of a completed randomized phase III trial. When unable to tolerate drug combinations because of unfavorable performance status, poor organ function (e.g., neuropathy, renal failure), and/or poor recovery from surgery, we would consider single-agent chemotherapy for our patients. Gemcitabine and a fluoropyrimidine (5-fluorouracil or capecitabine) are both acceptable agents. S1 is another option but is unavailable in most countries including the United States. Table 22.2 summarizes the data supporting our choices for adjuvant chemotherapy. In some patients who do not agree to intravenous (IV) chemotherapy, we would consider capecitabine alone to be a reasonable treatment option.

When to Start Chemotherapy
There are no randomized trials addressing the best timing for the initiation of adjuvant chemotherapy in pancreatic cancer. We start adjuvant chemotherapy within 6 to 12 weeks after resection, assuming adequate recovery from the surgery. In the case of delayed recovery, we still prefer delayed adjuvant chemotherapy over no chemotherapy. These preferences are based on available retrospective studies (11–13).

A Clinical Vignette ("How I Treat") is included at the end of the chapter.

TABLE 22.1 Select Clinical Trials for Adjuvant Therapy in Pancreatic Cancer That Are Either Ongoing or Completed Pending Outcome

Study Question	Study Design	Phase	Status	NCT
Adjuvant chemotherapy	Gemcitabine/Nab-paclitaxel vs. Gemcitabine	III	Completed	01964430
	FOLFOX/Nab-paclitaxel	II	Completed	02022033
Adjuvant therapy post neoadjuvant treatment	Gemcitabine/Nab-paclitaxel Adjuvant +/− Neoadjuvant	II	Ongoing	02047513
	Adjuvant Gemcitabine versus neoadjuvant+ adjuvant FOLFIRINOX	II/III	Ongoing	02172976
	Perioperative FOLFIRINOX	Pilot study	Ongoing	02782182
		II	Ongoing	02047474
Adjuvant chemoradiotherapy	Gemcitabine or combination therapy of choice+/− Chemoradiation[1] (RTOG-0848)	III	Ongoing	01013649
	Gemcitabine +/− SBRT in R0 with T3 or N1	II	Ongoing	02461836
	Gemcitabine +/− TS-1 chemoradiation in R1 or +lymph node	II		02754180

[1]This study also checked for the role of erlotinib and addition to gemcitabine. There was no significant benefit in the addition of erlotinib to gemcitabine.

FOLFIRINOX, 5-fluorouracil, leucovorin, irinotecan, and oxaliplatin; FOLFOX, folinic acid, fluorouracil, and oxaliplatin; SBRT, stereotactic body radiation therapy; TS-1, titanium silicate-1.

Duration of Chemotherapy

There is no prospective study comparing different durations of adjuvant treatment in pancreatic cancer. The preferred duration is 6 months, which is the length of time that was chosen in the landmark trials of adjuvant chemotherapy in pancreatic cancer.

ROLE OF RADIATION THERAPY

Indications

The role of radiation therapy as an adjuvant treatment in patients with resected localized or locally advanced pancreatic cancer remains controversial, largely because the disease is considered to have micrometastasis in the majority of patients at the outset. In patients who are considered at high risk of local recurrence after surgery (lymph node positive or R1 resection), addition of chemoradiation may be considered, though evidence behind this approach is limited in the era of modern management of localized pancreatic cancer. We utilize our multidisciplinary tumor board to discuss the need for radiation therapy in a given patient. We do not recommend adjuvant radiation therapy in patients with R2 resection or those with M1 disease. Of note, the decision whether to include chemoradiation in the management of a given patient does not influence our choice of adjuvant chemotherapy or its initiation. Select trials evaluating the role of chemoradiation are shown in Table 22.2.

Concomitant Chemotherapy Used With the Radiotherapy

We routinely use oral capecitabine on the days of radiation therapy except the weekends when radiation therapy will not be administered (14).

Timing of Radiation Therapy

There are no prospective data on the optimal timing of radiation therapy. Retrospective data suggest lack of difference in local or distant recurrence with early versus late application of

TABLE 22.2 Completed Adjuvant Therapy Trials in Patients With Resected Pancreatic Cancer

Study	Trial Outline				Median Overall Survival (Months (95% CI)	Estimated 5-year Survival	Toxicity
	Phase	Cohorts	Number of patients	Primary end point			
PRODIGE 24/CCTG PA.6 (4)	III	mFOLFIRINOX	247	Disease-free survival	54.4 (41.5–––)	–	(Grade 3–4) 75%
		Gemcitabine	246		34.8 (28.6–43.8)		(Grade 3–4) 51%
ESPAC-4 (3)	III	Gemcitabine+ Capecitabine	364	Overall survival	28.0 (23.5–31.5)	28.8% (22.9–35.2)	(Grade 3–4) 63%[1]
		Gemcitabine	366		25.5 (22.7–27.9)	16.3% (10.2–23.7)	(Grade 3–4) 54%[1]
ESPAC-3 (5)	III	Gemcitabine	537	Overall survival	23.6 (21.4–26.4)	17.5% (14.0–21.2)	SAE[2] 7.5%[3]
		Bolus 5-FU leucovorin	551		23.0 (21.1–25.0)	15.9% (12.7–19.4)	SAE 14%[3]
ESPAC-1 (6)[4]	III	Bolus 5-FU leucovorin	238	Overall survival	19.7 (16.4–22.4)	21.1% (14.6–28.5)	
		No chemo	235		14.0 (11.9–16.5)	8.0% (3.8–14.1)	
CONKO-001 (1,7)	III	Gemcitabine	179	Disease-free survival	22.8 (18.5–27.2)	20.7%(14.7–26.6)	SAE 14%
		No chemo	175		20.2 (17.7–22.8)	10.4% (5.9–15.0)	SAE 8%
JASPAC-01 (8)[5]	III	Gemcitabine	193	Overall survival	25.5 (22.5–29.6)	24.4% (18.6–30.8)	
		S1	192		46.5 (37.8–63.7)	44.1% (36.9–51.1)	

(continued)

TABLE 22.2 Completed Adjuvant Therapy Trials in Patients With Resected Pancreatic Cancer (*Continued*)

Study	Trial Outline				Median Overall Survival (Months (95% CI)	Estimated 5-year Survival	Toxicity
	Phase	Cohorts	Number of patients	Primary end point			
RTOG 9704 (9,10)	III	Gemcitabine[6]	221	Overall survival	20.5[7]	22% (16–29)[7]	(Grade 3–5) 79%[3]
		5-FU[6]	230		17.1[7]	18% (13–24)[7]	(Grade 3–5) 62%[3]

[1]Difference not statistically significant.
[2]SAE: serious adverse event.
[3]Difference is statistically significant.
[4]This trial also evaluated the role of chemoradiation; data presented here compares those with chemotherapy versus those without, regardless of the status of chemoradiation treatment.
[5]This study was performed exclusively in Japan.
[6]Both 3 weeks pre and 12 weeks post 5-FU based chemoradiation.
[7]Reported data are limited to those with pancreatic head tumors (n = 388).

chemoradiotherapy (15). However, in our practice we use chemoradiation at the conclusion of systemic adjuvant chemotherapy and we do not interrupt adjuvant chemotherapy to give the chemoradiation. The current intergroup trial RTOG 0848 has a similar schema of 6 months of chemotherapy followed by randomization to either chemoradiotherapy or none. We restage the patient at the conclusion of the adjuvant chemotherapy to rule out any metastatic disease that would preclude giving radiation therapy.

CHEMOTHERAPY POST NEOADJUVANT TREATMENT

The role of adjuvant chemotherapy in patients with prior neoadjuvant therapy is limited especially in patients who have significant residual disease at surgery. In general, patients who had received 2 to 3 months of neoadjuvant chemotherapy would be recommended to have an additional 2 to 3 months of adjuvant therapy using a similar regimen to the preoperative chemotherapy. There are ongoing trials addressing this question. Examples are presented in Table 22.1.

SUPPORTIVE CARE

Exocrine Insufficiency
Exocrine insufficiency is a common finding in patients who had surgery for pancreatic cancer, even without complete pancreatic resection (16). We routinely enlist the help of a nutritionist in managing patients postsurgery. We have a low threshold for pancreatic exocrine replacement therapy in patients experiencing weight loss and/or steatorrhea postsurgery. We initiate treatment with pancrelipase with each meal and each snack and adjust the dose based on weight gain and/or persistence of steatorrhea.

Endocrine Insufficiency
While diabetes mellitus is among the presenting symptoms of pancreatic cancer, postsurgical new onset diabetes is also seen in some of our patients. Adequate follow-up and treatment of this condition is therefore warranted.

Depression
High risk of recurrence imposes a significant emotional burden on patients. Depression is therefore not an uncommon finding in patients with resected pancreatic cancer and has to be actively explored. We therefore address the emotional aspect of management of our patients and ensure adequate referral to counselors, timely initiation of pharmacotherapy, or psychiatric referral as needed.

ROLE OF BIOMARKERS

hENT1
The nucleoside transporter for gemcitabine into the pancreatic cancer cells is human equilibrative nucleoside transporter 1(hENT1). While retrospective studies suggested the expression level of hENT1 (by immunohistochemistry) as a predictor of response to gemcitabine in the adjuvant setting (17,18), prospective evaluation in the CONKO-001 study did not confirm this finding (19). We therefore do not use hENT1 expression level in our practice.

SMAD4
Retrospective data suggested a role for SMAD4 as a predictor for biological behavior of pancreatic cancer. Patients with metastatic recurrence were more likely to have SMAD4 loss whereas those with local recurrence mostly had intact SMAD4 (20,21). SMAD4 is therefore a potential biomarker, especially in decision making about radiation treatment. We believe however that further prospective data is needed before the application of this biomarker. Therefore, SMAD4 is not part of our practice.

BRCA1/2

Detection of germline *BRCA1/2* mutations may influence the decision of using a platinum-based therapy in the adjuvant setting. However, it is still experimental, and we do not routinely check for these mutations or use such knowledge in designing adjuvant therapy for a given patient.

SURVEILLANCE

Though limited data is available on the role of surveillance post completion of adjuvant therapy, in our practice we follow some but not all of the National Comprehensive Cancer Network (NCCN) guidelines: we do history and physical, carbohydrate antigen 19-9 (CA 19-9) every 3 to 6 months for 2 years and every 6 to 12 months after that. We tend to do CT with contrast at the conclusion of the adjuvant therapy and then every 6 to 12 months (more likely 12) unless there is a clinical indication to do earlier. We make every attempt to explain to patients the goals of the follow-up and realistic expectations of the benefit from repeated CA19-9 measurements and imaging. The key message here is that a recurrence of the disease is incurable and earlier detection of recurrence in an asymptomatic phase is unlikely to alter overall survival.

Role of CA 19-9 in Relation to Managing Resectable Disease

Limitations

False-positive results

CA 19-9 measurements can pose clinical challenges because elevations can be seen in multiple noncancerous conditions including cholestasis and inflammatory/infectious processes of the pancreas or hepatobiliary system (22). It can also be elevated in other cancers including biliary, gastric, colon, uterine, ovarian, and breast cancer (23). Elevation of CA 19-9 should therefore be interpreted with caution and should not be relied on as the sole reason to restart treatment for pancreatic cancer. We also look for trends over time if the sole abnormality is an elevated CA19-9.

False-negative results

CA 19-9 can be undetectable in 5% to 10% of the general population with lack of Lewis antigen (23,24), and low levels are likely to be seen in small tumor burden. CA 19-9 therefore cannot be used universally in follow-up of patients.

Time to Check

We normally check CA 19-9 prior to the surgery, postsurgery, prior to the initiation of adjuvant therapy, and during surveillance follow-up (timing as mentioned earlier). If patients have normal or undetectable CA19-9 levels prior to surgery, we will probably not do further testing. We may also consider checking CA19-9 if the clinical picture during the adjuvant therapy is suggestive of disease recurrence.

Role of Imaging in Surveillance

While regular radiologic surveillance can detect pancreatic cancer before the appearance of symptoms (25), unless recurrence is purely localized earlier detection does not lead to better survival (26). Even when a localized recurrence is treated with either surgery or radiation therapy, it is not proven that it would either be curative or will result in significant improvement in survival because of the likelihood of associated micrometastatic disease.

Clinical Vignette 22.1

Case 1: A 66-year-old male with a history of localized adenocarcinoma of the head of the pancreas presents to you 7 weeks after the Whipple surgery. He has recovered well from the surgery. He has long-standing diabetic neuropathy with grade II neuropathy at baseline. He has chronic kidney disease with a creatinine clearance of 25 mL/minute. He has well-controlled heart failure with an ejection fraction of 50% on treatment. His Eastern Cooperative Oncology Group (ECOG) score at this time is 2. Which regimen would you recommend for adjuvant chemotherapy for this patient at this time?

Answer: Due to the presence of grade II peripheral neuropathy, FOLFIRINOX would not be a good option for this patient (due to oxaliplatin in the regimen). Considering the creatinine clearance of <30 mL/min, this patient would not be a candidate for capecitabine either. Single-agent chemotherapy (gemcitabine or fluorouracil) for 6 months is an acceptable option for this patient.

Case 2: A 69-year-old female with a history of localized adenocarcinoma of the head of the pancreas presents to you 8 weeks after successful Whipple surgery. Since the time of surgery, she has experienced diarrhea, bloating, and failure to gain weight despite good appetite. Diarrhea is worse after food ingestion and is associated with pale and oily appearing stool difficult to flush. What would you do at this time to control the diarrhea?

Answer: This patient has experienced steatorrhea due to pancreatic exocrine insufficiency. At this time, exocrine replacement (pancrelipase) with meals and snacks should be considered. New onset diabetes should be ruled out, especially in the case of uncontrolled blood sugars and continued weight loss despite adequate use of pancrelipase. Nutrition consult should be initiated, if already not performed.

REFERENCES

1. Oettle H, Neuhaus P, Hochhaus A, et al. Adjuvant chemotherapy with gemcitabine and long-term outcomes among patients with resected pancreatic cancer: the CONKO-001 randomized trial. *JAMA*. 2013;310(14):1473–1481. doi:10.1001/jama.2013.279201
2. Neoptolemos JP, Stocken DD, Friess H, et al. A randomized trial of chemoradiotherapy and chemotherapy after resection of pancreatic cancer. *N Engl J Med*. 2004;350(12):1200–1210. doi:10.1056/NEJMoa032295
3. Neoptolemos JP, Palmer DH, Ghaneh P, et al. Comparison of adjuvant gemcitabine and capecitabine with gemcitabine monotherapy in patients with resected pancreatic cancer (ESPAC-4): a multicentre, open-label, randomised, phase 3 trial. *Lancet*. 2017;389(10073):1011–1024. doi:10.1016/S0140-6736(16)32409-6
4. Conroy T, Hammel P, Hebbar M, et al. Unicancer GI PRODIGE 24/CCTG PA.6 trial: A multicenter international randomized phase III trial of adjuvant mFOLFIRINOX versus gemcitabine (gem) in patients with resected pancreatic ductal adenocarcinomas. *J Clin Oncol*. 2018;36(18_suppl):LBA4001. doi:10.1200/JCO.2018.36.18_suppl.LBA4001
5. Neoptolemos JP, Stocken DD, Bassi C, et al. Adjuvant chemotherapy with fluorouracil plus folinic acid vs gemcitabine following pancreatic cancer resection: a randomized controlled trial. *JAMA*. 2010;304(10):1073–1081. doi:10.1001/jama.2010.1275
6. Neoptolemos JP, Dunn JA, Stocken DD, et al. Adjuvant chemoradiotherapy and chemotherapy in resectable pancreatic cancer: a randomised controlled trial. *Lancet*. 2001;358(9293):1576–1585. doi:10.1016/S0140-6736(01)06651-X
7. Oettle H, Post S, Neuhaus P, et al. Adjuvant chemotherapy with gemcitabine vs observation in patients undergoing curative-intent resection of pancreatic cancer: a randomized controlled trial. *JAMA*. 2007;297(3):267–277. doi:10.1001/jama.297.3.267
8. Uesaka K, Boku N, Fukutomi A, et al. Adjuvant chemotherapy of S-1 versus gemcitabine for resected pancreatic cancer: a phase 3, open-label, randomised, non-inferiority trial (JASPAC 01). *Lancet*. 2016;388(10041):248–257. doi:10.1016/S0140-6736(16)30583-9
9. Regine WF, Winter KA, Abrams R, et al. Fluorouracil-based chemoradiation with either gemcitabine or fluorouracil chemotherapy after resection of pancreatic adenocarcinoma: 5-year analysis of the U.S. Intergroup/RTOG 9704 phase III trial. *Ann Surg Oncol*. 2011;18(5):1319–1326. doi:10.1245/s10434-011-1630-6
10. Regine WF, Winter KA, Abrams RA, et al. Fluorouracil vs gemcitabine chemotherapy before and after fluorouracil-based chemoradiation following resection of pancreatic adenocarcinoma: a randomized controlled trial. *JAMA*. 2008;299(9):1019–1026. doi:10.1001/jama.299.9.1019

11. Xia BT, Ahmad SA, Al Humaidi AH, et al. Time to initiation of adjuvant chemotherapy in pancreas cancer: a multi-institutional experience. *Ann Surg Oncol*. 2017;24(9):2770–2776. doi:10.1245/s10434-017-5918-z

12. Valle JW, Palmer D, Jackson R, et al. Optimal duration and timing of adjuvant chemotherapy after definitive surgery for ductal adenocarcinoma of the pancreas: ongoing lessons from the ESPAC-3 study. *J Clin Oncol*. 2014;32(6):504–512. doi:10.1200/JCO.2013.50.7657

13. Mirkin KA, Greenleaf EK, Hollenbeak CS, et a;. Time to the initiation of adjuvant chemotherapy does not impact survival in patients with resected pancreatic cancer. *Cancer*. 2016;122(19):2979–2987. doi:10.1002/cncr.30163

14. Mukherjee S, Hurt CN, Bridgewater J, et al. Gemcitabine-based or capecitabine-based chemoradiotherapy for locally advanced pancreatic cancer (SCALOP): a multicentre, randomised, phase 2 trial. *Lancet Oncol*. 2013;14(4):317–326. doi:10.1016/S1470-2045(13)70021-4

15. Patel AA, Nagarajan S2, Scher ED, et al. Early vs. Late chemoradiation therapy and the postoperative interval to adjuvant therapy do not correspond to local recurrence in resected pancreatic cancer. *Pancreat Disord Ther*. 2015;5(2):151. doi:10.4172/2165-7092.1000151

16. Sikkens EC, Cahen DL, de Wit J, et al. Prospective assessment of the influence of pancreatic cancer resection on exocrine pancreatic function. *Br J Surg*. 2014;101(2):109–113. doi:10.1002/bjs.9342

17. Morinaga S, Nakamura Y, Watanabe T, et al. Immunohistochemical analysis of human equilibrative nucleoside transporter-1 (hENT1) predicts survival in resected pancreatic cancer patients treated with adjuvant gemcitabine monotherapy. *Ann Surg Oncol*. 2012;19 Suppl 3:S558–S564. doi:10.1245/s10434-011-2054-z

18. Greenhalf W, Ghaneh P, Neoptolemos JP, et al. Pancreatic cancer hENT1 expression and survival from gemcitabine in patients from the ESPAC-3 trial. *J Natl Cancer Inst*. 2014;106(1):djt347. doi:10.1093/jnci/djt347

19. Sinn M, Riess H, Sinn BV, et al. Human equilibrative nucleoside transporter 1 expression analysed by the clone SP 120 rabbit antibody is not predictive in patients with pancreatic cancer treated with adjuvant gemcitabine - results from the CONKO-001 trial. *Eur J Cancer*. 2015;51(12):1546–1554. doi:10.1016/j.ejca.2015.05.005

20. Iacobuzio-Donahue CA, Fu B, Yachida S, et al. DPC4 gene status of the primary carcinoma correlates with patterns of failure in patients with pancreatic cancer. *J Clin Oncol*. 2009;27(11):1806–1813. doi:10.1200/JCO.2008.17.7188

21. Crane CH, Varadhachary GR, Yordy JS, et al. Phase II trial of cetuximab, gemcitabine, and oxaliplatin followed by chemoradiation with cetuximab for locally advanced (T4) pancreatic adenocarcinoma: correlation of Smad4(Dpc4) immunostaining with pattern of disease progression. *J Clin Oncol*. 2011;29(22):3037–3043. doi:10.1200/JCO.2010.33.8038

22. Maestranzi S, Przemioslo R, Mitchell H, et al. The effect of benign and malignant liver disease on the tumour markers CA19-9 and CEA. *Ann Clin Biochem*. 1998;35(Pt 1):99–103. doi:10.1177/000456329803500113

23. Lamerz R. Role of tumour markers, cytogenetics. *Ann Oncol*. 1999;10(Suppl 4):145–149. doi:10.1093/annonc/10.suppl_4.S145

24. Tempero MA, Uchida E, Takasaki H, et al. Relationship of carbohydrate antigen 19-9 and Lewis antigens in pancreatic cancer. *Cancer Res*. 1987;47(20):5501–5503.

25. Tzeng CW, Fleming JB, Lee JE, et al. Yield of clinical and radiographic surveillance in patients with resected pancreatic adenocarcinoma following multimodal therapy. *HPB (Oxford)*. 2012;14(6):365–372. doi:10.1111/j.1477-2574.2012.00445.x

26. Witkowski ER, Smith JK, Ragulin-Coyne E, et al. Is it worth looking? Abdominal imaging after pancreatic cancer resection: a national study. *J Gastrointest Surg*. 2012;16(1):121–128. doi:10.1007/s11605-011-1699-z

How I Treat Resectable Pancreatic Cancer With Neoadjuvant Therapy

Davendra P. S. Sohal

INTRODUCTION

Resectable pancreas cancer is defined as nonmetastatic cancer that does not involve the celiac axis vasculature. Beyond this definition, however, are various staging criteria for resectability of pancreatic cancer that are largely, but not completely, overlapping. These include definitions from the Americas Hepato-Pancreato-Biliary Association, Society of Surgical Oncology, MD Anderson Cancer Center, National Comprehensive Cancer Network, and the National Clinical Trials Network Intergroup (1–4). All these definitions are based on cross-sectional imaging, which is usually a contrast-enhanced CT scan of the chest, abdomen, and pelvis. An MRI scan with contrast is an acceptable alternative. Using such a scan, after metastatic disease in other organs and distant lymph nodes (i.e., lymph nodes outside the surgical basin) is ruled out, the relationship of the primary pancreatic tumor with the surrounding vasculature is evaluated carefully. A consensus is emerging toward the Intergroup definition, which is based on a geometric interface between tumor and various vessels, as opposed to subjective descriptors such as involvement, abutment, impingement, encasement, and so on, used in some of the other definitions (1). The Intergroup definition describes a resectable cancer as one where there is:

- No involvement of the celiac artery, common hepatic artery, and superior mesenteric artery (and, if present, replaced right hepatic artery)
- No involvement, or <180° interface between the tumor and the vessel wall, of the portal vein and/or superior mesenteric vein; and patent portal vein/splenic vein confluence

Of note, this definition applies mostly to the evaluation of tumors in the pancreatic head, which is where 70% to 75% of all cases originate. Some pancreatic body tumors may also grow to involve celiac axis vessels; pancreatic tail tumors rarely do so. Evaluation of resectability of body and tail tumors sometimes may include the assessment of adjacent organ involvement as well, such as invasion into the stomach or spleen. Using the Intergroup definition, approximately 15% to 20% of all cases of pancreatic cancer present as resectable disease.

CURRENT STANDARD OF CARE

The current standard of care for resectable pancreas cancer remains upfront surgical resection. This is followed by adjuvant therapy, as discussed in detail in the first portion of this chapter. Single-agent fluorouracil or gemcitabine with or without the addition of radiation remained the standard adjuvant therapy options until recently, when the combination of gemcitabine and capecitabine was shown to improve median overall survival to 28 months in the ESPAC-4 trial (5). Therefore, this combination, administered for 6 months, is now the standard adjuvant therapy recommendation.

RATIONALE FOR NEOADJUVANT THERAPY

Surgical resection followed by adjuvant therapy, however, still allows only suboptimal clinical outcomes. Long-term outcomes from the ESPAC-4 trial are not yet available; estimated 5-year

---

A Clinical Vignette ("How I Treat") is included at the end of the chapter.

overall survival in the gemcitabine–capecitabine arm appears to be approximately 25% at best (5). A new strategy—neoadjuvant therapy—is now being tested in this arena. This is based on the understanding that pancreatic cancer starts out as a systemic—not locoregional—disease (6). Preclinical studies indicate that pancreatic epithelial cells are present in systemic circulation without any histopathologic evidence of a primary tumor (7). Detailed genomic analyses focusing on the natural history of pancreatic cancer demonstrate that early pancreatic neoplastic lesions harbor mature genomic profiles, even prior to macroscopic metastases (8). This bears out in clinical experience as well. Most patients with pancreatic cancer that is resected die eventually of systemic disease, with or without meaningful locoregional recurrence, as noted in clinical and autopsy series (9,10). This is true even after margin-positive resections, where traditionally a locoregional problem is thought to be the culprit (11). Therefore, a therapeutic approach focusing on early systemic disease control may improve clinical outcomes. A key limitation to this approach had been the rather modest benefit from systemic chemotherapy—5-fluorouracil and gemcitabine, used as single agents in most adjuvant therapy trials (12). With the advent of multiagent regimens—namely, FOLFIRINOX (5-fluorouracil, irinotecan, and oxaliplatin) and Gem/nab-P (gemcitabine/nab-paclitaxel)—that have been shown to improve overall survival in the metastatic setting, that limitation can now be overcome (13,14).

An important additional benefit of the neoadjuvant approach is the delivery of planned therapy. Postoperative multiagent chemotherapy can be onerous; in the ESPAC-4 trial, adjuvant gemcitabine plus capecitabine could be completed in only 54% of patients (5). Furthermore, the neoadjuvant platform allows early identification of therapeutic failures. These could be due to either disease biology, where disease progresses despite aggressive systemic chemotherapy, or patient physiology, where such chemotherapy is not tolerated and leads to serious adverse events. In such cases, it is perhaps prudent to spare the patient aggressive surgery since the probability of cure is low, and alternative approaches to care may be pursued. Finally, the neoadjuvant platform allows prospective testing of serial biomarkers, either tissue based or blood based. Baseline diagnostic tissue specimens and resected surgical specimens and serial blood specimens collected on therapy can provide opportunities to evaluate such markers.

CURRENT EVIDENCE FOR NEOADJUVANT THERAPY

There are no randomized controlled trials published yet on the role of neoadjuvant therapy for resectable pancreatic cancer. A retrospective analysis from the National Cancer Database, a large surgical database across several hospitals in the United States, indicated that neoadjuvant therapy may improve clinical outcomes. In this propensity score-matched analysis of more than 8,000 patients, neoadjuvant therapy led to a median overall survival of 26 months, compared with 21 months with upfront resection (hazard ratio: 0.72, 95% confidence interval [CI]: 0.68–0.78, $p < .01$) (15). Similarly, a Markov decision analysis on 22 studies comprising more than 1,600 patients showed that life expectancy was 32.2 months with neoadjuvant therapy followed by resection, compared with 26.7 months with upfront resection followed by adjuvant therapy (16). Prospective studies in this arena are limited to small, mostly single-institution, phase II trials (Table 23.1). Two studies tested gemcitabine plus cisplatin, without the use of radiation. One enrolled 50 patients, with 70% undergoing resection in the gemcitabine plus cisplatin arm (compared with only 38% in the gemcitabine control arm), achieving a median overall survival of 15.6 months (compared with 9.9 months in the gemcitabine arm) (17). The other study was single-arm, enrolling 28 patients, with 89% undergoing resection, with a median overall survival of 26.5 months (18). A larger study on gemcitabine and cisplatin with the addition of radiation enrolled 90 patients, with a surprisingly lower resection proportion (58%) and median overall survival (17.4 months) (19). A more modern study of gemcitabine plus oxaliplatin, without radiation, showed a resection proportion of 71% and a median overall survival of 27.2 months (20).

It is evident from these results that meaningful conclusions are difficult to draw. The heterogeneity of results stems from various factors: exact definitions of resectability and methods to assess it vary across studies; the regimens used, including drugs, doses, schedules, and durations, are heterogeneous; and radiation use is similarly discrepant. Meta-analyses of these studies reveal some patterns, however. In resectable pancreatic cancer, approximately 65% to 80% of patients are able to undergo surgical resection after neoadjuvant therapy, with a median overall survival of 20 to 30 months (23,24). This compares favorably with the

TABLE 23.1 Selected Neoadjuvant Studies in Resectable Pancreatic Adenocarcinoma*

Author, Year, Reference	Number of Patients	Treatment Regimen	Primary Outcome	Primary Result	OS, If Not Primary Outcome
Palmer 2007 (17)	50	Gem + Cis	RR	70%	15.6
Heinrich 2008 (18)	28	Gem + Cis	RR	89%	26.5
Evans 2008 (21)	86	Gem + RT	NS		22.7
Varadhachary 2008 (19)	90	Gem + Cis + RT	NS		17.4
Van Buren 2013 (22)	59	Gem + Bev + RT	RR	73%	16.8
O'Reilly 2014 (20)	38	Gem + Ox	OS	27.2 months	

*All survival results are in months.

Bev, Bevacizumab; Cis, Cisplatin; Gem, gemcitabine; NS, not specified; OS, overall survival; Ox, Oxaliplatin; RR, resection rate; RT, radiation therapy.

surgery-first approach followed by single-agent adjuvant chemotherapy or chemoradiation, the contemporaneous standard of care when these neoadjuvant trials were conducted. Studies of more modern chemotherapy regimens are ongoing and are discussed in the next section.

The question of radiation therapy is also outstanding. As described earlier, many neoadjuvant studies used radiation, but doses and schedules varied. It is difficult to tease out the exact benefit of radiation since it is delivered alongside chemotherapy and there were no non-radiation control arms in these studies. Unfortunately, radiation therapy has not been shown to improve overall survival in any randomized controlled trial in pancreatic cancer. Modern methods of radiation, including intensity-modulated radiation therapy (IMRT) and stereotactic body radiation therapy (SBRT), are now being used and early studies show good safety and efficacy results (25). The exact role of radiation, if any, in the curative setting remains to be determined.

KEY ONGOING STUDIES OF NEOADJUVANT THERAPY

Questions described previously will hopefully be answered by ongoing studies of neoadjuvant/perioperative therapy for resectable pancreatic cancer (Table 23.2). The SWOG S1505 trial is a randomized phase II study of perioperative FOLFIRINOX versus Gem/nab-P, with a pick-the-winner design. The NEPAFOX study tests perioperative FOLFIRINOX versus adjuvant gemcitabine; the NEOPAC study tests the addition of neoadjuvant gemcitabine/oxaliplatin to adjuvant gemcitabine—these studies are testing regimens as well as timing. The NEONAX study tests perioperative versus adjuvant Gem/nab-P, and the PACT-15 study tests perioperative versus adjuvant gemcitabine/cisplatin/epirubicin/capecitabine combination—these studies are testing the timing of aggressive regimens. The NEOPA study tests neoadjuvant gemcitabine/radiation, in addition to adjuvant gemcitabine; RTOG0848 tests gemcitabine with or without radiation—these studies will provide evidence on the role of radiation.

SUMMARY

Resectable pancreatic cancer provides the best opportunity for cure of this otherwise deadly disease. Several ongoing clinical studies of neoadjuvant chemotherapy and chemoradiation will define the role and answer key questions in this setting: the preferred regimen; duration of neoadjuvant therapy; role of radiation; predictive biomarkers; eventual addition of immunotherapies and targeted therapies to the neoadjuvant platform.

TABLE 23.2 Selected Ongoing Neoadjuvant Studies for Resectable Pancreatic Adenocarcinoma

Study, Registration Number	Planned Sample Size	Treatment Arms	Primary Outcome
SWOG S1505 NCT02562716	150	Periop FOLFIRINOX Periop Gem/nab-P	2-yr OS
NEPAFOX NCT02172976	126	Periop FOLFIRINOX Adj Gem	OS
NEOPAC NCT01521702	310	Neoadj GemOx + Adj Gem Adj Gem	PFS
NEONAX NCT02047513	166	Periop Gem/nab-P Adj Gem/nab-P	18-mth DFS
PACT-15 NCT01150630	370	Periop Gem/Cis/Epi/Cape Adj Gem/Cis/Epi/Cape	1-yr DFS
NEOPA NCT01900327	410	Neoadj Gem/RT + Adj Gem Adj Gem	3-yr OS

Adj, adjuvant; Cape, Capecitabine; Cis, Cisplatin; DFS, disease-free survival; Epi, Epirubicin; FOLFIRI-NOX, 5-fluorouracil, irinotecan, and oxaliplatin; Gem, gemcitabine; mth, month; nab-P, nab-paclitaxel; Neoadj, neoadjuvant; OS, overall survival; Ox, Oxaliplatin; Periop, perioperative; PFS, progression-free survival; RT, radiation therapy; yr, year.

Clinical Vignette 23.1

A 66-year-old otherwise healthy male with no remarkable medical or surgical history is noted by his wife to have yellow discoloration of his skin, prompting a visit to his primary care physician. A review of systems yields nothing additional. Physical examination reveals icterus and no other findings—no abdominal tenderness or masses. Laboratory evaluation shows normal complete blood count and chemistries, except a total bilirubin of 8 mg/dl. A right upper quadrant ultrasound reveals common bile duct dilation to 20 mm. A CT scan is ordered next and reveals a pancreatic head mass, 3 cm, causing upstream pancreatic duct dilation and biliary tree dilation.

What Should Be the Next Intervention?
This is a classic presentation and appearance on imaging for a pancreatic head adeno-carcinoma. As discussed in Chapter 20, Diagnosis and Staging of Pancreatic Cancer, endoscopy with endoscopic ultrasound (EUS) and endoscopic retrograde cholan-giopancreatography (ERCP) is the most appropriate diagnostic and therapeutic inter-vention. An EUS-guided aspirate or biopsy can be obtained from the pancreatic head mass, and a biliary stent can relieve the obstruction.

EUS-guided fine-needle aspiration (FNA) of the pancreatic head mass confirms ade-nocarcinoma. ERCP-guided biliary stent begins to alleviate the jaundice.

What Should Be the Next Intervention?
Staging for pancreatic cancer is ideally performed with a contrast-enhanced pancreatic protocol CT scan. An MRI is an acceptable alternative. Neither PET scans nor EUS alone is sufficient to assess resectability.

A pancreatic protocol CT scan reveals no metastatic disease or adenopathy; the pancreatic head mass does not interface with any blood vessel.

How Would You Manage This Case?
This is an uncommon presentation, but fortunately for this patient, there is no vascu-lar involvement, making this a clearly resectable tumor. Only about 15% to 20% of

pancreatic cancers present as such. The patient is fit and healthy, making a curative approach the ideal plan.

The standard of care would be surgical resection (a Whipple procedure—pancreatoduodenectomy) followed by adjuvant therapy with gemcitabine and capecitabine.

As discussed earlier, there are several trials now investigating the neoadjuvant approach. In our institutional practice, this is our preferred approach. We present the standard-of-care option, as well as available clinical trials of neoadjuvant therapy. Pros and cons are discussed. The biggest concern with neoadjuvant therapy is delay of curative resection. Patients as well as doctors are usually concerned most about leaving a curable cancer unresected for several months. Most neoadjuvant trials incorporate chemotherapy or chemoradiation for 2 to 4 months prior to resection. A recovery period of 4 to 6 weeks after the end of neoadjuvant therapy is also required. More recent studies of neoadjuvant therapy, however, indicate that only a small proportion (less than 10%) of patients fail to undergo resection due to therapy side effects (20,22). These results are reassuring and can be used to provide further context to the discussion of risks and benefits.

REFERENCES

1. Katz MH, Marsh R, Herman JM, et al. Borderline resectable pancreatic cancer: need for standardization and methods for optimal clinical trial design. *Ann Surg Oncol.* 2013;20(8):2787–2795. doi:10.1245/s10434-013-2886-9
2. Callery MP, Chang KJ, Fishman EK, et al. Pretreatment assessment of resectable and borderline resectable pancreatic cancer: expert consensus statement. *Ann Surg Oncol.* 2009;16(7):1727–1733. doi:10.1245/s10434-009-0408-6
3. Varadhachary GR, Tamm EP, Abbruzzese JL, et al. Borderline resectable pancreatic cancer: definitions, management, and role of preoperative therapy. *Ann Surg Oncol.* 2006;13(8):1035–1046. doi:10.1245/ASO.2006.08.011
4. Tempero MA, Malafa MP, Al-Hawary M, et al. Pancreatic adenocarcinoma, version 2.2017, NCCN Clinical Practice Guidelines in Oncology. *J Natl Compr Cancer Netw.* 2017;15(8):1028–1061. doi:10.6004/jnccn.2017.0131
5. Neoptolemos JP, Palmer DH, Ghaneh P, et al. Comparison of adjuvant gemcitabine and capecitabine with gemcitabine monotherapy in patients with resected pancreatic cancer (ESPAC-4): a multicentre, open-label, randomised, phase 3 trial. *Lancet.* 2017;389(10073):1011–1024. doi:10.1016/S0140-6736(16)32409-6
6. Sohal DP, Walsh RM, Ramanathan RK, et al. Pancreatic adenocarcinoma: treating a systemic disease with systemic therapy. *J Natl Cancer Inst.* 2014;106(3):dju011. doi:10.1093/jnci/dju011
7. Rhim AD, Mirek ET, Aiello NM, et al. EMT and dissemination precede pancreatic tumor formation. *Cell.* 2012;148(1–2):349–361. doi:10.1016/j.cell.2011.11.025
8. Yachida S, Jones S, Bozic I, et al. Distant metastasis occurs late during the genetic evolution of pancreatic cancer. *Nature.* 2010;467(7319):1114–1117. doi:10.1038/nature09515
9. Iacobuzio-Donahue CA, Fu B, Yachida S, et al. DPC4 gene status of the primary carcinoma correlates with patterns of failure in patients with pancreatic cancer. *J Clin Oncol.* 2009;27(11):1806–1813. doi:10.1200/JCO.2008.17.7188
10. Hishinuma S, Ogata Y, Tomikawa M, et al. Patterns of recurrence after curative resection of pancreatic cancer, based on autopsy findings. *J Gastrointest Surg.* 2006;10(4):511–518. doi:10.1016/j.gassur.2005.09.016
11. Gnerlich JL, Luka SR, Deshpande AD, et al. Microscopic margins and patterns of treatment failure in resected pancreatic adenocarcinoma. *Arch Surg.* 2012;147(8):753–760. doi:10.1001/archsurg.2012.1126
12. Liao WC, Chien KL, Lin YL, et al. Adjuvant treatments for resected pancreatic adenocarcinoma: a systematic review and network meta-analysis. *Lancet Oncol.* 2013;14(11):1095–1103. doi:10.1016/S1470-2045(13)70388-7
13. Conroy T, Desseigne F, Ychou M, et al. FOLFIRINOX versus gemcitabine for metastatic pancreatic cancer. *N Engl J Med.* 2011;364(19):1817–1825. doi:10.1056/NEJMoa1011923
14. Von Hoff DD, Ervin T, Arena FP, et al. Increased survival in pancreatic cancer with nab-paclitaxel plus gemcitabine. *N Engl J Med.* 2013;369(18):1691–1703. doi:10.1056/NEJMoa1304369

15. Mokdad AA, Minter RM, Zhu H, et al. Neoadjuvant therapy followed by resection versus upfront resection for resectable pancreatic cancer: a propensity score matched analysis. *J Clin Oncol.* 2017;35(5):515–522. doi:10.1200/JCO.2016.68.5081

16. de Geus SW, Evans DB, Bliss LA, et al. Neoadjuvant therapy versus upfront surgical strategies in resectable pancreatic cancer: a Markov decision analysis. *Eur J Surg Oncol.* 2016;42(10):1552–1560. doi:10.1016/j.ejso.2016.07.016

17. Palmer DH, Stocken DD, Hewitt H, et al. A randomized phase 2 trial of neoadjuvant chemotherapy in resectable pancreatic cancer: gemcitabine alone versus gemcitabine combined with cisplatin. *Ann Surg Oncol.* 2007;14(7):2088–2096. doi:10.1245/s10434-007-9384-x

18. Heinrich S, Pestalozzi BC, Schafer M, et al. Prospective phase II trial of neoadjuvant chemotherapy with gemcitabine and cisplatin for resectable adenocarcinoma of the pancreatic head. *J Clin Oncol.* 2008;26(15):2526–2531. doi:10.1200/JCO.2007.15.5556

19. Varadhachary GR, Wolff RA, Crane CH, et al. Preoperative gemcitabine and cisplatin followed by gemcitabine-based chemoradiation for resectable adenocarcinoma of the pancreatic head. *J Clin Oncol.* 2008;26(21):3487–3495. doi:10.1200/JCO.2007.15.8642

20. O'Reilly EM, Perelshteyn A, Jarnagin WR, et al. A single-arm, nonrandomized phase II trial of neoadjuvant gemcitabine and oxaliplatin in patients with resectable pancreas adenocarcinoma. *Ann Surg.* 2014;260(1):142–148. doi:10.1097/SLA.0000000000000251

21. Evans DB, Varadhachary GR, Crane CH, et al. Preoperative gemcitabine-based chemoradiation for patients with resectable adenocarcinoma of the pancreatic head. *J Clin Oncol.* 2008;26(21):3496–3502. doi:10.1200/JCO.2007.15.8634

22. Van Buren G 2nd, Ramanathan RK, Krasinskas AM, et al. Phase II study of induction fixed-dose rate gemcitabine and bevacizumab followed by 30 Gy radiotherapy as preoperative treatment for potentially resectable pancreatic adenocarcinoma. *Ann Surg Oncol.* 2013;20(12):3787–3793. doi:10.1245/s10434-013-3161-9

23. Dhir M, Malhotra GK, Sohal DPS, et al. Neoadjuvant treatment of pancreatic adenocarcinoma: a systematic review and meta-analysis of 5520 patients. *World J Surg Oncol.* 2017;15(1):183. doi:10.1186/s12957-017-1240-2

24. Gillen S, Schuster T, Meyer zum Büschenfelde C, et al. Preoperative/neoadjuvant therapy in pancreatic cancer: a systematic review and meta-analysis of response and resection percentages. *PLoS Med.* 2010;7(4):e1000267. doi:10.1371/journal.pmed.1000267

25. Boyle J, Czito B, Willett C, et al. Adjuvant radiation therapy for pancreatic cancer: a review of the old and the new. *J Gastrointest Oncol.* 2015;6(4):436–444.

How I Treat Borderline Resectable and Locally Advanced Pancreatic Cancer

Hao Xie, Tanios Bekaii-Saab, and Wen Wee Ma

INTRODUCTION

Pancreatic ductal adenocarcinoma (PDAC) has poor prognosis even when diagnosed at its early stage. Borderline resectable and locally advanced PDAC accounts for approximately one-half of all newly diagnosed PDAC. The goal of disease-targeted treatment for patients with borderline resectable PDAC is to increase the margin-negative (R0) resection rate, which is associated with better survival. The treatment goal for patients with locally advanced PDAC is palliation, and conversion to surgically resectable disease occurs in very few patients (1). Contemporary combination chemotherapy regimens such as FOLFIRINOX (5-fluorouracil [5-FU], leucovorin, irinotecan, and oxaliplatin) and gemcitabine plus nab-paclitaxel from the metastatic setting were introduced to patients with borderline resectable or locally advanced PDAC as neoadjuvant therapy with or without chemoradiation. This chapter reviews the literature in the setting of a clinical vignette, and provides our approach to the management of borderline resectable and locally advanced PDAC.

BORDERLINE RESECTABLE PANCREATIC CANCER

Resectability of PDAC was determined by the degree of contact, encasement, or occlusion of surrounding arterial and venous structures. The definition of borderline resectable PDAC is in general with superior mesenteric artery (SMA) and celiac axis involvement <180° and potentially reconstructable superior mesenteric vein (SMV) and portal vein (PV). The detailed criteria defining borderline resectable PDAC are listed in Table 24.1 (2–4). Current guidelines advocate preoperative/neoadjuvant therapy in patients with borderline resectable PDAC though, to date, there are no published randomized trials that evaluate whether neoadjuvant approach has survival superiority over upfront surgery followed by adjuvant therapy. In addition, the optimal chemotherapy regimen and the role of radiation in neoadjuvant therapy remain unknown.

In a number of retrospective studies on patients with borderline resectable disease (5–8), neoadjuvant FOLFIRINOX or gemcitabine plus nab-paclitaxel with or without chemoradiation demonstrated a resection rate of 60% to 80% and an R0 resection rate of 80% to 90% (9). Patients who had surgical resection after neoadjuvant therapy had comparable survival to those who underwent upfront surgery historically (10).

The prospective, single-arm Alliance A021101 trial was designed to evaluate the use of preoperative modified FOLFIRINOX for four cycles followed by chemoradiation 50.4 Gy with capecitabine for borderline resectable PDAC. Patients who underwent pancreatectomy subsequently received two cycles of gemcitabine treatment adjuvantly. The overall response rate was 27% and the overall survival rate at 18 months was 55%. Fifteen (68%) of 22 patients had surgical resection, among whom 93% had R0 resection; 13% had complete pathologic response (11).

Based on the finding from the Alliance A021101 trial, the ongoing Alliance A021501 trial (NCT02839343), a phase II randomized trial, was designed to compare extended neoadjuvant modified FOLFIRINOX for eight cycles with modified FOLFIRINOX for seven cycles followed by stereotactic body radiation therapy (SBRT). Patients who have surgical resection will receive four cycles of adjuvant modified FOLFOX6. The primary end point is 18-month overall survival rate (12).

A Clinical Vignette ("How I Treat") is included at the end of the chapter.

TABLE 24.1 Definition of Borderline Resectable and Locally Advanced Pancreatic Adenocarcinoma

	Borderline Resectable PDAC	Locally Advanced PDAC
Extrapancreatic	Absence	Absence, lymph node metastases beyond field of resection
SMA	Contact ≤180°	Contact >180° or first jejunal branch
CHA	Contact without extension	
Celiac axis	Contact ≤180° (body/tail) or contact >180° without aorta or GDA involvement (body/tail)	Contact >180°
Aorta	No involvement	Involvement
SMV/PV	Contact >180° or contact ≤180° with contour irregularity or short thrombosis	Unreconstructable involvement or occlusion or contact with first draining jejunal branch into SMV
IVC	Contact	

CHA, common hepatic artery; GDA, gastroduodenal artery; IVC, inferior vena cava; PDAC, pancreatic ductal adenocarcinoma; PV, portal vein; SMA, superior mesenteric artery; SMV, superior mesenteric vein.

Patients with histologically confirmed borderline resectable PDAC should be evaluated for neoadjuvant therapy if they have good performance status. FOLFIRINOX and gemcitabine plus nab-paclitaxel are commonly used. The use of a specific chemotherapy regimen with or without radiation varies significantly among different institutions. But the principle of neoadjuvant therapy is to convert borderline resectable to resectable disease. Interval restaging scans should be utilized to evaluate disease response and resectability. Concurrent chemoradiation with fluoropyrimidine or gemcitabine can sometimes be introduced to patients who do not achieve resectable disease from neoadjuvant chemotherapy. Patients who had disease progression or found to have unresectable disease at the time of surgery should be managed as those with locally advanced or metastatic disease. Surgical resection is recommended for patients with a high likelihood of R0 resections. In addition, staging laparoscopy can be considered to clarify resectability prior to surgical resection. The application of adjuvant chemotherapy is similar to patients who have resectable disease at diagnosis. Additional chemotherapy options are based on the patient's postoperative recovery, choice, and response to neoadjuvant therapy (Figure 24.1).

LOCALLY ADVANCED PANCREATIC CANCER

Locally advanced PDAC is unresectable disease without distant metastasis. The definition of locally advanced PDAC is in general with SMA and celiac axis involvement ≥180° and unreconstructable SMV and PV. The detailed criteria defining locally advanced PDAC are listed in Table 24.1 (2,3).

A European phase III (FFCD-SFRO) trial randomized 119 patients with locally advanced pancreatic cancer to compare intensive induction chemoradiation 60 Gy with infusion 5-FU plus intermittent cisplatin versus induction gemcitabine alone and then followed by maintenance gemcitabine in both arms. The primary end point was overall survival. The intensive chemoradiation arm was more toxic and had significantly shorter median overall survival of 8.6 months compared to 13 months in the gemcitabine-alone arm (13).

The Eastern Cooperative Oncology Group (ECOG) 4201 trial evaluated the role of concurrent chemoradiation 50.4 Gy with gemcitabine in patients with localized unresectable pancreatic cancer. However, the study suffered from poor accrual and enrolled only 74 patients of the planned 316 patients, who were randomized to concurrent chemoradiation versus gemcitabine alone. The primary end point was overall survival, which was 11.1 months in the concurrent chemoradiation arm, significantly longer compared to 9.2 months in the gemcitabine-alone arm. The chemoradiation arm had a greater incidence of grade 4/5 toxicities (14).

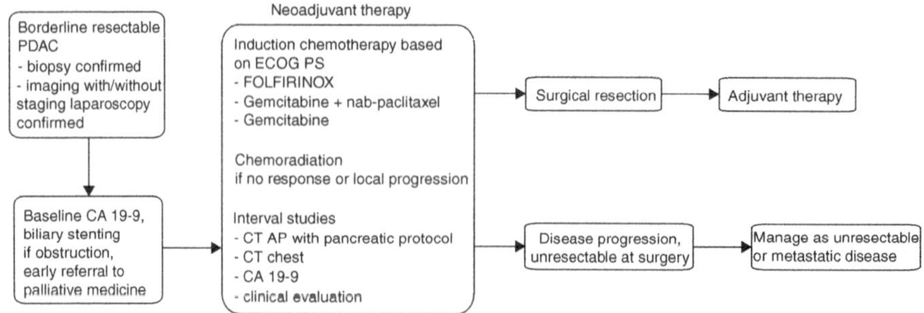

FIGURE 24.1   Treatment algorithm for borderline resectable pancreatic adenocarcinoma.

AP, anterior–posterior; CA 19-9, carbohydrate antigen 19-9; ECOG PS, Eastern Cooperative Oncology Group performance status; FOLFIRINOX, 5-fluorouracil, leucovorin, irinotecan, and oxaliplatin; PDAC, pancreatic ductal adenocarcinoma.

The LAP07 trial aimed to further investigate the role of chemoradiation in patients with locally advanced pancreatic cancer. 449 patients were first randomized to gemcitabine alone versus gemcitabine plus erlotinib. 269 patients who had disease control for 4 months on systemic therapy were then randomized to 2 months of the same chemotherapy versus chemoradiation 54 Gy with capecitabine. The median overall survivals of both chemotherapy and chemoradiation arms were 16.5 months and 15.2 months, respectively, not significantly different from each other. Erlotinib did not provide an additional survival benefit. Patients who received chemoradiation had significantly less local progression rate 32% versus 46% and longer treatment-free interval without significantly increased grade 3/4 toxicities (15).

A number of small nonrandomized or retrospective studies (6,9,16,17) evaluated the role of first-line FOLFIRINOX for patients with locally advanced pancreatic cancer given the high response rate in stage IV disease (18). A systemic review and patient-level meta-analysis included 315 patients with locally advanced disease from 11 studies. The pooled median overall survival was 24.2 months. In eight studies, 57% of the patients received radiotherapy or chemoradiation after FOLFIRINOX. The pooled proportion of patients who had resection was 25.9%, among whom 74% had R0 resection. It concluded that first-line FOLFIRINOX provided longer median overall survival to patients with locally advanced PDAC compared to gemcitabine (19).

Ongoing randomized clinical trials were designed to evaluate the role of chemoradiation compared with chemotherapy alone after contemporary induction chemotherapy with FOLFIRINOX (CONKO-007 NCT01827553) or gemcitabine plus nab-paclitaxel (SCALOP-2 NCT02024009, LAPACT NCT02301143), the role of SBRT in addition to modified FOLFIRINOX (NCT01926197, LAPC-1 NCT02292745), and also to directly compare FOLFIRINOX to gemcitabine in locally advanced PDAC (NEOPAN NCT02539537).

In summary, the use of systemic chemotherapy, local radiotherapy, or their combination in locally advanced unresectable PDAC is based on a patient's performance status (Figure 24.2). For patients with poor performance status, single-agent chemotherapy such as gemcitabine or palliative radiation therapy with best supportive care can potentially alleviate cancer-related pain, bleeding, or obstruction. For patients with ECOG performance status 0 or 1 and adequate organ functions, combination chemotherapy or induction chemotherapy followed by chemoradiation or SBRT is recommended. Systemic chemotherapy options include FOLFIRINOX and gemcitabine plus nab-paclitaxel. Patients should continue induction chemotherapy until achieving optimal response, up to 6 to 8 months. Chemoradiation with fluoropyrimidine or gemcitabine is usually reserved for patients with local progression on induction chemotherapy. Chemoradiation may improve local disease control but there is lack of survival benefit compared to continuation of gemcitabine monotherapy after induction chemotherapy, as per the LAP-07 trial. For patients with good performance status following induction therapy, surgical resection can be considered for those who have significant response to systemic therapy with the goal for margin-negative (R0) resection. For those who progressed, the chemotherapy options include gemcitabine-, fluoropyrimidine-, or liposomal irinotecan-containing chemotherapy regimens depending on previous treatment. Chemoradiation is typically reserved for patients with local disease progression and/or palliation.

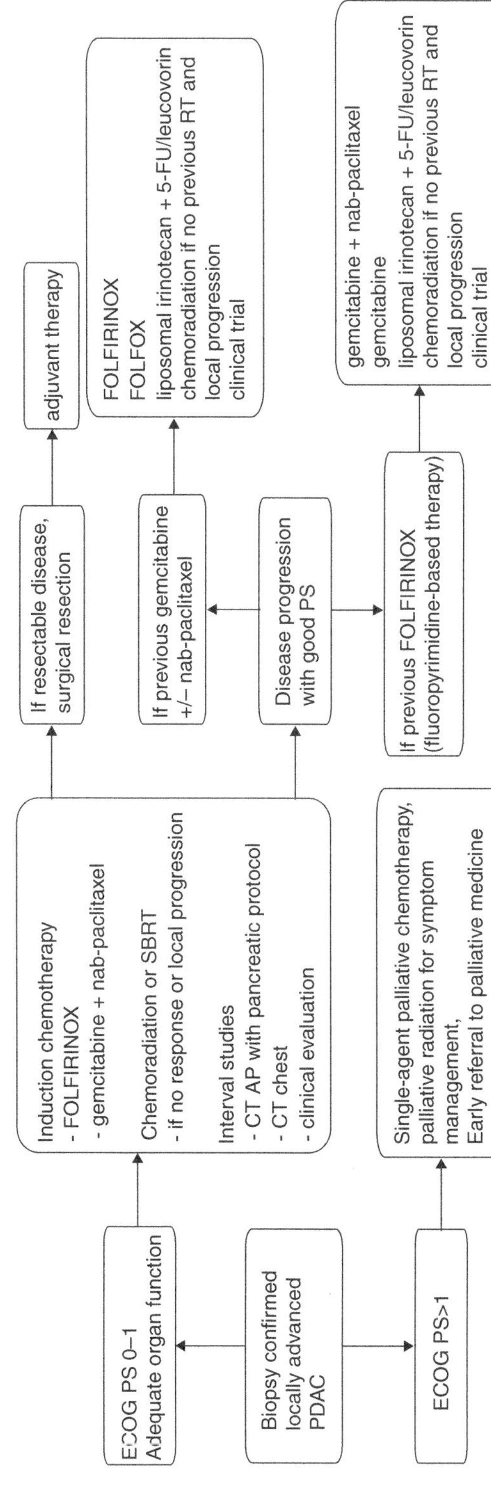

FIGURE 24.2 Treatment algorithm for locally advanced pancreatic adenocarcinoma.

5-FU, 5-fluorouracil; AP, anterior–posterior; ECOG PS, Eastern Cooperative Oncology Group performance status FOLFIRINOX, 5-fluorouracil, leucovorin, irinotecan, and oxaliplatin; FOLFOX, folinic acid, fluorouracil, and oxaliplatin; PDAC, pancreatic ductal adenocarcinoma; RT, radiation therapy; SBRT, stereotactic body radiation therapy.

In view of the poor prognosis, clinical trial enrollment and multimodality treatment approach are encouraged for patients with borderline resectable and locally advanced PDAC. Future studies should focus on defining the role of neoadjuvant combination chemotherapy and radiation therapy from randomized trials and the use of novel therapies such as biomarker-directed therapy, immune checkpoint inhibitors, cancer vaccines, and adoptive T-cell therapy.

Clinical Vignette 24.1

A 48-year-old gentleman initially presented with bilateral flank pain, anorexia, and weight loss. CT abdomen revealed an enhancing mass arising from the medial head of the pancreas, extending into mesenteric fat, measuring 3.5 cm, nearly completely encasing the superior mesenteric artery (SMA) and celiac trunk, and contacting the posterior aspect of the distal superior mesenteric vein (SMV). The portal vein and splenic vein were patent and uninvolved. Endoscopic ultrasound showed an ill-defined hypoechoic mass completely encasing the SMA and celiac trunk and encasement of portal confluence without evidence of nodal metastasis or biliary obstruction. Pathology from fine-needle aspiration was consistent with adenocarcinoma from the pancreas. Further imaging was negative for nodal or distant metastasis. Clinical staging was IIIA T4N0M0. His Eastern Cooperative Oncology Group (ECOG) performance status was 1 at the time of diagnosis. His carbohydrate antigen 19-9 (CA 19-9) was 1,990. He had adequate blood counts and organ functions. He was evaluated by multidisciplinary teams of medical oncology, radiation oncology, and surgery. Given the SMA and celiac axis involvement of >180°, his tumor was surgically unresectable and locally advanced (Figure 24.3A) as compared to the CT findings from another patient with borderline resectable pancreatic adenocarcinoma where the SMV was involved by the tumor but the SMA was not (Figure 24.3B). The use of induction chemotherapy with FOLFIRINOX or gemcitabine plus nab-paclitaxel was discussed. FOLFIRINOX was initiated by extrapolating the high response rate and survival data in the stage IV setting. The systemic chemotherapy was continued until the best response.

The LAP-07 study indicated that patients whose disease is controlled with induction chemotherapy would continue to benefit from systemic chemotherapy. Chemoradiation would benefit for patients with local progression during induction chemotherapy. Restaging CT abdomen after one cycle of FOLFIRINOX demonstrated stable disease but he experienced increasing CA 19-9 and progressive weight loss. At this time, gemcitabine plus nab-paclitaxel was introduced for patients like him who did not have optimal response and experienced clinical deterioration from FOLFIRINOX.

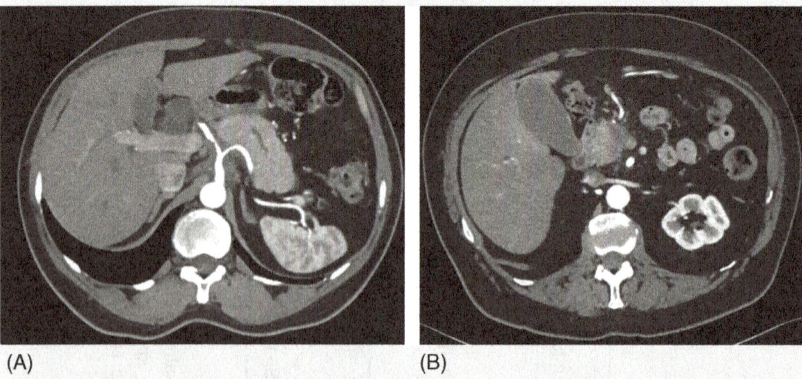

(A)   (B)

FIGURE 24.3   CT findings in (A) locally advanced pancreatic adenocarcinoma with encasement of the common hepatic artery and (B) borderline resectable pancreatic adenocarcinoma with tumor involvement of SMV but not SMA.

SMA, superior mesenteric artery; SMV, superior mesenteric vein.

REFERENCES

1. Shaib WL, Ip A, Cardona K, et al. Contemporary management of borderline resectable and locally advanced unresectable pancreatic cancer. *Oncologist.* 2016;21(2):178–187. doi:10.1634/theoncologist.2015-0316
2. National Comprehensive Cancer Network. Pancreatic Adenocarcinoma, Version 3.2017. https://www.nccn.org/professionals/physician_gls/pdf/pancreatic.pdf; 2018.
3. Al-Hawary MM, Francis IR, Chari ST, et al. Pancreatic ductal adenocarcinoma radiology reporting template: consensus statement of the Society of Abdominal Radiology and the American Pancreatic Association. *Radiology.* 2014;270(1):248–260. doi:10.1148/radiol.13131184
4. Katz MHG, Pisters PWT, Evans DB, et al. Borderline resectable pancreatic cancer: the importance of this emerging stage of disease. *J Am Coll Surg.* 2008;206(5):833–846; discussion 846–848. doi:10.1016/j.jamcollsurg.2007.12.020
5. Hosein PJ, Macintyre J, Kawamura C, et al. A retrospective study of neoadjuvant FOLFIRINOX in unresectable or borderline-resectable locally advanced pancreatic adenocarcinoma. *BMC Cancer.* 2012;12:199. doi:10.1186/1471-2407-12-199
6. Boone BA, Steve J, Krasinskas AM, et al. Outcomes with FOLFIRINOX for borderline resectable and locally unresectable pancreatic cancer. *J Surg Oncol.* 2013;108(4):236–241. doi:10.1002/jso.23392
7. Blazer M, Wu C, Goldberg RM, et al. Neoadjuvant modified (m) FOLFIRINOX for locally advanced unresectable (LAPC) and borderline resectable (BRPC) adenocarcinoma of the pancreas. *Ann Surg Oncol.* 2015;22(4):1153–1159. doi:10.1245/s10434-014-4225-1
8. Paniccia A, Edil BH, Schulick RD, et al. Neoadjuvant FOLFIRINOX application in borderline resectable pancreatic adenocarcinoma: a retrospective cohort study. *Medicine (Baltimore).* 2014;93(27):e198. doi:10.1097/MD.0000000000000198
9. Coveler AL, Herman JM, Simeone DM, et al. Localized pancreatic cancer: multidisciplinary management. *Am Soc Clin Oncol Educ Book.* 2016;35:e217–e226. doi:10.14694/EDBK_160827
10. Gillen S, Schuster T, Zum Meyer Buschenfelde C, et al. Preoperative/neoadjuvant therapy in pancreatic cancer: a systematic review and meta-analysis of response and resection percentages. *PLoS Med.* 2010;7(4):e1000267. doi:10.1371/journal.pmed.1000267
11. Katz MHG, Shi Q, Ahmad SA, et al. Preoperative modified FOLFIRINOX treatment followed by capecitabine-based chemoradiation for borderline resectable pancreatic cancer: alliance for clinical trials in oncology trial A021101. *JAMA Surg.* 2016;151(8):e161137. doi:10.1001/jamasurg.2016.1137
12. Katz MHG, Ou F-S, Herman JM, et al. Alliance for clinical trials in oncology (ALLIANCE) trial A021501: preoperative extended chemotherapy vs. chemotherapy plus hypofractionated radiation therapy for borderline resectable adenocarcinoma of the head of the pancreas. *BMC Cancer.* 2017;17(1):505. doi:10.1186/s12885-017-3441-z
13. Chauffert B, Mornex F, Bonnetain F, et al. Phase III trial comparing intensive induction chemoradiotherapy (60 Gy, infusional 5-FU and intermittent cisplatin) followed by maintenance gemcitabine with gemcitabine alone for locally advanced unresectable pancreatic cancer. Definitive results of the 2000-01 FFCD/SFRO study. *Ann Oncol.* 2008;19(9):1592–1599. doi:10.1093/annonc/mdn281
14. Loehrer PJ, Feng Y, Cardenes H, et al. Gemcitabine alone versus gemcitabine plus radiotherapy in patients with locally advanced pancreatic cancer: an Eastern Cooperative Oncology Group trial. *J Clin Oncol.* 2011;29(31):4105–4112. doi:10.1200/JCO.2011.34.8904
15. Hammel P, Huguet F, van Laethem J-L, et al. Effect of chemoradiotherapy vs chemotherapy on survival in patients with locally advanced pancreatic cancer controlled after 4 months of gemcitabine with or without erlotinib: the LAP07 randomized clinical trial. *JAMA.* 2016;315(17):1844–1853. doi:10.1001/jama.2016.4324
16. Faris JE, Blaszkowsky LS, McDermott S, et al. FOLFIRINOX in locally advanced pancreatic cancer: the Massachusetts General Hospital Cancer Center experience. *Oncologist.* 2013;18(5):543–548. doi:10.1634/theoncologist.2012-0435
17. Nanda RH, El-Rayes B, Maithel SK, et al. Neoadjuvant modified FOLFIRINOX and chemoradiation therapy for locally advanced pancreatic cancer improves resectability. *J Surg Oncol.* 2015;111(8):1028–1034. doi:10.1002/jso.23921
18. Conroy T, Desseigne F, Ychou M, et al. FOLFIRINOX versus gemcitabine for metastatic pancreatic cancer. *N Engl J Med.* 2011;364(19):1817–1825. doi:10.1056/NEJMoa1011923
19. Suker M, Beumer BR, Sadot E, et al. FOLFIRINOX for locally advanced pancreatic cancer: a systematic review and patient-level meta-analysis. *Lancet Oncol.* 2016;17(6):801–810. doi:10.1016/S1470-2045(16)00172-8

How I Treat Metastatic Pancreatic Cancer With Chemotherapy

Benjamin A. Krantz and Eileen M. O'Reilly

INTRODUCTION

The majority of patients with pancreatic ductal adenocarcinoma (PDAC) are diagnosed with advanced disease. In total, approximately 30% have locally advanced disease and 50% have metastases at presentation, with predominant sites of metastases by autopsy evaluation being liver (80%), lung (45%), peritoneum (48%), and abdominal lymph nodes (~20%) (1–3). Patients with advanced disease are ineligible for surgical resection and have treatable but incurable disease. The goals of treatment are symptom control, disease control, maximizing quality of life, and prolonging survival. The mainstay of PDAC treatment is systemic chemotherapy, but given overall challenging survival, clinical trials are recommended for eligible patients. This chapter focuses on the management of PDAC with currently approved therapies; Chapter 26, *How I Treat* Metastatic Pancreatic Cancer With Emerging Therapies, focuses on emerging targets and therapies.

INITIAL ASSESSMENT

In advance of determining treatment options, initial evaluations seek to confirm diagnosis, determine the extent of disease, and adjudicate ability to tolerate therapies. All patients are required to have a pathologic or cytologic diagnosis from the biopsy of the most accessible lesion. Increasingly molecular investigations including somatic tumor genome and germline sequencing may also be pursued. CT pancreas angiogram with pelvis and chest is the preferred imaging modality for baseline cross-sectional evaluation, and staging with MRI abdomen and pelvis with contrast and noncontrast chest CT is an alternative. Serologic tumor marker cancer antigen 19-9 (CA19-9) and carcinoembryonic antigen (CEA) should be evaluated and may be used as an adjunct to staging imaging.

During these initial meetings, prognosis should be discussed and goals of care and preferences related to advanced directives, support systems, and desired therapeutic intensity should be determined. A thorough evaluation of a patient's performance status, symptom burden, and comorbid conditions must be undertaken to gauge which therapies a patient may be able to tolerate physically and what palliative measures are necessary (4).

FRONTLINE TREATMENT

Current standards for initial therapy of advanced PDAC include gemcitabine and nab-paclitaxel and 5-fluorouracil (5-FU), leucovorin, and irinotecan with oxaliplatin (FOLFIRINOX); both regimens have shown superiority over gemcitabine monotherapy and have become the mainstays of frontline treatment for patients with good functional status (5–7).

FOLFIRINOX treatment is based on the PRODIGE IV trial in which 342 patients with untreated metastatic PDAC were randomized to receive fluorouracil 400 mg/m^2 followed by 2,400 mg/m^2 over 46 hours, irinotecan 180 mg/m^2, leucovorin 400 mg/m^2, oxaliplatin 85 mg/m^2 every 2 weeks or gemcitabine at 1,000 mg /m^2 for 7 weeks followed by a rest week and

---

A Clinical Vignette ("How I Treat") is included at the end of the chapter.

then on days 1, 8, and 15 of a 28-day cycle. Key inclusion criteria were Eastern Cooperative Oncology Group (ECOG) performance status of 0 or 1, bilirubin <1.5 upper limit of normal (ULN), and age 18 to 75. Overall survival (OS) and response rate were significantly improved in the FOLFIRINOX cohort (11.1 months vs. 6.8 months, hazard ratio [HR]: 0.57, p < .001 and 31.6% vs. 9.4%, p < .001, respectively). Grade 3 or 4 adverse events included neutropenia (46%), febrile neutropenia (5%), fatigue (24%), vomiting (15%), diarrhea (13%), and peripheral neuropathy (9%) with growth factor use in 43% of patients (5).

Gemcitabine and nab-paclitaxel are approved based on the results from the Metastatic Pancreatic Adenocarcinoma Clinical Trial (MPACT) study, which compared first-line gemcitabine 1,000 mg/m^2 and nab-paclitaxel 125 mg/m^2 on days 1, 8, and 15 of a 28-day cycle to gemcitabine at 1,000 mg /m^2 for 7 weeks followed by a rest week and then on days 1, 8, and 15 of a 28-day cycle. Patients were eligible if the Karnofsky performance status was 70 or greater and bilirubin was below the ULN. There was no upper age limit. OS in the gemcitabine and nab-paclitaxel was 8.5 months compared to 6.7 months in the gemcitabine-only arm (HR: 0.72, p < .001). Response rates were 23% versus 7% (HR: 3.19, p < .01), respectively. Notable adverse events included grade 3 or 4 neutropenia (43%), febrile neutropenia (3%), fatigue (17%), diarrhea (6%), and peripheral neuropathy (17%). Growth factors were used in 26% of patients (6).

In comparison to the PRODIGE IV study, it is notable that MPACT eligibility criteria allowed for older patients (10% were older than 75) and lower functional status (8% had ECOG performance status of 2).

For patients unable to tolerate frontline combination therapy or preference for lower therapeutic intensity, gemcitabine monotherapy continues to be a reasonable choice or gemcitabine and other cytotoxic combinations, for example, with capecitabine. Gemcitabine was approved in 1997 for the treatment of metastatic PDAC based on improved measures of quality of life along with a 1.2-month survival advantage for gemcitabine over 5-FU (OS 5.65 vs. 4.41 months) and improved 1-year survival rates (18% vs. 2%) (8).

Determining the Frontline Regimen

The four main factors in determining a patient's frontline therapy are patient preference for therapeutic intensity, functional status, presence of DNA damage repair deficiency, and comorbid conditions.

For patients desiring aggressive therapy, gemcitabine with nab-paclitaxel and FOLFIRINOX are the preferred options. There have been no head-to-head comparisons of these regimens, but as control group outcomes were comparable in both studies, FOLFIRINOX is generally believed to be the more active regimen. FOLFIRINOX, however, was administered to a younger cohort with better functional status and is potentially more challenging to tolerate with increased need for growth factors and higher rates of fatigue, myelosuppression, gastrointestinal toxicities, and neuropathy. Therefore, it is common practice to treat patients with more favorable performance status and support systems with FOLFIRINOX over gemcitabine and nab-paclitaxel. This is reflected in the American Society of Clinical Oncology (ASCO) clinical practice guidelines, which recommend FOLFIRINOX for patients with a favorable comorbidity profile loosely defined as ECOG 0 or 1, and good major organ functioning and absence of comorbid conditions that require ongoing active care. The ASCO clinical practice guidelines recommend gemcitabine and nab-paclitaxel for patients with a similar comorbidity profile as FOLFIRINOX, with comorbid conditions that are well controlled (4).

Additionally, common concerns that affect a patient's frontline therapeutic preference include alopecia secondary to gemcitabine (50%) and requirement for placement of central vascular access port and home infusional therapy for FOLFIRINOX.

As noted previously, for patients who are not considered good candidates for FOLFIRINOX or gemcitabine with nab-paclitaxel due to comorbidities or the desire to pursue less toxic regimens, single agent gemcitabine is a reasonable option or gemcitabine and capecitabine; the latter based on lower level evidence is a reasonable alternative (9).

Other options for frontline therapy can be considered on a case-by-case basis as there is not sufficient evidence to recommend any one regimen over another in unselected patients. These include gemcitabine with erlotinib, which was approved by the Food and Drug Administration (FDA) based on 2-week survival benefit over gemcitabine alone, gemcitabine with capecitabine, cisplatin or oxaliplatin, 5-FU with oxaliplatin (FOLFOX) or irinotecan (FOLFIRI), capecitabine with oxaliplatin, and capecitabine alone (10).

Specific comorbidities may also lend to specific treatment regimens. For example, 5-FU containing regimens may have an increased incidence of fluoropyrimidine related vasospasm in patients with underlying coronary artery disease. Nab-paclitaxel and oxaliplatin have to be carefully considered in patients with preexisting significant neuropathy, and irinotecan and taxanes should be avoided in patients with abnormal liver function/jaundice.

Specific Population: DNA Damage Repair Deficient Tumors

Patients with DNA damage repair deficiencies are a specific population that has demonstrated sensitivities to platinum agents in breast, ovarian, and pancreas cancers. DNA damage repair deficiencies include *BRCA 1 and 2*, *PALB2*, and *ATM*. In a cohort of 615 unselected patients with pancreas exocrine neoplasms, 8.1% of patients had *BRCA 1 or 2* mutations and 1.8% had *ATM* mutations. In the Ashkenazi Jewish subgroup, *BRCA 1 or 2* mutations were present in 18% versus 4.9% for non-Ashkenazi Jewish patients (11). Family histories of breast, ovarian, and pancreatic cancer alone may enrich for platinum sensitivity (12). The National Comprehensive Cancer Network (NCCN) guidelines recommend genetic risk evaluations for all individuals of Ashkenazi Jewish descent with pancreatic cancer, individuals with personal and/or family history of three or more cancers, an individual with a close relative with a known mutation in a cancer susceptibility gene, two or more relatives with breast cancer on the same side of the family with one diagnosed ≤50 years old, and a first- or second-degree relative with breast cancer ≤45 (13). Of note, more recent literature suggests that universal screening for germline testing for all individuals with PDAC may be warranted (11). For patients with DNA damage repair deficiencies and good functional status, FOLFIRINOX is an active regimen, with increasing data to support gemcitabine/cisplatin (14). Gemcitabine/oxaliplatin, FOLFOX, and capecitabine/oxaliplatin are alternatives that may be considered.

SECOND-LINE TREATMENT

The choice of second-line treatment for PDAC depends on similar factors to first-line therapy along with the choice of first-line therapy that was administered. Generally, a switch from 5-FU to gemcitabine-containing regimens or vice versa is recommended.

Patients with good functional status and favorable comorbidity profile who are able to tolerate additional frontline intensity therapy may be treated with second-line FOLFIRINOX if treated with gemcitabine and nab-paclitaxel as first-line or second-line gemcitabine and nab-paclitaxel after frontline FOLFIRINOX. A recent study evaluated second-line gemcitabine and nab-paclitaxel after progression on FOLFIRINOX or vice versa and found median OS of second-line therapy to be similar to the frontline therapy trials. The median OS was 10.8 months for gemcitabine and nab-paclitaxel and 10.4 months for FOLFIRINOX; however, response rates were notably lower at 10.5% and 16.6%, respectively. From initiation of first-line therapy, median OS was 20.6 for gemcitabine and nab-paclitaxel and 16.5 months for FOLFIRINOX. It should be noted that these results may not be generalizable as at the onset of second-line treatment, over 80% of patients had an ECOG performance status of 0, suggesting a more favorably fit population (15).

Nanoliposomal irinotecan with 5-FU was approved based on results of the NAPOLI-1 study, which compared beyond frontline nanoliposomal irinotecan with infusional 5-FU and leucovorin, nanoliposomal irinotecan alone, and infusional 5-FU and leucovorin alone, all after initial gemcitabine-containing therapy. Patients in the nanoliposomal irinotecan with 5-FU arm had improved outcome compared to 5-FU and leucovorin alone with median OS of 6.1 months versus 4.2 months (16). There was no significant difference in survival between nanoliposomal irinotecan alone and 5-FU with leucovorin alone. No head-to-head trials have been performed evaluating second-line nanoliposomal irinotecan with 5-FU/LV versus FOLFIRI or FOLFOX. Two recent meta-analyses have evaluated pyrimidines with the addition of oxaliplatin or irinotecan. One showed similar efficacies of oxaliplatin- and irinotecan-containing regimens, while the other showed improved progression-free survival (PFS) and OS for irinotecan-containing regimens and only a modest PFS with OS benefit for oxaliplatin-containing ones (17,18). If functional status is poor, 5-FU or capecitabine monotherapy along with optimal supportive care may be considered.

For patients who received frontline FOLFIRINOX who are not candidates for gemcitabine and nab-paclitaxel, gemcitabine combinations such as gemcitabine with oxaliplatin or capecitabine or gemcitabine monotherapy are options. There has not been a systematic study of second-line gemcitabine-based regimens, and any combination should be decided on an individual patient basis.

For all patients who are eligible, clinical trials in frontline and second-line settings are preferred options.

THIRD-LINE CHEMOTHERAPY

There are no approved agents beyond second-line therapy. Treatment should be individualized and may include two-agent combinations or monotherapy. For all patients who are eligible, clinical trials are a preferred approach. Somatic and germline profiling may inform possible matched trial options or off-label agent use (19).

SPECIFIC POPULATION: MICROSATELLITE INSTABILITY HIGH (MSI-H) AND DEFICIENT MISMATCH REPAIR (dMMR)

Patients with MSI-H and dMMR tumors represent a small but important subset of PDAC patients given the approval of pembrolizumab for patients with MSI-H or dMMR solid tumors agnostic to tissue of origin who have failed chemotherapy and have no satisfactory treatment options (20). dMMR is caused by biallelic inactivation of *MLH1, MSH2, MSH6,* or *PMS2* genes and results in the development of thousands of mutations that are easily identified at microsatellite, short tandem repeating DNA sequences. Methodologies for the identification of dMMR include immunohistochemical analysis for loss of mismatch repair protein expression, polymerase chain reaction (PCR) for microsatellites, and increasingly the use of next-generation sequencing bioinformatics analyses (e.g., MSISensor, mSINGs, etc.) (21).

The incidences of MSI-H/dMMR PDAC reported in the literature have varied widely; however, large series have demonstrated the rarity of these tumors. One of the largest series evaluations of dMMR tumors in PDAC, from Memorial Sloan Kettering Cancer Center, identified seven patients (0.8%) with dMMR tumors, all of whom had Lynch syndrome (21). Due to the rarity of these tumors in PDAC, limited data are available about response rates. In eight patients with PDAC and MSI-H tumors treated with pembrolizumab, two complete responses (CRs), three partial responses (PRs), and one stable disease (SD) were achieved with two being unevaluable (22). Although this set is small, the response rates compare favorably to the MSI-H noncolorectal cancer cohort in KEYNOTE 158, which had a 37.7% response rate (23). It is notable that pembrolizumab is the first approved biomarker selected therapy in PDAC, the approval of which may be the beginning of the age of biomarker-based therapy in PDAC (24).

Clinical Vignette 25.1

Case 1: A 55-year-old male with a past medical history significant for nonobstructive coronary artery disease and type 2 diabetes is found to have masses in the head of the pancreas, liver, and lung. Biopsy of a liver lesion reveals adenocarcinoma consistent with pancreas primary. He is ambulatory but restricted in his physical activity and able to carry out light work. He has two siblings with a history of breast cancer. He is interested in aggressive care.

Case 2: A 65-year-old female with a past medical history significant for stage II colon cancer at age 42 status posthemicolectomy and localized breast cancer at 50 status postmastectomy, with no evidence of either disease on last imaging 5 years ago re-presents and a workup identifies a diagnosis of pancreatic ductal adenocarcinoma with peritoneal metastases. Her disease has now progressed on first- and second-line therapy. She is no longer able to work but is active for most of the day. Her sister had colon and lung cancer and her mother had colon and renal cell carcinoma. She is interested in aggressive care.

Treating the Patient

Case 1: The patient has an ECOG performance status of 1 and desires aggressive therapy. Therefore, both FOLFIRINOX or gemcitabine and nab-paclitaxel should be considered as initial therapy. Family history is notable for two siblings with breast cancer supporting *BRCA* mutation testing. He has comorbidities of coronary artery disease and diabetes with neuropathy, suggesting prudent evaluation regarding the use of a fluoropyrimidine or oxaliplatin. If a germline or somatic *BRCA* mutation is detected and cardiac evaluation permits, cisplatin and gemcitabine is a rationale choice. If no DNA damage repair deficiency is found, gemcitabine and nab-paclitaxel would also be an appropriate frontline regimen.

Case 2: The patient has an ECOG performance status of 2 and has had disease progression on two lines of treatment and has a personal and family history of multiple malignancies. At this point, there are no further approved treatment options and her personal and family history of malignancy may be a signal of a genetic syndrome including Lynch syndrome. Her tumor should be tested, arguably via next-generation sequencing and if a microsatellite instability high/mismatch repair deficiency (MSI-H/dMMR) is identified, she would be a candidate for pembrolizumab. If not, single-agent chemotherapy or enrollment in a clinical trial could be considered.

REFERENCES

1. American Cancer Society. *Cancer Facts & Figures: 2018.* Atlanta, GA: American Cancer Society. https://www.cancer.org/research/cancer-facts-statistics/all-cancer-facts-figures/cancer-facts-figures-2018.html2018.
2. Surveillance, Epidemiology, and End Results (SEER) Program (www.seer.cancer.gov). *SEER*Stat Database: Incidence - SEER 18 Regs Research Data + Hurricane Katrina Impacted Louisiana Cases, Nov 2016 Sub (2000–2014).* National Cancer Institute D, Surveillance Research Program, Surveillance Systems Branch.
3. Iacobuzio-Donahue CA, Fu B, Yachida S, et al. DPC4 gene status of the primary carcinoma correlates with patterns of failure in patients with pancreatic cancer. *J Clin Oncol.* 2009;27(11):1806–1813. doi:10.1200/JCO.2008.17.7188
4. Sohal DP, Mangu PB, Khorana AA, et al. Metastatic pancreatic cancer: American Society of Clinical Oncology Clinical Practice Guideline. *J Clin Oncol.* 2016;34(23):2784–2796. doi:10.1200/JCO.2016.67.1412
5. Conroy T, Desseigne F, Ychou M, et al. FOLFIRINOX versus gemcitabine for metastatic pancreatic cancer. *N Engl J Med.* 2011;364(19):1817–1825. doi:10.1056/NEJMoa1011923
6. Von Hoff DD, Ervin T, Arena FP, et al. Increased survival in pancreatic cancer with nab-paclitaxel plus gemcitabine. *N Engl J Med.* 2013;369(18):1691–1703. doi:10.1056/NEJMoa1304369
7. National Comprehensive Cancer Network. NCCN Clinical Practice Guidelines in Oncology: Pancreatic Adenocarcinoma (Version 3.2017). 2017; https://www.nccn.org/professionals/physician_gls/pdf/pancreatic.pdf
8. Burris HA 3rd, Moore MJ, Andersen J, et al. Improvements in survival and clinical benefit with gemcitabine as first-line therapy for patients with advanced pancreas cancer: a randomized trial. *J Clin Oncol.* 1997;15(6):2403–2413. doi:10.1200/JCO.1997.15.6.2403
9. Herrmann R, Bodoky G, Ruhstaller T, et al. Gemcitabine plus capecitabine compared with gemcitabine alone in advanced pancreatic cancer: a randomized, multicenter, phase III trial of the Swiss Group for Clinical Cancer Research and the Central European Cooperative Oncology Group. *J Clin Oncol.* 2007;25(16):2212–2217. doi:10.1200/JCO.2006.09.0886
10. Moore MJ, Goldstein D, Hamm J, et al. Erlotinib plus gemcitabine compared with gemcitabine alone in patients with advanced pancreatic cancer: a phase III trial of the National Cancer Institute of Canada Clinical Trials Group. *J Clin Oncol.* 2007;25(15):1960–1966. doi:10.1200/JCO.2006.07.9525
11. Lowery MA, Wong W, Jordan EJ, et al. Prospective evaluation of germline alterations in patients with exocrine pancreatic neoplasms. *J Natl Cancer Inst.* 2018;110(10):1067–1074. doi:10.1093/jnci/djy024

12. Fogelman D, Sugar EA, Oliver G, et al. Family history as a marker of platinum sensitivity in pancreatic adenocarcinoma. *Cancer Chemother Pharmacol.* 2015;76(3):489–498. doi:10.1007/s00280-015-2788-6

13. National Comprehensive Cancer Network. Genetic/Familial High Risk Assessment: Breast and Ovarian (Version 1.2018). 2018; https://www.nccn.org/professionals/physician_gls/PDF/genetics_screening.pdf

14. O'Reilly EM, Lee JW, Lowery MA, et al. Phase 1 trial evaluating cisplatin, gemcitabine, and veliparib in 2 patient cohorts: germline BRCA mutation carriers and wild-type BRCA pancreatic ductal adenocarcinoma. *Cancer.* 2018;124(7):1374–1382. doi:10.1002/cncr.31218

15. Ozaka M, Sasaki T, Yamada I, et al. Second-line treatment of modified FOLFIRINOX or nab-paclitaxel plus gemcitabine for metastatic pancreatic adenocarcinoma. *J Clin Oncol.* 2018;36(4_suppl):458–458. doi:10.1200/jco.2018.36.4_suppl.458

16. Wang-Gillam A, Li CP, Bodoky G, et al. Nanoliposomal irinotecan with fluorouracil and folinic acid in metastatic pancreatic cancer after previous gemcitabine-based therapy (NAPOLI-1): a global, randomised, open-label, phase 3 trial. *Lancet.* 2016;387(10018):545–557. doi:10.1016/S0140-6736(15)00986-1

17. Petrelli F, Inno A, Ghidini A, et al. Second line with oxaliplatin- or irinotecan-based chemotherapy for gemcitabine-pretreated pancreatic cancer: a systematic review. *Eur J Cancer.* 2017;81:174–182. doi:10.1016/j.ejca.2017.05.025

18. Sonbol MB, Firwana B, Wang Z, et al. Second-line treatment in patients with pancreatic ductal adenocarcinoma: a meta-analysis. *Cancer.* 2017;123(23):4680–4686. doi:10.1002/cncr.30927

19. Lowery MA, Jordan EJ, Basturk O, et al. Real-time genomic profiling of pancreatic ductal adenocarcinoma: potential actionability and correlation with clinical phenotype. *Clin Cancer Res.* 2017;23(20):6094–6100. doi:10.1158/1078-0432.CCR-17-0899

20. FDA approves first cancer treatment for any solid tumor with a specific genetic feature [press release]. 2017; https://www.fda.gov/newsevents/newsroom/pressannouncements/ucm560167.htm; 2017.

21. Hu ZI, Shia J, Stadler ZK, et al. Evaluating mismatch repair deficiency in pancreatic adenocarcinoma: challenges and recommendations. *Clin Cancer Res.* 2018;24(6):1326–1336. doi:10.1158/1078-0432.CCR-17-3099

22. Le DT, Durham JN, Smith KN, et al. Mismatch repair deficiency predicts response of solid tumors to PD-1 blockade. *Science.* 2017;357(6349):409–413. doi:10.1126/science.aan6733

23. Diaz L, Marabelle A, Kim T, et al. Efficacy of pembrolizumab in phase 2 KEYNOTE-164 and KEYNOTE-158 studies of microsatellite instability high cancers. *Ann Oncol.* 2017;28:128–129 (suppl_5). doi:10.1093/annonc/mdx367.020

24. Krantz BA, O'Reilly EM. Biomarker-based therapy in pancreatic ductal adenocarcinoma: an emerging reality? *Clin Cancer Res.* 2017;24(10):2241–2250. doi:10.1158/1078-0432.ccr-16-3169

How I Treat Metastatic Pancreatic Cancer With Emerging Therapies

Benjamin A. Krantz and Eileen M. O'Reilly

INTRODUCTION

Outcomes in pancreas cancer remain challenging despite three new multiagent cytotoxic regimens becoming the mainstay of treatment over the past decade (1,2). Median overall survival (OS) times in the landmark clinical trials Metastatic Pancreatic Adenocarcinoma Clinical Trial (MPACT; gemcitabine and nab-paclitaxel vs. gemcitabine) and PRODIGE IV (FOLFIRINOX vs. gemcitabine) were 8.5 and 11.1 months, for gemcitabine and nab-paclitaxel and FOLFIRINOX, respectively (3,4). In NAPOLI-1, conducted in a beyond frontline setting, nanoliposomal irinotecan added to infusional 5-FU/LV increased survival by approximately 2 months (5). As such, 5-year survival for metastatic pancreatic ductal adenocarcinoma (PDAC) remains only 2.7% (6). There is a major unmet need for new therapies and improved outcomes in PDAC, and it is recommended that all patients consider enrollment in clinical trials at all stages of disease (7). Emerging targets in PDAC with drugs in development include the stroma, immune microenvironment, metabolomics, immunotherapy, and in selected patients, DNA damage repair mechanisms.

STROMA AND ENZYMATIC STROMAL DISRUPTION AND PEGPH20

The PDAC microenvironment is characterized by a dense hyaluronic acid (HA) rich, fibrotic stroma with immunosuppressive inflammatory cells including myeloid-derived suppressor cells (MDSCs), tumor-associated macrophages (TAMs), and T-regulatory cells (Tregs) (8). High HA levels in the stroma increase interstitial pressures causing collapse of vessels, impeding blood flow, and reducing drug delivery (9). High HA levels in the stroma are associated with worse outcomes (10).

PEGPH20 is a recombinant pegylated hyaluronidase enzyme designed to break down HA in the tumor microenvironment (TME) and therefore increase therapeutic delivery and cytotoxic effects. PEGPH20 has shown promising effects in a phase II study in combination with gemcitabine with nab-paclitaxel. Patients with high HA levels by immunohistochemical analysis treated with PEGPH20 in combination with gemcitabine and nab-paclitaxel had a greater median progression-free survival (mPFS) and objective response rate (ORR) compared to gemcitabine with nab-paclitaxel alone (mPFS: 9.2 vs. 5.2 months, p = .048, ORR: 45% vs. 31%). A trend toward improved OS was seen; however, it was not statistically significant (median OS: 11.5 vs. 8.5 months, hazard ratio [HR]: 0.96, 95% confidence interval: 0.57–1.61). An increased rate of thrombosis was found in the first half of the study, which was mitigated by primary prophylaxis with enoxaparin in the second half of the study (11). Alternate thrombosis mitigation with rivaroxaban is being studied in patients receiving combination PEGPH20 with gemcitabine and nab-paclitaxel. Safety and effectiveness of the combination was demonstrated with 1 thrombosis in 28 patients studied and a disease control rate of 86% (NCT02921022) (12). Surprisingly, PEGPH20 efficacy has not translated to benefit when combined with FOLFIRINOX and may even be detrimental. A phase II study evaluating modified FOLFIRINOX (mFOLFIRINOX) with or without PEGPH20 had a median OS of 15.1 months for mFOLFIRINOX alone and 7.6 months in the PEGPH20 arm (13). The median OS

A Clinical Vignette ("How I Treat") is included at the end of the chapter.

for mFOLFIRINOX in this study is the longest recorded to date; however, the PEGPH20 in combination with mFOLFIRINOX OS is lower than historical results. In addition, toxicity was higher on the experimental arm. Of note, this trial was conducted in the absence of biomarker selection for HA, and a retrospective analysis of tumor HA and clinical outcomes is ongoing. The reasons for the clinical observations reported remain to be fully understood and reconciled with the encouraging signal in the gemcitabine and nab-paclitaxel based triplet with PEGPH20. A phase III registration trial of PEGPH20 with gemcitabine and nab-paclitaxel versus gemcitabine and nab-paclitaxel is under way (NCT02715804).

IMMUNOTHERAPY

Strategies to harness the immune system against malignancy broadly seek to generate an immune response toward tumor cells or release inhibition of an existing immune response. Strategies to generate an immune response include cancer vaccines, immune stimulating antibodies, and adoptive cell therapy, whereas methods to release a suppressed immune response include immune checkpoint blockade or reducing immunosuppressive cells in the TME.

Immune Checkpoint Blockade

Given the revolutionary effects of immune checkpoint inhibition in melanoma, non–small cell lung cancer, renal cell carcinoma, and others, immune checkpoint blockade has been actively studied in PDAC. T-cells in the PDAC microenvironment express PD-1 and CTLA-4, which when stimulated generate immune tolerance (14). Unfortunately, early study with anti-PD-1 and anti-CTLA-4 monotherapy and combination therapy with gemcitabine has not yielded significant clinical benefit in PDAC nor has the combination of two immune checkpoint inhibitors yielded benefit (15). Despite the early challenges, there is strong belief that the right combinatorial strategies will yield improved results (16,17). Combinations with more active cytotoxic backbones are being pursued utilizing the anti-PD-1 agents, nivolumab with gemcitabine and nab-paclitaxel (NCT02309177) and pembrolizumab with gemcitabine and nab-paclitaxel (NCT02331251). The anti-PD-L1 antibody, atezolizumab, is being studied with gemcitabine and nab-paclitaxel (NCT02715531).

Immune Checkpoint Agonism

Data has demonstrated that patients with greater T-cell expansion to tumor neoantigen stimulation have longer survival in PDAC (18). Therefore, it follows that stimulating endogenous T-cell expansion and activation through activating checkpoint agonism may improve responses in PDAC. CD40 is an immune activating receptor in the tumor necrosis factor super family with broad expression on immune cells including B-cells, dendritic cells, and monocytes. CD40 stimulation is important for generating an immune response through improvement in antigen processing and presentation, and through the release of cytokines from activated antigen presenting cells. Thus, CD40 is a critical regulator of both humoral and cellular immunity. CD40 ligand is also expressed on some malignant cells, including 25% of pancreas adenocarcinomas, with stimulation that leads to apoptosis (19). Multiple CD40 antibodies have been studied in lymphomas and solid tumors. In pancreas cancer specifically, a small study of 21 patients receiving CP870-893 with gemcitabine had 5 partial responses and 11 stable diseases (20). Combining immune stimulation with checkpoint inhibition is a two-pronged approach that may prime the immune system against tumor antigens and prevent tolerance. The CD40 agonist, APX005M, is being evaluated in combination with nivolumab and gemcitabine and nab-paclitaxel in a phase I dose finding study with planned randomized phase II assessment once safety is demonstrated (NCT03214250).

T-Cell Recruitment and Bispecific T-Cell Engagers (BiTEs)

Tumor infiltration by immune cells is a critical element in the cellular response to malignancy. Bispecific antibodies that target CD3 on T-cells and tumor associated antigens are an exciting approach to direct and activate effector cells in the proximity of tumor cells. Currently, one bispecific antibody is approved for use in cancer. Blinatumomab is a CD3/CD19 bispecific antibody for the treatment of acute B-cell lymphoblastic leukemia. Many, however, are currently under investigation. RO6958688 is a CEA/CD3 bispecific antibody which colocalizes T-cells to tissues that express CEA. CEA is expressed in at least 70% of PDAC patients (21). RO6958688 is being studied in combination with atezolizumab in a phase IB study in patients with unresectable CEA-expressing malignancies (NCT02324257). Another permutation of this strategy is arming T-cells with bispecific antibodies. In this strategy, T-cells are collected, expanded ex vivo, and activated with a bispecific antibody before readministering cells to a patient. A phase I/II study is under way evaluating activated T-cells armed with an EGFR/CD3 bispecific antibody (NCT03269526). This methodology bypasses the need for genetic modification of the cells and, therefore, has a faster production time than other methods of adoptive cell transfer.

Adoptive Cell Transfer

Adoptive cell therapy is the process of collecting cells from a patient, expanding, and often modifying them in the laboratory and reinfusing them into a patient. Chimeric antigen receptor T-cells (CARTs) are the most successful adoptive therapy approach to date with two approved therapeutics: tisagenlecleucel in children and adults up to 25 years old with B-cell acute lymphoblastic leukemia and axicabtagene ciloleucel for B-cell non-Hodgkin lymphoma.

CARTs express antibody-like receptors linked to a T-cell receptor transmembrane domain and intracellular signaling domains. When the antibody is engaged, CART activation occurs and a cytotoxic response is initiated. Despite the phenomenal results in hematologic malignancies, CART results have been more tempered in solid tumors including PDAC. Data to date is limited. A phase I trial evaluating feasibility of generating mesothelin-directed CARTs in PDAC administered CARTs to six patients, two of whom achieved stable disease as their best response (22). Anecdotally, a single PDAC patient who received anti-CEA CARTs by hepatic artery infusion had no residual liver disease at 11 months posttreatment (23).

Other CARTs in clinical trials for PDAC are directed toward mesothelin (NCT01583686), epidermal growth factor receptor (EGFR; NCT02873390), MUC1 (NCT02587689), prostate stem cell antigen (NCT02744287), and NK receptors (NCT03018405). CARTs directed toward CA 19-9 and MUC16 are in preclinical development.

Cancer Vaccines

Cancer vaccines deliver antigen to the immune system in order to generate an immune response toward the shared antigen on cancer cells. GVAX is the most well-studied PDAC vaccine, composed of allogenic irradiated PDAC cells that have been transfected to express GM-CSF. Early study of GVAX in combination with ipilimumab showed improved outcome with the combination compared to ipilimumab alone with median OS of 5.7 versus 3.6 months and 1-year OS of 27% versus 7% (24). A phase I/II of GVAX with or without nivolumab in resectable PDAC and a phase II of GVAX with pembrolizumab and stereotactic body radiation therapy in locally advanced disease are both recruiting (NCT02451982, NCT02648282).

IMMUNE MICROENVIRONMENT MODULATION

The immune microenvironment is characterized by effector CD8+ and CD4+ helper T-cells as well as immunosuppressive MDSCs, TAMs, and Tregs (25). Cancer-associated fibroblasts (CAFs) and PDAC cells secrete a number of chemokines including CXCL1/2/5/12 and CCL2, which lead to migration of immunosuppressive cells into the microenvironment and exclusion of effector cells from the vicinity of tumor cells (26). Chemokine antagonists are in development to inhibit migration of immunosuppressive cells and mitigate inhibition of effector cells.

CXCR4

CXCR4 is a chemokine receptor expressed on effector T-cells. Antagonism of CXCL12 binding to CXCR4 induces accumulation of tumor infiltrating lymphocytes (27). BL-8040 is an inhibitor of CXCR4 being studied in combination with pembrolizumab (NCT02826486) and atezolizumab (NCT03193190). Early biomarker results from NCT02826486 utilizing biopsies and blood collection on day 1 and after a 5-day BL-8040 monotherapy lead in have been published. Results demonstrated reductions in circulating Tregs without effect on T-cells, NKT cells, or B-cell populations, and CD3+ and CD8+ cell abundance in the tumor core was increased in 43% of patients (28). Plerixafor is another CXCR4 inhibitor that is currently being studied in phase I dose finding study (NCT02179970). Despite promising preclinical data and early positive correlative data for BL-8040, CXCR4-targeting has had a mixed development. Ulocuplumab, a blocking monoclonal antibody targeting CXCR4, was studied in combination with nivolumab with the trial terminated for lack of efficacy (NCT02472977).

CCR2

CCR2 is a promigratory receptor on macrophages whose ligand CCL2 is secreted by PDAC cells. CCR2 blockade reduces MDSCs and TAM migration into tumors, which has led to a number of CCR2 inhibitors entering the clinic (29,30). CCX872-B was administered to an unresectable PDAC patient population in combination with FOLFORINOX and achieved an ORR of 30% to 37%, 12-week tumor control rate of 78%, and 18-month OS of 29% (31,32). BMS-813160 is a combined CCR2/5 inhibitor that is being evaluated in combination with gemcitabine and nab-paclitaxel in untreated patients and in combination with nivolumab in previously treated patients (NCT03184870). CCR5 is expressed on T-cells, Tregs, and PDAC cells and is believed to play a role in immune tolerance and metastatic progression (33,34). PF04136309 has also demonstrated early efficacy in combination with FOLFIRINOX (ORR = 49%) and gemcitabine and nab-paclitaxel (ORR 60%) in phase I study (30,35). Phase II study of gemcitabine and nab-paclitaxel, however, was terminated early, and no further study is being pursued at this time.

Macrophage Colony Stimulating Factor-1 (CSF-1)
CSF-1 is secreted by PDAC cells and is crucial for survival of TAMs. Inhibition of CSF-1 receptor (CSF1-R) decreases TAMs in the TME and leads to increased expression of PD-L1 and CTLA-4 (36). Cabiralizumab, a monoclonal antibody against CSF1-R6, is designed to deplete TAMs in the TME. Early study in combination with nivolumab in heavily treated patients (45% ≥3 prior regimens) found 3/21 PDAC patients with partial responses of 293, 275+, and 168+ days duration, 1 prolonged stable disease of 182 days, and 1 patient treated beyond disease progression who experienced a >40% reduction in baseline target lesions with 247 days on study (37). Cabiralizumab is being studied in a randomized phase II trial in combination with nivolumab with and without chemotherapy (NCT03336216). CSF1R inhibition in combination with checkpoint blockade is an active area of study with multiple trials recruiting: AMG820 in combination with pembrolizumab (NCT02713529), pexidartinib with durvalumab (NCT02777710), and MCS110 in combination with PDR001 (NCT02807844).

Focal Adhesion Kinase (FAK)
FAK is a nonreceptor tyrosine kinase whose activity is upregulated in PDAC cells. It is an important regulator of desmoplasia and creation of an immunosuppressive microenvironment through regulation of certain chemokine expressions including CXCL12 and CCL5 (38). Preclinical models have shown that FAK inhibition decreases infiltration of fibroblast activation protein (+) fibroblasts, MDSCs, TAMs, and Tregs and sensitizes previously resistant PDAC models to PD-1 therapy (39). Multiple studies of FAK inhibitors are under way. GSK2256098 is in phase II study in combination with the MEK inhibitor trametinib (NCT02428270), and defactinib is being studied in phase I in combination with gemcitabine and pembrolizumab (NCT02546531) and in phase I/II with pembrolizumab (NCT02758587).

TARGETED THERAPIES

Despite extensive study of EGFR, PDGFR, and KRAS/MAPK pathway antagonists, targeted therapy for the major part has not been a successful endeavor in PDAC. Cell cycle inhibition is a novel therapeutic target that is under extensive evaluation in PDAC. Cell cycle dysregulation is a hallmark of malignancy and in PDAC specifically critical cell cycle regulator genes, *TP53* and *CDKN2*, are among the most common mutations. Inactivation of *TP53* and *CDKN2* products, p16 and p21, leads to cell cycle dysregulation through downstream disinhibition of cyclin/cyclin dependent kinase (CDK) cell cycle progression. CDK inhibitors are approved in breast cancer including first line in HER2 negative hormone receptor positive cancers in combination with antihormonal therapy (40). In PDAC, CDK inhibitors have shown efficacy in xenograft models and multiple CDK inhibitors are in clinical trials in combination with targeted agents and chemotherapeutics (41). Palbociclib is being studied with nab-paclitaxel (NCT02501902) and carboplatin or cisplatin (NCT02897375), whereas ribociclib and abemaciclib are in clinical study in combination with MEK inhibitors, PI3K/AKT/MTOR inhibitors, and TGF-B antagonists (NCT02985125, NCT02703571, NCT02981342).

METABOLIC TARGETING

The PDAC microenvironment is a relatively acellular, avascular, hypoxic environment. Tumor metabolic adaptations to this environment include a reliance on anaerobic metabolism, glutamate metabolism, and autophagy. Additionally, PDAC cells have been found to be deficient in certain enzymes required for amino acid generation. These characteristics may allow for targeting tumor metabolism with minimal off-target effects. ADI-PEG 20 is a pegylated form of arginine deiminase designed to deplete arginine in cells with low arginine succinate synthetase. It has been evaluated in a dose finding study with expansion cohort receiving ADI-PEG in combination with gemcitabine and nab-paclitaxel. Response rate for patients treated with the recommended phase II dose in first-line setting was 45.5% (5/11) with median PFS of 6.1 months and median OS of 11.3 months (42). Further development is planned. Eryaspase, a red blood cell encapsulated L-asparaginase, aims to deplete asparagine in tumors impairing protein synthesis. In a phase II study of second-line therapy with eryaspase in combination with either gemcitabine or fluorouracil, leucovorin, and oxaliplatin (FOLFOX), a survival advantage of 7.1 weeks was seen in the eryaspase treated group (26.1 vs. 19.0 weeks, HR: 0.57, *p* = .03) (43). CPI-613 targets pyruvate dehydrogenase and alpha-ketoglutarate in the tricarboxylic acid cycle, leading to decreased mitochondrial export of anabolic intermediates necessary for resistance and recovery from chemotherapy. In a phase I dose finding study in combination with FOLFIRINOX, metastatic patients treated at the maximum dose of CPI-613 had an ORR of 61% including 17% with complete responses. Median OS had not been reached but was at least 12.4 months (44).

TARGETING DNA DAMAGE REPAIR DEFICIENCY

Pathogenic germline alterations occur in approximately 20% of PDAC patients, half of which occur in homologous recombination genes *BRCA1/2* (8.1%) and *ATM* (1.8%). However, in this cohort 41.8% of patients with pathogenic germline alterations did not meet current guidelines for germline testing. Given the underdiagnosis and actionability of these mutations, universal germline screening may be warranted (45).

As discussed in Chapter 25, *How I Treat* Metastatic Pancreatic Cancer With Chemotherapy, patients with DNA damage repair deficits, specifically in homologous recombination, have improved responses to platinum-based therapy. Platinum agents create DNA cross-links, which lead to double-strand DNA breaks, which are repaired through homologous recombination. Poly ADP-ribose polymerase is required for repair of single-strand breaks, which if not repaired, become double-strand DNA breaks, which if not repaired, for example due to homologous combination deficiency, leads to apoptosis (46). Multiple PARP inhibitors are approved for the treatment of *BRCA* mutant ovarian cancers and are under investigation in pancreas cancer. Olaparib monotherapy was evaluated in a phase II study in 23 patients with PDAC who had previous gemcitabine therapy. Patients had a 22% response rate and 35% stable disease rate with 1-year survival of 41% (47). Olaparib is being investigated in a phase III registration trial as maintenance therapy versus placebo in patients with *BRCA* mutations who have been stable on platinum therapy for 16 weeks (POLO study, NCT02184195). It is also being studied in patients with "BRCAness" defined as no *BRCA* mutation, but a family history of *BRCA* related malignancies (NCT02677038). Veliparib monotherapy was evaluated in patients with known germline *BRCA1/2* or *PALB2* mutations whose disease had progressed on one or two lines of treatment. Response rates were modest with no confirmed responses and 25% stable disease in a 16-patient cohort, with modest results likely due in major part to prior platinum exposure and resistance (48). In combination with gemcitabine and cisplatin in a phase I dose finding study, seven out of nine patients with *BRCA* mutations had an objective response and median OS was 23.3 months, compared to 11 months for *BRCA* (–) patients (49). Veliparib is being studied in *BRCA 1/2* and *PALB2* mutations in combination with gemcitabine/cisplatin versus gemcitabine/cisplatin as first-line therapy or alone in previously treated patients (NCT01585805) and as second line with FOLFIRI versus FOLFIRI without requirement for *BRCA* mutation (NCT02890355).

Clinical Vignette 26.1

Case 1: A 68-year-old male presents with newly diagnosed metastatic pancreatic ductal adenocarcinoma (PDAC) to the liver. He has no personal history of cancer. He has one sister with breast cancer and his mother had ovarian cancer. He is in excellent health with no medical comorbidities and no limitations in functional status. He would like to pursue aggressive therapy and is interested in investigational clinical trials.

Case 2: A 72-year-old female with metastatic PDAC to liver and lung whose disease has now progressed on first-line 5-fluorouracil, leucovorin, irinotecan, and oxaliplatin (FOLFIRINOX). She has no personal or family history of malignancy. She has no comorbidities and continues to work as an accountant. She is interested in investigational therapy.

Treating the Patient

Case 1: The patient has a good performance status without medical comorbidities and is therefore an appropriate candidate for enrollment in a clinical trial for frontline investigational therapy. He has two family members with *BRCA*-associated cancers and therefore would benefit for genetic testing for DNA damage repair deficiency (dDDR). If he has a mutation in a DNA damage repair gene (*BRCA 1/2, ATM, PALB2*), he would be a candidate for combination therapy with a platinum agent and PARP inhibitor, currently being evaluated in a prospective trial or a trial evaluating the role of olaparib as maintenance therapy. If he does not have a dDDR tumor, first-line clinical trials utilizing a cytotoxic backbone in combination with immunotherapeutics or stromal disrupting therapy may be pursued. A few examples include the CCR 2/5 inhibitor, BMS-813160, on a backbone of gemcitabine and nab-paclitaxel (NCT03184870); the CD40 agonist, APX005M, with nivolumab, gemcitabine, and nab-paclitaxel (NCT03214250); and PEGPH20 also with gemcitabine and nab-paclitaxel (NCT02715804).

Case 2: The patient has an Eastern Cooperative Oncology Group (ECOG) performance status of 0 or 1, no medical comorbidities, and her disease has progressed on frontline FOLFIRINOX. She is therefore a candidate for second-line investigational therapies. Many investigational strategies are available for patients whose disease has progressed on frontline therapy, and enrollment depends on patient preference and study availability. Several relevant trials have been outlined earlier and in Table 26.1 and include studies of checkpoint inhibitors with cytotoxic chemotherapy, checkpoint inhibitors with chemokine inhibitors, bispecific antibodies, adoptive cell transfer, and targeted therapies.

TABLE 26.1 Selected Ongoing Clinical Trials for Patients With Metastatic PDAC

Clinical Trial Identifier/ Status	Therapeutic Agents	Mechanism of Action	Treatment Line	Phase	Outcome Measures
NCT02715804	GN +/− PEGPH20	PEGPH20: pegylated recombinant hyaluronidase	1st line	III	PFS, OS
NCT02715531	Atezolizumab and GN	Atezolizumab: anti-PD-L1 antibody	1st line	I	AE
NCT03214250	GN with nivolumab, APX005M, or both	Nivolumab: anti-PD-1 antibody, APX005M: CD40 agonist antibody	1st line	I/II	AEs, OS

(continued)

TABLE 26.1 Selected Ongoing Clinical Trials for Patients With Metastatic PDAC (*continued*)

Clinical Trial Identifier/ Status	Therapeutic Agents	Mechanism of Action	Treatment Line	Phase	Outcome Measures
NCT02309177 Active, not recruiting	Nivolumab with nab-paclitaxel +/− gemcitabine	Nivolumab: anti-PD-1 antibody	1st line and previously treated	I	DLTs, AEs
NCT03184870	BMS-813160 with GN, nivolumab or alone	BMS-813160: CCR2/5 inhibitor	1st line with GN 2nd line with nivolumab, alone	I/II	AEs, DLTs, ORR, PFS
NCT02331251 Active, not recruiting	Pembrolizumab with GN	Pembrolizumab: anti-PD-1 antibody	No prior GN	I/II	1b: RP2D 2: AEs, RR, OS, PFS
NCT03374852 Not yet recruiting	CPI-1613 with mFOLFIRINOX	CPI-1613: pyruvate dehydrogenase and alpha-ketoglutarate inhibitor	1st line	II	OS
NCT01585805	1st line: gemcitabine, cisplatin +/− veliparib; Previously treated: velaparib	Velaparib: PARP inhibitor	1st line in combination, previously treated in monotherapy	II	Part I: RP2D, ORR combination Part II: ORR veliparib alone
NCT03193190	Intervention: Atezolizumab with cobimetinib, PEGPH20, or BL-8040 Control: GN or FOLFOX	Atezolizumab: anti-PD-L1 antibody, cobimetinib: MEK inhibitor, PEGPH20: pegylated recombinant hyaluronidase, BL-8040: CXCR4 inhibitor	2nd line	I/II	ORR, AEs
NCT02890355	mFOLFIRI and veliparib	Veliparib: PARP inhibitor	2nd line	II	OS
NCT03269526	Anti-CD3 x anti-EGFR-bispecific antibody armed activated T-cells		Any treatment line after one dose of chemotherapy	I/II	AEs, OS
NCT01583686	Anti-mesothelin CART and aldesleukin with cyclophosphamide and fludarabine preconditioning	Aldesleukin: IL-2	Previously treated	I/II	Safety
NCT02587689	anti-MUC1 CART		Previously treated	I/II	Phase I: AE

(*continued*)

TABLE 26.1 Selected Ongoing Clinical Trials for Patients With Metastatic PDAC (*continued*)

Clinical Trial Identifier/ Status	Therapeutic Agents	Mechanism of Action	Treatment Line	Phase	Outcome Measures
NCT02826486	BL-8040 and pembrolizumab	BL-8040: CXCR4 inhibitor pembrolizumab: anti-PD-L1 antibody	Previously treated	II	ORR
NCT02179970	Plerixafor	Plerixafor: CXCR4 antagonist	Previously treated	I	AE
NCT03336216	Intervention: cabiralizumab with nivolumab with GN, FOLFOX, or alone Control: GN or 5-FU/LV/ nanoliposomal irinotecan	Cabiralizumab: CSF1R inhibitor	Previously treated	II	PFS
NCT02713529	AMG820 and pembrolizumab	AMG820: anti-CSF1R antibody, pembrolizumab: anti-PD-1 antibody	Previously Treated	I/II	Phase I: AE Phase II: ORR
NCT02777710	Durvalumab and pexidartinib	Durvalumab: anti-PD-L1 antibody, pexidartinib: CSF-1 receptor antagonist	Previously treated	I	Part 1: DLT Part 2: ORR
NCT02807844	MCS110 and PDR001	MCS110: anti-macrophage CSF Mab, PDR001: anti-PD-1 antibody	Previously treated	I/II	Phase I: AE Phase II: ORR
NCT02703571	Ribociclib with trametinib	Ribociclib: CDK4/6 inhibitor	Previously treated	I/II	DLTs, ORR
NCT02981342	Intervention: abemaciclib with LY3023414 or galunisertib Control: gemcitabine or capecitabine	Abemaciclib: CDK4/6 inhibitor LY3023414: dual PI3K/mTOR inhibitor galunisertib: TGF-β receptor antagonist	Previously treated	II	Part I: DCR Part II: PFS
NCT02184195	Olaparib	Olaparib: PARP inhibitor	Stable on platinum x 16 weeks, germline *BRCA* mutation	III	PFS

(*continued*)

TABLE 26.1 Selected Ongoing Clinical Trials for Patients With Metastatic PDAC (*continued*)

Clinical Trial Identifier/ Status	Therapeutic Agents	Mechanism of Action	Treatment Line	Phase	Outcome Measures
NCT02677038	Olaparib	Olaparib: PARP inhibitor	Previously treated "*BRCA*ness"	II	ORR
NCT02501902	Palbociclib with nab-paclitaxel	Palbociclib CDK4/6 inhibitor	No prior treatment with study agents	I w/ expansion	DLT
NCT02897375	Palbociclib with cisplatin or carboplatin	Pabociclib: CDK4/6 inhibitor	No treatment in preceding 4 weeks	I w/ expansion	AEs, DLTs, RP2D
NCT02546531	Defactinib, pembrolizumab, and gemcitabine	Defactinib: FAK inhibitor, Pembrolizumab: anti-PD-1 antibody	I: Failed SOC Expansion: 2nd line, Maintenance if stable on frontline	I w/ expansion	MTD
NCT02324257	RO6958688 +/–obinutuzumab	RO6958688: CD3/CEA bispecific antibody Obinutuzumab: anti-CD20 antibody	Failed SOC	I	AEs, DLTs, pharmaco-kinetics
NCT02758587	Defactinib with pembrolizumab	Defactinib: FAK inhibitor, Pembrolizumab: anti-PD-1 antibody	Failed SOC	I/II	AEs
NCT02985125	Ribociclib with everolimus	Ribociclib: CDK4/6 inhibitor	Failed 5-FU and gemcitabine-containing regimens	I/II	PFS
NCT02744287	BPX-601, rimiducid	BPX-601: antiprostate stem cell antigen CART	Failed SOC	I	MTD, DLTs
NCT03018405	NKR-2 cells	NK receptor CART	Refractory	I/II	AEs

AE, adverse events; CART, chimeric antigen receptor T-cell; CDK, cyclin dependent kinase; CSF1R, macrophage colony stimulating factor-1 receptor; DCR, disease control rate; DLT, dose limiting toxicity; FAK, focal adhesion kinase; FOLFIRI, fluorouracil/leucovorin/irinotecan; FOLFIRINOX, fluorouracil/leucovorin/irinotecan/oxaliplatin; FOLFOX, fluorouracil/leucovorin/ oxaliplatin; GN, gemcitabine/nab-paclitaxel; MTD, maximum tolerated dose; ORR, objective response rate; OS, overall survival; PARP, poly-ADP ribose reductase; PDAC, pancreatic ductal adenocarcinoma; PFS, progression-free survival; RP2D, recommended phase 2 dose; SOC, standard of care.

REFERENCES

1. American Cancer Society. Cancer facts & figures: 2018. Atlanta, GA: American Cancer Society. https://www.cancer.org/research/cancer-facts-statistics/all-cancer-facts-figures/cancer-facts-figures-2018.html2018

2. National Comprehensive Cancer Network. NCCN Clinical Practice Guidelines in Oncology: Pancreatic Adenocarcinoma (Version 3.2017). 2017; https://www.nccn.org/professionals/physician_gls/pdf/pancreatic.pdf

3. Von Hoff DD, Ervin T, Arena FP, et al. Increased survival in pancreatic cancer with nab-paclitaxel plus gemcitabine. *N Engl J Med.* 2013;369(18):1691–1703. doi:10.1056/NEJMoa1304369

4. Conroy T, Desseigne F, Ychou M, et al. FOLFIRINOX versus gemcitabine for metastatic pancreatic cancer. *N Engl J Med.* 2011;364(19):1817–1825. doi:10.1056/NEJMoa1011923

5. Wang-Gillam A, Li CP, Bodoky G, et al. Nanoliposomal irinotecan with fluorouracil and folinic acid in metastatic pancreatic cancer after previous gemcitabine-based therapy (NAPOLI-1): a global, randomised, open-label, phase 3 trial. *Lancet.* 2016;387(10018):545–557. doi:10.1016/S0140-6736(15)00986-1

6. Surveillance, Epidemiology, and End Results (SEER) Program (www.seer.cancer.gov). *SEER*Stat Database: Incidence - SEER 18 Regs Research Data + Hurricane Katrina Impacted Louisiana Cases, Nov 2016 Sub (2000–2014).* National Cancer Institute D, Surveillance Research Program, Surveillance Systems Branch.

7. Sohal DP, Mangu PB, Khorana AA, et al. Metastatic pancreatic cancer: American Society of Clinical Oncology clinical practice guideline. *J Clin Oncol.* 2016;34(23):2784–2796. doi:10.1200/JCO.2016.67.1412

8. Moffitt RA, Marayati R, Flate EL, et al. Virtual microdissection identifies distinct tumor- and stroma-specific subtypes of pancreatic ductal adenocarcinoma. *Nat Genet.* 2015;47(10):1168–1178. doi:10.1038/ng.3398

9. Provenzano PP, Cuevas C, Chang AE, et al. Enzymatic targeting of the stroma ablates physical barriers to treatment of pancreatic ductal adenocarcinoma. *Cancer Cell.* 2012;21(3):418–429. doi:10.1016/j.ccr.2012.01.007

10. Whatcott CJ, Diep CH, Jiang P, et al. Desmoplasia in primary tumors and metastatic lesions of pancreatic cancer. *Clin Cancer Res.* 2015;21(15):3561–3568. doi:10.1158/1078-0432.CCR-14-1051

11. Hingorani SR, Bullock AJ, Seery TE, et al. Randomized phase II study of PEGPH20 plus nab-paclitaxel/gemcitabine (PAG) vs AG in patients (Pts) with untreated, metastatic pancreatic ductal adenocarcinoma (mPDA). *J Clin Oncol.* 2017;35(15_suppl):4008–4008. doi:10.1200/jco.2017.35.15_suppl.4008

12. Yu KH, Mantha S, Tjan C, et al. Pilot study of gemcitabine, nab-paclitaxel, PEGPH20, and rivaroxaban for advanced pancreatic adenocarcinoma: an interim analysis. *J Clin Oncol.* 2018;36(4_suppl):405–405. doi:10.1200/jco.2018.36.4_suppl.405

13. Ramanathan RK, McDonough S, Philip PA, et al. A phase IB/II randomized study of mFOLFIRINOX (mFFOX) + pegylated recombinant human hyaluronidase (PEGPH20) versus mFFOX alone in patients with good performance status metastatic pancreatic adenocarcinoma (mPC): SWOG S1313 (NCT #01959139). *J Clin Oncol.* 2018;36(4_suppl):208–208. doi:10.1200/jco.2018.36.4_suppl.208

14. Loos M, Giese NA, Kleeff J, et al. Clinical significance and regulation of the costimulatory molecule B7-H1 in pancreatic cancer. *Cancer Lett.* 2008;268(1):98–109. doi:10.1016/j.canlet.2008.03.056

15. O'Reilly EM, Oh D-Y, Dhani N, et al. A randomized phase 2 study of durvalumab monotherapy and in combination with tremelimumab in patients with metastatic pancreatic ductal adenocarcinoma (mPDAC): ALPS study. *J Clin Oncol.* 2018;36(4_suppl):217–217. doi:10.1200/jco.2018.36.4_suppl.217

16. Kalyan A, Kircher SM, Mohindra NA, et al. Ipilimumab and gemcitabine for advanced pancreas cancer: A phase Ib study *J Clin Oncol* 2016;34(15_suppl):e15747–e15747. doi:10.1200/jco.2016.34.15_suppl.e15747

17. Aglietta M, Barone C, Sawyer MB, et al. A phase I dose escalation trial of tremelimumab (CP-675,206) in combination with gemcitabine in chemotherapy-naive patients with metastatic pancreatic cancer. *Ann Oncol.* 2014;25(9):1750–1755. doi:10.1093/annonc/mdu205

18. Balachandran VP, Luksza M, Zhao JN, et al. Identification of unique neoantigen qualities in long-term survivors of pancreatic cancer. *Nature.* 2017;551(7681):512–516. doi:10.1038/nature24462

19. Vonderheide RH, Bajor DL, Winograd R, et al. CD40 immunotherapy for pancreatic cancer. *Cancer Immunol Immunother.* 2013;62(5):949–954. doi:10.1007/s00262-013-1427-5

20. Beatty GL, Torigian DA, Chiorean EG, et al. A phase I study of an agonist CD40 monoclonal antibody (CP-870,893) in combination with gemcitabine in patients with advanced pancreatic ductal adenocarcinoma. *Clin Cancer Res.* 2013;19(22):6286–6295. doi:10.1158/1078-0432.CCR-13-1320

21. Heyderman E, Larkin SE, O'Donnell PJ, et al. Epithelial markers in pancreatic carcinoma: immunoperoxidase localisation of DD9, CEA, EMA and CAM 5.2. *J Clin Pathol.* 1990;43(6):448–452. doi:10.1136/jcp.43.6.448

22. Beatty GL, O'Hara MH, Nelson AM, et al. Safety and antitumor activity of chimeric antigen receptor modified T cells in patients with chemotherapy refractory metastatic pancreatic cancer. *J Clin Oncol.* 2015;33(15_suppl):3007–3007.

23. Sorrento Therapeutics Autologous Anti-CEA CAR-T Cell Therapy for Liver Metastases Demonstrates Therapeutic Activity in Stage IV Pancreas Cancer in a Phase 1b HITM-SURE Trial (NCT02850536) [press release]. 2018; http://investors.sorrentotherapeutics.com/news-releases/news-release-details/sorrento-therapeutics-autologous-anti-cea-car-t-cell-therapy

24. Le DT, Lutz E, Uram JN, et al. Evaluation of ipilimumab in combination with allogeneic pancreatic tumor cells transfected with a GM-CSF gene in previously treated pancreatic cancer. *J Immunother.* 2013;36(7):382–389. doi:10.1097/CJI.0b013e31829fb7a2

25. Sanford DE, Belt BA, Panni RZ, et al. Inflammatory monocyte mobilization decreases patient survival in pancreatic cancer: a role for targeting the CCL2/CCR2 axis. *Clin Cancer Res.* 2013;19(13):3404–3415. doi:10.1158/1078-0432.CCR-13-0525

26. Steele CW, Karim SA, Leach JD, et al. CXCR2 Inhibition profoundly suppresses metastases and augments immunotherapy in pancreatic ductal adenocarcinoma. *Cancer Cell.* 2016;29(6):832–845. doi:10.1016/j.ccell.2016.04.014

27. Feig C, Jones JO, Kraman M, et al. Targeting CXCL12 from FAP-expressing carcinoma-associated fibroblasts synergizes with anti-PD-L1 immunotherapy in pancreatic cancer. *Proc Natl Acad Sci U S A.* 2013;110(50):20212–20217. doi:10.1073/pnas.1320318110

28. Hidalgo MM, Epelbaum R, Semenisty V, et al. Evaluation of pharmacodynamic (PD) biomarkers in patients with metastatic pancreatic cancer treated with BL-8040, a novel CXCR4 antagonist. *J Clin Oncol.* 2018;36(4_suppl):276–276. doi:10.1200/jco.2018.36.4_suppl.276

29. Wang-Gillam A, Noel MS, Sleijfer S, et al. The inhibition of CCR2 to modify the microenvironment in pancreatic cancer mouse model and to support the profiling of the CCR2 inhibitor CCX872-B in patients. *J Clin Oncol.* 2016;34(15_suppl):e15743–e15743. doi:10.1200/jco.2016.34.15_suppl.e15743

30. Nywening TM, Wang-Gillam A, Sanford DE, et al. Targeting tumour-associated macrophages with CCR2 inhibition in combination with FOLFIRINOX in patients with borderline resectable and locally advanced pancreatic cancer: a single-centre, open-label, dose-finding, non-randomised, phase 1b trial. *Lancet Oncol.* 2016;17(5):651–662. doi:10.1016/s1470-2045(16)00078-4

31. Noel MS, Hezel AF, Linehan D, et al. Orally administered CCR2 selective inhibitor CCX872-b clinical trial in pancreatic cancer. *J Clin Oncol* 2017;35(4_suppl):276–276. doi:10.1200/jco.2017.35.4_suppl.276

32. Linehan D, Noel MS, Hezel AF, et al. Overall survival in a trial of orally administered CCR2 inhibitor CCX872 in locally advanced/metastatic pancreatic cancer: Correlation with blood monocyte counts. *J Clin Oncol.* 2018;36(5_suppl):92–92. doi:10.1200/jco.2018.36.5_suppl.92

33. Singh SK, Banerjee S, Lillard JW, et al. Expression of CCR5 and its ligand CCL5 in pancreatic cancer. *J Immunol.* 2016;196(1 Supplement):51.53–51.53.

34. Ward ST, Li KK, Hepburn E, et al. The effects of CCR5 inhibition on regulatory T-cell recruitment to colorectal cancer. *Br J Cancer.* 2014;112:319. doi:10.1038/bjc.2014.572

35. Noel M, Lowery M, Ryan D, et al. Phase Ib study of PF-04136309 (an oral CCR2 inhibitor) in combination with nab-paclitaxel/gemcitabine in first-line treatment of metastatic pancreatic adenocarcinoma. *Ann Oncol.* 2017;28(suppl_5):257–257. doi:10.1093/annonc/mdx369.132

36. Zhu Y, Knolhoff BL, Meyer MA, et al. CSF1/CSF1R blockade reprograms tumor-infiltrating macrophages and improves response to T-cell checkpoint immunotherapy in pancreatic cancer models. *Cancer Res.* 2014;74(18):5057–5069. doi:10.1158/0008-5472.CAN-13-3723

37. Wainberg Z, Piha-Paul S, Luke J, et al. First-in-human phase 1 dose escalation and expansion of a novel combination, anti–CSF-1 receptor (cabiralizumab) plus anti–PD-1 (nivolumab), in patients with advanced solid tumors. *J Immunother Cancer.* 2017;5(Suppl 3_O42):89.

38. Symeonides SN, Anderton SM, Serrels A. FAK-inhibition opens the door to checkpoint immunotherapy in pancreatic cancer. *J Immunother Cancer.* 2017;5:17. doi:10.1186/s40425-017-0217-6

39. Jiang H, Hegde S, Knolhoff BL, et al. Targeting focal adhesion kinase renders pancreatic cancers responsive to checkpoint immunotherapy. *Nat Med.* 2016;22(8):851–860. doi:10.1038/nm.4123

40. FDA Approves Abemaciclib as Initial Therapy for HR-Positive, HER2-Negative Metastatic Breast Cancer [press release]. 2018; https://www.fda.gov/Drugs/InformationOnDrugs/ApprovedDrugs/ucm598404.htm

41. Feldmann G, Mishra A, Bisht S, et al. Cyclin-dependent kinase inhibitor dinaciclib (SCH727965) inhibits pancreatic cancer growth and progression in murine xenograft models. *Cancer Biol Ther.* 2011;12(7):598–609. doi:10.4161/cbt.12.7.16475

42. Lowery MA, Yu KH, Kelsen DP, et al. A phase 1/1B trial of ADI-PEG 20 plus nab-paclitaxel and gemcitabine in patients with advanced pancreatic adenocarcinoma. *Cancer.* 2017;123(23):4556–4565. doi:10.1002/cncr.30897

43. Hammel P, Bachet J, Portales F, et al. A Phase 2b of eryaspase in combination with gemcitabine or FOLFOX as second-line therapy in patients with metastatic pancreatic adenocarcinoma (NCT02195180). *Ann Oncol.* 2017;28(suppl_5):211-211. doi:10.1093/annonc/mdx369.005

44. Alistar A, Morris BB, Desnoyer R, et al. Safety and tolerability of the first-in-class agent CPI-613 in combination with modified FOLFIRINOX in patients with metastatic pancreatic cancer: a single-centre, open-label, dose-escalation, phase 1 trial. *Lancet Oncol.* 2017;18(6):770–778. doi:10.1016/S1470-2045(17)30314-5

45. Lowery MA, Wong W, Jordan EJ, et al. Prospective evaluation of germline alterations in patients with exocrine pancreatic neoplasms. *J Natl Cancer Inst.* 2018;110(10):1067–1074. doi:10.1093/jnci/djy024

46. Ashworth A. A synthetic lethal therapeutic approach: poly(ADP) ribose polymerase inhibitors for the treatment of cancers deficient in DNA double-strand break repair. *J Clin Oncol.* 2008;26(22):3785–3790. doi:10.1200/JCO.2008.16.0812

47. Kaufman B, Shapira-Frommer R, Schmutzler RK, et al. Olaparib monotherapy in patients with advanced cancer and a germline BRCA1/2 mutation. *J Clin Oncol.* 2015;33(3):244–250. doi:10.1200/JCO.2014.56.2728

48. Lowery MA, Kelsen DP, Capanu M, et al. Phase II trial of veliparib in patients with previously treated BRCA-mutated pancreas ductal adenocarcinoma. *Eur J Cancer.* 2018;89:19–26. doi:10.1016/j.ejca.2017.11.004

49. O'Reilly EM, Lee JW, Lowery MA, et al. Phase 1 trial evaluating cisplatin, gemcitabine, and veliparib in 2 patient cohorts: Germline BRCA mutation carriers and wild-type BRCA pancreatic ductal adenocarcinoma. *Cancer.* 2018;124(7):1374–1382. doi:10.1002/cncr.31218

Hepatocellular Cancer

Epidemiology of Hepatocellular Cancer

Safi Shahda and Bert H. O'Neil

INTRODUCTION

According to the International Agency for Research on Cancer, liver cancer is the fifth most common cancer in men and the ninth in women; and it is largely a problem of the less developed regions (1). Worldwide, liver cancer is responsible for 782,000 new cases, with 83% of these cases occurring in underdeveloped regions (50% in China alone). Of this total number, 554,000 occurred in men (7.5% of all cancer cases in men) and 228,000 occurred in women (3.4% of all cancer cases in women). Gender disparity is not fully understood biologically, but has been attributed to sex hormones' role in interleukin-6 (IL-6) production in the liver as mediated by Kupffer cells (2).

Hepatocellular carcinoma (HCC) represents the most common primary liver malignancy; in approximately 80% of cases, it is associated with chronic hepatitis B or C (3). The etiology of HCC varies based on geographic location and endemic diseases. For example, while immunization for hepatitis B virus (HBV) is a common practice in the United States and other developed countries, HBV continues to be a leading cause for HCC in sub-Saharan Africa and East Asia (4). This affects the variability of age at diagnosis from country to country, due to time of exposure to HBV and age at contracting the infection. HCC is rarely seen during the first four decades of life except in populations where HBV infection is endemic and HBV is contracted at birth. While HCC is on the decline among the world's highest incidence regions, it has been on the rise in the past two decades in regions with low incidence rates (e.g., United States) (5). Moreover, the most common cause of HCC in the West is cirrhosis associated with hepatitis C virus (HCV) and alcohol abuse. The development of effective, well-tolerated therapy to eradicate HCV will likely shift the incidence rate of HCV-related HCC over the next two decades (6). However, the rapid increase in the obesity epidemic has given rise to increased diagnosis of nonalcoholic fatty liver disease (NAFLD) and nonalcoholic steatohepatitis (NASH). In turn, these disorders have increased rates of HCC unrelated to alcohol or viral hepatitis.

In the United States, the incidence of HCC has increased from 1.4 per 100,000 between 1975 and 1977 to 4.8 per 100,000 in 2005–2007, and the greatest increase was observed in Blacks and Hispanics (1). The rising incidence continued as of 2012, and this increase was observed across all ethnic and racial groups, although it is higher in men between the ages of 55 and 59 (7). Approximately half of the increase in HCC cases was attributed to the aging cohort with chronic HCV infection. HBV accounts for 10% to 15% of HCC cases in the United States; less than 5% are infected with both viruses and 30% to 35% have neither HCV nor HBV. Hereby, we review risk factors of HCC and their role in hepatocarcinogenesis.

HEPATITIS B VIRUS

HBV is a member of the hepadnaviridae virus family, and it is a small, partially double-stranded DNA. It specifies a small number of known gene products, including a reverse transcriptase/DNA polymerase, capsid protein, envelope proteins (L, M, and S) as well as proteins of uncertain function such as "X" and "e."

HBV is the leading risk factor for HCC globally, which contributes to more than 50% of all cases worldwide (8). In endemic areas where the prevalence is high and HBV vaccine is not readily available, HBV is acquired vertically during birth where >90% of exposed infants become chronic carriers. While HBV is known to cause HCC in the absence of cirrhosis, the majority (70%–90%) of HBV-related HCCs occur in the context of underlying liver cirrhosis. HBV likely contributes directly to hepatocarcinogenesis by integrating viral DNA into previously normal hepatocytes—where HBV DNA has been isolated from human HCC as well as HCC cell lines (9). Several factors are associated with increased incidence including: demographics (male gender, Asian and African ancestry), viral related (higher HBV viral load, coinfection with HCV, HIV, and hepatitis D virus [HDV]), and environmental (smoking, heavy alcohol intake, and exposure to aflatoxin). In the Western world, estimates of incidence of HCC in the setting of HBV are 0.02 per 100 person-years in inactive carriers, 0.3 in chronic carriers without cirrhosis, and 2.2 in subjects with compensated cirrhosis (3).

HEPATITIS C VIRUS

HCV is classified in the Hepacivirus genus within the Flaviviridae family. HCV infection is a highly dynamic process with a viral half-life of only a few hours. This high replicative activity, together with the lack of a proofreading function of the viral RdRp, is the basis of the high genetic variability of HCV (10). There are six major genotypes that differ in their nucleotide sequence by 30% to 35%. In the United States and Western Europe, genotypes 1a and 1b are most common followed by genotypes 2 and 3. The other genotypes are virtually never found in these countries but are common in other areas, such as Egypt (genotype 4), South Africa (genotype 5), and Southeast Asia (genotype 6) (11). This provides the foundation for drug development and understanding resistance patterns for HCV therapy (12).

HCV is most prevalent in persons with history of injection drug use and recipients of blood products before the 1990s (when routine testing for HCV became widely available). Sexual transmission of the virus is not common, and tends to co-occur in subjects who are coinfected with HIV. However, coinfection with HIV increases the risk of sexual and maternal–fetal transmission of HCV. Patients are typically asymptomatic during the acute phase, and chronic infection is generally silent until cirrhosis develops. The duration between acute infection and cirrhosis generally exceeds a decade (13). In contrast to HBV, most patients who become infected with HCV develop chronic infection. This is because clearance of viremia is rare due to the ability of HCV to evade the immune system (14,15).

The model of natural progression of HCV infection is well established. Progression from acute to chronic infection occurs in 80% of patients, which in turn leads to cirrhosis in nearly 20% leading to HCC risk of 1% to 4% per year (16). Co-occurrence of HIV, HBV, or alcohol abuse can accelerate this progression to cancer (17).

IMPACT OF EFFECTIVE ANTI-HCV THERAPY ON HCC

Due to the direct correlation between HCV infection and the development of cirrhosis and HCC, one would anticipate that eliminating HCV would lead to decreased incidence of HCC. However, several factors need to be taken into account when addressing this question. The presence of other risk factors known to contribute to HCC development, the presence of already established cirrhosis, and other medical comorbidities such as obesity, diabetes, and smoking affect risk of HCC even after HCV eradication. Unfortunately, most studies that address these questions (and have adequate follow-up) date to the era of less effective therapy such as interferon. These older studies demonstrated decreased risk of HCC in patients with sustained viral response (SVR); however, the risk continues in subjects with cirrhosis even after eradicating HCV (18–20).

The development of direct antiviral agents (DAA) that have favorable toxicity profile and a higher "cure" rate holds the promise to eliminate HCV (21) and HCV-related HCC. Unfortunately, recent small studies have reported alarming results of *increased* incidence of HCC, and also increased recurrence after curative resection following successful anti-HCV therapy utilizing DAA (22–24). However, these studies have several limitations including inadequate sample size, lack of control, retrospective nature, and heterogeneous populations. In contrast, a large retrospective study evaluating 22,500 subjects treated across the Veterans Affairs Medical Centers in the United States receiving DAA was conducted (25). Compared to subjects without SVR, achieving SVR was associated with a *lower* incidence of de novo HCC: 0.90 versus 3.45 HCC/100 person-years; adjusted HR: 0.28, 95% confidence interval (CI): 0.22–0.36. This study supports that effective treatment for HCV would likely minimize HCV-related HCC, and therefore, screening for persons at risk for HCV with a goal to treat and cure prior to developing HCV-related liver disease would be of great value.

ALCOHOL-RELATED HCC

The relation between HCC and heavy alcohol intake is also well established (26). Alcohol-related cirrhosis and HCC are more commonly seen in the Western world and certain Asian countries. Heavy drinking is defined as drinking more than 60 to 80 gm of alcohol per day. Data suggest that even smaller amounts of alcohol have an impact on increased risk of HCC compared to never drinkers (27); however, a steep increase is observed in incidence for amounts >60 gm/day. Furthermore, there is a synergistic effect when viral hepatitis is present in conjunction with heavy alcohol intake. There appears to be a twofold increase for each viral (HCV or HBV) hepatitis (28). The working hypothesis is that alcohol contributes to the development of HCC via stepwise liver cirrhosis, but other mechanisms have been proposed including chromosomal loss, oxidative stress, modulation of retinoid turnover, DNA methylation, and alteration of the innate immune response (29). Prior to identifying hepatitis C, many studies have claimed a high rate of incidence of HCC in patients with alcoholic cirrhosis. However, epidemiologic studies have demonstrated that HCV infection is more prevalent in people with alcohol abuse.

NONALCOHOLIC STEATOHEPATITIS/NONALCOHOLIC FATTY LIVER DISEASE

NASH and NAFLD are associated with obesity and metabolic disorder, which in the light of the obesity pandemic are both on the rise (30). Reports indicate that nearly 25% of the U.S. population has NAFLD, and a subset of these patients will develop NASH (31). In one study of 328 patients, prevalences of NAFLD and NASH were 46% and 12%, respectively. Diabetics and Hispanics are at a higher risk for developing NAFLD and NASH (32). The distinction between these two conditions is challenging with noninvasive measures. Population-based studies suggest that nearly 6% to 8% of the U.S. population has NASH and 1.5% to 2% has NASH-related cirrhosis, twice as many as those with HCV-related cirrhosis. NASH with or without cirrhosis is a well-known risk factor for HCC, with increased risk when combined with underlying HCV infection or alcohol intake (33). NAFLD induces HCC via complex mechanisms. Preclinical models demonstrate several deregulated pathways in patients with NAFLD-associated HCC, including NFkB, PI3K-AKT-PTEN, and dysregulated microRNAs (34,35).

There are clinically distinct features of NAFLD-associated HCC, including older age, more women, and lesser degree of cirrhosis compared with viral hepatitis mediated HCC. Additionally, serum alpha-fetoprotein (AFP) is more modestly elevated in NAFLD-related HCC compared with virally mediated HCC. Despite these differences, patients with NASH-related HCC appear to have similar survival rates in comparison to other HCC etiologies.

REFERENCES

1. Mittal S, El-Serag HB. Epidemiology of hepatocellular carcinoma: consider the population. *J Clin Gastroenterol*. 2013;47 Suppl:S2–S6. doi:10.1097/MCG.0b013e3182872f29
2. Naugler WE, Sakurai T, Kim S, et al. Gender disparity in liver cancer due to sex differences in MyD88-dependent IL-6 production. *Science*. 2007;317(5834):121–124. doi:10.1126/science.1140485
3. El-Serag HB. Epidemiology of viral hepatitis and hepatocellular carcinoma. *Gastroenterology*. 2012;142(6):1264–1273.e1. doi:10.1053/j.gastro.2011.12.061
4. Lavanchy D. Hepatitis B virus epidemiology, disease burden, treatment, and current and emerging prevention and control measures. *J Viral Hepat*. 2004;11(2):97–107. doi:10.1046/j.1365-2893.2003.00487.x
5. El-Serag HB, Kanwal F. Epidemiology of hepatocellular carcinoma in the United States: where are we? where do we go? *Hepatology*. 2014;60(5):1767–1775. doi:10.1002/hep.27222
6. Lieberman J, Sarnow P. Micromanaging hepatitis C virus. *N Engl J Med*. 2013;368(18):1741–1743. doi:10.1056/NEJMe1301348
7. White DL, Thrift AP, Kanwal F, et al. Incidence of hepatocellular carcinoma in all 50 United States, from 2000 through 2012. *Gastroenterology*. 2017;152(4):812–820.e5. doi:10.1053/j.gastro.2016.11.020
8. Perz JF, Armstrong GL, Farrington LA, et al. The contributions of hepatitis B virus and hepatitis C virus infections to cirrhosis and primary liver cancer worldwide. *J Hepatol*. 2006;45(4):529–538. doi:10.1016/j.jhep.2006.05.013

9. Brechot C, Pourcel C, Louise A, et al. Presence of integrated hepatitis B virus DNA sequences in cellular DNA of human hepatocellular carcinoma. *Nature*. 1980;286(5772):533–535. doi:10.1038/286533a0

10. Moradpour D, Penin F, Rice CM. Replication of hepatitis C virus. *Nat Rev Microbiol*. 2007;5(6):453–463. doi:10.1038/nrmicro1645

11. Bukh J, Miller RH, Purcell RH. Genetic heterogeneity of hepatitis C virus: quasispecies and genotypes. *Semin Liver Dis*. 1995;15(1):41–63. doi:10.1055/s-2007-1007262

12. Lauer GM, Walker BD. Hepatitis C virus infection. *N Engl J Med*. 2001;345(1):41–52. doi:10.1056/NEJM200107053450107

13. Hajarizadeh B, Grebely J, Dore GJ. Epidemiology and natural history of HCV infection. *Nat Rev Gastroenterol Hepatol*. 2013;10(9):553–562. doi:10.1038/nrgastro.2013.107

14. Gale M Jr, Foy EM. Evasion of intracellular host defence by hepatitis C virus. *Nature*. 2005;436(7053):939–945. doi:10.1038/nature04078

15. Li XD, Sun L, Seth RB, et al. Hepatitis C virus protease NS3/4A cleaves mitochondrial antiviral signaling protein off the mitochondria to evade innate immunity. *Proc Natl Acad Sci U S A*. 2005;102(49):17717–17722. doi:10.1073/pnas.0508531102

16. Kiyosawa K, Sodeyama T, Tanaka E, et al. Interrelationship of blood transfusion, non-A, non-B hepatitis and hepatocellular carcinoma: analysis by detection of antibody to hepatitis C virus. *Hepatology*. 1990;12(4 Pt 1):671–675. doi:10.1002/hep.1840120409

17. Pineda JA, Romero-Gómez M, Díaz-García F, et al. HIV coinfection shortens the survival of patients with hepatitis C virus-related decompensated cirrhosis. *Hepatology*. 2005;41(4):779–789. doi:10.1002/hep.20626

18. Aleman S, Rahbin L, Weiland O, et al. A risk for hepatocellular carcinoma persists long-term after sustained virologic response in patients with hepatitis C-associated liver cirrhosis. *Clin Infect Dis*. 2013;57(2):230–236. doi:10.1093/cid/cit234

19. El-Serag HB, Kanwal F, Richardson P, et al. Risk of hepatocellular carcinoma after sustained virological response in veterans with hepatitis C virus infection. *Hepatology*. 2016;64(1):130–137. doi:10.1002/hep.28535

20. van der Meer AJ, Feld JJ, Hofer H, et al. Risk of cirrhosis-related complications in patients with advanced fibrosis following hepatitis C virus eradication. *J Hepatol*. 2017;66(3):485–493. doi:10.1016/j.jhep.2016.10.017

21. Chung RT, Baumert TF. Curing chronic hepatitis C—the arc of a medical triumph. *N Engl J Med*. 2014;370(17):1576–1578. doi:10.1056/NEJMp1400986

22. Conti F, Buonfiglioli F, Scuteri A, et al. Early occurrence and recurrence of hepatocellular carcinoma in HCV-related cirrhosis treated with direct-acting antivirals. *J Hepatol*. 2016;65(4):727–733. doi:10.1016/j.jhep.2016.06.015

23. Ravi S, Axley P, Jones D, et al. Unusually high rates of hepatocellular carcinoma after treatment with direct-acting antiviral therapy for hepatitis C related cirrhosis. *Gastroenterology*. 2017;152(4):911–912. doi:10.1053/j.gastro.2016.12.021

24. Reig M, Mariño Z, Perelló C, et al. Unexpected high rate of early tumor recurrence in patients with HCV-related HCC undergoing interferon-free therapy. *J Hepatol*. 2016;65(4):719–726. doi:10.1016/j.jhep.2016.04.008

25. Kanwal F, Kramer J, Asch SM, et al. Risk of hepatocellular cancer in HCV patients treated with direct-acting antiviral agents. *Gastroenterology*. 2017;153(4):996–1005.e1. doi:10.1053/j.gastro.2017.06.012

26. Stickel F, Schuppan D, Hahn EG, et al. Cocarcinogenic effects of alcohol in hepatocarcinogenesis. *Gut*. 2002;51(1):132–139. doi:10.1136/gut.51.1.132

27. LoConte NK, Brewster AM, Kaur JS, et al. Alcohol and cancer: a statement of the American Society of Clinical Oncology. *J Clin Oncol*. 2018;36(1):83–93. doi:10.1200/JCO.2017.76.1155

28. Hassan MM, Hwang L-Y, Hatten CJ, et al. Risk factors for hepatocellular carcinoma: synergism of alcohol with viral hepatitis and diabetes mellitus. *Hepatology*. 2002;36(5):1206–1213. doi:10.1053/jhep.2002.36780

29. Seitz HK, Stickel F. Molecular mechanisms of alcohol-mediated carcinogenesis. *Nat Rev Cancer*. 2007;7(8):599–612. doi:10.1038/nrc2191

30. Loomba R, Sanyal AJ. The global NAFLD epidemic. *Nat Rev Gastroenterol Hepatol*. 2013;10(11):686–690. doi:10.1038/nrgastro.2013.171

31. Michelotti GA, Machado MV, Diehl AM. NAFLD, NASH and liver cancer. *Nat Rev Gastroenterol Hepatol*. 2013;10(11):656–665. doi:10.1038/nrgastro.2013.183

32. Williams CD, Stengel J, Asike MI, et al. Prevalence of nonalcoholic fatty liver disease and nonalcoholic steatohepatitis among a largely middle-aged population utilizing ultrasound and liver biopsy: a prospective study. *Gastroenterology*. 2011;140(1):124–131. doi:10.1053/j.gastro.2010.09.038

33. Ascha MS, Hanouneh IA, Lopez R, et al. The incidence and risk factors of hepatocellular carcinoma in patients with nonalcoholic steatohepatitis. *Hepatology*. 2010;51(6):1972–1978. doi:10.1002/hep.23527
34. Stiles B, Wang Y, Stahl A, et al. Liver-specific deletion of negative regulator Pten results in fatty liver and insulin hypersensitivity [corrected]. *Proc Natl Acad Sci U S A*. 2004;101(7):2082–2087. doi:10.1073/pnas.0308617100
35. Baker RG, Hayden MS, Ghosh S. NF-kappaB, inflammation, and metabolic disease. *Cell Metab*. 2011;13(1):11–22. doi:10.1016/j.cmet.2010.12.008

Diagnosis and Staging of Hepatocellular Cancer

Safi Shahda and Bert H. O'Neil

INTRODUCTION

A hepatocellular carcinoma (HCC) diagnosis is established based on a combination of tests including alpha-fetoprotein (AFP), radiographic findings, and (perhaps, less commonly) histology. AFP is neither specific nor sensitive enough to be pathognomonic for a diagnosis of HCC; AFP is elevated in nonmalignant liver disorders and in intrahepatic cholangiocarcinoma (IHCCA). Therefore, the presence of a liver mass suspicious for HCC with elevated AFP does not adequately establish a diagnosis of HCC unless the radiographic findings are consistent with those of HCC. Radiographic diagnosis of HCC requires contrast-enhanced dynamic imaging such as CT or MRI (e.g., a dual- or triple-phase CT or MRI with dynamic contrast imaging). A "typical-appearing" HCC enhances during the arterial phase (the remaining of the liver lacks contrast during the arterial phase) and exhibits "washout" during the venous or delayed phase. The presence of arterial uptake followed by washout is highly specific for HCC in the setting of underlying liver disease. An unenhanced sequence is also important to distinguish proteinaceous fluid or blood from tumor (1).

On occasion, histologic diagnosis of HCC is necessary. Characteristic microscopic morphologic features of HCC include wide trabeculae, a prominent acinar pattern, small cell changes, cytologic atypia, mitotic activity, vascular invasion, absence of Kupffer cells, and the loss of the reticulin network (2). Immunohistochemical markers of HCC include positive staining for glypican 3, HSP 70, and glutamine synthetase. Cytokeratin 7 and 19, typically markers of biliary endothelium, should be negative (3).

HCC is a multifocal disease in 75% of cases at diagnosis. The diagnosis is established based on history and physical, imaging, and serologic markers (AFP > 400 ng/ml). AFP is only elevated in 50% to 75% of cases; therefore, a suspicious lesion on ultrasound in the presence of normal AFP requires a second imaging modality to confirm the diagnosis (4).

SCREENING

It is recommended that high-risk individuals undergo screening for HCC to enable early detection and effective therapy. The only two studies that attempted to address HCC screening in a randomized, controlled manner had substantial limitations in study design and compliance, and interventions once cancer was identified, limiting the ability to definitively develop a conclusion (5,6). Several challenges would be encountered when conducting a prospective randomized clinical trial at this point, precluding such a study. Foremost, a very large sample size is required. Additionally, controlling for variables associated with HCC (e.g., extent of cirrhosis, HCC etiology, active alcohol abuse, smoking, diabetes, geographic region) is difficult.

Screening guidelines have been endorsed by several societies including the American Association of Study of Liver Disease, U.S. Veterans Affairs, World Gastroenterology Association, European Association of the Study of the Liver, and the National Comprehensive Cancer Network (7–9). The screening guidelines include considering active surveillance in a programmatic approach. This would identify patients with high-risk behavior and risk factors for HCC and provide counseling alongside the screening. For individuals with hepatitis B virus (HBV) and hepatitis C virus (HCV), therapeutic interventions as appropriate are recommended. Counseling and alcohol rehab referrals should be offered for patients with alcohol abuse. With the increase in incidence of nonalcoholic fatty liver disease (NAFLD), targeting the root cause such as obesity, hyperlipidemia, poorly controlled diabetes, or other modifiable risk factors should be actively managed.

DEFINITION FOR AT-RISK POPULATION THAT MAY BENEFIT FROM SURVEILLANCE

Population at Risk	Incidence of HCC
Asian male hepatitis B carriers over age 40	0.4%–0.6%/year
Asian female hepatitis B carriers over age 50	0.3%–0.6%/year
Hepatitis B carrier with family history of HCC	Unknown; higher than without a family history
Cirrhotic hepatitis B carriers	3%–8%/year
African/North American Blacks with hepatitis B	Incidence is early in life
Hepatitis C cirrhosis	3%–5%/year
Genetic hemochromatosis and cirrhosis	Unknown, likely >1.5%/year
Alpha-1 antitrypsin deficiency and cirrhosis	Unknown, likely >1.5%/year

HCC, hepatocellular carcinoma.

Due to the incidence rate in HBV carriers, it is recommended to start screening Asian men at age 40 and Asian women at age 50. However, African Americans tend to develop HBV-related HCC at a younger age, and therefore, it is recommended to start screening at age 20. All HBV carriers with cirrhosis, regardless of age should be screened for HCC. There is strong correlation between HBV viral load and risk of HCC (10). In the case of a family history of HCC, surveillance should start at an age younger than 40, although the appropriate age has not been defined. In Caucasian HBV carriers with no cirrhosis and with inactive hepatitis, as determined by a long-term normal ALT and low HBV DNA viral load, the incidence of HCC is probably too low to justify active surveillance. However, there are additional risk factors that have to be taken into account, including older age, persistence of viral replication and coinfection with hepatitis C or HIV, or the presence of other underlying liver diseases. Nonetheless, even in the absence of cirrhosis, adult Caucasian patients with active disease are likely to be at risk for HCC and should be screened.

The risk of HCC in patients with chronic HCV is highest and has been best studied in patients who have established cirrhosis, in whom the incidence of HCC is between 2% and 8% per year. A prospective, population-based study of the risk of HCC in patients with anti-HCV antibodies demonstrated a 20-fold increased risk of HCC compared to anti-HCV-negative subjects (11). The presence or absence of cirrhosis was not evaluated in this study. HCV infected individuals who do not have cirrhosis have a much lower risk of developing HCC. Based on current knowledge, all patients with HCV and liver cirrhosis should undergo surveillance.

Patients who are coinfected with HIV and either HBV or HCV may have more rapidly progressive liver disease and (12) when they reach cirrhosis, they are also at increased risk of HCC (13). The MORTAVIC study indicated that HCC was responsible for 25% of all liver-related deaths in the post-HAART era in HIV infected individuals (14). The criteria for entering coinfected patients into programs for HCC screening are the same as for monoinfected patients.

The rate of HCC related to alpha-1 antitrypsin deficiency or autoimmune hepatitis is unknown, and there are insufficient data from epidemiologic studies to accurately assess the rate of HCC and support screening recommendations.

STAGING

HCC represents a unique malignancy in which the extent of cancer is not the only determinant of therapeutic options. Commonly used functional measures such as Karnofsky Performance Score (KPS) and Eastern Cooperative Oncology Group (ECOG) score are very relevant measurements; but equally important is the liver function impairment commonly seen in patients with HCC due to underlying cirrhosis. Therefore, several staging systems attempted to address these variables. Hereby, we review commonly used systems.

Tumor, Node, and Metastasis (TNM)

It takes into account the tumor size, location, nodal status, and the presence or absence of metastases. The recently published updated TNM staging system varies from prior versions by further characterizing T stage. This newly proposed system clearly demonstrates differences across T stages (T1a, T1b, T2, and T3) in patients who undergo resection. However, this system does not take into account the extent of cirrhosis or tumor histology. It is the only staging system that has been validated prospectively in patients treated with liver resection or transplantation.

Okuda Staging System

This system was developed based on retrospective analysis of 850 patients describing the natural history of HCC in untreated patients based on tumor size and simplified liver function analysis of ascites, bilirubin, and albumin. For patients with Okuda stage I, II, and III, median survival was 8.3, 2.0, and 0.7 months, respectively. This system does not take into account the vascular involvement or the presence of extrahepatic disease including organ and nodal metastases. Therefore, it is used for patients who are not surgical candidates, and it is purely a clinical scoring system (15).

Cancer of the Liver Italian Program (CLIP) Score

This prognostic score accounts for tumor-related factors such as tumor marker (AFP), vascular invasion, single versus multinodular disease, and the extent of liver involvement. It additionally accounts for liver function by incorporating the Child–Pugh score and portal vein thrombosis (16). Several studies have suggested the superiority of the CLIP scoring system when compared to others, in which based on a CLIP score ranging from 0 to 6, prognosis varied significantly (31 to 2 months) (17).

Barcelona Clinic Liver Cancer (BCLC) Staging System

This system constitutes four stages incorporating the underlying liver disease, performance status, and the presence of extrahepatic disease and vascular involvement (18). Unlike previously discussed systems, it provides an algorithmic approach to patients' care as opposed to a patient-centered approach. Studies evaluating the prognostic value of HCC staging systems determined that the BCLC staging model provides the most accurate prognostic assessment. This is by and large due to the elements involved in this modeling, which include liver-specific, tumor-specific, and patient-specific assessments (19).

REFERENCES

1. Jelic S, Sotiropoulos GC, on behalf of the ESMO Guidelines Working Group. Hepatocellular carcinoma: ESMO clinical practice guidelines for diagnosis, treatment and follow-up. *Ann Oncol.* 2010;21 Suppl 5:59–64. doi:10.1093/annonc/mdq166
2. Schlageter M, Terracciano LM, D'Angelo S, et al. Histopathology of hepatocellular carcinoma. *World J Gastroenterol.* 2014;20(43):15955–15964. doi:10.3748/wjg.v20.i43.15955
3. Libbrecht L, Severi T, Cassiman D, et al. Glypican-3 expression distinguishes small hepatocellular carcinomas from cirrhosis, dysplastic nodules, and focal nodular hyperplasia-like nodules. *Am J Surg Pathol.* 2006;30(11):1405–1411. doi:10.1097/01.pas.0000213323.97294.9a
4. Bruix J, Sherman M, American Association for the Study of Liver Diseases. Management of hepatocellular carcinoma: an update. *Hepatology.* 2011;53(3):1020–1022. doi:10.1002/hep.24199
5. Zhang BH, Yang BH, Tang ZY. Randomized controlled trial of screening for hepatocellular carcinoma. *J Cancer Res Clin Oncol.* 2004;130(7):417–422. doi:10.1007/s00432-004-0552-0
6. Chen JG, Parkin DM, Chen Q-G, et al. Screening for liver cancer: results of a randomised controlled trial in Qidong, China. *J Med Screen.* 2003;10(4):204–209. doi:10.1258/096914103771773320
7. Ferenci P, Fried M, Labrecque D, et al. World Gastroenterology Organisation Guideline. Hepatocellular carcinoma (HCC): a global perspective. *J Gastrointestin Liver Dis.* 2010;19(3):311–317. doi:10.1097/MCG.0b013e3181d46ef2
8. Garcia-Tsao G, Lim JK, Members of the Veterans Affairs Hepatitis C Resource Center Program. Management and treatment of patients with cirrhosis and portal hypertension: recommendations from the Department of Veterans Affairs Hepatitis C Resource Center Program and the National Hepatitis C Program. *Am J Gastroenterol.* 2009;104(7):1802–1829. doi:10.1038/ajg.2009.191

9. European Association for the Study of the Liver, European Organisation for Research and Treatment of Cancer. EASL-EORTC clinical practice guidelines: management of hepatocellular carcinoma. *J Hepatol.* 2012;56(4):908–943. doi:10.1016/j.jhep.2011.12.001

10. Chen CJ, Yang H-I, Su J, et al. Risk of hepatocellular carcinoma across a biological gradient of serum hepatitis B virus DNA level. *JAMA.* 2006;295(1):65–73. doi:10.1001/jama.295.1.65

11. Sun CA, Wu DM, Lin C-C, et al. Incidence and cofactors of hepatitis C virus-related hepatocellular carcinoma: a prospective study of 12,008 men in Taiwan. *Am J Epidemiol.* 2003;157(8):674–682. doi:10.1093/aje/kwg041

12. Bica I, McGovern B, Dhar R, et al. Increasing mortality due to end-stage liver disease in patients with human immunodeficiency virus infection. *Clin Infect Dis.* 2001;32(3):492–497. doi:10.1086/318501

13. Salmon-Ceron D, Lewden C, Morlat P, et al. Liver disease as a major cause of death among HIV infected patients: role of hepatitis C and B viruses and alcohol. *J Hepatol.* 2005;42(6):799–805. doi:10.1016/j.jhep.2005.01.022

14. Lewden C, May T, Rosenthal E, et al. Changes in causes of death among adults infected by HIV between 2000 and 2005: the "Mortalite 2000 and 2005" surveys (ANRS EN19 and Mortavic). *J Acquir Immune Defic Syndr.* 2008;48(5):590–598. doi:10.1097/QAI.0b013e31817efb54

15. Okuda K, Ohtsuki T, Obata H, et al. Natural history of hepatocellular carcinoma and prognosis in relation to treatment. Study of 850 patients. *Cancer.* 1985;56(4):918–928. doi:10.1002/1097-0142(19850815)56:4<918::AID-CNCR2820560437>3.0.CO;2-E

16. The Cancer of the Liver Italian Program (CLIP) Investigators. Prospective validation of the CLIP score: a new prognostic system for patients with cirrhosis and hepatocellular carcinoma. *Hepatology.* 2000;31(4):840–845. doi:10.1053/he.2000.5628

17. Farinati F, Rinaldi M, Gianni S, et al. How should patients with hepatocellular carcinoma be staged? Validation of a new prognostic system. *Cancer.* 2000;89(11):2266–2273. doi:10.1002/1097-0142(20001201)89:11<2266::AID-CNCR15>3.0.CO;2-0

18. Llovet JM, Bru C, Bruix J. Prognosis of hepatocellular carcinoma: the BCLC staging classification. *Semin Liver Dis.* 1999;19(3):329–338. doi:10.1055/s-2007-1007122

19. Marrero JA, Fontana RJ, Barrat A, et al. Prognosis of hepatocellular carcinoma: comparison of 7 staging systems in an American cohort. *Hepatology.* 2005;41(4):707–716. doi:10.1002/hep.20636

Cellular and Molecular Pathology of Hepatocellular Cancer

Safi Shahda and Bert H. O'Neil

INTRODUCTION

Hepatocellular carcinoma (HCC) is a clinically heterogeneous disease that frequently arises in a liver with underlying cirrhosis; however, occasionally HCC is discovered in a liver without underlying pathology. The various causes of HCC lead to cancer via different mechanisms, which are likely associated with specific molecular patterns (1). The hepatitis B virus (HBV) genome is commonly identified in HCC when compared to its adjacent noncancer liver tissue. Additionally, HBV-associated HCC is frequently associated with mutations such as *TERT*, *MLL4*, and *CCNE1*.The extent of HBV genomic integration has been reportedly associated with survival (2). In contrast, hepatitis C virus (HCV) leads to defined molecular events along the progression from cirrhosis to dysplasia to HCC. Pathway analysis of microarray data has revealed dysregulation of the Notch and Toll-like receptor pathways in cirrhosis, followed by deregulation of the JAK/STAT pathway in early carcinogenesis, followed by upregulation of genes involved in DNA replication and repair and cell cycle once cancer is established (3).

HCC is the product of chronic and active inflammation associated with viral hepatitis or chronic inflammation associated with fatty infiltration or alcohol exposure. HCC formation is heavily dependent on the tumor immune microenvironment. In patients with resected HCC (4), the balance between regulatory T (Treg) cells and cytotoxic T-lymphocytes (CTLs) may influence prognosis. In one study of this question, 5-year overall survival (OS) and disease-free survival (DFS) rates were only 24.1% and 19.8% for resected patients with intratumoral high Tregs and low activated CTLs, compared with 64.0% and 59.4% for the group with intratumoral low Tregs and high activated CTLs. Preclinical models demonstrated that developing resistance to standard-of-care tyrosine kinase inhibitors (TKIs) is associated with tumor immune evasion and could be reversed by immunotherapeutic approaches (5). Additionally, overexpression of programmed death ligand (PD-L) receptors on resected HCC is associated with worse prognosis, underscoring the role of the immune surveillance/evasion in HCC recurrence after curative therapies (6).

Defining molecular pathways and genomic alterations in HCC could lead to effective therapy and individualized treatment selection. The long-standing challenge has been that HCC is frequently diagnosed based on radiographic and serologic findings without the need for tissue confirmation. Additionally, since HCC tends to be a vascular tumor, it created a challenge regarding the amount of tissue that could safely be obtained to allow for molecular analysis. In such cases, surgically resected samples, while having limitations, present a resource to understand drivers of HCC.

In one study (7), 243 surgically resected tumors underwent whole codon sequencing across HCC with variable underlying liver disease: cirrhosis (n = 118), fibrosis (n = 46), and none fibrotics (n = 79). Additional risk factors were noted including alcohol abuse (41%), HCV infection (26%), nonalcoholic steatohepatitis (NASH; 18%), HBV infection (14%), hemochromatosis (7%), and others (11%). In this study, 28,478 somatic mutations were identified, of which 6,184 occurred in one tumor with hypermutated phenotype. Excluding this sample, the investigators identified a median of 21 silent and 64 nonsilent mutations per tumor (ranging from 1 to 706 mutations in total), corresponding to a mean somatic mutation rate in coding sequences of 1.3 mutations per megabase. Alterations with frequency >5% could be grouped into 11 pathways: telomere maintenance (60%), Wnt-B-catenin (54%), PI3K-AKT-mTOR (51%), p53/cell cycle (49%), MAPK (43%), hepatic differentiation (34%), epigenetic regulators (32%), chromatic remodeling (28%), oxidative stress (12%), IL-6/JAK-STAT (9%), and TGFb (5%). These investigators went on to explore mutational signatures associated with pathogenesis of HCC. In a subset of patients, co-exposure to alcohol and tobacco was associated with higher mutation rates, presence of alterations in B-catenin pathway, and the absence of cirrhosis, suggesting that a genotoxic effect could be the culprit in hepatocarcinogenesis. Furthermore, this analysis revealed that 28% of genomic alterations could be targeted with currently Food and Drug Administration (FDA) approved drugs and 86% by drugs in clinical trials.

The Cancer Genome Atlas network has conducted a comprehensive integrative analysis of HCC: 363 samples were analyzed by whole-exome sequencing; a subset of them, 196 samples, underwent comprehensive analysis including DNA methylation, RNA, miRNA, and proteomic analysis. In total, 12,136 genes had nonsilent mutations, and 26 genes were determined to be significantly mutated genes (SMGs) by the MutSigCV algorithm. Of these 26 genes, 18 were reported as SMGs previously, which included TP53, WNT pathway, and the chromatin remodeling genes. Among the 26 MutSigCV-identified SMGs were eight genes not previously considered HCC drivers. *LZTR1* encodes an adaptor of CUL3-containing E3 ligase complexes and was mutated in 10 of 377 HCC (3%). Other genes identified as significantly mutated by MutSigCV included *AZIN1*, *RP1L1*, *EEF1A1*, *GPATCH4*, *CREB3L3*, *AHCTF1*, and *HIST1H1C*. None of these genes have been reported as drivers in HCC previously.

CHARACTERIZING MUTATIONAL SIGNATURE

Applying algorithmic analysis to enrich for mutational signatures, specific patterns were identified; one signature is associated with aristolochic acid, and another is associated with aflatoxin B1 (AFB1) exposure, which is associated with the point mutation *R249S* in the *TP53* gene. Recurrent *TP53-R249S* mutant samples had significant enrichment of AFB1 signature activity in comparison to other *TP53* mutants or WT samples. HBV-positive samples had much higher AFB1 activity than HBV-negative HCC, indicating a likely synergy in hepatocarcinogenesis.

Comparison of genome-scale DNA methylation profiles in normal tissue and HCC revealed significant amounts of both hypo- and hypermethylation in the tumors. Unsupervised clustering of HCC using CpG sites that showed cancer-specific DNA hypermethylation identified four hypermethylation clusters. Two clusters exhibited elevated hypermethylation. One in particular contained all of the tumors with *IDH1/2* mutations. A third cluster disproportionately enriched for CDKN2A epigenetic silencing, *TERT* promoter mutations, and *CTNNB1* mutations. Analysis of copy number variations identified reoccurring amplifications in driver oncogenes, such as CCND1, FGF19, MYC, MET, VEGFA, MCL1, and TERT; and deletions in tumor suppressor genes were apparent for RB1, CDKN2A, ERRFI1, and NCOR1.

When comparing molecular findings to the hepatitis etiology, HCC samples associated with HBV were significantly more likely to be mutated in TP53 and significantly less likely to harbor *TERT* promoter mutations than HBV-negative HCC. In contrast, HCV-related HCC displayed significantly increased frequency of *CDKN2A* promoter silencing and *TERT* promoter mutation.

Heterogeneity is a concept that has long been recognized in cancer evolution; however, a recent study demonstrated intratumor heterogeneity in regard to genomic and epigenetic changes in HCC (8). This study highlighted the role hepatocarcinogenesis plays, including the early stages of mutation evolution affecting the development of HCC. Utilizing noninvasive tools such as circulating tumor cells may enable further quantitative and qualitative analysis of HCC-associated circulating tumor cells, which also could be utilized as a surrogate marker for response to therapy (9).

These analyses highlight the variable drivers across HCC pathologies and therefore, molecular signatures. This will likely affect future drug development to select treatment based on genomic aberrations, utilizing newer technologies including liquid biopsies to further assign patients to matched therapeutic options.

REFERENCES

1. Thorgeirsson SS, Grisham JW. Molecular pathogenesis of human hepatocellular carcinoma. *Nat Genet*. 2002;31(4):339–346. doi:10.1038/ng0802-339
2. Sung WK, Zheng H, Li S, et al. Genome-wide survey of recurrent HBV integration in hepatocellular carcinoma. *Nat Genet*. 2012;44(7):765–769. doi:10.1038/ng.2295
3. Wurmbach E, Chen Y-b, Khitrov G, et al. Genome-wide molecular profiles of HCV-induced dysplasia and hepatocellular carcinoma. *Hepatology*. 2007;45(4):938–947. doi:10.1002/hep.21622

4. Gao Q, Qiu S-J, Fan J, et al. Intratumoral balance of regulatory and cytotoxic T cells is associated with prognosis of hepatocellular carcinoma after resection. *J Clin Oncol*. 2007;25(18):2586–2593. doi:10.1200/JCO.2006.09.4565

5. Chen YC, Ramjiawan RR, Reiberger T, et al. CXCR4 inhibition in tumor microenvironment facilitates anti-programmed death receptor-1 immunotherapy in sorafenib-treated hepatocellular carcinoma in mice. *Hepatology*. 2015;61(5):1591–1602. doi:10.1002/hep.27665

6. Gao Q, Wang X-Y, Qiu S-J, et al. Overexpression of PD-L1 significantly associates with tumor aggressiveness and postoperative recurrence in human hepatocellular carcinoma. *Clin Cancer Res*. 2009;15(3):971–979. doi:10.1158/1078-0432.CCR-08-1608

7. Schulze K, Imbeaud S, Letouzé E, et al. Exome sequencing of hepatocellular carcinomas identifies new mutational signatures and potential therapeutic targets. *Nat Genet*. 2015;47(5):505–511. doi:10.1038/ng.3252

8. Lin DC, Mayakonda A, Dinh HQ, et al. Genomic and epigenomic heterogeneity of hepatocellular carcinoma. *Cancer Res*. 2017;77(9):2255–2265. doi:10.1158/0008-5472.CAN-16-2822

9. Kalinich M, Bhan I, Kwan TT, et al. An RNA-based signature enables high specificity detection of circulating tumor cells in hepatocellular carcinoma. *Proc Natl Acad Sci U S A*. 2017;114(5):1123–1128. doi:10.1073/pnas.1617032114

How I Treat Early-Stage Hepatocellular Cancer Through Transplant

Emmanouil Giorgakis and Amit K. Mathur

INTRODUCTION

Hepatocellular carcinoma (HCC) is an aggressive malignancy and represents the most common primary hepatic malignancy worldwide, with high prevalence in Eastern and Southeast Asia, and sub-Saharan Africa. In the United States, HCC incidence has tripled over the past three decades, likely related to the growth in incidence of chronic liver disease (1). HCC survival is poor, with an estimated 10% to 15% overall 5-year survival, likely related to advanced stage at diagnosis (2).

Perhaps the greatest advancement in the treatment of HCC has been the development of the Barcelona Clinic Liver Cancer (BCLC) staging and treatment algorithm (Figure 30.1) (3,4). It has served as a clinical guide for HCC management in Western countries for several years, and also frames the clinical investigation of novel locoregional and systemic treatments in clinical trials. Curative treatments for HCC are applicable to very early stage, early-stage, and possibly intermediate-stage disease. There are three potentially curative HCC treatment strategies: liver resection, liver transplantation, and ablative strategies followed by resection or transplantation. Cirrhotics with HCC are candidates for liver transplantation, and in select cases for resection. For those patients not eligible for curative resection or transplant due to tumor burden, underlying hepatic disease, or organ shortage, an array of locoregional and systemic treatments are available to treat patients up front as a bridge to resection and/or transplantation, or as a destination therapy through serial or concurrent therapies. While this has been seen on a limited basis in previous years, new therapeutic strategies have emerged that may transform the clinical management of early- and advanced-stage HCC.

SURVEILLANCE FOR HCC

In order to reduce cancer-related mortality, HCC screening is applied to the at-risk population to detect disease at earlier stages (5). Screening is recommended universally in cirrhotic patients and is applied to those with chronic liver disease including viral hepatitis and non-alcoholic fatty liver disease (NAFLD) (4,6–8). Ultrasound at 6-month intervals is the recommended imaging method for surveillance, with or without alpha-fetoprotein (AFP) levels (9). AFP might improve the performance of ultrasound-based screening, but its cost-effectiveness is the subject of debate (6). When surveying patients for HCC, current guidelines suggest if the ultrasound is positive (identification of a suspicious nodule with size ≥10 mm), in the presence of AFP >100 ng/ml, the patient should undergo further workup with cross-sectional imaging, especially MRI (5,10–12). Indeterminate nodules identified at ultrasound (nodules <10 mm), repeat ultrasound ± AFP should be repeated in 3 to 6 months (Figure 30.2). These guidelines also shape the evaluation of lesions greater than 10 mm.

Once a nodule is identified and cross-sectional imaging is obtained, multiple criteria have been established to make a radiological diagnosis of HCC (12–14). The most specific radiological findings to establish the diagnosis include arterial phase hyperenhancement and delayed (portal) venous phase hypoattenuation, or "washout" with the presence of a coronal pseudocapsule; see Figure 30.3 (12,15). MRI imaging is the preferred radiological method for

---

A Clinical Vignette ("How I Treat") is included at the end of the chapter.

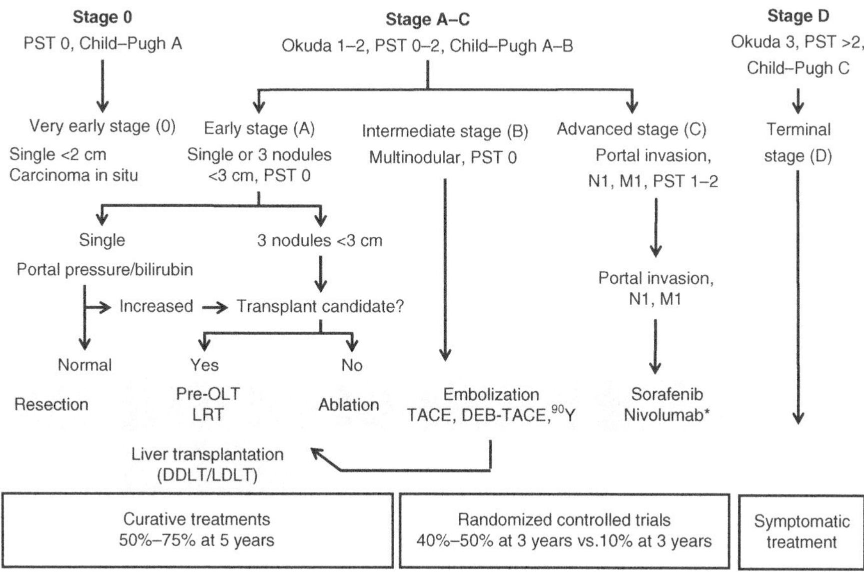

FIGURE 30.1 Adapting the BCLC staging classification and treatment algorithm to current practice.

BCLC, Barcelona Clinic Liver Cancer; DDLT, deceased donor liver transplantation; DEB-TACE, drug-eluting beads transarterial chemoembolization; HVWP, hepatic venous wedge pressure; LDLT, living donor liver transplantation; LRT, locoregional therapy; OLT, orthotopic liver transplantation; PST, performance status test; RFA, radiofrequency ablation; TACE, transarterial chemoembolization.

Adapted Barcelona Clinic Liver Cancer Staging and Treatment Algorithm. The broadly adapted BCLC staging classification for the management of hepatocellular carcinoma incorporates both staging and stratified evidence-based treatment strategies. Very early and early-stage patients with normal bilirubin and HVWP <10 mmHg are suitable for curative treatments such as resection. Liver transplantation is applied in early-stage patients where resection is not possible, and classically, offered to HCC patients within Milan criteria. Most recently, efforts to downstage intermediate HCC patients toward Milan criteria using LRT have been utilized to test tumor biology over time and to offer transplantation to patients who were declined in the past. RFA is the preferred locoregional approach for early-stage lesions provided anatomic considerations are met. Patients with multinodular lesions benefit from TACE, and increasingly with other complementary transarterial therapies including TACE with DEB-TACE and selective ^{90}Y radioembolization. Patients with macroscopic vascular invasion and extrahepatic spread have a first-line treatment with sorafenib, with an expected 3-year survival of 10% to 40%. Immunotherapy with nivolumab and similar drugs has shown benefit in patients who have failed sorafenib and are now the subject of clinical trials in multiple HCC stage subgroups. End-stage patients receive symptomatic and palliative treatments, and have survival less than 3 months. Novel systemic therapy strategies in current clinical trials including checkpoint inhibitors and other immunotherapy strategies may alter this algorithm in years to come.

assessing suspicious hepatic nodules in chronic liver disease patients; its per-lesion sensitivity is superior to CT for lesions ≥10 mm (80% vs. 68%; p = .0023) (16). For lesions <10 mm, per-lesion sensitivity is low with either modality (16). An additional advancement in MR imaging is the addition of gadoxetic acid in protocols to enhance sensitivity in detecting HCC in at-risk patients. Gadoxetic acid–enhanced MRI has higher per-lesion sensitivity versus MRI with other contrast agents (87% vs. 74 %, p = .03) (17). Importantly, these criteria are applied in the at-risk population, as defined, to maintain modest sensitivity but high specificity of the test. Lesions that do not meet these HCC imaging criteria warrant further investigation, including characterization with serial imaging or biopsy.

In high-risk patients who meet radiologic criteria for HCC, no biopsy is needed prior to curative treatment. However, biopsy is indicated if a lesion is highly suspicious but does not meet imaging criteria for HCC, or meets the criteria in circumstances where the individual is not an at-risk individual, or another diagnosis is likely. For example, biopsy would be warranted

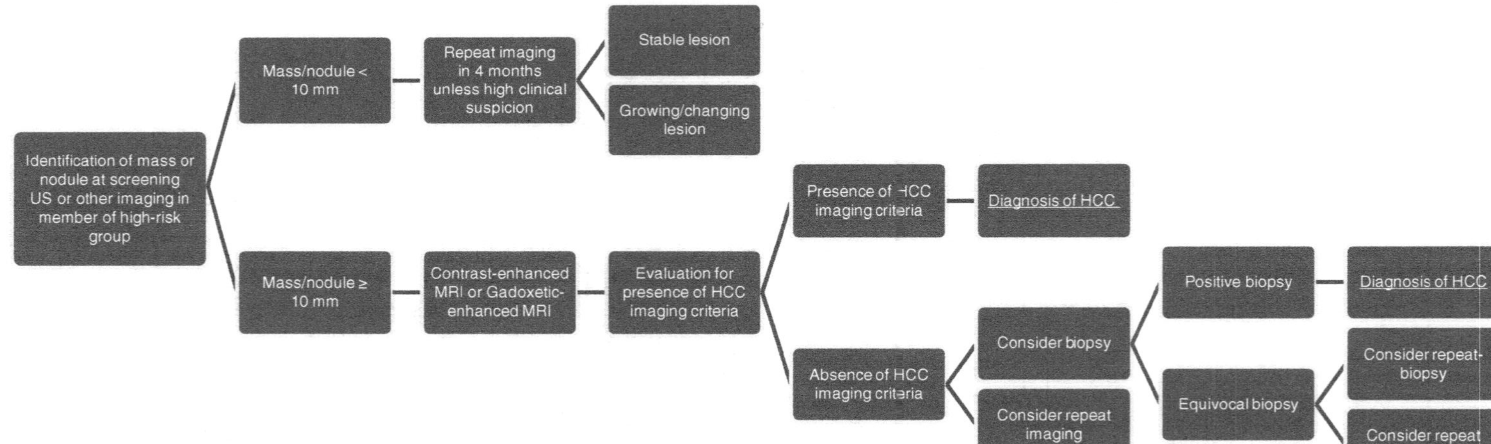

FIGURE 30.2   Algorithm to establish diagnosis of HCC after screening in a high-risk population. This algorithm has been adapted from guidelines published by the European Association for the Study of the Liver and the American Association for the Study of Liver Disease and applied to our current practice. Individuals are considered to be members of a high-risk population for HCC when they have an established diagnosis of cirrhosis and are strongly recommended to be enrolled in an HCC surveillance program. Other members with chronic liver disease may also be screened, but the association between HCC surveillance and mortality reduction is unclear at this time. Screening may be performed with ultrasound with or without the use of AFP as a biomarker. Decision making on the pursuit of an HCC diagnostic evaluation is based on the size of nodule detected at screening; larger lesions require cross-sectional imaging. MRI is our imaging modality of choice, which has higher sensitivity per lesion compared to CT. Imaging allows us to establish the diagnosis of HCC based on validated imaging criteria. In the absence of clear imaging findings to "rule in" HCC, we utilize biopsy to establish a tissue diagnosis.

AFP, alpha-fetoprotein; HCC, hepatocellular carcinoma.

Class 0
- Technically inadequate imaging exam

Class 1
- No evidence of HCC by imaging criteria

Class 2
- Benign appearing lesion or parenchymal abnormality

Class 3
- Indeterminate lesion

Class 4
- Indeterminate lesion with some criteria identified in HCC

Class 5A
- ≥10 mm and <20 mm on late arterial or portal venous phase imaging
- Contrast enhancement in arterial phase with "washout" during delayed phase and peripheral rim enhancement to suggest a "pseudocapsule"

Class 5A–g
- Same size criteria as in 5A but lesion grows in size
- Contrast enhancement in arterial phase and 50% increase in diameter on serial CT/MRI imaging over ≤ 6 months

Class 5B
- ≥20 mm and ≤50 mm
- Contrast enhancement in arterial phase and either 1) washout in delayed phase 2) pseudocapsule development in delayed phase 3) growth by 50% or more on serial CT/MRI ≤6 months s apart or 4) positive tissue diagnosis of HCC

Class 5T
- Previous OPTN 5 or biopsy-proven lesion treated with locoregional therapy

Class 5X
- Size ≥50 mm
- Contrast enhancement in arterial phase and either washout in delayed phase or pseudocapsule enhancement

FIGURE 30.3 OPTN imaging criteria for HCC. In order to standardize the awarding of MELD exception points for HCC in the United States, the OPTN established criteria for HCC based on consensus imaging interpretation guidelines. These criteria allow for standardized reporting of imaging findings and provide clinical context for defining the extent of HCC disease.

OPTN, Organ Procurement and Transplantation Network; HCC, hepatocellular carcinoma; MELD, Model of End-Stage Liver Disease.

if a lesion meets imaging criteria in a noncirrhotic patient, or in the presence of intrahepatic structural or vascular abnormalities such as patients with hepatic congestion from cardiac dysfunction, presence of multifocal focal nodular hyperplasia (FNH), Budd–Chiari syndrome, hereditary hemorrhagic telangiectasia (Osler–Weber–Rendu syndrome), or in patients with concurrent elevations of carcinoembryonic antigen (CEA) or CA19-9, which may indicate other malignant conditions including intrahepatic cholangiocarcinoma, mixed HCC–cholangiocarcinoma, or metastatic disease from other tumors.

DIAGNOSTIC EVALUATION AND STAGING

Once the diagnosis is established, patients require further imaging for extrahepatic staging. HCC frequently metastasizes to the lungs, adrenal glands, bone, and lymph nodes. AFP should be obtained during screening or at the time of diagnosis. Contrast-enhanced chest CT assists in the evaluation of lung metastases. Bone scans are performed selectively during the initial assessment on symptomatic patients or for disease monitoring while on the transplant wait list or posttreatment. Assessment of liver function is critical to guide treatment strategies. Referral to specialty hepatology care is also warranted. Serological tests to evaluate for the presence of viral hepatitis, classification of chronic liver disease severity by Child–Pugh–Turcotte score (Table 30.1) and Model of End-Stage Liver Disease (MELD) score are warranted (18,19). Liver disease severity is an important indicator of survival, and aggressive therapy of moribund patients is discouraged. In the absence of metastatic disease, clinicians should assess performance status and comorbidities.

TABLE 30.1 Child–Turcotte–Pugh Scoring for Severity of Chronic Liver Disease

Clinical and Laboratory Criteria	Points		
	1	2	3
Encephalopathy	None	Grade 1–2	Grade 3–4
Ascites	None	Mild–moderate (diuretic responsive)	Severe (refractory to diuretics)
Bilirubin	<2	2–3	>3
Albumin	>3.5	2.8–3.5	<2.8
Prothrombin time or INR	<4 <1.7	4–6 1.7–2.3	>6 >2.3
CTP Class	**1-Yr Survival**	**2-Yr Survival**	
Class A = Total of 5–6 points	100%	85%	
Class B = Total of 7–9 points	81%	57%	
Class C = Total of 10–15 points	45%	35%	

CTP, Child–Turcotte–Pugh; INR, international normalized ratio.

RESECTION FOR VERY EARLY AND EARLY HCC

The BCLC criteria (Figure 30.1) outline treatment options based on the extent of liver involvement.

Very early (single lesion HCC < 2 cm) and early-stage (single lesion HCC or up to 3 nodules <3 cm) HCCs are amenable to curative treatment. Only 20% to 30% of HCC patients present at this stage, with an estimated 5-year survival of 50% to 70% after therapy (20). Our current approach follows the trajectory of the BCLC algorithm, with some exceptions in intermediate HCC and in developing individualized treatment approaches based on clinical judgment.

Resection of HCC is the treatment of choice in noncirrhotic patients. Assessment of hepatic reserve, the presence of portal hypertension, and cholestasis are critical to identifying whether patients are candidates for resection. In select patients with cirrhosis, namely those without signs of decompensated liver function, resection for HCC has been shown to be a viable treatment option (21–23). Our approach to assessment of portal hypertension includes clinical evaluation of liver reserve, performance status, comorbidities, presence of stigmata of chronic liver disease, laboratory testing to evaluate synthetic liver function, and select application of hepatic venous wedge pressure gradient (portal hypertension is defined by >10 mmHg). Resection is typically reserved for Child's A and B patients with favorable tumor location, suitability of liver remnant, unifocal disease, and good predicted postoperative liver function. Recent data also intimate that central resections on cirrhotic patients with HCC are feasible (24). Tumor anatomy relative to Couinaud sectoral involvement (Figure 30.4) and the preservation and/or reconstruction of vascular and biliary structures are major considerations (25).

In patients with nondiseased livers as much as 75% of the liver may be safely excised. Critics of the use of resection for HCC management in cirrhotic patients cite the potential for de novo carcinogenesis due to a "field defect" related to ongoing inflammation, fibrosis, and regeneration in the remnant liver (26). However, in areas with poor liver donor supply, absence of living donors, or unsuitable transplant candidacy, resection is the treatment of choice provided postoperative liver function will remain preserved. We typically aim for resection when patients fit within this profile: adequate liver function Child–Pugh Class A or B with limited portal hypertension; single mass with no major vascular invasion; adequate vascular and biliary inflow and outflow; and the presence of an adequate future liver remnant (FLR).

Assessing and optimizing FLR are critical to judging the feasibility of resection for HCC. In the United States, volumetric assessment of the liver by cross-sectional imaging is the mainstay of FLR assessment. We define adequate FLR as ≥25% volume without cirrhosis, and ≥40% volume in well-compensated cirrhosis. We apply multiple techniques to induce FLR

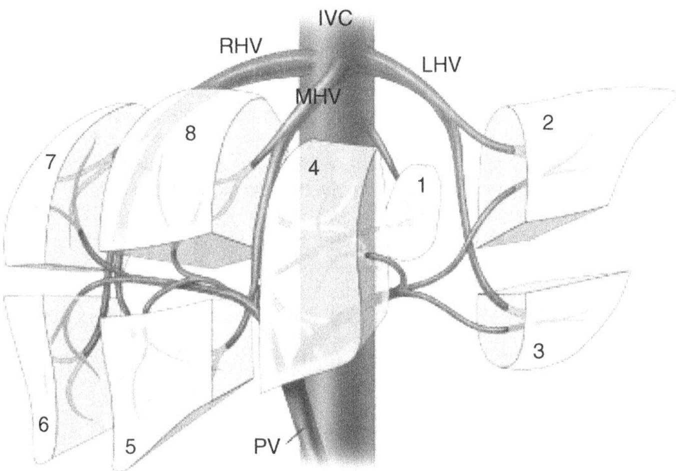

FIGURE 30.4   Segmental anatomy of the liver by the Couinaud classification. Identification of the location of an HCC in the liver is critical to determining the appropriate treatment strategy. When evaluating surgical resectability of an HCC tumor, the Couinaud segmental anatomy is analyzed critically using cross-sectional imaging, typically MR and/or CT, to evaluate vascular inflow and outflow, as well as relevant biliary anatomy.

HCC, hepatocellular carcinoma; IVC, inferior vena cava; LHV, left hepatic vein; MHV, middle hepatic vein; RHV, right hepatic vein.

Source: Reprinted with permission from Brown RS, Jr. Live donors in liver transplantation. *Gastroenterology.* 2008;134(6):1802–1813. doi:10.1053/j.gastro.2008.02.092

hypertrophy. Portal vein embolization (PVE) and ^{90}Y radioembolization are strongly considered prior to major hepatectomy on patients with chronic liver disease to induce hypertrophy of the FLR (27,28). For patients requiring major hepatectomy who fail to gain significant hypertrophy in the FLR, resection should be considered carefully as there may be a higher risk of post-resection hepatic insufficiency and death. An additional approach to inducing FLR that has developed significantly in the past decade has been associating liver partition with portal vein ligation (ALPPS). For staged hepatectomy ALPPS has been primarily applied in the metastatic colorectal metastasis setting but has been applied in the HCC setting as well, albeit with higher mortality (29). We approach the use of these technologies to induce FLR in a multidisciplinary fashion with hepatologists, body radiologists, interventional radiologists, and oncologists.

Traditional teaching suggests that anatomic resections may be the ideal approach for HCC, but this is evolving due to surgical and imaging technological innovations. Laparoscopic techniques have been increasingly applied in hepatobiliary malignancies, with good outcomes. Previous resistance to the use of laparoscopic liver resections was related to fear of catastrophic hemorrhage without direct vascular control, carbon dioxide gas embolization, inadequate control of bile ducts, increased operative time, lack of adequate margins, and other concerns. Several recent technological advances, such as the laparoscopic staplers, thermal coagulative devices, and ultrasonic dissectors, allow for safe ligation and division of the hepatic vasculature, parenchymal transection, hemostasis, and biliary duct ligation. Additional application of hand ports through minilaparotomy incisions facilitates resection, specimen extraction, and improves safety in major resections. A recent large-scale meta-analysis of laparoscopic versus open liver resection for HCC on a total of 5,889 patients showed that laparoscopic hepatectomies were associated with favorable outcomes in operative blood loss, blood transfusion requirements, pathologic resection margins, R0 resection rate, and length of hospital stay, without differences in overall and progression-free survival (30). Numerous single-center reports and recent meta-analysis of long-term survival outcomes of laparoscopic versus open hepatectomy for HCC on cirrhotics showed similar perioperative and oncologic outcomes in selected patients (31).

LOCOREGIONAL THERAPY

We utilize locoregional therapy for HCC as a bridge to curative treatment (resection or transplantation), for those patients who are not considered candidates for surgical curative treatment, or for tumor downstaging. Locoregional therapies may also be considered for unresectable disease, but this is controversial. These treatments encompass a variety of technologies and are most often administered by interventional radiologists, with special interests in the oncological treatment of liver tumors. Notably, there is significant variation in expertise and practice patterns of these evolving technologies.

Selection of the appropriate locoregional therapy is made in a multidisciplinary fashion. Multiple options exist, including ablation, arterially directed therapy including chemoembolization and radioembolization, as well as radiation therapy. Considerations in the selection process include tumor size, location, previous treatment strategies applied, and goals of treatment.

Ablation

Ablation encompasses a vast array of techniques, including monopolar radiofrequency ablation (RFA), multipolar RFA, microwave ablation (MWA), cryoablation, and irreversible electroporation (IRE). RFA is considered one of the principal HCC curative options on cirrhotic patients, along with resection and transplantation (26). RFA may be applied percutaneously, laparoscopically, or via an open surgical approach, and may represent a curative option for small lesions, less than 3 cm in size (32). Larger lesions (3–5 cm in size) are often treated with ablation and arterially directed therapies in combination to prolong survival (33). Classical (monopolar) RFA causes thermal ablation and coagulation necrosis through induction of Joule effect and heat production (reaching 60°C–100°C) from electric current. Given that heat propagates from the energy source (centrifugal ablation), selection of this modality for local tumor control must account for "heat sink effect" related to vascular flow in nearby blood vessels and tumor size, as centrifugal ablation precludes equal tissue necrosis at the periphery versus the center. In order to mitigate these issues and other procedural complications, novel ablation techniques including multibipolar RFA, MWA, and IRE have evolved (26). Results of ablation are excellent. Small HCCs can expect a complete radiological response in more than 95% of the cases and up to 90% pathological response with multipolar ablation (34). HCC recurrence after RFA for lesions within the Milan criteria is 10% to 30% and can be treated with repeated ablation. Local recurrence is likely related to tumor biology or inadequate local treatment, as tumor size and proximity of major vessels are risk factors for relapse (26). Adjuvant systemic therapy with sorafenib after ablation was associated with increased patient harms and no survival benefit in the STORM trial (35).

Arterial-Directed Therapies

Transarterial therapies for HCC employ selective catheterization of branch hepatic arteries that supply the tumor. These are optimally applied to intermediate-stage HCC, although several groups opine that resection may be applied safely to select patients in this group. When resection is not feasible, multiple transarterial options exist. These therapies include bland transarterial embolization (TAE), chemoembolization (TACE), TACE with drug-eluting beads (DEB-TACE), and radioembolization (TARE) with yttrium-90 microspheres (36–39). Selection of modality is considered complementary, but each modality has technical and clinical nuances that must be considered. Local center expertise is paramount to preserving patient safety (40). Most HCC contained by the liver may be amenable to such treatments, but may be contraindicated based on target vessel anatomy and liver function. Relative contraindications include preexisting cholestasis and decompensated liver function (38,39). "Radiation lobectomy" is the term that has emerged to describe selective ^{90}Y radioembolization of Couinaud sectoral arteries and sparing of remaining parenchyma. This has significant promise for BCLC-B HCC treatment as a bridge to curative treatment with resection or transplant (41,42). Additional studies of adjuvant or concomitant sorafenib treatment have not been associated with benefit in two randomized trials (43–45). The utilization of arterial-directed therapies at our center is driven by a multidisciplinary approach. Multispecialty engagement in the care of HCC patients is applied, with technical expertise for TACE, DEB-TACE, and TARE residing in the practices of high-volume interventional radiologists.

Radiation Treatment

The use of external body radiation therapy (EBRT) or stereotactic body radiation therapy (SBRT) is a treatment option in patients with unresectable or inoperable disease, or when intermediate-stage patients cannot be treated with ablation or arterially directed therapies. SBRT is recommended in order to reduce radiation-induced toxicity and optimize treatment accuracy. SBRT is considered an alternative to other ablation techniques since it delivers large ablative doses of radiation; it should therefore be considered when other therapies are contraindicated or have failed (46,47). We typically consider SBRT when treating a limited number of lesions with the goal of sparing as much uninvolved liver as possible. Recently, proton beam therapy has emerged as an additional tool for the treatment of HCC (48), although large-scale dissemination is limited due to the availability of the technology.

LIVER TRANSPLANTATION FOR EARLY AND INTERMEDIATE HCC

Liver transplantation for HCC is reserved for patients with unresectable tumors due to location, inadequate hepatic reserve from chronic liver disease, or high burden of tumor reserve. Conceptually, transplantation as an HCC treatment has inherent appeal—it cures the underlying cirrhosis, thus ridding of the "field defect," and provides maximal locoregional control. In early clinical transplantation, liver transplantation was initially regarded as a failed therapy for HCC due to high recurrence. This persisted into the 1980s due to the lack of sophisticated understanding of appropriate patient selection for liver transplantation. In 1996, Mazzaferro and colleagues from Milan, Italy, initially described excellent outcomes in 48 patients with small unresectable HCC who underwent liver transplantation (49), which heralded the creation of the Milan criteria to guide liver transplantation. These were adopted worldwide. In the United States, the Organ Procurement and Transplantation Network (OPTN), the policy-making body for U.S. transplantation, has adopted Milan Criteria for liver transplantation for the treatment of HCC. These include a single tumor 2 to 5 cm, up to three tumors ≤3 cm each, and the absence of macrovascular involvement or extrahepatic disease. Milan criteria have been validated in multiple studies in subsequent years, and serves as the basis of most modern clinical liver transplant protocols for HCC treatment (50–52).

Presently, there has been reasonable clinical data supporting not just the transplantation of patients within Milan Criteria but also select patients with HCC tumor burden beyond Milan criteria. These evolved due to some inherent limitations of the Milan criteria, including lack of inclusion of important prognostic data such as vascular invasion, tumor differentiation, and the understaging misclassification of HCC patients by imaging versus explant pathology (with retention of good long-term survival) (53–57). The most prominent "beyond Milan" staging systems in North America have been those proposed and utilized by the University of California San Francisco (UCSF) group (58) and by the Baylor group in Dallas, Texas (59,60), and more recently, revised "up-to-seven" criteria by the MetroTicket study group based in Milan (61). Multiple centers have proposed staging criteria based on the tumor size and number of lesions, but few have accounted for additional prognostic signs in transplant patient selection. Sapisochin et al. proposed the extended Toronto criteria that de-emphasize tumor size and number and emphasize differentiation, vascular invasion, cancer symptoms, and hepatic decompensation (62). Their study indicated up to 72% 5-year survival in patients meeting these criteria who were also beyond Milan, and similar prognosis as those within Milan.

Locoregional therapy is typically applied in transplantable patients as a bridge to definitive therapy with total hepatectomy. Success with and advances in locoregional therapy have ushered in a new era of liver transplantation for HCC, where BCLC-B patients can be downstaged into Milan criteria with reasonable overall and progression-free survival after transplantation (63–66). These protocols involve set eligibility criteria, focused locoregional strategy, a waiting period to assess tumor biology, defined end points to determine timeliness of transplant, and dropout from treatment failure. Transplant as the definitive treatment for HCC in this context may be advanced using total hepatectomy followed by deceased donor liver transplantation (DDLT) or living donor liver transplantation (LDLT). This paradigm has many parallels to the ideas advanced in the treatment of other gastrointestinal tumor types, allowing for individualized patient treatment based on tumor biology, patient performance status, therapeutic morbidity, and likelihood of durable long-term survival.

Organ allocation and distribution policies have a significant effect on the development of treatment algorithms for transplant-eligible patients with HCC. Currently, HCC patients in the

United States can be wait-listed for DDLT at any point in time based on their native, biological MELD score. After locoregional therapy for T2 HCC and a mandatory 6-month wait to assess tumor biology, these patients may receive additional MELD exception points to enable them to "compete" for livers with non-HCC patients. These exception points begin at MELD 22 and cap at MELD 34. These cutoffs are the subject of significant ongoing national policy debate at present. This debate is related to variation in deceased donor organ utilization, local organ availability, HCC and non-HCC liver transplant wait-list mortality, and the distribution of scarce resources based on assigned societal value.

In order to maximize opportunities for timely transplantation of HCC patients, our center has taken an egalitarian approach to donor allograft utilization. Besides standard criteria deceased donor livers, we also use marginal deceased donor livers such as those from donors after circulatory death (donation after circulatory death [DCD]), steatotic donor livers, and older donor livers. Well-compensated liver disease recipients—the typical HCC patients listed for transplant—can tolerate early allograft dysfunction associated with DCD and other extended criteria grafts, with comparable oncological outcomes (67,68). Our center also utilizes LDLT using right- and left-lobe allografts for HCC therapy with and without downstaging, as has been described (69,70).

TECHNICAL CONSIDERATIONS IN LIVER TRANSPLANTATION

The technical approach to total hepatectomy and liver replacement has been well described (71). Total hepatectomy offers the most radical approach to tumor eradication. Careful review of preoperative imaging will assist in tumor burden assessment, as well as planning for vascular and biliary reconstruction. Abdominal exploration should ensure no extrahepatic spread of disease at the time of transplantation. Unexpected lymphatic spread or metastatic disease during abdominal exploration is an indication to abandon the transplant. Assessment of venous thrombi in the portal and hepatic veins is also important. Graft options include deceased donor and living donor allografts.

Vascular reconstructive options have not been shown to affect HCC recurrence or survival, but the pros and cons of each should be well understood by the operating surgeon. Caval replacement is typically used in the presence of caudate tumors, but caval preservation techniques have demonstrated excellent outcomes overall with less postoperative renal insufficiency. Right dome capsular lesions often abut the right hemidiaphragm. On such occasions, resection of the liver en bloc with the infiltrated portion of the diaphragm should be considered. Portal vein reconstruction is typically performed in the standard fashion unless otherwise precluded by flow-related phenomena. Previous transarterial therapy may also affect the quality of hepatic arteries for reconstruction and should be a consideration when evaluating arterial reconstruction options. Biliary reconstruction options may include choledochocholedochostomy or biliary-enteric drainage (71).

POSTTREATMENT MONITORING AND EVALUATION FOR HCC RECURRENCE

After transplantation, there are multiple factors that drive the risk of recurrence. Recent data by Mehta et al. has led to the development of RETREAT prognostic scoring at Mayo Clinic and UCSF, which models HCC recurrence risk and attempts to stratify recurrence risk (72,73). AFP at the time of definitive treatment, tumor size and tumor number, and the presence of microvascular invasion are independently associated with recurrence (Exhibit 30.1). The RETREAT model performed well during validation, with good discrimination (C-statistic = 0.82) and superior recurrence risk classification versus Milan criteria alone. This model has been validated using United Network for Organ Sharing (UNOS) explant pathology as well (72). These studies hold significant promise in standardizing HCC surveillance after liver transplantation, provide the framework for staging algorithms, and help select patients for novel adjuvant therapies.

FUTURE DIRECTIONS

The treatment of HCC requires a multidisciplinary approach involving surgical oncology, transplant surgery, hepatology, oncology, interventional radiology, body radiology, radiation

EXHIBIT 30.1 RETREAT Criteria for Risk of Post–Liver Transplant Recurrence of HCC

Factors Associated With HCC Recurrence
AFP at time of resection/transplantation
Tumor size
Tumor number
Microvascular invasion

AFP, alpha-fetoprotein; HCC, hepatocellular carcinoma.

oncology, and other specialists. The success of treatments in recent years has brought on the evolution of "transplant oncology" as its own field and the cross-application of clinical tools developed in the care of HCC patients across clinical oncological care (74). Further advancements in the treatment of HCC patients must continue with the highest levels of multidisciplinary engagement to develop valid studies and achieve the best outcomes for patients.

Perhaps the most promising avenues for HCC treatment are in further refinement of locoregional therapies and in the use of developing adjuvant and neoadjuvant treatments including immunotherapy. Recent approval for nivolumab and other similar drugs in advanced HCC will inevitably lead to trials for its use in early-stage, early, and intermediate HCC. These trials hold significant promise for improved outcomes for patients with HCC.

Clinical Vignette 30.1

Case 1: The patient has no known history of chronic liver disease and is diagnosed with an incidental 9 cm mass in the upper abdomen after undergoing a diagnostic evaluation for kidney stones. MRI reveals a 9 cm × 5 cm × 4 cm tumor with arterial enhancement but no clear evidence of washout or pseudocapsule on delayed images, consistent with an OPTN 4 lesion. In the case of a suspicious-appearing liver mass without the presence of strong imaging criteria for HCC, biopsy can be considered. Biopsy indicates well-differentiated HCC without microvascular invasion. AFP is 400 ng/ml. In the setting of normal liver function and absence of portal hypertension, this patient should be considered for hepatic resection. In select patients with cirrhosis without significant portal hypertension, resection can be considered.

Case 2: The patient has a known diagnosis of cirrhosis related to NAFLD, and three lesions are identified on screening ultrasound as being suspicious for HCC. AFP is 75 ng/ml. MRI confirms the presence of three suspicious-appearing OPTN 5B lesions (all display arterial enhancement, and delayed washout with a pseudocapsule): lesion 1 is deep within segment 5 and is 2.5 cm × 2.5 cm × 2 cm; lesion 2 is in segment 7 and is 2.2 cm × 2.1 cm × 1.9 cm; and lesion 3 is 1.9 cm × 2.1 cm × 1.8 cm in segment 3, consistent with T2 HCC within Milan Criteria. The patient has diuretic-controlled ascites, varices, and medication-controlled encephalopathy. The MELD score is 10. He has an Eastern Cooperative Oncology Group (ECOG) performance status of 1. He has excellent family support, and financial/insurance coverage for all therapies is available. Locoregional therapy followed by liver transplantation should be considered. Locoregional therapy and liver transplant evaluation can occur simultaneously. Locoregional therapy with a combination of ablation and arterial-directed therapies could be considered after multidisciplinary discussion. If liver transplant evaluation yields that the patient is not a candidate for transplant, locoregional therapies could be considered with serial imaging to evaluate response to therapy.

Case 3: A 71-year-old patient with Child's C cirrhosis is referred for the presence of a 6 cm liver mass in the right lobe of the liver with multiple satellite nodules. MRI confirms the presence of the primary mass and satellite nodules, and imaging criteria are met for the diagnosis of HCC. AFP is 1,050 ng/ml. The patient has uncontrolled encephalopathy, massive ascites, and poor performance status. The MELD score is 30. While some providers may be tempted to consider liver transplantation for this patient, this patient has tumor burden beyond Milan Criteria, contraindications to locoregional therapy (advanced portal hypertension) that would preclude downstaging, and poor performance status that may limit transplant candidacy independent of the HCC-related risks. This patient should not be considered for curative therapies and palliative care could be considered.

REFERENCES

1. De Angelis R, Sant M, Coleman MP, et al. Cancer survival in Europe 1999–2007 by country and age: results of EUROCARE--5-a population-based study. *Lancet Oncol.* 2014;15(1):23–34. doi:10.1016/S1470-2045(13)70546-1
2. Bruix J, Reig M, Sherman M. Evidence-based diagnosis, staging, and treatment of patients with hepatocellular carcinoma. *Gastroenterology.* 2016;150(4):835–853. doi:10.1053/j.gastro.2015.12.041
3. Llovet JM, Fuster J, Bruix J, et al. The Barcelona approach: diagnosis, staging, and treatment of hepatocellular carcinoma. *Liver Transpl.* 2004;10(2 Suppl 1):S115–S120. doi:10.1002/lt.20034
4. Bruix J, Sherman M, Llovet JM, et al. Clinical management of hepatocellular carcinoma. Conclusions of the Barcelona-2000 EASL conference. European Association for the Study of the Liver. *J Hepatol.* 2001;35(3):421–430. doi:10.1016/S0168-8278(01)00130-1
5. Heimbach JK, Kulik LM, Finn RS, et al. AASLD guidelines for the treatment of hepatocellular carcinoma. *Hepatology.* 2018;67(1):358–380. doi:10.1002/hep.29086
6. Bruix J, Llovet JM. Hepatocellular carcinoma: is surveillance cost effective? *Gut.* 2001;48(2):149–150. doi:10.1136/gut.48.2.149
7. Bruix J, Sherman M, American Association for the Study of Liver Diseases. Management of hepatocellular carcinoma: an update. *Hepatology.* 2011;53(3):1020–1022. doi:10.1002/hep.24199
8. Reig M, Gambato M, Man NK, et al. Should patients with NAFLD/NASH be surveyed for HCC? *Transplantation.* 2019;103(1):39–44. doi:10.1097/TP.0000000000002361
9. European Association for the Study of the Liver, European Organisation for Research and Treatment of Cancer. EASL-EORTC clinical practice guidelines: management of hepatocellular carcinoma. *J Hepatol.* 2012;56(4):908–943. doi:10.1016/j.jhep.2011.12.001
10. Galle PR, Forner A, Llovet JM, et al. EASL clinical practice guidelines: management of hepatocellular carcinoma. *J Hepatol.* 2018;69(1):182–236. doi:10.1016/j.jhep.2018.03.019
11. Pomfret EA, Washburn K, Wald C, et al. Report of a national conference on liver allocation in patients with hepatocellular carcinoma in the United States. *Liver Transpl.* 2010;16(3):262–278. doi:10.1002/lt.21999
12. Chernyak V, Fowler KJ, Kamaya A, et al. Liver Imaging Reporting and Data System (LI-RADS) Version 2018: imaging of hepatocellular carcinoma in at-risk patients. *Radiology.* 2018;289(3):816–830. doi:10.1148/radiol.2018181494
13. Abd Alkhalik Basha M, Abd El Aziz El Sammak D, El Sammak AA. Diagnostic efficacy of the Liver Imaging-Reporting and Data System (LI-RADS) with CT imaging in categorising small nodules (10-20 mm) detected in the cirrhotic liver at screening ultrasound. *Clin Radiol.* 2017;72(10):901.e901–901.e911. doi:10.1016/j.crad.2017.05.019
14. Bae JS, Kim JH, Yu MH, et al. Diagnostic accuracy of gadoxetic acid-enhanced MR for small hypervascular hepatocellular carcinoma and the concordance rate of Liver Imaging Reporting and Data System (LI-RADS). *PLoS One.* 2017;12(5):e0178495. doi:10.1371/journal.pone.0178495
15. Wald C, Russo MW, Heimbach JK, et al. New OPTN/UNOS policy for liver transplant allocation: standardization of liver imaging, diagnosis, classification, and reporting of hepatocellular carcinoma. *Radiology.* 2013;266(2):376–382. doi:10.1148/radiol.12121698
16. Fowler KJ, Potretzke TA, Hope TA, et al. LI-RADS M (LR-M): definite or probable malignancy, not specific for hepatocellular carcinoma. *Abdom Radiol.* 2018;43(1):149–157. doi:10.1007/s00261-017-1196-2
17. Kim BR, Lee JM, Lee DH, et al. Diagnostic performance of gadoxetic acid-enhanced liver MR Imaging versus multidetector CT in the detection of dysplastic nodules and early hepatocellular carcinoma. *Radiology.* 2017;285(1):134–146. doi:10.1148/radiol.2017162080

18. Child CG, Turcotte JG. Surgery and portal hypertension. *Major Probl Clin Surg*. 1964;1:1–85.
19. Kamath PS, Wiesner RH, Malinchoc M, et al. A model to predict survival in patients with end-stage liver disease. *Hepatology*. 2001;33(2):464–470. doi:10.1053/jhep.2001.22172
20. Bruix J. Hepatocellular carcinoma: paving the road for further developments. *Semin Liver Dis*. 2014;34(4):361. doi:10.1055/s-0034-1395181
21. Beard RE, Wang Y, Khan S, et al. Laparoscopic liver resection for hepatocellular carcinoma in early and advanced cirrhosis. *HPB (Oxford)*. 2018;20(6):521–529. doi:10.1016/j.hpb.2017.11.011
22. Belghiti J. Resection of hepatocellular carcinoma complicating cirrhosis. *Br J Surg*. 1991;78(3):257–258. doi:10.1002/bjs.1800780302
23. Poon RT, Fan ST, Lo CM, et al. Long-term prognosis after resection of hepatocellular carcinoma associated with hepatitis B-related cirrhosis. *J Clin Oncol*. 2000;18(5):1094–1101. doi:10.1200/JCO.2000.18.5.1094
24. Kim WJ, Kim KH, Kim SH, et al. Laparoscopic versus open liver resection for centrally located hepatocellular carcinoma in patients with cirrhosis: a propensity score-matching Analysis. *Surg Laparosc Endosc Percutan Tech*. 2018;28(6):394–400. doi:10.1097/SLE.0000000000000569
25. Brown RS Jr. Live donors in liver transplantation. *Gastroenterology*. 2008;134(6):1802–1813. doi:10.1053/j.gastro.2008.02.092
26. Nault JC, Sutter O, Nahon P, et al. Percutaneous treatment of hepatocellular carcinoma: State of the art and innovations. *J Hepatol*. 2017;68(4):783–797. doi:10.1016/j.jhep.2017.10.004
27. Sun JH, Zhang YL, Nie CH, et al. Effects of liver cirrhosis on portal vein embolization prior to right hepatectomy in patients with primary liver cancer. *Oncol Lett*. 2018;15(2):1411–1416.
28. Edeline J, Lenoir L, Boudjema K, et al. Volumetric changes after (90)y radioembolization for hepatocellular carcinoma in cirrhosis: an option to portal vein embolization in a preoperative setting? *Ann Surg Oncol*. 2013;20(8):2518–2525. doi:10.1245/s10434-013-2906-9
29. D'Haese JG, Neumann J, Weniger M, et al. Should ALPPS be used for liver resection in intermediate-stage HCC? *Ann Surg Oncol*. 2016;23(4):1335–1343. doi:10.1245/s10434-015-5007-0
30. Jiang B, Yan XF, Zhang JH. Meta-analysis of laparoscopic versus open liver resection for hepatocellular carcinoma. *Hepatol Res*. 2018;48(8):635–663. doi:10.1111/hepr.13061
31. Goh EL, Chidambaram S, Ma S. Laparoscopic vs open hepatectomy for hepatocellular carcinoma in patients with cirrhosis: a meta-analysis of the long-term survival outcomes. *Int J Surg*. 2018;50:35–42. doi:10.1016/j.ijsu.2017.12.021
32. Salati U, Barry A, Chou FY, et al. State of the ablation nation: a review of ablative therapies for cure in the treatment of hepatocellular carcinoma. *Future Oncol*. 2017;13(16):1437–1448. doi:10.2217/fon-2017-0061
33. Peng ZW, Zhang YJ, Liang HH, et al. Recurrent hepatocellular carcinoma treated with sequential transcatheter arterial chemoembolization and RF ablation versus RF ablation alone: a prospective randomized trial. *Radiology*. 2012;262(2):689–700. doi:10.1148/radiol.11110637
34. Cho YK, Kim JK, Kim MY, et al. Systematic review of randomized trials for hepatocellular carcinoma treated with percutaneous ablation therapies. *Hepatology*. 2009;49(2):453–459. doi:10.1002/hep.22648
35. Bruix J, Takayama T, Mazzaferro V, et al. Adjuvant sorafenib for hepatocellular carcinoma after resection or ablation (STORM): a phase 3, randomised, double-blind, placebo-controlled trial. *Lancet Oncol*. 2015;16(13):1344–1354. doi:10.1016/S1470-2045(15)00198-9
36. Llovet JM, Real MI, Montana X, et al. Arterial embolisation or chemoembolisation versus symptomatic treatment in patients with unresectable hepatocellular carcinoma: a randomised controlled trial. *Lancet*. 2002;359(9319):1734–1739. doi:10.1016/S0140-6736(02)08649-X
37. Malagari K, Pomoni M, Kelekis A, et al. Prospective randomized comparison of chemoembolization with doxorubicin-eluting beads and bland embolization with BeadBlock for hepatocellular carcinoma. *Cardiovasc Intervent Radiol*. 2010;33(3):541–551. doi:10.1007/s00270-009-9750-0
38. Kulik LM, Carr BI, Mulcahy MF, et al. Safety and efficacy of 90Y radiotherapy for hepatocellular carcinoma with and without portal vein thrombosis. *Hepatology*. 2008;47(1):71–81. doi:10.1002/hep.21980
39. Salem R, Lewandowski RJ, Mulcahy MF, et al. Radioembolization for hepatocellular carcinoma using Yttrium-90 microspheres: a comprehensive report of long-term outcomes. *Gastroenterology*. 2010;138(1):52–64. doi:10.1053/j.gastro.2009.09.006
40. Sangro B, Salem R. Transarterial chemoembolization and radioembolization. *Semin Liver Dis*. 2014;34(4):435–443. doi:10.1055/s-0034-1394142
41. Gaba RC, Lewandowski RJ, Kulik LM, et al. Radiation lobectomy: preliminary findings of hepatic volumetric response to lobar yttrium-90 radioembolization. *Ann Surg Oncol*. 2009;16(6):1587–1596. doi:10.1245/s10434-009-0454-0
42. Siddiqi NH, Devlin PM. Radiation lobectomy-a minimally invasive treatment model for liver cancer: case report. *J Vasc Interv Radiol*. 2009;20(5):664–669. doi:10.1016/j.jvir.2009.01.023

43. Pawlik TM, Reyes DK, Cosgrove D, et al. Phase II trial of sorafenib combined with concurrent transarterial chemoembolization with drug-eluting beads for hepatocellular carcinoma. *J Clin Oncol*. 2011;29(30):3960–3967. doi:10.1200/JCO.2011.37.1021

44. Kudo M, Imanaka K, Chida N, et al. Phase III study of sorafenib after transarterial chemoembolisation in Japanese and Korean patients with unresectable hepatocellular carcinoma. *Eur J Cancer*. 2011;47(14):2117–2127. doi:10.1016/j.ejca.2011.05.007

45. Lencioni R, Llovet JM, Han G, et al. Sorafenib or placebo plus TACE with doxorubicin-eluting beads for intermediate stage HCC: the SPACE trial. *J Hepatol*. 2016;64(5):1090–1098. doi:10.1016/j.jhep.2016.01.012

46. Hoffe SE, Finkelstein SE, Russell MS, et al. Nonsurgical options for hepatocellular carcinoma: evolving role of external beam radiotherapy. *Cancer Control*. 2010;17(2):100–110. doi:10.1177/107327481001700205

47. Wahl DR, Stenmark MH, Tao Y, et al. Outcomes after stereotactic body radiotherapy or radiofrequency ablation for hepatocellular carcinoma. *J Clin Oncol*. 2016;34(5):452–459. doi:10.1200/JCO.2015.61.4925

48. Yoo GS, Yu JI, Park HC. Proton therapy for hepatocellular carcinoma: current knowledges and future perspectives. *World J Gastroenterol*. 2018;24(28):3090–3100. doi:10.3748/wjg.v24.i28.3090

49. Mazzaferro V, Regalia E, Doci R, et al. Liver transplantation for the treatment of small hepatocellular carcinomas in patients with cirrhosis. *N Engl J Med*. 1996;334(11):693–699. doi:10.1056/NEJM199603143341104

50. Bismuth H, Majno PE, Adam R. Liver transplantation for hepatocellular carcinoma. *Semin Liver Dis*. 1999;19(3):311–322. doi:10.1055/s-2007-1007120

51. Llovet JM, Fuster J, Bruix J. Intention-to-treat analysis of surgical treatment for early hepatocellular carcinoma: resection versus transplantation. *Hepatology*. 1999;30(6):1434–1440. doi:10.1002/hep.510300629

52. Jonas S, Bechstein WO, Steinmuller T, et al. Vascular invasion and histopathologic grading determine outcome after liver transplantation for hepatocellular carcinoma in cirrhosis. *Hepatology*. 2001;33(5):1080–1086. doi:10.1053/jhep.2001.23561

53. Zavaglia C, De Carlis L, Alberti AB, et al. Predictors of long-term survival after liver transplantation for hepatocellular carcinoma. *Am J Gastroenterol*. 2005;100(12):2708–2716. doi:10.1111/j.1572-0241.2005.00289.x

54. Llovet JM, Bruix J, Fuster J, et al. Liver transplantation for small hepatocellular carcinoma: the tumor-node-metastasis classification does not have prognostic power. *Hepatology*. 1998;27(6):1572–1577. doi:10.1002/hep.510270616

55. Libbrecht L, Bielen D, Verslype C, et al. Focal lesions in cirrhotic explant livers: pathological evaluation and accuracy of pretransplantation imaging examinations. *Liver Transpl*. 2002;8(9):749–761. doi:10.1053/jlts.2002.34922

56. Burrel M, Llovet JM, Ayuso C, et al. MRI angiography is superior to helical CT for detection of HCC prior to liver transplantation: an explant correlation. *Hepatology*. 2003;38(4):1034–1042. doi:10.1002/hep.1840380430

57. Marsh JW, Dvorchik I. Liver organ allocation for hepatocellular carcinoma: are we sure? *Liver Transpl*. 2003;9(7):693–696. doi:10.1053/jlts.2003.50086

58. Yao FY, Ferrell L, Bass NM, et al. Liver transplantation for hepatocellular carcinoma: comparison of the proposed UCSF criteria with the Milan criteria and the Pittsburgh modified TNM criteria. *Liver Transpl*. 2002;8(9):765–774. doi:10.1053/jlts.2002.34892

59. Guiteau JJ, Cotton RT, Washburn WK, et al. An early regional experience with expansion of Milan Criteria for liver transplant recipients. *Am J Transplant*. 2010;10(9):2092–2098. doi:10.1111/j.1600-6143.2010.03222.x

60. Onaca N, Klintmalm GB. Liver transplantation for hepatocellular carcinoma: the Baylor experience. *J Hepatobiliary Pancreat Sci*. 2010;17(5):559–566. doi:10.1007/s00534-009-0163-x

61. Mazzaferro V, Llovet JM, Miceli R, et al. Predicting survival after liver transplantation in patients with hepatocellular carcinoma beyond the Milan criteria: a retrospective, exploratory analysis. *Lancet Oncol*. 2009;10(1):35–43. doi:10.1016/S1470-2045(08)70284-5

62. Sapisochin G, Goldaracena N, Laurence JM, et al. The extended Toronto criteria for liver transplantation in patients with hepatocellular carcinoma: a prospective validation study. *Hepatology*. 2016;64(6):2077–2088. doi:10.1002/hep.28643

63. Yao FY, Fidelman N. Reassessing the boundaries of liver transplantation for hepatocellular carcinoma: where do we stand with tumor down-staging? *Hepatology*. 2016;63(3):1014–1025. doi:10.1002/hep.28139

64. Yao FY, Mehta N, Flemming J, et al. Downstaging of hepatocellular cancer before liver transplant: long-term outcome compared to tumors within Milan criteria. *Hepatology*. 2015;61(6):1968–1977. doi:10.1002/hep.27752

65. Majno PE, Adam R, Bismuth H, et al. Influence of preoperative transarterial lipiodol chemoembolization on resection and transplantation for hepatocellular carcinoma in patients with cirrhosis. *Ann Surg*. 1997;226(6):688–701; discussion 701–683.

66. Yao FY, Breitenstein S, Broelsch CE, et al. Does a patient qualify for liver transplantation after the down-staging of hepatocellular carcinoma? *Liver Transpl*. 2011;17 Suppl 2:S109–S116. doi:10.1002/lt.22335

67. Battula N, Reichman TW, Amiri Y, et al. Outcomes utilizing imported liver grafts for recipients with hepatocellular carcinoma. *Liver Transpl*. 2017;23(3):299–304. doi:10.1002/lt.24709

68. Khorsandi SE, Yip VS, Cortes M, et al. Does donation after cardiac death utilization adversely affect hepatocellular cancer survival? *Transplantation*. 2016;100(9):1916–1924. doi:10.1097/TP.0000000000001150

69. Llovet JM, Pavel M, Rimola J, et al. Pilot study of living donor liver transplantation for patients with hepatocellular carcinoma exceeding Milan Criteria (Barcelona Clinic Liver Cancer extended criteria). *Liver Transpl*. 2018;24(3):369–379. doi:10.1002/lt.24977

70. Azoulay D, Audureau E, Bhangui P, et al. Living or brain-dead donor liver transplantation for hepatocellular carcinoma: a multicenter, western, intent-to-treat cohort study. *Ann Surg*. 2017;266(6):1035–1044. doi:10.1097/SLA.0000000000001986

71. Busuttil RW, Klintmalm GB. *Transplantation of the Liver*. Amsterdam, Elsevier Inc. 2013.

72. Mehta N, Dodge JL, Roberts JP, et al. Validation of the prognostic power of the RETREAT score for hepatocellular carcinoma recurrence using the UNOS database. *Am J Transplant*. 2018;18(5):1206–1213. doi:10.1111/ajt.14549

73. Mehta N, Heimbach J, Harnois DM, et al. Validation of a Risk Estimation of Tumor Recurrence After Transplant (RETREAT) score for hepatocellular carcinoma recurrence after liver transplant. *JAMA Oncol*. 2017;3(4):493–500. doi:10.1001/jamaoncol.2016.5116

74. Hibi T, Sapisochin G. What is transplant oncology? *Surgery*. 2019;165(2):281–285. doi:10.1016/j.surg.2018.10.024

How I Treat Early-Stage Hepatocellular Cancer Through Surgery

Rachel M. Lee and Kenneth Cardona

INTRODUCTION

Hepatocellular carcinoma (HCC) is the most common primary liver malignancy in adults (1). Once largely considered a disease of sub-Saharan Africa and East Asia, the incidence and mortality rates of HCC in the United States have increased significantly such that, from 1992 to 2010, the incidence of HCC in the United States increased from 3.1 to 5.9 per 100,000 persons (2,3). There were 42,200 new cases of primary liver cancer in the United States in 2018, as well as 30,200 deaths, making primary liver cancer the fifth most common cause of cancer-related death for men and the eighth most common cause of cancer-related death for women in the United States (4). To date, surgical resection, either in the form of liver trans-plantation or hepatic resection, has been considered the primary curative treatment modality for HCC, with tumor burden and the degree of underlying liver dysfunction predominantly dictating which surgical intervention to pursue (5,6). From an oncologic perspective, four major prognostic indicators (tumor size, number of tumors, major vascular invasion, and extrahepatic disease) have been identified and are the basis for prognostic models and clinical staging systems currently available for HCC (7,8). While implementation of such models (e.g., Milan Criteria and University of California Expanded Criteria) in patients undergoing liver transplan-tation has resulted in reproducible, favorable outcomes, these models or staging systems have not been able to predict similar, consistent outcomes in patients undergoing hepatic resection (9,10). This difference in outcomes is primarily related to the fact that HCC presents a unique challenge when considering surgical resection as the malignancy is usually associated with considerable underlying liver parenchymal disease, which significantly increases the risks associated with hepatic resection, emphasizing the importance of appropriate patient selec-tion. The recently updated Barcelona Clinic Liver Cancer (BCLC) staging system is unique in that the assessment of underlying liver disease and patient performance status are included in the prognostic and treatment strategy. In the BCLC system, hepatic resection is only recom-mended for patients with early-stage HCC with preserved liver function and good performance status to obtain optimal outcomes (11). In the subsequent sections of this chapter, we focus on hepatic resection for early HCC, with a specific focus on patient selection.

EVALUATION FOR HEPATIC RESECTION: TUMOR AND STAGING CHARACTERISTICS

Initial evaluation of patients for surgical resection of HCC begins with the assessment of tumor burden and extent of disease. Diagnosis of HCC is largely based on imaging—the hallmark of HCC on cross-sectional imaging is hypervascularity and enhancement on the arterial phase with washout in the portal and delayed venous phases seen on triphasic CT or MRI (12). These characteristics, in the context of underlying liver disease, present in one imaging modality are sufficient to establish the diagnosis of HCC for lesions >2 cm (13). For lesions between 1 and 2 cm, the classic enhancement pattern needs to be present on two different imaging modalities to establish the diagnosis of HCC, with tissue biopsy indicated for lesions not exhibiting the classic enhancement pattern or observed on only one imaging modality (13). In regard to the

---

A Clinical Vignette ("How I Treat") is included at the end of the chapter.

quality of cross-sectional imaging, CT scan is slightly less sensitive (68% vs. 81%) yet more specific (93% vs. 85%) than MRI; however, MRI is more accurate in differentiating regenerative/dysplastic nodules commonly seen in cirrhotic livers from HCC (14,15).

Apart from establishing the diagnosis of HCC, cross-sectional imaging of the abdomen and pelvis allows for assessment of tumor burden, vascular invasion, evidence of portal hypertension, presence of intra-abdominal metastases, and provides an estimate of the future liver remnant (FLR) in patients being considered for resection. Extrahepatic metastases for HCC most commonly occur in the lung, abdominal lymph nodes, and bone; thus, complete staging for HCC should include a CT of the chest (16). Routine bone scan is not indicated unless clinical symptoms suggest involvement (15). Finally, serum alpha-fetoprotein (AFP) is the most commonly used biomarker for screening and diagnosis of HCC, with a value of >400 ng/mL considered diagnostic in the context of a liver mass. However, AFP alone should not be used to guide treatment decisions as serum levels vary widely among individuals and are not elevated at all in 10% to 30% of patients with HCC (17,18).

Tumor size, number, location within the liver, and the presence of vascular invasion are important factors to consider when evaluating a patient for hepatic resection. Historically, larger tumors (particularly >5 cm in diameter) present considerable technical challenges during resection, have been shown to be inversely correlated with survival, and are considered to be higher risk for intra- and extrahepatic recurrences (19). Nevertheless, surgical resection is the only viable treatment option and chance for cure for such patients as transplantation is only offered to select patients with specific size restrictions (Milan criteria: 1 lesion <5 cm or up to 3 lesions <3 cm each) (9,20), and locoregional ablative therapies are not effective for such large tumors (19). To this end, several groups have shown favorable outcomes with resection of large and even *giant* (>10 cm) hepatic tumors. However, it is important to note that recent studies have demonstrated a link between increasing tumor size and increasing rates of vascular invasion (21–23). Thus, increasing tumor size may be associated with more aggressive tumor biology (i.e., vascular invasion) and should be taken into account when considering a patient for hepatic resection.

The presence of multiple hepatic tumors is an independent prognostic factor for patients with HCC, and has traditionally been seen as a relative contraindication for hepatic resection due to the significantly worse prognosis appreciated in these patients when compared to patients with solitary tumors (21,24,25). However, due to limited availability of organs for transplantation and the large number of patients with multifocal disease who do not meet criteria for transplantation, surgical resection offers the only chance for potential cure in this cohort of patients (19). In select series, acceptable rates of survival (1-year 74% and 5-year 39%) for resection of multifocal tumors have been reported. However, in these series the 5-year recurrence rate has also been reported to be quite high (>70%) and therefore, consideration of neoadjuvant or preoperative therapy may be advisable in this cohort of patients (26,27).

Absolute contraindications to hepatic resection include the presence of extrahepatic disease, as well as inadequate or compromised vascular inflow, outflow (i.e., invasion of the main portal trunk, inferior vena cava, and/or the common hepatic artery), and biliary drainage of the FLR. However, in carefully selected patients, hepatic resection combined with tumor thrombectomy or vena cava resection has been reported with acceptable perioperative outcomes and modest oncological outcomes though early recurrence rates have been shown to be high. Therefore, our understanding of the role of hepatic resection in these circumstances of major vascular invasion needs to be further investigated (28,29).

EVALUATION FOR SURGICAL RESECTION: PATIENT AND HEPATIC CHARACTERISTICS

Critical components in the evaluation of the patient for hepatic resection involve assessment of the patient's functional status, underlying liver function, and FLR (Figure 31.1). Currently, there are a plethora of scales, tools, and models that can be used to assess a patient's functional status or frailty. A routinely used scale across clinical specialties is the Eastern Cooperative Oncology Group (ECOG) performance scale (0 "fully active, able to carry on all pre-disease performance without restriction" to 5 "dead"). This scale is a broadly used and accepted measure of characterizing a patient's functional status. While initially intended to document and assess the performance status of patients receiving therapy on a clinical trial (30), more recently, it has been used as a preoperative risk stratification tool. In a study of 375 hepatectomy patients in

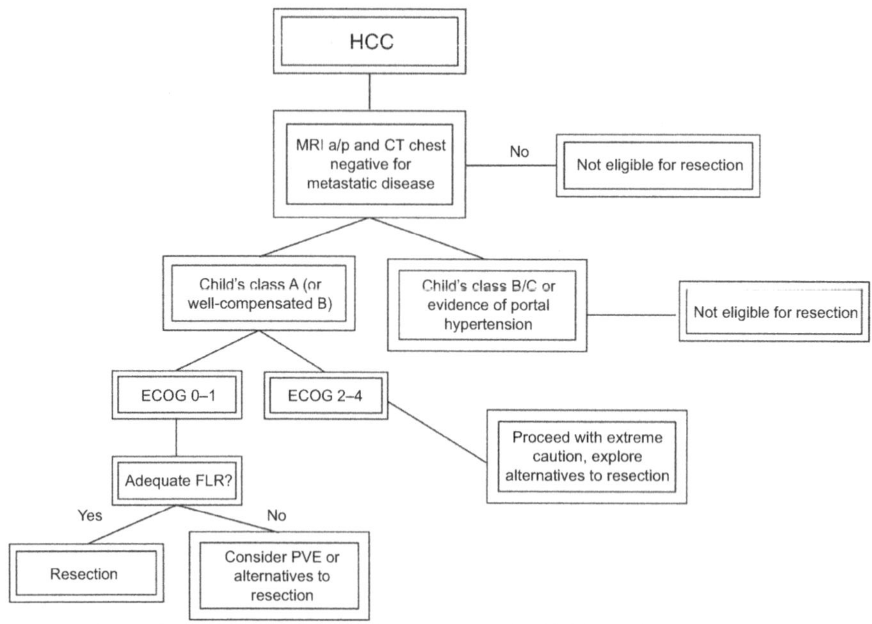

FIGURE 31.1 Algorithm approach to early HCC.

ECOG, Eastern Cooperative Oncology Group; FLR, future liver remnant; HCC, hepatocellular carcinoma; PVE, portal vein embolization.

California, a worse ECOG status was found to be associated with a significantly increased risk of 30-day postoperative complication, readmission, and mortality (31). In another study of over 7,000 hepatectomy cases in Japan, partial or total assistance with activity of daily living (consistent with an ECOG performance status of 3 or 4: "capable of only limited self-care; confined to bed or chair more than 50% of waking hours" or "completely disabled; cannot carry on any self-care; totally confined to bed or chair") was found to be significantly associated with an increased risk of 30-day mortality and 90-day in-hospital mortality (30,32).

The leading cause of death after hepatic resection is acute liver failure, making determination of the severity and degree of underlying liver dysfunction paramount in evaluating a patient for surgery (33). The Child–Turcotte–Pugh (CTP) and Model of End-Stage Liver Disease (MELD) scores are two major clinical scoring systems used to classify and risk-stratify patients based on underlying liver dysfunction. The CTP score uses physical exam measures of ascites and encephalopathy, and laboratory studies of total bilirubin, international normalized ratio (INR), and serum albumin to divide patients into three classes—A, B, and C. Patients with Child's class A cirrhosis (score of 5–6) are generally well compensated and can tolerate up to a 50% hepatic resection with acceptable rates of perioperative morbidity and mortality, and thus are generally considered appropriate candidates, from a liver standpoint, for hepatic resection. Patients with Child's class B cirrhosis (score of 7–9) can potentially tolerate up to a 25% hepatic resection; however, this carries a 30% risk of operative mortality. Child's class C cirrhosis (score of 10 or greater) is associated with an 80% risk of operative mortality and is considered an absolute contraindication to any hepatic resection. Based on this data, the majority of Child's class B and all Child's class C cirrhotic patients are referred for liver transplantation or other modes of liver-directed therapies such as ablation or embolization, rather than hepatic resection (15,33). The MELD score, an objective value composed of INR, total bilirubin, and serum creatinine, is used primarily to predict survival of patients awaiting liver transplantation; however, recent studies have used the score to risk-stratify patients being considered for hepatic resection. A MELD score ≥ 9 has been shown to be associated with a significantly increased risk of morbidity and mortality after hepatic resection—23% 5-year survival and 29% perioperative mortality versus 51% and 0% in patients with MELD of 8 or less (34).

Additionally, an indirect measurement of considerable underlying liver dysfunction is the presence of portal hypertension and thus patients need to be evaluated for its presence prior to proceeding with surgery. A clinical history of previous variceal bleeding (upper gastrointestinal bleeding requiring esophageal variceal banding), radiographic evidence of portal hypertension (splenomegaly, esophagogastric varices, and ascites), and thrombocytopenia (<100,000/mcL) can all be used as surrogate markers for portal hypertension and have been shown to be associated with increased morbidity and mortality after hepatic resection (35–38).

While CTP and MELD scores as well as evidence of portal hypertension are passive measures of liver function, the indocyanine green (ICG) clearance is an active measure of global liver function. Although not routinely used in the United States, it has been extensively studied and used in Asia and Europe. The test uses ICG clearance from the bloodstream after 15 minutes as a measure of hepatocyte function. Less than 10% of ICG remains in the blood in a normal liver after 15 minutes. Above 15% to 20% of ICG retained in the blood indicates impaired liver function, and >40% indicates severe liver dysfunction. A retention of 7.3% ± 3.4% has been found to correlate with Child's class A cirrhosis, 13.7% ± 2.3% with Child's class B cirrhosis, and 45.1% ± 7.5% with Child's class C cirrhosis (39). The ICG clearance rate, rather than retention at 15 minutes, has also been used to predict outcomes after hepatic resection; patients with a clearance rate of under 5 mL/min/kg were found to have significant perioperative mortality and should not be considered for hepatic resection (40).

Finally, the FLR must be appropriately assessed at the time of consideration for surgical resection, as a small or inadequate liver remnant poses a greater risk for postoperative liver dysfunction/failure and is associated with higher overall postoperative complication and mortality rates (33). A healthy, noncirrhotic liver can tolerate resection of up to 80%, leaving an FLR of 20%, due to the liver's ability to regenerate and compensate functionally for volume loss (41). A cirrhotic liver, however, cannot tolerate as aggressive of a resection and requires an FLR of at least 40% to 50% (42–44). Evaluation of the FLR can be done in various ways. CT volumetry may be performed to estimate the total liver volume (TLV) and volume of the proposed FLR via three-dimensional imaging. This has been shown to be accurate and reproducible; however, large tumors may falsely increase the TLV calculation, and no evaluation of underlying liver disease or function is included in the analysis (45–47). The TLV can also be calculated using a formula based on body surface area (TLV in cm^3 = −794.41 + 1267.28 × body surface area in m^2), which is unaffected by tumor volume and considered a standardized calculation (48). A combination of the two methods can also be used—calculation of TLV using body surface area and of the FLR using CT volumetry.

Patients in whom there is a concern about the size and/or quality of the FLR can be considered for portal vein embolization (PVE) to induce preoperative liver hypertrophy of the FLR. Additionally, this will also provide important information about the FLR regenerative capacity. The extent of hypertrophy is affected by many factors, including age, receipt of chemotherapy, recanalization of the portal vein after embolization, and hepatic steatosis in addition to underlying liver function (49–53). PVE has been shown to increase resectability rates in patients with primary hepatic malignancies. A systematic review of the literature on PVE in patients with primary hepatic malignancies reported a median resection rate of 90% after PVE (range 52%–100%) (54). Response to PVE can also be used to guide further treatment. In patients with normal background liver, hypertrophy of greater than 5% of the original FLR volume is associated with a low perioperative risk. However, in patients with background severe liver dysfunction a greater degree of hypertrophy is needed; hypertrophy of the FLR by greater than 10% of its original size is associated with a low risk for perioperative complications. However for both groups, total FLR volume after PVE must also be considered prior to resection (55). The absence of meaningful hypertrophy after PVE indicates low or absent regenerative capacity and should be considered as a contraindication to hepatic resection (33).

OPERATIVE CONSIDERATIONS

Once hepatic resection is determined to be an appropriate treatment strategy for a patient with HCC, operative considerations include laparoscopic versus open approach, anatomic versus nonanatomic resection, and appropriate surgical margins.

Laparoscopic hepatectomy has become increasingly common. A randomized clinical trial comparing laparoscopic versus open approaches for left lateral sectionectomies was attempted in the Netherlands and was stopped early due to slow accrual; however, no significant differences were found regarding length of stay, readmission, morbidity, or mortality (56). Numerous retrospective reviews have shown that laparoscopic hepatic resection is associated with decreased intraoperative blood loss, lower blood transfusion requirement, and decreased length of hospital stay with no differences found in overall survival, disease-free survival, and recurrence when compared to open hepatic resections (57,58). Laparoscopic liver resection appears to be safe and oncologically sound when performed by experienced surgeons. Without strong data indicating one approach to be superior to the other, from an oncologic or outcomes perspective, the technique with which to approach each case therefore must be individualized and factors such as tumor location, the patient's ability to tolerate laparoscopy, and the surgeon's expertise and comfort level must all be considered.

In regard to the type of hepatic resection, anatomic resections have been shown in several series to offer improved, recurrence-free and overall survival advantages than nonanatomic (wedge) resections (59–61). However, the degree of underlying liver dysfunction may not allow for major anatomical resections on all patients with HCC, and thus nonanatomic resection is typically performed in patients with increased hepatic dysfunction in order to minimize the amount of *normal* hepatic parenchyma resected and therefore maximizing the size of the FLR (33).

The optimal width of surgical margins remains controversial. A prospective randomized trial comparing narrow (1 cm) to wide (2 cm) margins found improved survival in patients with wide surgical margins with all recurrences at the margins of liver resection occurring in patients with narrow surgical margins (62). Additionally, a recent meta-analysis comparing narrow (0.5–1 cm) to wide (>1 cm) margins showed improved 5-year recurrence-free and overall survival rates (odds ratio [OR]: 1.69, 95% confidence interval [CI]: 1.37–2.08 and OR: 1.76, 95% CI: 1.20–2.59, respectively) with wider margins (63). However, another meta-analyses showed no difference in recurrence or survival between 1 cm and >1 cm margins (64). Thus, the true optimal surgical margin is unknown and warrants further investigation.

OUTCOMES

Perioperative rates of major complications and mortality after hepatic resection for early-stage HCC have decreased in recent decades, largely due to improvements in patient selection, surgical technique, perioperative care, and regionalization to high-volume centers. Overall postoperative complication rates have been shown to range from 21% to 48%, with the most common complications including biliary leakage, intra-abdominal abscess, and surgical site infection. Serious complication rates (Clavien–Dindo classification of 3 or higher) have been reported to be 15% to 17%. Reported rates of postoperative liver failure vary widely from 0.9% to 14% across studies (65–67). Perioperative mortality rates in recent series are less than 4% (68,69). Furthermore, overall survival has also improved in recent decades, with 5-year overall survival rates of 39% to 55% reported in recent series (68,70,71). However, recurrence rates remain high, in large part because the remaining liver continues to harbor malignant potential in the context of the underlying cirrhosis. Macrovascular tumor invasion, macronodular cirrhosis, and a larger tumor diameter (>5 cm) have been shown to be independent predictors of decreased recurrence-free survival and need to be taken into consideration when considering hepatic resection (72,73).

SUMMARY

Surgical treatment of early-stage HCC continues to evolve with improvements in surgical technique and perioperative care of patients with chronic liver disease. Surgical resection remains a critical tool in the treatment of early HCC, and is the only potential option for cure in select patients. Patient selection is complex, yet paramount for successful outcomes, and will continue to be refined as techniques and therapies continue to improve and evolve.

Clinical Vignette 31.1

Ms. Smith is a 76-year-old woman with multiple comorbidities, including coronary artery disease, atrial fibrillation, hypertension, diabetes mellitus, hypothyroidism, systemic lupus erythematosus, and obesity (body mass index of 45) who presented to clinic with abdominal discomfort and a 20-pound weight loss. Cross-sectional imaging of the abdomen revealed an incidental liver lesion, which was further evaluated with an MRI of the liver (Figure 31.2). The MRI showed significant hepatic steatosis with no stigmata of chronic liver disease or cirrhosis with a 4 cm exophytic mass in the right lobe of the liver adjacent to the gallbladder demonstrating arterial enhancement and washout on delayed sequences, consistent with hepatocellular carcinoma with no evidence of metastatic disease within the abdomen or pelvis. Staging CT of the chest was remarkable for interstitial lung disease, but had no evidence of metastasis. Her alpha-fetoprotein tumor marker level was 45 ng/ml. She was presented at a multidisciplinary tumor board where surgical therapy (transplant vs. resection), locoregional therapies, and clinical trial opportunities were discussed. She was not deemed a transplant candidate and thus hepatic resection was recommended. She underwent an open resection of segments 5 and 6. Final surgical pathology showed a margin-negative, 4 cm well-differentiated hepatocellular carcinoma with no lymphovascular or perineural invasion and background liver with steatosis.

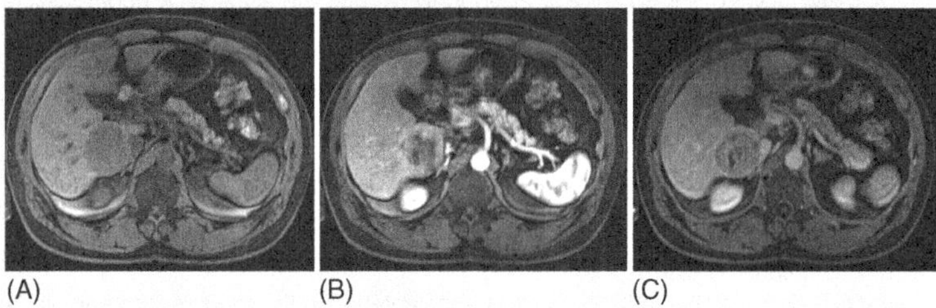

(A)   (B)   (C)

FIGURE 31.2 MRI of the abdomen revealing imaging findings compatible with HCC (LI-RADS-5). (A) Segment 6 mass is mildly hypointense to adjacent hepatic parenchyma on precontrast imaging; (B) late hepatic arterial phase image shows heterogeneous mass with APHE; (C) the mass demonstrates "washout" or hypoenhancement relative to adjacent liver on 3-minute delayed images, as well as a "pseudocapsule."

APHE, arterial phase hyperenhancement; HCC, hepatocellular carcinoma.

REFERENCES

1. Wallace MC, Preen D, Jeffrey GP, et al. The evolving epidemiology of hepatocellular carcinoma: a global perspective. *Expert Rev Gastroenterol Hepatol.* 2015;9(6):765–779. doi:10.1586/174741 24.2015.1028363
2. Altekruse SF, Henley SJ, Cucinelli JE, et al. Changing hepatocellular carcinoma incidence and liver cancer mortality rates in the United States. *Am J Gastroenterol.* 2014;109(4):542–553. doi:10.1038/ajg.2014.11
3. Altekruse SF, McGlynn KA, Reichman ME. Hepatocellular carcinoma incidence, mortality, and survival trends in the United States from 1975 to 2005. *J Clin Oncol.* 2009;27(9):1485–1491. doi:10.1200/JCO.2008.20.7753
4. Siegel RL, Miller KD, Jemal A. Cancer statistics, 2018. *CA Cancer J Clin.* 2018;68(1):7–30. doi:10.3322/caac.21442
5. Forner A, Llovet JM, Bruix J. Hepatocellular carcinoma. *Lancet.* 2012;379(9822):1245–1255. doi:10.1016/S0140-6736(11)61347-0
6. Jarnagin W, Chapman WC, Curley S, et al. Surgical treatment of hepatocellular carcinoma: expert consensus statement. *HPB (Oxford).* 2010;12(5):302–310. doi:10.1111/j.1477-2574.2010.00182.x

7. Vauthey JN, Lauwers GY, Esnaola NF, et al. Simplified staging for hepatocellular carcinoma. *J Clin Oncol*. 2002;20(6):1527–1536. doi:10.1200/JCO.2002.20.6.1527

8. American Joint Committee on Cancer. Liver. In: Edge SB, Byrd DR, Compton CC, et al, eds. *AJCC Cancer Staging Manual*. 7th ed. New York, NY: Springer Publishing; 2010:191–194.

9. Mazzaferro V, Regalia E, Doci R, et al. Liver transplantation for the treatment of small hepatocellular carcinomas in patients with cirrhosis. *N Engl J Med*. 1996;334(11):693–699. doi:10.1056/NEJM199603143341104

10. Mazzaferro V, Bhoori S, Sposito C, et al. Milan criteria in liver transplantation for hepatocellular carcinoma: an evidence-based analysis of 15 years of experience. *Liver Transpl*. 2011;17 Suppl 2:S44–S57. doi:10.1002/lt.22365

11. Forner A, Reig M, Bruix J. Hepatocellular carcinoma. *Lancet*. 2018;391(10127):1301–1314. doi:10.1016/S0140-6736(18)30010-2

12. Bruix J, Sherman M, Practice Guidelines Committee AAftSoLD. Management of hepatocellular carcinoma. *Hepatology*. 2005;42(5):1208–1236. doi:10.1002/hep.20933

13. Benson AB 3rd, Abrams TA, Ben-Josef E, et al. NCCN clinical practice guidelines in oncology: hepatobiliary cancers. *J Natl Compr Canc Netw*. 2009;7(4):350–391. doi:10.6004/jnccn.2009.0027

14. Colli A, Fraquelli M, Casazza G, et al. Accuracy of ultrasonography, spiral CT, magnetic resonance, and alpha-fetoprotein in diagnosing hepatocellular carcinoma: a systematic review. *Am J Gastroenterol*. 2006;101(3):513–523. doi:10.1111/j.1572-0241.2006.00467.x

15. Fong ZV, Tanabe KK. The clinical management of hepatocellular carcinoma in the United States, Europe, and Asia: a comprehensive and evidence-based comparison and review. *Cancer*. 2014;120(18):2824–2838. doi:10.1002/cncr.28730

16. Katyal S, Oliver JH 3rd, Peterson MS, et al. Extrahepatic metastases of hepatocellular carcinoma. *Radiology*. 2000;216(3):698–703. doi:10.1148/radiology.216.3.r00se24698

17. Wang K, Bai Y, Chen S, et al. Genetic correction of serum AFP level improved risk prediction of primary hepatocellular carcinoma in the Dongfeng-Tongji cohort study. *Cancer Medicine*. 2018;7(6):2691–2698. doi:10.1002/cam4.1481

18. Jelic S, Sotiropoulos C. Hepatocellular carcinoma: ESMO Clinical Practice Guidelines for diagnosis, treatment, and follow-up. *Ann Oncol*. 2010;21(5):59–64. doi:10.1093/annonc/mdq166

19. Truty MJ, Vauthey JN. Surgical resection of high-risk hepatocellular carcinoma: patient selection, preoperative considerations, and operative technique. *Ann Surg Oncol*. 2010;17(5):1219–1225. doi:10.1245/s10434-010-0976-5

20. Yokoyama I, Todo S, Iwatsuki S, et al. Liver transplantation in the treatment of primary liver cancer. *Hepatogastroenterology*. 1990;37(2):188–193.

21. Pawlik TM, Delman KA, Vauthey JN, et al. Tumor size predicts vascular invasion and histologic grade: implications for selection of surgical treatment for hepatocellular carcinoma. *Liver Transpl*. 2005;11(9):1086–1092. doi:10.1002/lt.20472

22. Pawlik TM, Poon RT, Abdalla EK, et al. Critical appraisal of the clinical and pathologic predictors of survival after resection of large hepatocellular carcinoma. *Arch Surg*. 2005;140(5):450–457; discussion 457–458. doi:10.1001/archsurg.140.5.450

23. Tsai TJ, Chau GY, Lui WY, et al. Clinical significance of microscopic tumor venous invasion in patients with resectable hepatocellular carcinoma. *Surgery*. 2000;127(6):603–608. doi:10.1067/msy.2000.105498

24. Nagasue N, Kohno H, Chang YC, et al. Liver resection for hepatocellular carcinoma. Results of 229 consecutive patients during 11 years. *Ann Surg*. 1993;217(4):375–384. doi:10.1097/00000658-199304000-00009

25. Wang BW, Mok KT, Liu SI, et al. Is hepatectomy beneficial in the treatment of multinodular hepatocellular carcinoma? *J Formos Med Assoc*. 2008;107(8):616–626. doi:10.1016/S0929-6646(08)60179-5

26. Ishizawa T, Hasegawa K, Aoki T, et al. Neither multiple tumors nor portal hypertension are surgical contraindications for hepatocellular carcinoma. *Gastroenterology*. 2008;134(7):1908–1916. doi:10.1053/j.gastro.2008.02.091

27. Ng KK, Vauthey JN, Pawlik TM, et al. Is hepatic resection for large or multinodular hepatocellular carcinoma justified? Results from a multi-institutional database. *Ann Surg Oncol*. 2005;12(5):364–373. doi:10.1245/ASO.2005.06.004

28. Wakayama K, Kamiyama T, Yokoo H, et al. Surgical management of hepatocellular carcinoma with tumor thrombi in the inferior vena cava or right atrium. *World J Surg Oncol*. 2013;5(11):259. doi:10.1186/1477-7819-11-259

29. Jibiki M, Inoue Y, Kudo T, et al. Combined resection of a tumor and the inferior vena cava: report of two cases. *Surg Today*. 2014;44(1):166–170. doi:10.1007/s00595-012-0337-z

30. Oken M, Creech R, Tormey D, et al. Toxicity and response criteria of the Eastern Cooperative Oncology Group. *Am J Clin Oncol (CCT).* 1982;5:649–655. doi:10.1097/00000421-198212000-00014
31. Abbass M, Slezak J, D'iFronzo A. Predictors of early postoperative outcomes in 375 consecutive hepatectomies: a single-institution experience. *Am Surg.* 2013;79:961–967.
32. Kenjo A, Miyata H, Gotoh M, et al. Risk stratification of 7,732 hepatectomy cases in 2011 from the National Clinical Database for Japan. *J Am Coll Surg.* 2013;218(3):412–422. doi:10.1016/j.jamcollsurg.2013.11.007
33. Fonseca A, Cha C. Hepatocellular carcinoma: a comprehensive overview of surgical therapy. *J Surg Oncol.* 2014;110(6):712–719. doi:10.1002/jso.23673
34. Teh S, Christein J, Donohue J. Hepatic resection of hepatocellular carcinoma in patients with cirrhosis: model of end-stage liver disease (MELD) score predicts perioperative mortality. *J Gastrointest Surg.* 2005;9:1207–1215. doi:10.1016/j.gassur.2005.09.008
35. Cucchetti A, Ercolani G, Vivarelli M. Is portal hypertension a contraindication to hepatic resection? *Ann Surg.* 2009;250(6):922–928. doi:10.1097/SLA.0b013e3181b977a5
36. Jarnigin W, Gonen M, Fong Y. Improvement in perioperative outcome after hepatic resection: analysis of 1,803 consecutive cases over the past decade. *Ann Surg.* 2002;236(4):397–406. doi:10.1097/00000658-200210000-00001
37. Poon R, Fan S, Lo C. Improving perioperative outcome expands the role of hepatectomy in management of benign and malignant hepatobiliary diseases: analysis of 1222 consecutive patients from a prospective database. *Ann Surg.* 2004;240(4):698–708.
38. Kaneko K, Shirai Y, Wakai T. Low preoperative platelet counts predict a high mortality after partial hepatectomy in patients with hepatocellular carcinoma. *World J Gastroenterol.* 2005;11(37):5888–5892. doi:10.3748/wjg.v11.i37.5888
39. Sheng Q, Lang R, He Q, et al. Indocyanine green clearance test and model for end-stage liver disease score of patients with liver cirrhosis. *Hepatobilliary Pancreat Dis Int.* 2009;8(1):46–49.
40. Hemming A, Scudamore C, Shackleton C. Indocyanine green clearance as a predictor of successful hepatic resection in cirrhotic patients. *Am J Surg.* 1992;163:515–518. doi:10.1016/0002-9610(92)90400-L
41. Nagasue N, Yukaya H, Ogawa Y. Human liver regeneration after major hepatic resection. *Ann Surg.* 1987;206:30–39. doi:10.1097/00000658-198707000-00005
42. Breitenstein S, Apestegui C, Petrowsky H. "State of the art" in liver resection and living donor transplantation: a worldwide survey of 100 liver centers. *World J Surg.* 2009;33:797–803. doi:10.1007/s00268-008-9878-0
43. Farges O, Malassagne B, Flejou J. Risk of major liver resection in patients with underlying chronic liver disease: a reappraisal. *Ann Surg.* 1999;229:210–215. doi:10.1097/00000658-199902000-00008
44. Shirabe K, Shimada M, Gion T. Postoperative liver failure after major hepatic resection for hepatocellular carcinoma in the modern era with special reference to remnant liver volume. *J Am Coll Surg.* 1999;188(3):304–309. doi:10.1016/S1072-7515(98)00301-9
45. Heymsfield S, Fulenwider T, Nordlinger B. Accurate measurement of liver, kidney, and spleen volume and mass by computerized axial tomography. *Ann Intern Med.* 1979;90(2):185–187. doi:10.7326/0003-4819-90-2-185
46. Saito S, Yamanaka J, Miura K. A novel 3D hepatectomy simulation based on liver circulation: application to liver resection and transplantation. *Hepatology.* 2005;41(6):1297–1304. doi:10.1002/hep.20684
47. Yamanaka J, Saito S, Fujimoto J. Impact of preoperative planning using virtual segmental volumetry on liver resection for hepatocellular carcinoma. *World J Surg.* 2007;31(6):1249–1255. doi:10.1007/s00268-007-9020-8
48. Vauthey J, Abdalla E, D'oherty D, M. I. Body surface area and body weight predict total liver volume in Western adults. *Liver Transpl.* 2002;8(3):233–240. doi:10.1053/jlts.2002.31654
49. Kageyama Y, Kokudo T, Amikura K, et al. Impaired liver function attenuates liver regeneration and hypertrophy after portal vein embolization. *World J Hepatol.* 2016;8:1200–1204. doi:10.4254/wjh.v8.i28.1200
50. Kasai Y, Hatano E, Iguchi K. Prediction of the remnant liver hypertrophy ratio after preoperative portal vein embolization. *Eur Surg Res.* 2013;51:129–137. doi:10.1159/000356297
51. de Baere T, Teriitehau C, Deschamps F. Predictive factors for hypertrophy of the future remnant liver after selective portal vein embolization. *Ann Surg Oncol.* 2010;17:2081–2089. doi:10.1245/s10434-010-0979-2
52. Malinowski M, Stary V, Lock J. Factors influencing hypertrophy of the left lateral liver lobe after portal vein embolization. *Lagenbecks Arch Surg.* 2015;400:237–246. doi:10.1007/s00423-014-1266-7

53. Tanaka K, Kumamoto T, Matsuyama R, et al. Influence of chemotherapy on liver regeneration induced by portal vein embolization or first hepatectomy of a staged procedure for colorectal liver metastases. *J Gastrointest Surg.* 2010;14:359–368. doi:10.1007/s11605-009-1073-6

54. Glantzounis G, Tokidis E, Basourakos S, et al. The role of portal vein embolization in the surgical management of primary hepatobiliary cancers. A systematic review. *Eur J Surg Oncol.* 2017;43(1):32–41. doi:10.1016/j.ejso.2016.05.026

55. Abdalla E. Portal vein embolization (prior to major hepatectomy) effects on regeneration, resectability, and outcome. *J Surg Oncol.* 2010;102(8):960–967. doi:10.1002/jso.21654

56. Wong-Lun-Hing E, van Dam R, van Breukelen G, et al. Randomized clinical trial of open versus laparoscopic left lateral hepatic sectionectomy within an enhanced recovery after surgery programme (ORANGE II study). *Br J Surg.* 2017;104(5):525–535. doi:10.1002/bjs.10438

57. Jiang B, Yan X, Zhang J. Meta-analysis of laparoscopic versus open liver resection for hepatocellular carcinoma. *Hepatol Res.* 2018;48(8):635–663. doi:10.1111/hepr.13061

58. Guro H, Cho J, Han H, et al. Outcomes of major laparoscopic liver resection for hepatocellular carcinoma. *Surg Oncol.* 2018;27(1):31–35. doi:10.1016/j.suronc.2017.11.006

59. Kaibori M, Kon M, Kitawaki T, et al. Comparison of anatomic and non-anatomic hepatic resection for hepatocellular carcinoma. *J Hepatobiliary Pancreat Sci.* 2017;24(11):616–626. doi:10.1002/jhbp.502

60. Cucchetti A, Qiao G, Cescon M, et al. Anatomic versus nonanatomic resection in cirrhotic patients with early hepatocellular carcinoma. *Surgery.* 2014;155(3):512–521. doi:10.1016/j.surg.2013.10.009

61. Cucchetti A, Cescon M, Ercolani G, et al. A comprehensive meta-regression analysis on outcome of anatomic resection versus nonanatomic resection for hepatocellular carcinoma. *Ann Surg Oncol.* 2012;19(12):3697–3705. doi:10.1245/s10434-012-2450-z

62. Shi M, Guo R, Lin X, et al. Partial hepatectomy with wide versus narrow resection margin for solitary hepatocellular carcinoma: a prospective randomized trial. *Ann Surg.* 2007;245(1):36–43. doi:10.1097/01.sla.0000231758.07868.71

63. Zhong F, Zhang Y, Liu Y, et al. Prognostic impact of surgical margin in patients with hepatocellular carcinoma: a meta-analysis. *Medicine (Baltimore).* 2017;96(37):e8043. doi:10.1097/MD.0000000000008043

64. Tang Y, Wen T, Chen X. Resection margin in hepatectomy for hepatocellular carcinoma: a systematic review. *Hepatogastroenterology.* 2012;59(117):1393–1397.

65. Harimoto N, Shirabe K, Ikegami T, et al. Postoperative complications are predictive of poor prognosis in hepatocellular carcinoma. *J Surg Res.* 2015;199:470–477. doi:10.1016/j.jss.2015.06.012

66. Pravisani R, Baccarani U, Isola M, et al. Impact of surgical complications on the risk of hepatocellular carcinoma recurrence after hepatic resection. *Updates Surg.* 2018;70(1):57–66. doi:10.1007/s13304-017-0486-0

67. Tranchart H, Gaillard M, Chirica M, et al. Multivariate analysis of risk factors for postoperative complications after laparoscopic liver resection. *Surg Endosc.* 2015;29(9):2538–2544. doi:10.1007/s00464-014-3965-0

68. Fan S, Mau Lo C, Poon R, et al. Continuous improvement of survival outcomes of resection of hepatocellular carcinoma: a 20 year experience. *Ann Surg.* 2011;253(4):745–758. doi:10.1097/SLA.0b013e3182111195

69. Li G, Speicher P, Lidsky M, et al. Hepatic resection for hepatocellular carcinoma: do contemporary morbidity and mortality rates demand a transition to ablation as first line treatment? *J Am Coll Surg.* 2014;218(4):827–834. doi:10.1016/j.jamcollsurg.2013.12.036

70. Nathan H, Schulick R, Choti M, et al. Predictors of survival after resection of early hepatocellular carcinoma. *Ann Surg.* 2009;249(5):799–805. doi:10.1097/SLA.0b013e3181a38eb5

71. Pandey D, Lee K, Wai C, et al. Long term outcome and prognostic factors for large hepatocellular carcinoma (10 cm or more) after surgical resection. *Ann Surg Oncol.* 2007;14(10):2817–2823. doi:10.1245/s10434-007-9518-1

72. Gan W, Huang J, Zhang M, et al. New normogram predicts the recurrence of hepatocellular carcinoma in patients with negative preoperative serum AFP subjected to curative resection. *J Surg Oncol.* 2018;117;1540–1547. doi:10.1002/jso.25046

73. You D, Kim D, Sec C, et al. Prognostic factors after curative resection for hepatocellular carcinoma and the surgeon's role. *Ann Surg Treat Res.* 2017;93(5):252–259. doi:10.4174/astr.2017.93.5.252

How I Treat Early-Stage Hepatocellular Cancer With Local Nonsurgical Approaches (IO)

Junaid Raja and Hyun S. Kim

LOCOREGIONAL AND TRANSCATHETER APPROACHES

Over the past 20 years, locoregional therapies (LRTs) offered by interventional oncology (IO) have redefined the treatment algorithm for hepatocellular carcinoma (HCC). Next to the gold standard of an orthotopic liver transplant, LRT has become a preferential therapy for the management of patients with oligometastatic HCC or those who are candidates for bridging therapy. This is in large part due to limited offerings with high toxicity in conventional chemotherapy. Moreover, given the minimally invasive and frequently effective approach LRT has to offer, it has become a mainstay in the antineoplastic arsenal and has been incorporated into the National Comprehensive Cancer Network (NCCN) guidelines. To follow, we discuss the role of LRT in the treatment of HCC including four main topics: patient selection for LRT, periprocedural details for different types of LRT, safety considerations, and a discussion on LRT selection.

PATIENT SELECTION

Scoring Tools for LRT
Patient selection for LRT is broader than for many other treatment modalities. There are many potential options for LRT in HCC that depend primarily on the intent of therapy. Locoregional techniques may be used as primary therapy or as an adjuvant and may be employed for cure, bridge, or palliation. Consequently, the decision as to candidacy for therapy depends on the individual patient's goal.

One of the patient populations in whom LRT is employed is patients who are poor surgical candidates due to inadequate functional or anatomic liver reserve, tumor distribution, or comorbid conditions. In addition, a select group in whom LRT is also preferred to therapy is that with presumed less aggressive malignancies to optimally avoid repeat hepatectomies.

There are at present more than eight prognostic scoring tools for HCC of which the most widely used are the Barcelona Clinic Liver Cancer (BCLC) staging criteria and Hong Kong Liver Cancer (HKLC); see Table 32.1. Nearly all of these scales incorporate the tumor, node, and metastasis (TNM) stage as well as Child–Pugh cirrhosis mortality prognostication characteristics into their predictive model as well as serologic markers including bilirubin and transaminases. Two of the scales (HKLC and Chinese University Prognostic Index [CUPI]) have been primarily validated in a specific cross-section of HCC patients, chiefly Asian patients with hepatitis B virus (HBV) associated HCC, whereas the majority of patients in the Western world with virally induced HCC are via the hepatitis C virus (HCV).

The significance of these scoring mechanisms is stratification not only of the disease severity but also evidence-guided treatment recommendations (Figure 32.1). In specific, BCLC recommends LRT in the form of ablation (radiofrequency, microwave, cryoablation, etc.) for patients who have very early stage (0), small (<2 cm), singular, primary tumors with Child–Pugh A, and excellent performance status but who are not candidates for liver transplantation. Similarly ablation is advised for patients with early-stage (A) HCC with up to three lesions measuring ≤3 cm maximally who are Child–Pugh A and have excellent performance status and have either increased portal venous pressure, bilirubin, and/or associated diseases. Additionally, BCLC recommends transarterial chemoembolization (TACE) for intermediate stage (B) HCC

A Clinical Vignette ("How I Treat") is included at the end of the chapter.

TABLE 32.1 Prognostication Scoring Systems in Hepatocellular Carcinoma

Scoring System	Abbreviation	Original Reference
Barcelona Clinic Liver Cancer	BCLC	Llovet JM, Brú C, Bruix J. Prognosis of hepatocellular carcinoma: the BCLC staging classification. *Semin Liver Dis*. 1999;19:329–338. doi:10.1055/s-2007-1007122 (1)
Hong Kong Liver Cancer	HKLC	Yau T, Tang VYF, Yao TJ. et al. Development of Hong Kong Liver Cancer Staging System with treatment stratification for patients with hepatocellular carcinoma. *Gastroenterology*. 2014;146:1691–1700.e3. doi:10.1053/j.gastro.2014.02.032 (2)
Modified Japan Integrated Staging	JIS	Ikai I, Takayasu K, Omata M. et al. A modified Japan Integrated Stage score for prognostic assessment in patients with hepatocellular carcinoma. *J Gastroenterol*. 2006;41:884–892. doi:10.1007/s00535-006-1878-y (3)
Cancer of the Liver Italian Program	CLIP	Daniele B, Annunziata M, Barletta, E. et al. Cancer of the Liver Italian Program (CLIP) score for staging hepatocellular carcinoma. *Hepatol Res*. 2007;37:S206–S209. doi:10.1111/j.1872-034x.2007.00186.x (4)
Chinese University Prognostic Index	CUPI	Leung TW, Tang AM, Zee B. et al. Construction of the Chinese University Prognostic Index for hepatocellular carcinoma and comparison with the TNM staging system, the Okuda staging system, and the Cancer of the Liver Italian Program staging system: a study based on 926 patients. *Cancer*. 2002;94:1760–1769. doi:10.1002/cncr.10384 (5)
French	GRETCH	Chevret S, Trinchet JC, Mathieu D, et al. A new prognostic classification for predicting survival in patients with hepatocellular carcinoma. Groupe d'Etude et de Traitement du Carcinome Hépatocellulaire. *J Hepatol*. 1999;31:133–141. doi:10.1016/s0168-8278(99)80173-1 (6)
Okuda	Okuda	Okuda K, Ohtsuki T, Obata H, et al. Natural history of hepatocellular carcinoma and prognosis in relation to treatment. Study of 850 patients. *Cancer*.1985;56:918–928. doi:10.1002/1097-0142(19850815)56:4<918::aid-cncr2820560437>3.0.co;2-e (7)
Taipei	Taipei	Hsu CY, Huang YH, Hsia CY, et al. A new prognostic model for hepatocellular carcinoma based on total tumor volume: the Taipei Integrated Scoring System. *J Hepatol*. 2010;53:108–117. doi:10.1016/j.jhep.2010.01.038 (8)
BCHP Staging System	BCHP	Prajapati HJ, Kim HS. Treatment algorithm based on the multivariate survival analyses in patients with advanced hepatocellular carcinoma treated with trans-arterial chemoembolization. *PloS One*. 2017;12(2):e0170750 . doi:10.1371/journal.pone.0170750

with large, multinodular disease in patients with up to Child–Pugh B and excellent performance status but without extrahepatic metastasis.

The HKLC system is slightly broader in its recommendations to consider ablation, liver transplantation, or resection in patients with an "early tumor" and Eastern Cooperative Oncology Group (ECOG) performance status 0 or 1 with Child–Pugh A or B cirrhosis, and up to three tumors measuring ≤5 cm maximally without intrahepatic venous or extrahepatic vascular metastasis (stage I or IIa). TACE is advised by HKLC for stage III patients who are ECOG

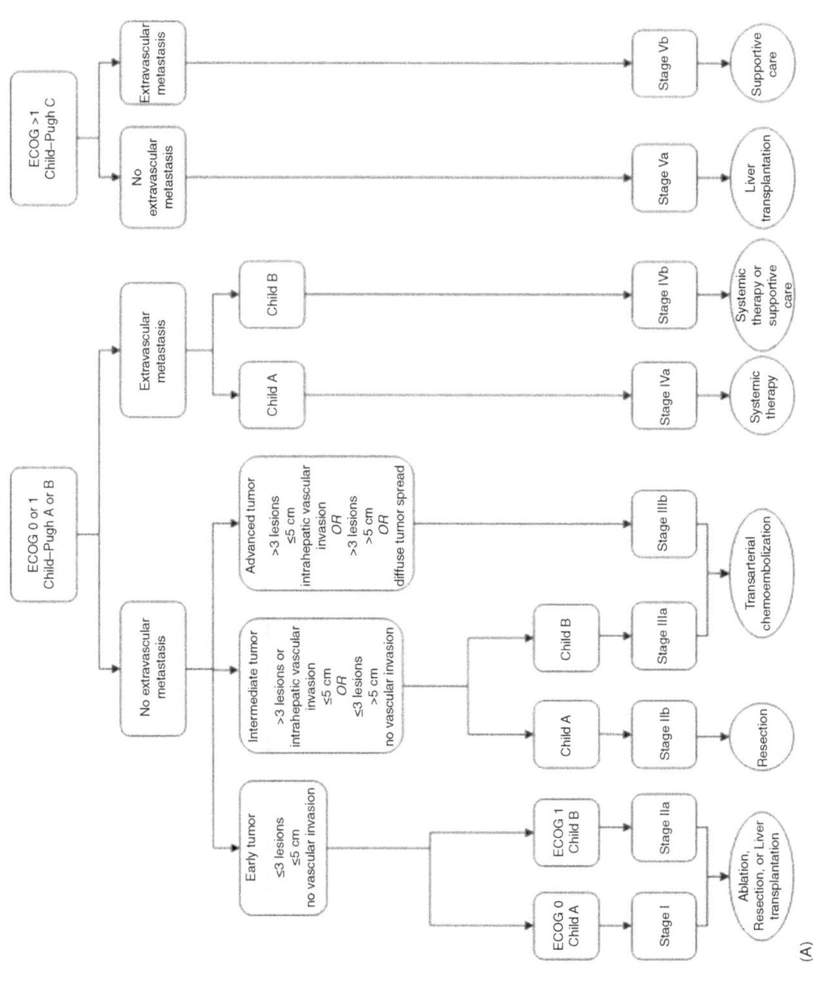

FIGURE 32.1 Hepatocellular cancer staging criteria. (A) Hong Kong Liver Cancer staging criteria (*continued*)

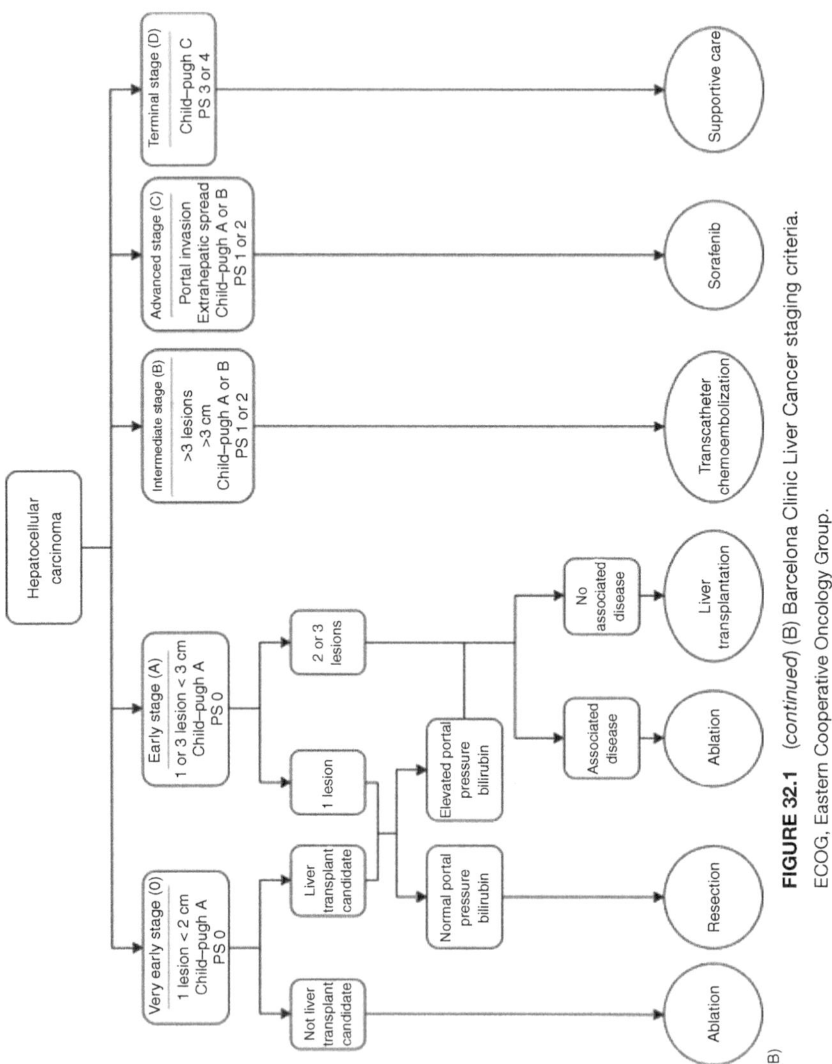

FIGURE 32.1 *(continued)* (B) Barcelona Clinic Liver Cancer staging criteria. ECOG, Eastern Cooperative Oncology Group.

0 or 1 with Child–Pugh B cirrhosis without extrahepatic vascular invasion and who either have more than three lesions that are <5 cm in size or intrahepatic vascular invasion, or patients with less than three lesions and no intrahepatic vascular invasion but a lesion measuring >5 cm (stage IIIa). Additionally, TACE is also recommended for patients who are ECOG 0 or 1 with Child–Pugh A or B cirrhosis without extrahepatic vascular invasion with locally advanced tumors with more than three lesions that are <5 cm but locally invasive of vasculature, more than three lesions that are >5 cm, or diffuse hepatic spread of tumor (stage IIIb).

An additional group that is not specifically defined in the prognostication scores but frequently benefits from LRT by ablation or TACE in HCC is advanced staged patients with refractory pain or symptoms from bulky or peripheral/subcapsular metastases. A subpopulation of patients with HCC who benefit from LRT, though again, not for curative intent for malignancy are patients who have had rupture of the liver and HCC and require embolic therapy to stop intraperitoneal hemorrhage.

Last, a discussion on scoring systems for LRT in HCC would be incomplete without a mention of transplantation guidelines. As further elaborated on the "bridging" and "downstaging" section to follow, LRT has a critical role in expanding the candidacy pool for liver transplantation for patients with HCC. The impact of expanding the pool is immense as patients who were otherwise borderline or ineligible for potentially curative therapy now have an opportunity to successfully undergo liver transplantation instead of being relegated to supportive care measures alone.

Predictors for Disease Recurrence or Survival

There are limited studies prognosticating likelihood of HCC recurrence and overall survival following LRT. Though these studies considered multiple variables, the greatest predictor for overall and disease-free survival following LRT was severity of cirrhosis at baseline using the Child–Pugh or Model of End-Stage Liver Disease (MELD; though this is not a typical metric calculated for HCC patients) scores or liver elastography. Additionally, systemic hypertension was suggested to be a predictor for overall survival in patients who received LRT, and both alpha-fetoprotein and visceral obesity were associated with a higher likelihood of disease recurrence.

LOCOREGIONAL AND TRANSCATHETER THERAPIES

Curative Intent Ablation

Perhaps the most widely used interventional oncologic technique for LRT in HCC is percutaneous ablation. Percutaneous ablation uses image guidance for probe placement in or surrounding the targeted lesion(s) before directly inducing cell lysis via thermal, mechanical, or electric mechanisms. There are six major types of ablation modalities: radiofrequency ablation (RFA), microwave ablation (MWA), cryoablation, high-intensity focused ultrasound (HIFU), laser, and irreversible electroporation (IRE).

RFA is the longest used and most well-described LRT for HCC with its first related use in 1996. The physical principles underpinning this technique is the use of a radiofrequency electrical current (between 100 kHz and 500 kHz) via an image-guided needle to induce local hyperthermia between 60°C and 100°C and cause coagulation necrosis with a surrounding ring of thermally ablated tissue. Optimally 0.5 cm to 1.0 cm of peripherally ablated normal liver parenchyma is preferred to ensure adequacy of treatment margins (Figure 32.2). However, though this approach is extremely effective at its specified target, there can be challenges in obtaining a sufficiently large ablation zone. In particular, the thermal effect during RFA in the region of the probe can induce tissue boiling and charring, which dampens electrothermal transmission. This of course is in part beneficial in limiting field effects to excess normal parenchyma but can result in complex geothermal ablation cavities that may require retreatment or additional probe placement to ensure adequacy of the therapy. Furthermore, this complex geometry can be further compounded by the "heat sink" effect wherein dispersed thermal energy in the liver transmitted to blood vessels can be lost due to blood flow away from the liver. Still patients with HCC are more likely to benefit from percutaneous RFA in the liver in comparison to patients with metastatic lesions as a pseudocapsule insulates the HCC lesions and the fibrotic liver allowing for higher achieved temperatures and longer duration of exposure to therapy in what is referred to as the "oven effect."

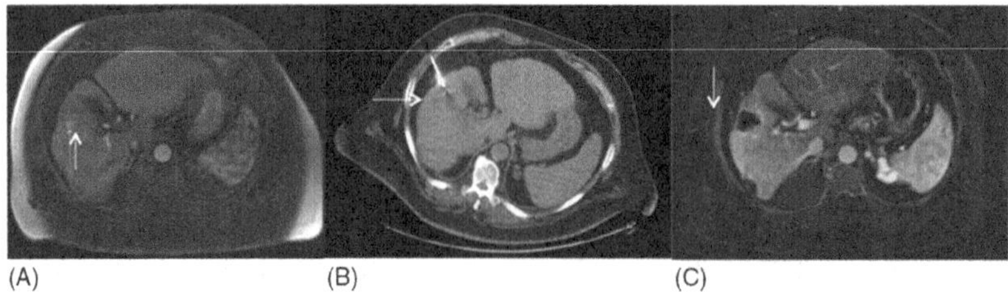

FIGURE 32.2 Radiofrequency ablation. (A) Preprocedural MRI of a hepatoma; (B) intraprocedural CT during radiofrequency ablation; (C) postprocedural MRI of the resultant ablation cavity.

The next most classical percutaneous LRT technique in HCC is MWA. Microwave ablation has been shown to be equally efficacious in smaller HCC lesions and potentially more efficacious in preventing local progression in larger target lesions. MWA therapy consists of image-guided placement of an antenna through which low-frequency or, more typically, high-frequency (2.45 GHz) microwave impulses can be transmitted (Figure 32.3). These impulses then induce heating of polar molecules including water in the targeted region to achieve increased heat. Given the high thermal effect in short spurts MWA is able to achieve a cooling mechanism has now become nearly universally incorporated with the antenna probe shaft. The overall result is similar to RFA in that coagulative necrosis is induced by thermal effect on the tissues. However, in contrast to RFA a larger ablation zone can be produced as microwaves can transmit through charred tissue and tissue with poor conductivity or high impedance and are less impacted by "heat sink" effects. Moreover, the effect of MWA can be monitored in real time by concomitant Doppler ultrasonography of the target lesions. Here too an ideal peripheral margin of ablating 0.5 cm to 1.0 cm of normal hepatic tissue is employed to ensure adequacy of margin.

The third most commonly utilized ablative LRT in HCC is cryoablation. Whereas RFA and MWA use hyperthermia for cytotoxicity, cryoablation is a hypothermic technique in which a compressed gas, most commonly argon or less commonly nitrogen, is deployed across a probe typically placed by CT into target lesions (Figure 32.4). Consequently, the probe tip is able to achieve temperatures as low as −160°C far surpassing the toxic range of −40°C. The initial step of the three-stage process is typically a 10-minute freeze. As a consequence extracellular water freezes inducing an osmotic fluid shift extracellularly dehydrating and damaging the integrity of the cell, which is exacerbated in the subsequent 8-minute thaw step during which the now hypertonic intracellular compartment is flooded, and the cell membrane bursts. Thereafter another 10-minute freeze cycle follows resulting in maximal direct cytotoxic injury to the target. In addition to tumor parenchymal injury, cryoablation induces vascular injury by thermal induced vasoconstriction and stasis as well as endothelial damage locally achieving Virchow's triad and augmenting coagulative necrosis. A unique attribute of cryoablation is the formation of gradient ablation zone, or "ice ball," in which the centermost aspect has undergone coagulative necrosis, adjacent tissue has undergone direct hypothermic cytotoxicity, and more peripheral tissue undergoes apoptosis. The significance of this effect as further discussed in the following is increased immunogenicity against the tumor and potential for

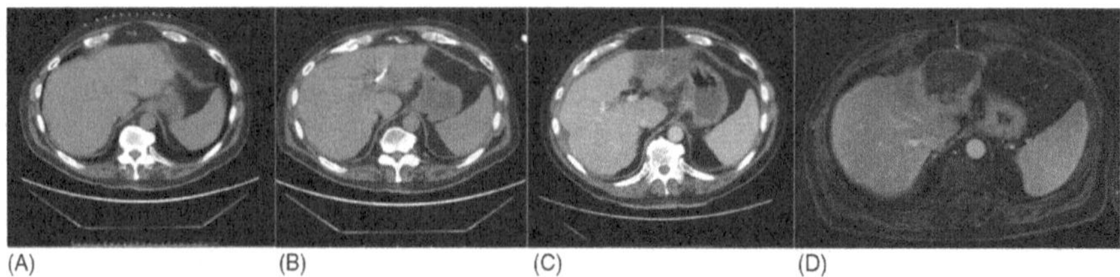

FIGURE 32.3 Microwave ablation. (A) Preprocedural CT of a hepatoma; (B) intraprocedural CT during microwave ablation; (C) postprocedural CT of the resultant ablation cavity; (D) postprocedural MRI of the resultant ablation cavity.

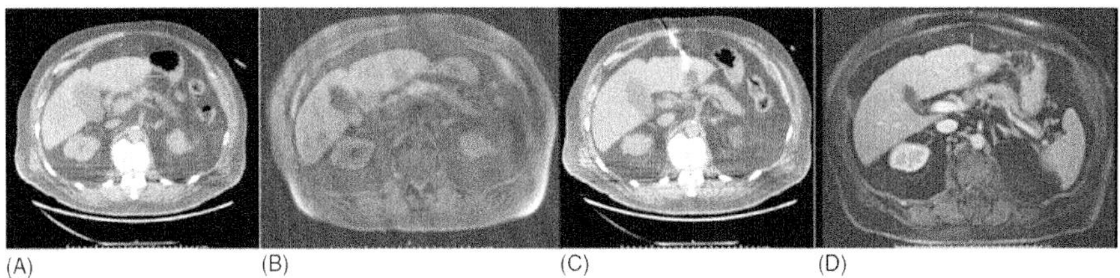

FIGURE 32.4   Cryoablation. (A) Preprocedural CT of a hepatoma; (B) preprocedural MRI of a hepatoma; (C) intraprocedural CT during cryoablation demonstrating an ice ball; (D) postprocedural MRI of the resultant ablation cavity.

abscopal effects. It is also given this gradient that at least 1.0 cm of normal parenchyma is also required for a satisfactory ablation cavity.

The ablation technique gaining increasing popularity and promise in interventional oncology generally and more specifically in HCC is irreversible electroporation (IRE). IRE uses high-voltage direct current pulses between polar electrodes placed by image guidance to induce the formation of a sufficient quantity of nanopores along the cellular membrane, which results in apoptosis. Most typically there are 90 pulses lasting 100 microseconds delivering 3kV across the targeted ablation zone. The ablation zone in IRE is much more precise in comparison to the thermal ablation cavities, which allows for safely ablating near vital structures including vasculature and the biliary tree. Moreover, the more controlled induction of apoptosis prevents the formation of fibrosis and limits the local inflammatory reaction that results as a consequence of the procedure. Optimally with this technique, 0.5 cm of normal parenchyma should also be included in the ablation zone to ensure adequacy of margins. One key difference in the technical aspect of this technique is the need for two parallel probes to allow polarization of current. This is in contrast to other thermal ablative techniques in which a solitary probe may be used. Many studies regarding its scope of use for IRE remain to be performed. However, early clinical evidence already demonstrates IRE may be safely and successfully performed in patients with Child–Pugh B HCC with results equally efficacious as MWA. Additionally, a significant limitation of this modality is the need for general anesthesia as well as a paralytic and cardiac monitoring to mitigate the risks of inadvertent delivery of current to other tissues.

Additional techniques for ablation including laser and HIFU are less commonly employed due to their limited therapeutic scope. Briefly, laser ablation uses high-intensity monochromatic electromagnetic radiation to precisely thermally ablate target tissue via coagulative necrosis. One of the major limitations with this modality is extremely high scatter and absorption of radiation limiting its distribution to approximately 2 cm maximally from the probe tip. HIFU uses acoustic radiation focused to a specific target to deliver pressure waves that expand/contract tissue (acoustic cavitation) and percutaneously induce coagulative necrosis. Unsurprisingly, this technique is limited by tissue penetration and requisite depth to the target lesion. There is also less specificity in creating defined ablation margins.

Curative or Palliative Intent Transcatheter Therapy (TACE and Transarterial Radioembolization [TARE])

In addition to or in lieu of percutaneous ablative techniques, transarterial delivery of chemotherapeutics and radioembolics can be used to effectively target and kill tumor cells. The fundamental principle of catheter-directed chemoembolization and radioembolization is similar in that by selectively administering toxic therapies to a tumor's vasculature, a higher dose of drug may be delivered to the target site without concern for systemic metabolism and/or related toxicities. Of course, there are still toxicities and adverse effects associated with any therapy, locoregional or systemic, and precautionary measures must be taken. Moreover, in the case of HCC and the liver, HCC tends to be fed via an arterial supply while the majority of the liver parenchyma is otherwise supplied by the portal venous system, a fact that can be exploited by TACE/TARE.

The conception of transcatheter oncolytic therapies originated with the use of gelatin sponge blocks soaked In chemotherapeutics and administered into the hepatic artery along with contrast media in Japan in the late 1970s. Subsequently, multiple iterations of refinements

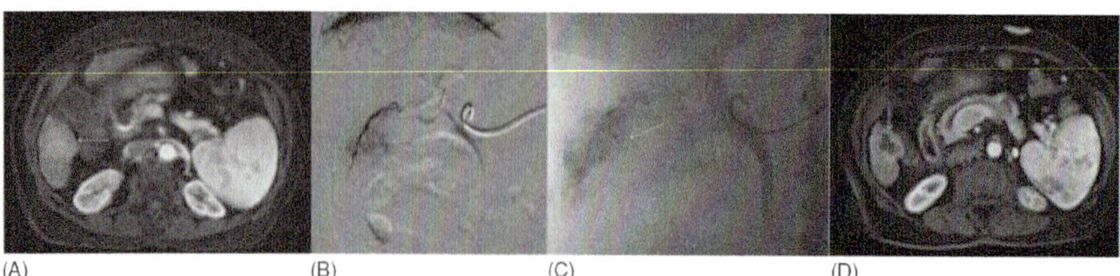

(A)   (B)   (C)   (D)

FIGURE 32.5   Transcatheter arterial chemoembolization. (A) Preprocedural MRI of a hepatoma; (B) diagnostic angiogram demonstrating hepatoma tumor blush; (C) intraprocedural angiogram following chemoembolization delivery; (D) postprocedural MRI of the resultant ablation cavity.

have ensued with a shared mechanistic approach of superselectively inoculating branch(es) of the hepatic artery with chemotherapy to induce local ischemia mechanically and cytotoxic damage chemically. The conventional form of this technique (cTACE) includes the use of an iodized poppy seed oil (lipiodol) along with chemotherapy such as doxorubicin or cisplatin. One benefit of using lipiodol is that the embolized vessel can be imaged via CT several weeks postprocedurally to ensure adequate effect.

Additionally, a newer approach includes the use of drug-eluting beads with chemotherapy (drug-eluting beads transarterial chemoembolization [DEB-TACE]) and water-soluble radiopaque contrast to further increase the degree of local ischemia inducing by the procedure. The drug-eluting beads or microspheres can vary in size from 40 μm to 75 μm or 100 μm depending on the clinical target. It is consequently essential to perform adequate contrast-enhanced cross-sectional imaging preprocedurally so that vascular variants and the entire vascular supply to the lesion(s) including potential secondary feeding vessels can be satisfactorily identified and planned for (Figure 32.5). The patient populations in whom the greatest efficacy of TACE has been demonstrated are BCLC stage B and HKLC stage III HCC who generally have large and bulky lesions. Last, the selection of chemotherapy for HCC in TACE is generally doxorubicin though cisplatin is also used. Though there is an increasing pool of research on using irinotecan for DEB-TACE, the primary focus has been on colorectal metastases to the liver rather than HCC. One factor that must be weighed with doxorubicin use though is the maximum lifetime dose of 450 mg/m^2 given the risk for cardiotoxicity beyond this limit.

The other major transcatheter therapy for HCC is the use of radioactive particles, in particular Yttrium-90 (^{90}Y), for TARE. Conceptually, this is similar to TACE in that superselection of a feeding hepatic arterial branch for an HCC lesion is performed; however, a few more steps and considerations must be taken with TARE. Specifically, given the nature of the radioembolics and potential consequence of nontarget embolization, a nuclear medicine shunt study using ^{99m}Tc-MAA to assess pulmonary shunting must be performed (Figure 32.6). The maximal allowable hepatopulmonary shunt is 20% or a maximal treatment lung dose by dosimetry of 30 Gy or cumulative lung dose of 50 Gy. The procedure itself consists of disbursing microspheres coated with the radioisotope into the hepatic arterial vasculature

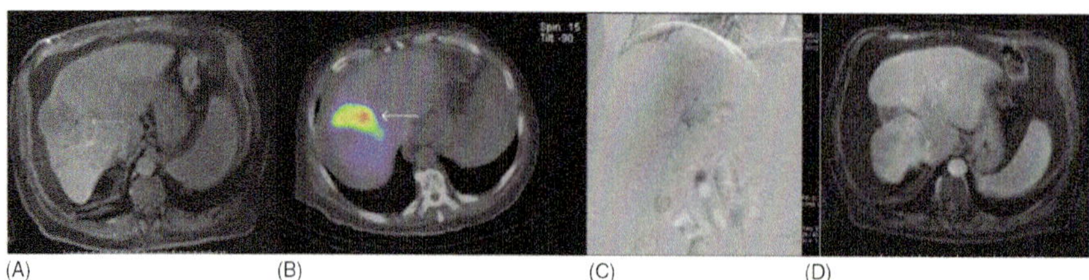

(A)   (B)   (C)   (D)

FIGURE 32.6   Transcatheter arterial radioembolization. (A) Preprocedural MRI of a hepatoma; (B) preprocedural SPECT/CT demonstrating ^{99}Tc macroaggregated albumin accumulation within the hepatoma; (C) intraprocedural angiogram following radioembolization delivery; (D) postprocedural MRI of the resultant ablation cavity.

SPECT, single-photon emission computed tomography.

with a target destination of tumor capillaries. ^{90}Y is a emitter with a half-life of 64.2 hours and given its direct proximity to the tumor is able to deliver a tumor toxic dose directly to the neoplasm. ^{166}Ho and ^{188}Rh have also been studied as alternative radionuclides though neither has yet been approved. Some of the unique strengths of this technique include lower rates of postembolization fatigue syndrome, abdominal pain, and nausea in comparison to TACE. Consequently, patients who underwent TARE had shorter postintervention hospitalization time and required fewer treatment sessions. An additional benefit of this approach in these cirrhotic patients with cancer is that it can be safely used in patients who have portal vein thrombus. A benefit of TARE in comparison to TACE is also a longer time to progression, though overall survival rates remain comparable. As a result of its better tolerability, TARE is frequently used for older patients and those with comorbid conditions. Furthermore, trials also demonstrate that in select populations TARE with adjuvant sorafenib may improve overall survival, though evidence for improvement in overall survival in TACE with adjuvant sorafenib remains controversial.

Bridging and Downstaging Therapy
A unique scope in which LRT is able to benefit patients with HCC is by serving as a bridge or to partially treat, or "downstage," lesions to enable or maintain candidacy for definitive cure by orthotopic liver transplant. To better understand this principle, it is important to understand the role of prognostication and formulation of candidacy for orthotopic liver transplantation. As with all other solid organ transplantation, there is a donor and receiving pool mismatch with more patients in need for transplant than organs available. Moreover, the emotional, physical, and mental strain imposed by organ transplantation and subsequent lifelong immunosuppressants, frequent follow-ups, and potential for complications or graft failure impose an immense challenge to patients. However, in the case of patients who are able to satisfy additional requirements for candidacy for liver transplantation, there remains the need to screen for objective likelihood of transplant success. For this aim, one of the two major criteria is employed depending on institutional preference to assess candidacy for transplant (Table 32.2).

The most classic tool is the Milan criteria, which described favorable tumor characteristics for patients undergoing liver transplantation as those with a single lesion of ≤5 cm or up to three lesions ≤3 cm. This approach demonstrated a 4-year statistically significant overall survival benefit of 85% versus 50% and recurrence-free survival of 92% versus 59% in patients meeting and not meeting criteria, respectively. However, as alluded to previously, availability of liver transplants can be variable and patients who are otherwise candidates at times must endure months to years on the waiting list during which time their disease may progress. Consequently, in certain cases LRT may be performed on the upper limit of acceptable sized or growing tumors to maintain candidacy and help "bridge" the time on the waiting list. Furthermore, subsequent studies assessed the impact of LRT in "downstaging" patients who initially had Milan criteria exclusive disease but following therapy met the classical criteria. These patients originally had HCC with a single lesion of ≤6 cm in size, two lesions of ≤5 cm each in size, or six lesions ≤4 cm in size and a cumulative disease burden measuring ≤12 cm in diameter. It was found that these patients too are beneficial candidates for orthotopic liver transplantation with LRT serving as a bridge.

The other major scale for liver transplantation in HCC is the San Francisco criteria, which is slightly more liberal and allows for transplantation in HCC patients with a lesion of ≤6.5 cm and

TABLE 32.2 Liver Transplantation Candidacy Scoring Systems in Hepatocellular Carcinoma

	Milan Criteria	San Francisco Criteria
Classical candidates	• 1 lesion ≤5 cm • 3 lesions each ≤3 cm	• 1 lesion ≤6.5 cm • 3 lesions each ≤4.5 cm, but cumulatively ≤8 cm
Downstaging candidates	• 1 lesion ≤6 cm • 2 lesions each ≤5 cm • 6 lesion each ≤4 cm, but cumulatively ≤12 cm	• 1 lesion ≤8 cm • 3 lesions each ≤5 cm, but cumulatively ≤8 cm • 5 lesion each ≤3 cm, but cumulatively ≤8 cm

up to three lesions measuring equal to or <4.5 cm maximally with a cumulative size of 8 cm. Here too "bridging" and "downstaging" techniques have also been shown to be successful in prolonging or improving candidacy and success for liver transplantation in patients with a solitary lesion of ≤8 cm, up to three lesions with a cumulative size of ≤8 cm and no single lesion >5 cm, and up to five lesions with a cumulative size of <8 cm and no lesion >3 cm. Typically the majority of the LRT tool kit is available for downstaging therapy, and secondary factors including size and location are generally instructive in the approach most likely to be successful. Perhaps the only contraindicated approach for downstaging therapy would be radioembolics, such as yttrium-90, as using this technique might unnecessarily increase the radiation risk to a surgical team during an open approach.

Finally, preoperative LRT in patients who subsequently underwent liver transplant has shown noninferiority in subsequent survival in multiple studies. In fact, other preliminary studies suggest there may be a survival benefit in patients with United Network for Organ Sharing (UNOS) stage T2 and T3 HCC who undergo preoperative LRT, though further studies are still required.

Recovery

One of the distinct advantages of LRT in comparison to operative procedures is the general well tolerability of therapy and short recovery interval. In fact, interventional techniques have become so refined and sufficient experience has been gained such that at our institution the vast majority of LRT procedures are performed as an outpatient with no overnight observation period. Still, a postprocedural observation period is necessary in a postanesthesia care unit, as most LRT procedures require at least moderate sedation and IRE requires general anesthesia. Additionally, depending on institutional and interventionalist preference immediate postprocedural imaging may be obtained, which can range from a chest x-ray to exclude pneumothorax to cross-sectional imaging with CT to more closely assess the ablated region for immediate postprocedural effects or complications. Once an adequate observational period has lapsed with stable hemodynamics and no serious adverse events, patients are frequently discharged to the care of an adult accompanying and providing transportation for them (e.g., a spouse or another family member).

Predictors for Disease Recurrence or Survival

There are limited studies prognosticating likelihood of HCC recurrence and overall survival following LRT. Though these studies considered multiple variables, the greatest predictor for overall and disease-free survival following LRT was severity of cirrhosis at baseline using the Child–Pugh or MELD (though this is not a typical metric calculated for HCC patients) scores or liver elastography. Additionally, systemic hypertension was suggested to be a predictor for overall survival in patients who received LRT and both alpha-fetoprotein and visceral obesity were associated with a higher likelihood of disease recurrence.

WHAT TO LOOK OUT FOR

Contraindications

In addition to theoretical candidacy for LRT procedures, individual patients must also be evaluated from a general preprocedural standpoint that may at times require cardiac, pulmonary, and/or anesthesiological clearance. Generally the necessity to obtain additional clearances is dependent on individual patients and their comorbidities (e.g., congestive heart failure, obstructive lung disease, morbid obesity). Additionally other parameters that generally contraindicate LRT include unstable hemodynamics, sepsis, severe and irreversible coagulopathy (e.g., platelets <30,000, international normalized ratio [INR] >2.0), current use of direct oral anticoagulants, and encephalopathy.

In regard to the actual HCC target itself, lesions accounting for >40% of the liver is contraindicated for LRT. Lesions in high-risk locations such as adjacent to vasculature, the biliary tree, diaphragm, pericardium, or lung are relative contraindications for most LRT for which an additional technique such as hydrodissection or balloon displacement can sometimes be considered. A significant tumoral arteriovenous shunt and portal vein thrombus are also relative contraindications to most LRT.

Additionally, specific techniques also have additional restrictions: IRE patients who are not candidates for general anesthesia are contraindicated for this modality as are patients with pacemakers and many dysthymias given the high electric voltage delivered. Pulmonary shunting of >20% is a contraindication for ^{90}Y TARE therapy given the potential of systemic distribution of the radiotherapeutic.

Patients should also be nil per os (NPO) at least 6 hours and preferably 8 hours prior to LRT given the likelihood of moderate sedation or higher. For this reason, an adult in whose care they can be discharged postprocedurally should also accompany them. The patient must be consentable and consented as to general risks of interventional procedures (e.g., bleeding, infection, inadvertent puncture) in addition to more procedure specific discussion of risks and benefits. As with all procedures, a preprocedural checklist including a time-out confirming correct patient, site, and procedure should be performed. Cleaning and draping of the percutaneous access site is subsequently performed with aseptic technique before the procedure is performed with sterility.

Potential Adverse Events and Management

Potential adverse events are possible with all procedures including LRT. The general risks of interventional procedures include infection, vascular injury, and nontarget treatment or injury. Each LRT modality additionally carries more specific risks. For all ablative therapies in HCC, an inherent risk includes damage to nearby structures. In particular in the liver this certainly includes normal parenchyma but also the portal vasculature and biliary tree. Some modalities such as IRE and laser therapy are more adept to sharper margins for ablation zones with nearly no extension beyond positioned probes whereas other techniques such as the thermal modalities and especially cryoablation are dependent on specific dose and duration of therapy and create a more indiscreet ablation zone. In the case of cryoablation, the imprecise transitions between cold necrosis, induced apoptosis, and reversible cellular injury are in part why a more generous margin must be included in the ablation zone in comparison to other techniques. Moreover, the most common adverse event for many locoregional techniques and in particular ablations and RFA includes postembolization syndrome (PES). PES consists of postprocedural fatigue and abdominal pain that is generally associated with necrosis of larger lesions. Additionally capsular necrosis, subcapsular hematoma, biloma, cholecystitis, abscess formation, and rare self-limiting intraperitoneal hemorrhage are other potential complications. For each of these, diligent technique in performing the procedure can dramatically reduce the propensity for complication. Furthermore, for the majority of these adverse events, conservative management and observation are the mainstays of therapy though certainly in the event of infection antibiotic therapy is obviously indicated.

The risk of adverse events when using LRT ablative techniques has been previously described in a very broad range with the general consensus that generally <10% have any adverse effects. The most common adverse events include PES that includes lethargy and abdominal pain. These symptoms generally are self-limiting, and patients may generally be observed on the order of hours to a day. The next most common adverse effects include abdominal infection, biliary injury, liver or pulmonary injury and rarely visceral injury, cardiac events, and rarely tumor seeding. The potential of tumor seeding from the ablation probe tract remains a controversial possibility with a wide range of incidences reported in the literature ranging from less than 1 in 100 to nearly 1 in 8 with the majority of studies favoring the lower percentage risk. Also, two overall agreed upon findings are that tumor seeding does not alter the overall survival for a patient and multiple needle passes (e.g., for biopsy prior to therapy) increase the risk. Consequently, certain interventionalists have adapted their own techniques to minimize their risk for seeding the tumor track though overall this has not been a tremendous concern. With regard to cryotherapy, a unique but potentially life-threatening complication is known as "cryoshock." Cryoshock consists of a spectrum that consists of systemic inflammatory response syndrome (SIRS), disseminated intravascular coagulopathy (DIC), or multiorgan failure. The population most at risk for this complication is patients with large lesions. It is proposed that the necrosed hepatocytes release debris that is phagocytosed by the liver's unique macrophages known as the Kupffer cells. Consequently, these cells can reduce cytokines and other inflammatory peptides to cause systemic inflammation. The population at greatest risk for cryoshock is patients with lesions that occupy greater than one third of the liver.

IRE includes two main sources of risk: the procedure itself and general anesthesia. The risk of general anesthesia in IRE is comparable to that in all LRTs and operative procedures with the key exception that neuromuscular blockade is required. The primary reason for the need for a paralytic is to prevent the risk of the delivered electrical dose stimulating the musculature and causing rhabdomyolysis or other injury from severe muscle spasm. This risk to specifically cardiac muscle is the reason there is restrictive eligibility criteria for patients with prior cardiac histories. Moreover, the risk of dysrhythmia is another reason the procedure is performed under general anesthesia, optimally with an attending anesthesiologist present. Additionally, paralytics themselves carry a risk of causing electrolyte abnormality and malignant hyperthermia. As the treatment zone for IRE is strictly defined between the placed electrodes, lesions may be targeted that abut vital structures. However, in order to adequately treat these lesions the risk for injuring a vital structure is higher. Similarly, lesions >5 cm in size are difficult to treat given the distance between electrodes, which may be facilitated by additional or repositioning probes but this can again increase the risk of inadvertent puncture.

In regard to TACE and TARE, the most dreaded adverse events would be nontarget embolization. Generally the two mechanisms by which this occurs is hyposelective delivery and shunting. Hyposelective delivery is typically the result of reaching maximum length of the microcatheter system or encountering a selective branch with a physically impossible angle to navigate. In this setting it is known that the delivered therapeutic may not only target the neoplastic lesion for which reason monitoring for untoward effects such as PES and transaminitis/liver injury is indicated. The other mechanism, shunting, can ultimately induce the same adverse events of PES, damage to normal parenchyma, and biochemical abnormalities. However, the process by which this occurs is by a series of accessory vasculature in the region of the lesion and vascular malformations that lead to nontarget delivery of the therapeutic. Overall the most common adverse effects with TACE/TARE are PES and transaminitis.

SELECTION OF LOCOREGIONAL TECHNIQUES

The core question when to use which LRT modality remains one of debate and expert opinion. Whereas in many other forms of oncology a strict algorithm may be followed for determining treatment selection and at times dose, LRT is more flexible. There are certainly case scenarios in which certain modalities are contraindicated or not likely to be beneficial (e.g., IRE in a patient with cardiac dysrhythmia, TARE in patients with a shunt, laser ablation in a large lesion); however, a multitude of other scenarios have treatment guidance from institutional preferences and operator experience.

For instance, local disease of one or two peripheral intraparenchymal lesions ≤3 to 4 cm in size would likely be best treated with ablation. Additionally, as the most experience and research is with thermal ablation and MWA is less limited by a heat sink effect, this may be the preferred modality for most (though certainly RFA or cryoablation would also be medically sound options). In contrast, local disease with a lesion adjacent to the portal vein may also benefit from ablation but given the higher risk of vascular or biliary damage from thermal ablation would require a more defined distribution of the ablation zone and thus IRE may be a safer and more effective option for that particular patient. A patient on adjuvant immunotherapy with slightly central lesions may in comparison be best suited for cryotherapy. Similarly, patients with more advanced disease who are not candidates for curative ablation or have multifocal disease may benefit from TACE or TARE. Younger patients and those with few comorbidities and seeking downstaging or bridging therapy for imminent transplantation may benefit from cTACE or DEB-TACE. On the other hand, patients who are older or who have portal venous thrombus or in whom adjuvant sorafenib is being considered may benefit from TARE.

However, as alluded to previously the selection of LRT can at times become an art form in which the patient's needs must be balanced with individual risks of the procedure, and novel palliative combination therapies may need to be considered. For instance, in the case of a patient with advanced-stage disease but a high pulmonary hepatic shunt fraction, TACE with or without systemic chemotherapy may be considered. Furthermore if the aforementioned patient has multiple smaller lesions that are fed by vasculature that is too small to canalize with a microcatheter, less selective TACE or TARE may be considered or else using ablative techniques with multiple probes is another option. Another option depending on the level of individual complexity that can be and is considered in patients who do not neatly conform to general practice options is multimodality and multistage options. That is, to use a combination of systemic, embolic, and ablative modalities to control symptoms caused by HCC ranging from capsular pain to mass effect inducing vascular or biliary compromise, and so on. Dividing ablations to multiple sessions for larger lesion can be beneficial and more likely to avoid cryoshock and PES.

As suggested earlier, ultimate selection of specific LRTs for individual patients with HCC depends on more than just the histologic subtype. Each of the LRT modalities has unique strengths and weaknesses in different populations that require multidisciplinary communication and cooperation and thoughtful consideration. In our experience, key considerations for treatment selection should include size and number of lesions, location of lesions and nearby structures, targeted outcome, adjuvant systemic therapies, performance status, and transplant candidacy (Figure 32.7).

FUTURE DIRECTIONS

The most exciting facet of LRT in HCC is the future. There are frequently new ideas and discoveries in an expanding literature growing the therapeutic offerings by interventionalists. These include new drug and radiation delivery platforms, combination therapies with immunotherapeutics, and the aspirational goal of an LRT with abscopal effects.

One concept of expanding the current scope of transcatheter embolic therapy is innovating the microspheres used for delivery. In particular, early evidence supports the concept of combining the concept of DEB-TACE and TARE to formulate chemotherapy and radioisotope coated beads that may be directly inoculated into a tumor's vasculature. Additionally, other designs include biodegradable delivery vehicles, expanding the type of drugs or chemotherapies used, and targeting cell surface glycoproteins or other molecular markers with a carrier bead or molecule to deliver the oncotherapy.

Moreover, the prospects of adjuvancy with immunotherapeutics including immune checkpoint inhibitors and oncoviruses are among the most intriguing and potentially promising therapies that will usher in the new wave of interventional oncology for HCC. The predicated concept is LRT may either treat immunotherapy refractory disease, or more excitingly, augment the immune system or the therapeutic response to immunotherapy. Although any of the LRT techniques may offer benefit, the use of cryotherapy has shown encouraging results in animal and early human studies in terms of facilitating tumor immunogenicity and priming the immune system against neoplastic antigens. In the case of cryotherapy, it has been proposed this modality may even hold the potential to induce abscopal effects. Serum from nonhuman primate and leporine models post cryoablation has shown tumor-specific antibodies. Moreover, cryoablation is able to induce a high degree of inflammation with proinflammatory cytokines including interleukins 1 and 6, nuclear factor κB and TNF and antigen accumulation in dendritic cells. In comparison to other LRT modalities such as RFA and MWA, cryotherapy is also able to elicit a greater lesional infiltration by neutrophils and either macrophages or tumor killing CD8$^+$ cells. One proposed mechanistic advantage that has been proposed for cryotherapy versus hyperthermic ablations is that hyperthermic ablations may denature proteins and cellular structures while cryotherapy more selectively disrupts the plasma membrane. It is thought that as a consequence the immune cells are able to sample and develop antibodies against intracytoplasmic proteins. However, there are still limitations as there is also an apparent counter immunosuppressive mechanism that cryotherapy induces that is not well understood but hypothesized to perhaps be related to whether cells are killed by necrosis or apoptosis.

The notion of oncoviral LRT is a specific burgeoning area of interest in interventional immuno-oncotherapy. Recent translational and clinical studies have shown promise with different approaches. For instance, a clinical trial in a Chinese study assessed TACE adjuvant intra-arterial oncolytic human adenovirus 5 (H101) administration for HCC and found improved progression-free and overall survival in comparison to TACE monotherapy. Additional animal model studies demonstrated in non-HCC models that intralesional inoculation improves recruitment of tumor infiltrating cells and may improve immunogenicity to checkpoint inhibitor immunotherapy. Perhaps most stirringly, evidence of abscopal effects was also seen in the animal models treated with intratumoral oncoviral therapy. Certainly in regard to the scope, technology, and curative possibilities for LRT in HCC, the best is yet to come.

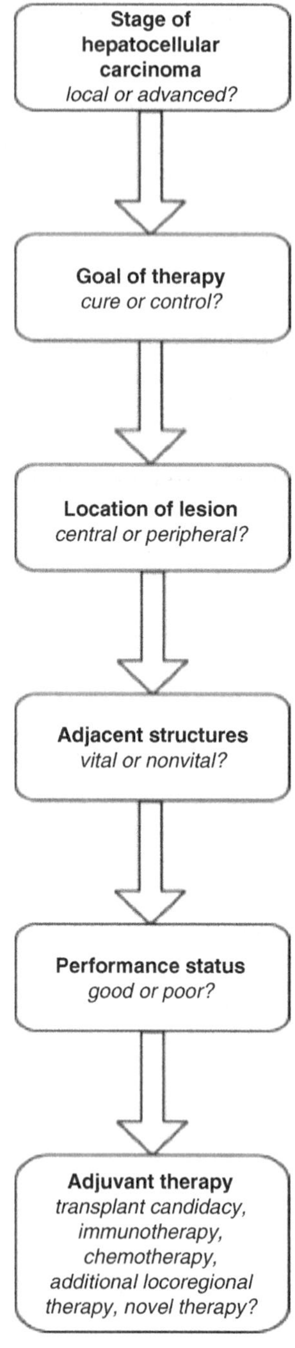

FIGURE 32.7 Logic flowchart.

Clinical Vignette 32.1

A 55-year-old male with hepatitis C cirrhosis and a new diagnosis of multifocal hepatocellular carcinoma presented for evaluation for locoregional therapy after a staging MRI demonstrated 1.0 cm segment VI, 3.0 cm segment IV, 0.7 cm segment II, and 6.2 cm segment VIII arterially enhancing lesions with washout compatible with hepatoma. The patient is on Lasix and Aldactone only for medications, and completed a course of Harvoni with sustained viral response six months earlier. He works as a cashier and stockroom attendant at a local grocery store. He is also happily married and has two children who are all healthy. He quit smoking 5 years ago and is a never-drinker. The key clinical questions for this case are what would be the role or goal of locoregional therapy in this patient and what type(s) of locoregional therapy can be offered and what would be the level of response required for transplant candidacy.

The patient has newly diagnosed oligometastatic hepatocellular carcinoma with four lesions with the largest measuring ≤6.2 cm and cumulatively measuring 10.9 cm. He has an excellent performance status and an established support system. He would be a candidate for downstaging therapy with a goal of achieving transplant candidacy. He would in principle be a candidate for transcatheter for palliative purposes, though in this circumstance his barrier to transplant candidacy is the 6.2 cm segment VIII lesion. For this reason, thermal ablative therapy such as with microwave ablation (provided sufficient distance of the superior margin of the tumor from the diaphragm) targeting at least the segment VIII lesion would be preferred. As long as the segment VIII lesion at least decreases in size by 30% the patient would become a transplant candidate, though it is expected the tumor may in fact demonstrate complete response to the ablation.

ADDITIONAL READINGS

Adhoute X, Penaranda G, Castellani P, et al. Recommendations for the use of chemoembolization in patients with hepatocellular carcinoma: usefulness of scoring system? *World J Hepatol.* 2015;7(3):521. doi:10.4254/wjh.v7.i3.521

Bhutiani N, Philips P, Scoggins CR, et al. Evaluation of tolerability and efficacy of irreversible electroporation (IRE) in treatment of Child-Pugh B (7/8) hepatocellular carcinoma (HCC). *HPB.* 2016;18(7):593–599. doi:10.1016/j.hpb.2016.03.609

Blümmel J, Reinhardt S, Schäfer M, et al. Drug-eluting beads in the treatment of hepatocellular carcinoma and colorectal cancer metastases to the liver. *Eur Oncol Haematol.* 2012;3:162–166. doi:10.17925/EOH.2012.08.3.162

Brace CL. Radiofrequency and microwave ablation of the liver, lung, kidney, and bone: what are the differences? *Curr Probl Diagn Radiol.* 2009;38(3):135–143. doi:10.1067/j.cpradiol.2007.10.001

Cannon R, Ellis S, Hayes D, et al. Safety and early efficacy of irreversible electroporation for hepatic tumors in proximity to vital structures. *J Surg Oncol.* 2013;107(5):544–549. doi:10.1002/jso.23280

Cescon M, Cucchetti A, Ravaioli M, et al. Hepatocellular carcinoma locoregional therapies for patients in the waiting list. Impact on transplantability and recurrence rate. *J Hepatol.* 2013;58(3):609–618. doi:10.1016/j.jhep.2012.09.021

Chinnaratha MA, Chuang MA, Fraser RJL, et al. Percutaneous thermal ablation for primary hepatocellular carcinoma: a systematic review and meta-analysis. *J Gastroenterol Hepatol.* 2016;31(2):294–301. doi:10.1111/jgh.13028

Chu KF, Dupuy DE. Thermal ablation of tumours: biological mechanisms and advances in therapy. *Nat Rev Cancer.* 2014;14(3):199. doi:10.1038/nrc3672

de Baère T, Risse O, Kuoch V, et al. Adverse events during radiofrequency treatment of 582 hepatic tumors. *Am J Roentgenol.* 2003;181(3):695–700. doi:10.2214/ajr.181.3.1810695

Dong B, Liang P, Yu X, et al. Percutaneous sonographically guided microwave coagulation therapy for hepatocellular carcinoma: results in 234 patients. *Am J Roentgenol.* 2003;180(6):1547–1555. doi:10.2214/ajr.180.6.1801547

Dong H, Strome SE, Salomao DR, et al. Tumor-associated B7-H1 promotes T-cell apoptosis: a potential mechanism of immune evasion. *Nat Med.* 2002;8(8):793–800. doi:10.1038/nm730

El Fouly A, Ertle J, El Dorry A, et al. In intermediate stage hepatocellular carcinoma: radioembolization with yttrium 90 or chemoembolization? *Liver Int.* 2015;35(2):627–635. doi:10.1111/liv.12637

Facciorusso A, Di Maso N, Muscatiello N. Microwave ablation versus radiofrequency ablation for the treatment of hepatocellular carcinoma: a systematic review and meta-analysis. *Int J Hyperthermia.* 2016;32(3):339–344. doi:10.3109/02656736.2015.1127434

Forner A, Llovet JM, Bruix J. Hepatocellularcarcinoma. *Lancet.* 2012;379(9822):1245. doi:10.1016/S0140-6736(11)61347-0

Gallo G, Carucci P, Veltri A, et al. Predictive factors of tumor recurrence and death in patients with hepatocellular carcinoma treated by locoregional therapies: results of a retrospective cohort study. *J Hepatol.* 2017;66(1):S217. doi:10.1016/S0168-8278(17)30731-6

Ganne-Carrié N, Nault JC, Ziol M, et al. Predicting recurrence following radiofrequency percutaneous ablation for hepatocellular carcinoma. *Hepat Oncol.* 2014;1(4):395–408. doi:10.2217/hep.14.22

Gervais DA, Arellano RS. Percutaneous tumor ablation for hepatocellular carcinoma. *Am J Roentgenol.* 2011;197(4):789–794. doi:10.2214/AJR.11.7656

Gervais DA, Goldberg SN, Brown DB, et al. Society of Interventional Radiology position statement on percutaneous radiofrequency ablation for the treatment of liver tumors. *J Vasc Interv Radiol.* 2009;20(7):S342–S347. doi:10.1016/j.jvir.2009.04.029

Govindarajan N, Froud T, Suthar R, Barbery K. Irreversible electroporation of hepatic malignancy. *Semin Intervent Radiol.* 2013;30(01):067–073. doi:10.1055/s-0033-1333655

Heckman JT, deVera MB, Marsh JW, et al. Bridging locoregional therapy for hepatocellular carcinoma prior to liver transplantation. *Ann Surg Oncol.* 2008;15(11):3169–3177. doi:10.1245/s10434-008-0071-3

Hilgard P, Hamami M, El Fouly A, et al. Radioembolization with yttrium-90 glass microspheres in hepatocellular carcinoma: European experience on safety and long-term survival. *Hepatology.* 2010;52(5):1741–1749. doi:10.1002/hep.23944

Kim H-C. Radioembolization for the treatment of hepatocellular carcinoma. *Clin Mol Hepatol.* 2017;23(2):109. doi:10.3350/cmh.2017.0004

Kudo M, Chung H, Osaki Y. Prognostic staging system for hepatocellular carcinoma (CLIP score): its value and limitations, and a proposal for a new staging system, the Japan Integrated Staging Score (JIS score). *J Gastroenterol.* 2003;38(3):207–215. doi:10.1007/s005350300038

Lee SH, Kim SU, Jang JW, et al. Use of transient elastography to predict de novo recurrence after radiofrequency ablation for hepatocellular carcinoma. *Onco Targets Ther.* 2015;8:347. doi:10.2147/OTT.S75077

Lencioni R, de Baere T, Soulen MC, et al. Lipiodol transarterial chemoembolization for hepatocellular carcinoma: a systematic review of efficacy and safety data. *Hepatology.* 2016;64(1):106–116. doi:10.1002/hep.28453

Lencioni R. Loco-regional treatment of hepatocellular carcinoma. *Hepatology.* 2010;52(2):762–773. doi:10.1002/hep.23725

Lin X-j, Li Q-j, Lao X-m, et al. Transarterial injection of recombinant human type-5 adenovirus H101 in combination with transarterial chemoembolization (TACE) improves overall and progressive-free survival in unresectable hepatocellular carcinoma (HCC). *BMC Cancer.* 2015;15(1):707. doi:10.1186/s12885-015-1715-x

Liu L, Chen H, Wang M, et al. Combination therapy of sorafenib and TACE for unresectable HCC: a systematic review and meta-analysis. *PloS One.* 2014;9(3):e91124. doi:10.1371/journal.pone.0091124

Livraghi T, Goldberg SN, Lazzaroni S, et al. Small hepatocellular carcinoma: treatment with radio-frequency ablation versus ethanol injection. *Radiology.* 1999;210(3):655–661. doi:10.1148/radiology.210.3.r99fe40655

Llovet JM, Vilana R, Brú C, et al. Increased risk of tumor seeding after percutaneous radiofrequency ablation for single hepatocellular carcinoma. *Hepatology.* 2001;33(5):1124–1129. doi:10.1053/jhep.2001.24233

Lu DS, Yu NC, Raman SS, et al. Percutaneous radiofrequency ablation of hepatocellular carcinoma as a bridge to liver transplantation. *Hepatology.* 2005;41(5):1130–1137. doi:10.1002/hep.20688

Lu W, Zhang J, Yang C. Recent Advances in Hepatocellular Cancer. In: *Interventional Techniques to Hepatocellular Carcinoma.* 2016.

Lubner MG, Brace CL, Ziemlewicz TJ, et al. Microwave ablation of hepatic malignancy. *Semin Interv Radiol.* 2013;30(1):56–66. doi:10.1055/s-0033-1333654

Ludwig JM, Xing M, Gai Y, et al. Targeted Yttrium 89-Doxorubicin Drug-Eluting Bead – a safety and feasibility pilot study in a rabbit liver cancer model. *Mol Pharm.* 2017;14(8):2824–2830. doi:10.1021/acs.molpharmaceut.7b00336

Lyu T, Wang X, Su Z, et al. Irreversible electroporation in primary and metastatic hepatic malignancies: a review. *Medicine*. 2017;96(17):e6386. doi:10.1097/MD.0000000000006386

Majno PE, Adam R, Bismuth H, et al. Influence of preoperative transarterial lipiodol chemoembolization on resection and transplantation for hepatocellular carcinoma in patients with cirrhosis. *Ann Surg*. 1997;226(6):688. doi:10.1097/00000658-199712000-00006

Mazzaferro V, Regalia E, Doci R, et al. Liver transplantation for the treatment of small hepatocellular carcinomas in patients with cirrhosis. *N Engl J Med*. 1996;334(11):693–700. doi:10.1056/NEJM199603143341104

Mulier S, Mulier P, Ni Y, et al. Complications of radiofrequency coagulation of liver tumours. *Br J Surg*. 2002;89(10):1206–1222. doi:10.1046/j.1365-2168.2002.02168.x

Prajapati H, Spivey JR, Hanish SI, et al. mRECIST and EASL responses at early time point by contrast-enhanced dynamic MRI predict survival in patients with unresectable hepatocellular carcinoma (HCC) treated by doxorubicin drug-eluting beads transarterial chemoembolization (DEB TACE). *Ann Oncol*. 2012;24(4):965–973. doi:10.1093/annonc/mds605

Prajapati HJ, Kim HS. Treatment algorithm based on the multivariate survival analyses in patients with advanced hepatocellular carcinoma treated with trans-arterial chemoembolization. *PloS One*. 2017;12(2):e0170750. doi:10.1371/journal.pone.0170750

Prajapati HJ, Dhanasekaran R, El-Rayes BF, et al. Safety and efficacy of doxorubicin drug-eluting bead transarterial chemoembolization in patients with advanced hepatocellular carcinoma. *J Vasc Interv Radiol*. 2013;24(3):307–315. doi:10.1016/j.jvir.2012.11.026

Prajapati HJ, Rafi S, El-Rayes BF, et al. Safety and feasibility of same-day discharge of patients with unresectable hepatocellular carcinoma treated with doxorubicin drug-eluting bead transcatheter chemoembolization. *J Vasc Interv Radiol*. 2012;23(10):1286–1293.e1.

Ramanathan M, Shroads M, Choi M, et al. Predictors of intermediate-term survival with destination locoregional therapy of hepatocellular cancer in patients either ineligible or unwilling for liver transplantation. *J Gastrointest Oncol*. 2017;8(5):885. doi:10.21037/jgo.2017.07.05

Ravaioli M, Grazi GL, Piscaglia F, et al. Liver transplantation for hepatocellular carcinoma: results of down-staging in patients initially outside the Milan selection criteria. *Am J Transplant*. 2008;8(12):2547–2557. doi:10.1111/j.1600-6143.2008.02409.x

Russell SJ, Peng K-W, Bell JC. Oncolytic virotherapy. *Nat Biotechnol*. 2012;30(7):658–670. doi:10.1038/nbt.2287

Salem R, Gordon AC, Mouli S, et al. Y90 radioembolization significantly prolongs time to progression compared with chemoembolization in patients with hepatocellular carcinoma. *Gastroenterology*. 2016;151(6):1155–1163.e2. doi:10.1053/j.gastro.2016.08.029

Scheffer HJ, Nielsen K, de Jong MC, et al. Irreversible electroporation for nonthermal tumor ablation in the clinical setting: a systematic review of safety and efficacy. *J Vasc Interv Radiol*. 2014;25(7):997–1011. doi:10.1016/j.jvir.2014.01.028

Sherman M. Staging for hepatocellular carcinoma: complex and confusing. *Gastroenterology*. 2014;146(7):1599–1602. doi:10.1053/j.gastro.2014.04.026

Song JE. Conventional vs drug-eluting beads transarterial chemoembolization for hepatocellular carcinoma. *World J Hepatol*. 2017;9(18):808. doi:10.4254/wjh.v9.i18.808

Vauthey J, Klimstra D, Blumgart L. A simplified staging system for hepatocellular carcinomas. *Gastroenterology*. 1995;108(2):617–618. doi:10.1016/0016-5085(95)90109-4

Violi NV, Duran R, Guiu B, et al. Efficacy of microwave ablation versus radiofrequency ablation for the treatment of hepatocellular carcinoma in patients with chronic liver disease: a randomised controlled phase 2 trial. *Lancet Gastroenterol Hepatol*. 2018;3(5):317–325. doi:10.1016/s2468-1253(18)30029-3

Yamada R, Sato M, Kawabata M, et al. Hepatic artery embolization in 120 patients with unresectable hepatoma. *Radiology*. 1983;148(2):397–401. doi:10.1148/radiology.148.2.6306721

Yao FY, Kerlan RK, Hirose R, et al. Excellent outcome following down-staging of hepatocellular carcinoma prior to liver transplantation: an intention-to-treat analysis. *Hepatology*. 2008;48(3):819–827. doi:10.1002/hep.22412

Yao FY, Kinkhabwala M, LaBerge JM, et al. The impact of pre-operative loco-regional therapy on outcome after liver transplantation for hepatocellular carcinoma. *Am J Transplant*. 2005;5(4):795–804. doi:10.1111/j.1600-6143.2005.00750.x

Yao FY. Expanded criteria for liver transplantation in patients with hepatocellular carcinoma. *Hepatol Res*. 2007;37(s2):S267–S274. doi:10.1111/j.1872-034X.2007.00195.x

Zamarin D, Holmgaard RB, Subudhi SK, et al. Localized oncolytic virotherapy overcomes systemic tumor resistance to immune checkpoint blockade immunotherapy. *Sci Transl Med*. 2014;6(226):226ra32. doi:10.1126/scitranslmed.3008095

Zhang L, Hu P, Chen X, Bie P. Transarterial chemoembolization (TACE) plus sorafenib versus TACE for intermediate or advanced stage hepatocellular carcinoma: a meta-analysis. *PloS One*. 2014;9(6):e100305. doi:10.1371/journal.pone.0100305

REFERENCES

1. Llovet JM, Brú C, Bruix J. Prognosis of hepatocellular carcinoma: the BCLC staging classification. *Semin Liver Dis*. 1999;19:329–338. doi:10.1055/s-2007-1007122
2. Yau T, Tang VYF, Yao TJ. et al. Development of Hong Kong Liver Cancer Staging System with treatment stratification for patients with hepatocellular carcinoma. *Gastroenterology*. 2014;146:1691–1700.e3. doi:10.1053/j.gastro.2014.02.032
3. Ikai I, Takayasu K, Omata M. et al. A modified Japan Integrated Stage score for prognostic assessment in patients with hepatocellular carcinoma. *J Gastroenterol*. 2006;41:884–892. doi:10.1007/s00535-006-1878-y
4. Daniele B, Annunziata M, Barletta, E. et al. Cancer of the Liver Italian Program (CLIP) score for staging hepatocellular carcinoma. *Hepatol Res*. 2007;37:S206–S209. doi:10.1111/j.1872-034x.2007.00186.x
5. Leung TW, Tang AM, Zee B. et al. Construction of the Chinese University Prognostic Index for hepatocellular carcinoma and comparison with the TNM staging system, the Okuda staging system, and the Cancer of the Liver Italian Program staging system: a study based on 926 patients. *Cancer*. 2002;94:1760–1769. doi:10.1002/cncr.10384
6. Chevret S, Trinchet JC, Mathieu D, et al. A new prognostic classification for predicting survival in patients with hepatocellular carcinoma. Groupe d'Etude et de Traitement du Carcinome Hépatocellulaire. *J Hepatol*. 1999;31:133–141. doi:10.1016/s0168-8278(99)80173-1
7. Okuda K, Ohtsuki T, Obata H, et al. Natural history of hepatocellular carcinoma and prognosis in relation to treatment. Study of 850 patients. *Cancer*.1985;56:918–928. doi:10.1002/1097-0142(19850815)56:4<918::aid-cncr2820560437>3.0.co;2-e
8. Hsu CY, Huang YH, Hsia CY, et al. A new prognostic model for hepatocellular carcinoma based on total tumor volume: the Taipei Integrated Scoring System. *J Hepatol*. 2010;53:108–117. doi:10.1016/j.jhep.2010.01.038

How I Treat Early-Stage Hepatocellular Cancer With Local Nonsurgical Approaches (Radiation)

Jonathan B. Ashman

INTRODUCTION

Managing patients with hepatocellular carcinoma (HCC) is complex and requires multidisciplinary coordination. Factors that are critical to decision making include the number and size of primary tumors, vascular invasion, extrahepatic spread, performance status, and liver function typically in the setting of cirrhosis. In order to appropriately stage and treat patients, these disease and patient factors have been incorporated into various prognostic tools such as the Barcelona Clinic Liver Cancer (BCLC) system. A recent review from the BCLC group discusses resection, transplantation, percutaneous thermal ablation, transarterial chemoembolization (TACE), and transarterial radioembolization (TARE) as treatment options but makes no mention of radiation therapy in their algorithm (1). The role of radiation therapy historically has been limited by the technical ability to deliver safe and effective doses to patients with underlying liver disease. However, HCC is a radiosensitive disease, and the modern era of image-guided photon therapy and charged particle therapy offers new opportunities for incorporation of radiation therapy into the care of these patients. The challenge is to appropriately define those patients who will optimally benefit from radiation.

RADIATION TOLERANCE OF THE LIVER

The ability to deliver a safe and meaningful dose of radiation to a tumor in the liver underpins both the past limitations of radiation therapy in the treatment of HCC and the capabilities of modern photon and particle therapy. The hepatic lobule is the functional subunit of the liver. As each lobule is independent, the health of the overall organ is dependent on the number of intact lobules. This organization is termed "parallel" architecture and implies that radiation sensitivity is strongly related to the volume of the organ treated rather than to maximum point doses. The tolerance of the liver to whole-organ radiation is in the range of 30 to 35 Gy in 1.8 to 2.0 Gy per fraction (2). Dawson and colleagues modeled the normal tissue complication probability (NTCP) and demonstrated the volume effect with complication risk rising sharply above a mean dose of approximately 30 Gy (3). Moreover, tolerances were dependent on the health of the underlying liver when comparing patients with primary liver tumors to ones with metastatic disease. However, primary liver tumors require higher doses for optimum local control, and, therefore, there was limited role for radiotherapy prior to the era of three-dimensional conformal radiation therapy (3DCRT).

CONFORMAL RADIATION THERAPY

Dose escalation trials at the University of Michigan established that 3DCRT techniques could safely deliver ablative doses to small volumes of liver for the treatment of HCC (4). A phase I/II trial for patients with both primary (35 of 128 patients with HCC) and metastatic liver tumors escalated the dose up to 90 Gy in twice-daily fractions of 1.5 Gy each with concurrent hepatic artery floxuridine. The median survival for the HCC cohort was 15 months, and

---

A Clinical Vignette ("How I Treat") is included at the end of the chapter.

radiation-induced liver disease (RILD) was detected in only 4% of patients. A Japanese study used a similar hyperfractionated regimen of 45 to 75 Gy in 1.5 Gy twice-daily fractions with concurrent thalidomide and reported a 2-year survival of 45% (5). A third phase II trial from France delivered 66 Gy in 2 Gy per fraction and reported a local control rate of 78% at 29 months (6). No grade 4–5 toxicity was detected among patients with Child–Pugh (CP) class A, while 3 of 11 patients with CP class B developed grade 4 toxicity. A multicenter phase I dose escalation trial was able to reach 62 Gy in 2 Gy fractions without identifying a dose-limiting toxicity but closed after treating 19 patients due to poor accrual and could not reach the highest dose level planned to 70 Gy (7).

STEREOTACTIC BODY RADIATION THERAPY (SBRT)

SBRT (now often referred to as stereotactic ablative radiotherapy [SABR]) delivers large doses per fraction ranging from 5 to 20 Gy in a hypofractionated approach to extracranial tumors. Based on the experience of intracranial stereotactic radiosurgery, these regimens are biologically more potent but require high precision delivery with image guidance and motion management to limit exposure to normal surrounding tissue. In the United States, SBRT is defined for regulatory purposes as 1 to 5 fractions but elsewhere regimens up to 10 fractions have been considered SBRT. The first publication describing SBRT for liver tumors was in 1995 (8). A small prospective phase I–II trial in 2006 with eight HCC patients and 17 metastatic patients reported 75% local control (9). One patient with CP class B died of hepatic toxicity within the first month of treatment. A larger phase I trial was reported by Tse et al. from Princess Margaret Hospital, which included 41 HCC patients limited to CP class A liver function (10). A six-fraction regimen was delivered with a median total dose of 36 Gy. The prescription dose was tailored for each individual patient in order to maintain normal tissue tolerance based on the University of Michigan NTCP model. Local control was 65% and overall survival at 1 year was 48%. A decline in alpha-fetoprotein (AFP) was observed in 16 of 21 patients. Five patients progressed from CP class A to class B, but this appeared to be correlated to larger tumors, less radiation dose, and ultimately disease progression. A dose-limiting toxicity was not reached. The results of this trial were extended with the report of an additional 102 patients treated on an expanded phase I/II trial and an immediately subsequent phase II trial (11). Overall local control at 1 year was 87%, and the median overall survival was 17 months. With regard to toxicity, treatment potentially contributed to seven deaths, of which five were due to liver failure, one was secondary to cholangitis, and one secondary to gastrointestinal bleed after reirradiation. Hepatic deterioration was defined by advancement in CP class in the absence of clear progressive disease and occurred in 29% of patients at 3 months post-SBRT but only in 6% at 12 months, which suggested the possibility of recovery after acute injury.

The results of these prospective trials were buttressed by a large Japanese retrospective experience of 185 patients (15% CP class B) treated to 35 to 40 Gy in five fractions (12). Local control and overall survival at 3 years were 91% and 70%, respectively, with 10% of patients experiencing CP class decline by two points and only two cases of grade 5 liver failures. A French retrospective study of 77 patients treated to 45 Gy in three fractions report local control and overall survival at 2 years of 99% and 56%, respectively (13). Only one patient experienced grade 3 acute RILD and one patient experienced grade 3 chronic ascites, although there were two cases of grade 3–4 gastric ulcer and one case of grade 2 colic ulcer. Patients with preserved liver function may also benefit from SBRT even if the tumors are large and exceed 10 cm (14). Taken together, these prospective and retrospective studies established a favorable profile of safety and efficacy for SBRT in HCC, but interpretation of the survival results was limited by a patient population with advanced disease.

More recently, a prospective phase II trial delivered SBRT with curative intent in a cohort of patients with intact liver function and a solitary tumor less than 4 cm in size (15). The prescription dose was 35 to 40 Gy in five fractions. With a median follow-up of 41.7 months in 90 evaluable patients, the 3-year local control was 96.3%. Moreover, in this favorable population, median overall survival was 54.7 months and 66.7% at 3 years. Only eight patients (8.9%) progressed to worse CP score of at least two points, and six of the eight recovered baseline liver function within 6 months. Another recent phase II trial has explored an adaptive SBRT approach using indocyanine green retention before and after three fractions of treatment to determine the dose delivered for the last two fractions (16). Of the 90 patients who were enrolled, there were 69 patients (77%) with HCC. Outstanding 1-year and 2-year local control rates of 99% and 95%, respectively, were achieved with only 7% of patients experiencing a 2-point decline in CP score.

Patients with more advanced liver disease can be treated with SBRT, but the majority of patients experienced a decline of CP score by at least two points by 3 months and any survival benefit appeared to be largely limited to patients with CP class B7 cirrhosis (17). A retrospective review of 65 patients treated to 48 Gy in four fractions demonstrated local control and overall survival at 2 years of 100% and 76%, respectively (18). However, grade 3 or higher toxicity was observed in 23% of patients, and the incidence of toxicity was significantly higher in CP class B patients. A prospective phase I–II trial from Washington University included 26 patients (12 with HCC; 12 with intrahepatic cholangiocarcinoma; two with mixed tumors) treated to a median dose of 55 Gy in five fractions (19). While local control was 91% at 1 year, nine patients (35%) experienced decline in CP class and two patients died from hepatic failure. Therefore, while both retrospective and prospective studies demonstrate consistently high tumor control, caution must be maintained especially for patients with cirrhosis advanced beyond CP class A. A recent analysis identified CP class, mean liver dose, and dose to 700–900 cubic centimeters of liver as most strongly associated with hepatic toxicity along with thrombocytopenia and portal vein thrombosis (PVT) (20).

A major question is how to integrate SBRT into the HCC treatment algorithm along with other local-regional therapies such as TACE and percutaneous ablation (21). A single-institution retrospective analysis comparing radiofrequency ablation (RFA) and SBRT reported good local control with either technique for tumors less than 2 cm, but SBRT appeared superior for larger tumors (22). A more recent analysis using the National Cancer Database questions this conclusion that SBRT is superior to RFA (23). Moreover, Markov modeling found that SBRT was not cost-effective compared to RFA as initial treatment for inoperable HCC but was favored as salvage for recurrence after RFA (24). SBRT has additional benefits of maintenance of quality of life (25). For patients undergoing TACE, a meta-analysis suggested an overall survival benefit for patients receiving a combination of TACE and radiation therapy compared to TACE alone (26). A consensus statement released after the 7th Annual Asia-Pacific Primary Liver Cancer Expert Meeting endorsed SBRT as a safe and effective treatment option for small HCC (27).

PORTAL VEIN THROMBOSIS

PVT is a high-risk feature when detected in HCC, which often precludes TACE. Radiotherapy can be used to treat HCC when PVT is present and can also be directed at the PVT itself. A recent meta-analysis compared 3DCRT with SBRT or radioembolization. While overall survival was similar among patients treated with each technique, SBRT yielded a response rate of 71%, which was statistically significantly higher than the other modalities and appeared to have a more favorable toxicity profile (28).

PROTON BEAM THERAPY (PBT)

Charged particles such as protons have significantly different dose distributions within tissue compared to photons. The Bragg peak describes the narrow range of maximal dose deposition beyond which the charged particles stop. By using a mixture of particle energies, the Bragg peak effectively can be spread out to cover the target while delivering smaller doses to tissues in the entrance path and no exit dose. Our facility employs only pencil-beam scanning technology in which small spheres ("spots") of dose are painted within the target layer by layer from deep to shallow depths. Although particle therapy introduces additional uncertainties into treatment planning and delivery especially with respect to organ motion, the integral dose to nontarget tissue is typically superior to photon planning. When considering the parallel organization of the liver and the need to spare as much functional tissue as possible, the physical properties of proton therapy suggest a clinical advantage over photon treatment for patients with HCC

One of the largest experiences with proton beam for HCC was reported from Tsukuba University in Japan (29). This retrospective study included 318 patients of which approximately 75% were CP class A and 25% CP class B. Long-term overall survival at 5 years was 44.6% and 55.9% for CP class A patients. There were no grade 4/5 toxicities and no significant liver toxicity. The same group replicated these results in a prospective study of 51 patients treated to 66 Gy radiobiological equivalent (RBE) in 10 fractions (30). Local control and overall survival at 5 years were 87.8% and 38.7%, respectively.

Initial prospective data supporting the use of PBT was reported by Loma Linda University (31). Seventy-six patients were treated to 63 Gy (RBE) in 15 fractions. The patient cohort represented a high-risk and advanced disease population with 54% of patients outside Milan criteria, 24% of patients with CP class C, 16% of patients with Model of End-Stage Liver Disease (MELD) >15, and 48% of the tumors were larger than 5 cm. Survival at 3 years was 70% and 10% for patients who did or did not undergo liver transplantation, and liver toxicity was minimal.

The same group has reported interim results of a prospective randomized trial comparing PBT to TACE (32). With a median follow-up of 28 months, nonsignificant trends in favor of proton beam were observed for local control and progression-free survival. Patients treated with PBT had significantly fewer days of hospitalization within 30 days of the procedure.

Most significantly, a multi-institutional phase II trial studied proton beam for primary liver tumors, including 44 patients with HCC, 37 patients with intrahepatic cholangiocarcinoma, and two patients with mixed tumors (33). In the HCC cohort, 72.7% of the patients had CP class A and 29.5% had tumor vascular thrombus. The median dose was 58 Gy (RBE) in 15 fractions with peripheral lesions treated to 67.5 Gy (RBE) and central tumors within 2 cm of the porta hepatis treated to 58.05 Gy (RBE). Local control was 94.8%, and median progression-free survival and overall survival were 13.9 and 49 months, respectively. No grade 4 or 5 toxicities were observed, and only three patients progressed from CP class A to class B within 6 months.

CHOOSING PROTONS OR PHOTONS

Protons and photons have not been compared directly, and it appears that many cases can be treated well with either photon SBRT or proton beam. For centers such as ours with both technologies, the question then arises as to how to select the optimal treatment in any particular case. A dosimetry study was performed to compare intensity-modulated radiation therapy (IMRT) or proton beam for 13 tumors in 10 patients, and the risk of RILD was then modeled based on liver exposure (34). A rapid rise in the calculated risk of RILD was found in the IMRT plans compared to PBT for tumors greater than 6 cm. A second study sought to look at both tumor size and location. Comparison plans were systematically generated for different size mock spherical tumors in different locations within the liver, and then the model was verified for 10 patients (35). First, the model showed no benefit from protons compared to photons for tumors less than 3 cm at any location or for tumors of any size in a caudal or left medial location. Improved liver sparing was achieved with protons when the tumor size was greater than or equal to 3 cm and was located in the dome or central liver.

A meta-analysis was performed to compare conformal radiation, SBRT, and charged particle therapy (36). Outcomes were inferior for conformal radiation, but statistically significant differences for overall survival, progression-free survival, local control, and acute toxicity were not found when comparing SBRT with particle therapy. Late toxicity favored particle therapy compared with either photon-based technique.

In practice, each case is approached individually. Typically, patients present with baseline cirrhosis, and proton beam would be preferred to maximize sparing of functional liver parenchyma. However, photon SBRT may be preferred in order to optimize image guidance. In our facility, we treat patients with proton beam in a free-breathing mode if target motion is less than 1 cm or we utilize a deep inspiration breath-hold technique for patients with motion exceeding 1 cm. Patients with cirrhosis may have altered breathing patterns or may not be able to hold their breath, and these patient therefore may be more suitable to treat with active respiratory gating using photon SBRT. Treatment times are generally longer with proton therapy, and patients who are older or more frail also may benefit from the faster treatment delivery on certain photon units with high output modes. Photon SBRT also may be preferred for patients with implantable cardiac devices such as pacemakers or defibrillators. Even with pencil-beam scanning, internally scattered neutron production occurs with proton beam and may lead to device malfunction (37). We carefully evaluate each of these patients to determine the degree to which their cardiac function is dependent on the device and work closely with our colleagues in cardiac electrophysiology to assess the risks and benefits of proton beam or photon therapy.

CONCLUSIONS

Our case highlights many of the issues concerning radiation therapy for HCC. In current practice, radiation therapy often is considered only after other local therapies have failed or are not technically feasible. Nevertheless, radiation therapy can effectively control HCC. Substantial prospective and retrospective data supports the safety and efficacy of radiation therapy in the management of HCC. Both photon SBRT and proton beam should be considered as options. As in our case, smaller tumors in patients with well-compensated liver cirrhosis can be treated with both modalities, but proton beam may be preferred for larger and more central lesions and in patients with more advanced liver disease. In my opinion, the key question is not proton versus photon, but instead the appropriate place for radiation therapy in the treatment algorithm alongside other local-regional therapies (38). Clinical trials should continue to test the role of radiation prospectively either against or in combination with TACE or ablation. Also, there will likely be an increasing role for TARE as internally direct brachytherapy as another alternative local-regional treatment option. In the meantime, radiation oncologists must attend liver tumor boards to actively participate in the multidisciplinary care of their patients with this complex disease.

Clinical Vignette 33.1

A 75-year-old woman presented with nonalcoholic steatohepatitis (NASH)-related cirrhosis. A surveillance liver MRI demonstrated a 2 cm mass in segment VIII consistent with HCC. Her past medical history included a diagnosis of gastric B cell lymphoma successfully treated more than 10 years earlier with rituximab, cyclophosphamide, doxorubicin, vincristine, and prednisone (R-CHOP) followed by radiotherapy. It was felt that the chemotherapy was most likely the etiology of cirrhosis. The case was reviewed at the multidisciplinary tumor board. TACE with drug-eluting beads was performed with initial favorable radiographic response. Ten months after this initial treatment, a local recurrence and a bland, nonoccluding thrombus in the portal vein were detected on follow-up MRI (Figure 33.1). These findings correlated with a rise in the AFP from 5.7 to 9.0 ng/ml. The patient's cirrhosis was well compensated with a CP class A and MELD score of 7. The case was reviewed again at the multidisciplinary tumor board. Repeat TACE was not recommended, and the location in the dome was not favorable for percutaneous ablation. Therefore, SBRT was recommended.

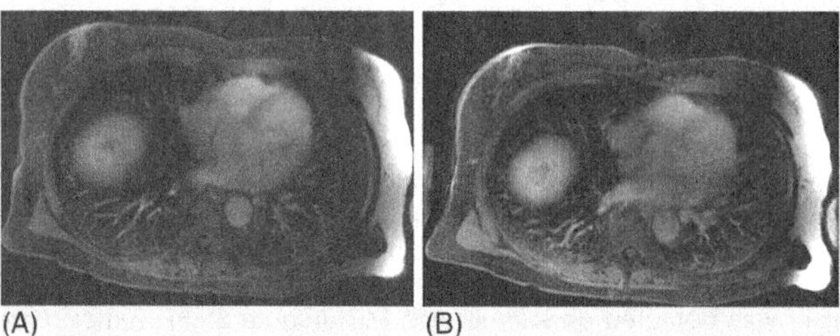

FIGURE 33.1   Axial IV contrast enhanced dynamic T1-weighted MRI demonstrating new hypervascularity in the segment VIII lesion on arterial phase imaging (A) and washout on delayed phase (B).

IV, intravenous.

Prior to radiation simulation, the patient was referred for ultrasound-guided placement of fiducial markers. The gold markers are most commonly placed under percutaneous ultrasound guidance, but CT or endoscopic ultrasound guidance techniques are alternatives depending on the tumor location and local expertise. Ideally, four markers are placed at least well spaced around the tumor in different planes (three are required for stereotaxis and the fourth as a backup in case of fiducial migration). Fiducial markers can improve the accuracy of motion assessment during treatment planning and image guidance during radiation treatment delivery. However, the markers may introduce added uncertainty during target definition because of the metal CT artifact, especially when markers are placed too close together. Therefore, good communication is necessary between the radiation oncologist and the interventional radiology team as to optimal localization. Other relative or absolute contraindications to fiducial placement include the tumor location, patient's general health and degree of cirrhosis, anticoagulation status, and local technical expertise. In our department, image-guided photon SBRT is performed using cone-beam CT, which does not require fiducial markers when the whole liver and diaphragm can act as localization surrogate and the patient is treated in a free-breathing state. When photon liver SBRT is performed with motion management techniques such as deep inspiration breath hold or respiratory gating, fiducial markers significantly increase confidence and efficiency of treatment delivery.

After fiducial marker placement, the patient was simulated supine, arms up, with a thermoplastic body mask for immobilization. A four-dimensional CT was performed and determined that the tumor excursion in the superior/inferior dimension was approximately 1.5 cm. Since this was greater than our departmental threshold of 1 cm of motion in which treatment in free breathing is acceptable, it was determined to use respiratory gating. Using a window gated around the end-expiratory phase of breathing, target motion was reduced to approximately 0.2 cm in all dimensions. Treatment planning CT scans were obtained with and without intravenous (IV) contrast. IV contrast and image protocols designed to capture multiple contrast phases are critical to the precise definition of HCC for SBRT, since many of these tumors appear isodense to surrounding liver on noncontrast CT. Diagnostic MRI sequences were fused with the CT simulation images to improve target definition.

In the planning phase, the gross tumor volume (GTV) was defined using the IV contrast CT images and the appropriate MRI images. The GTV was expanded to create an internal target volume (ITV) encompassing only the motion between the 20% to 60% phases of the respiratory cycle. A 5 mm planning target volume (PTV) was then added symmetrically to account for any patient setup error. Planning then commenced to deliver a prescription dose of 50 Gy over five fractions designed with IMRT using a volumetric-modulated arc therapy (VMAT) technique (Figure 33.2). Image-guided radiation therapy (IGRT) was performed with on-board cone-beam CT. Dose volume histogram analysis was performed to assess for target coverage and dose to normal organs at risk (OARs). The volume of the PTV receiving 100% of the dose was set at 95%. The mean liver dose was 5.0 Gy and the volume of liver excluded from receiving 15 Gy was 1,209 cubic centimeters (cc). The mean heart dose was 3.9 Gy, and no heart was exposed to 20 Gy or more.

The patient tolerated SBRT well with no acute side effects. At three months post-SBRT, the patient continued to do well without any decline in her liver function. No residual hyperenhancement or washout was detected on surveillance MRI, and the AFP decreased to 4.3 ng/ml. The patient did well until 2 years after SBRT, when the AFP rose to 421 ng/ml and a new OPTN5 lesion measuring 3.9 × 3.7 × 5.3 cm located in segment IV was detected on surveillance MRI (Figure 33.3). Tumor thrombus was also detected in the left portal vein extending medially from the mass. Liver function had been maintained at CP class A. Again, the patient was discussed at our multidisciplinary tumor board. Radiation therapy was the only treatment option felt to be appropriate; proton therapy was preferred based on the tumor size and location and prior radiation exposure.

Simulation for proton therapy is performed in a similar fashion to photon SBRT. Fiducial markers are required for proton therapy in our facility because IGRT is accomplished using kilovoltage (kV) x-ray imaging at isocenter with matched flat-panel detectors. Cone-beam CT at the treatment isocenter is not available on our proton therapy unit. Simulation was performed with the patient in the supine position with arms up and

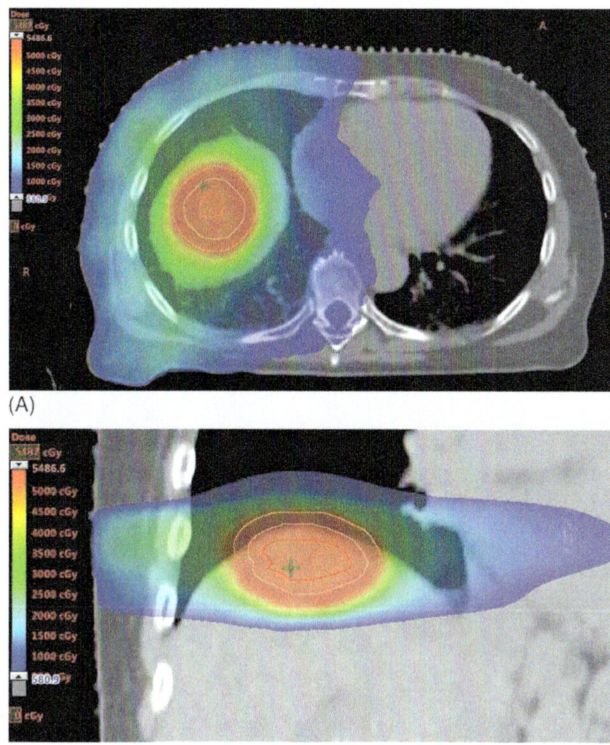

FIGURE 33.2　Colorwash dose distribution in axial (A) and coronal (B) imaging planes for SBRT plan to a prescription dose of 50 Gy using IMRT with VMAT technique. Target volumes indicated as GTV (red); ITV (pink); PTV (orange).

GTV, gross tumor volume; IMRT, intensity-modulated radiation therapy; ITV, internal target volume; PTV, planning target volume; SBRT, stereotactic body radiation therapy; VMAT, volumetric-modulated arc therapy.

in a thermoplastic body mask. Noncontrast and IV contrast planning CT scans were obtained as before and again fused with diagnostic MRI for target delineation. Motion was measured at only 0.6 cm in the superior–inferior direction and minimal anterior–posterior or right–left directions. Therefore, an ITV-based technique was used with the patient free-breathing. Pencil-beam scanning proton therapy plan using a three-field single-field optimization (SFO) technique was designed to deliver 52.5 Gy RBE in 15 fractions of 3.5 Gy each (Figure 33.4). A 15-fraction regimen is currently preferred over a 5-fraction SBRT regimen due to these increased uncertainties in proton planning and image-guidance systems. Typically, our plans utilize two or three fields to balance the incremental improvements in dose distribution with the efficiency of treatment delivery. Because protons are more susceptible than photons to uncertainties in setup and range, multiple-field design can improve the robustness of proton plans. In addition, multiple-field design reduces the entrance dose and therefore potential skin toxicity as well as mitigating possible increased radiobiologic effects at the end of proton range. The mean liver dose was 9.9 Gy and liver volume excluded from 15 Gy was 1,019 cc . The cumulative mean liver dose from both treatments was 21 Gy and the total liver volume excluded from 15 Gy was 720 cc. No acute toxicities were noted during proton therapy, and the patient continues on surveillance.

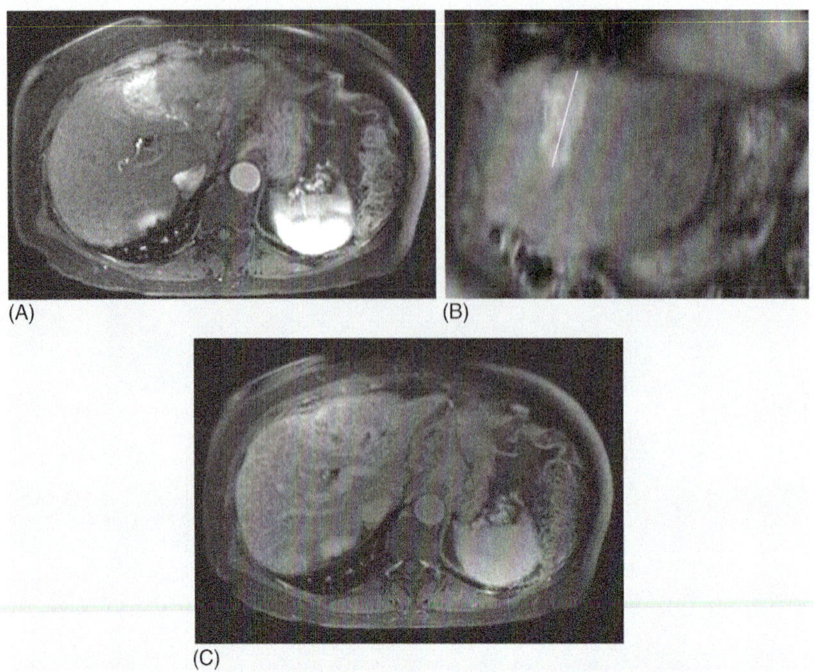

FIGURE 33.3 Follow-up IV contrast enhanced dynamic T1-weighted MRI demonstrating new hypervascular lesion in the segment IVa and IVb lesion on arterial phase imaging in axial (A) and coronal (B) planes and washout on axial delayed phase (B).

IV, intravenous.

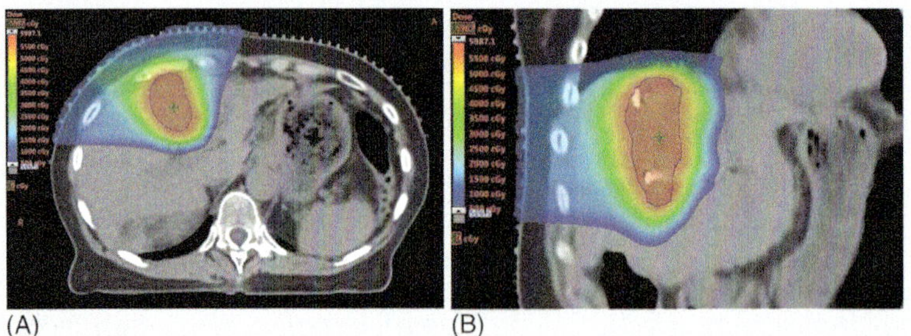

FIGURE 33.4 Colorwash dose distribution in axial (A) and coronal (B) imaging planes for pencil-beam scanning proton plan to a prescription dose of 52.5 Gy (RBE) using three-field SFO technique. Target volumes indicated as ITV (red).

ITV, internal target volume; RBE, radiobiological equivalent; SFO, single-field optimization.

REFERENCES

1. Forner A, Reig M, Bruix J. Hepatocellular carcinoma. *Lancet*. 2018;391:1301–1314. doi:10.1016/S0140-6736(18)30010-2
2. Lawrence TS, Robertson JM, Anscher MS, et al. Hepatic toxicity resulting from cancer treatment. *Int J Radiat Oncol Biol Phys*. 1995;31(5):1237–1248. doi:10.1016/0360-3016(94)00418-K

3. Dawson LA, Normolle D, Balter JM, et al. Analysis of radiation-induced liver disease using the Lyman NTCP model. *Int J Radiat Oncol Biol Phys*. 2002;53(4):810–821. doi:10.1016/S0360-3016(02)02846-8

4. Ben-Josef E, Normolle D, Ensminger WD, et al. Phase II trial of high-dose conformal radiation therapy with concurrent hepatic artery floxuridine for unresectable intrahepatic malignancies. *J Clin Oncol*. 2005;23(34):8739–8747. doi:10.1200/JCO.2005.01.5354

5. Hsu WC, Chan SC, Ting LL, et al. Results of three-dimensional conformal radiotherapy and thalidomide for advanced hepatocellular carcinoma. *Jpn J Clin Oncol*. 2006;36(2):93–99. doi:10.1093/jjco/hyi242

6. Mornex F, Girard N, Beziat C, et al. Feasibility and efficacy of high-dose three-dimensional-conformal radiotherapy in cirrhotic patients with small-size hepatocellular carcinoma non-eligible for curative therapies—mature results of the French Phase II RTF-1 trial. *Int J Radiat Oncol Biol Phys*. 2006;66(4):1152–1158. doi:10.1016/j.ijrobp.2006.06.015

7. Herrmann E, Naehrig D, Sassowsky M, et al. External beam radiotherapy for unresectable hepatocellular carcinoma, an international multicenter phase I trial, SAKK 77/07 and SASL 26. *Radiat Oncol*. 2017;12(1):12. doi:10.1186/s13014-016-0745-0

8. Blomgren H, Lax I, Naslund I, et al. Stereotactic high dose fraction radiation therapy of extracranial tumors using an accelerator. Clinical experience of the first thirty-one patients. *Acta Oncol*. 1995;34(6):861–870. doi:10.3109/02841869509127197

9. Mendez Romero A, Wunderink W, Hussain SM, et al. Stereotactic body radiation therapy for primary and metastatic liver tumors: a single institution phase i-ii study. *Acta Oncol*. 2006;45(7):831–837. doi:10.1080/02841860600897934

10. Tse RV, Hawkins M, Lockwood G, et al. Phase I study of individualized stereotactic body radiotherapy for hepatocellular carcinoma and intrahepatic cholangiocarcinoma. *J Clin Oncol*. 2008;26(4):657–664. doi:10.1200/JCO.2007.14.3529

11. Bujold A, Massey CA, Kim JJ, et al. Sequential phase I and II trials of stereotactic body radiotherapy for locally advanced hepatocellular carcinoma. *J Clin Oncol*. 2013;31(13):1631–1639. doi:10.1200/JCO.2012.44.1659

12. Sanuki N, Takeda A, Oku Y, et al. Stereotactic body radiotherapy for small hepatocellular carcinoma: a retrospective outcome analysis in 185 patients. *Acta Oncol*. 2014;53(3):399–404. doi:10.3109/0284186X.2013.820342

13. Huertas A, Baumann AS, Saunier-Kubs F, et al. Stereotactic body radiation therapy as an ablative treatment for inoperable hepatocellular carcinoma. *Radiother Oncol*. 2015;115(2):211–216. doi:10.1016/j.radonc.2015.04.006

14. Que JY, Lin LC, Lin KL, et al. The efficacy of stereotactic body radiation therapy on huge hepatocellular carcinoma unsuitable for other local modalities. *Radiat Oncol*. 2014;9:120. doi:10.1186/1748-717X-9-120

15. Takeda A, Sanuki N, Tsurugai Y, et al. Phase 2 study of stereotactic body radiotherapy and optional transarterial chemoembolization for solitary hepatocellular carcinoma not amenable to resection and radiofrequency ablation. *Cancer*. 2016;122(13):2041–2049. doi:10.1002/cncr.30008

16. Feng M, Suresh K, Schipper MJ, et al. Individualized adaptive stereotactic body radiotherapy for liver tumors in patients at high risk for liver damage: a phase 2 clinical trial. *JAMA Oncol*. 2018;4(1):40–47. doi:10.1001/jamaoncol.2017.2303

17. Culleton S, Jiang H, Haddad CR, et al. Outcomes following definitive stereotactic body radiotherapy for patients with Child-Pugh B or C hepatocellular carcinoma. *Radiother Oncol*. 2014;111(3):412–417. doi:10.1016/j.radonc.2014.05.002

18. Kimura T, Aikata H, Takahashi S, et al. Stereotactic body radiotherapy for patients with small hepatocellular carcinoma ineligible for resection or ablation therapies. *Hepatol Res*. 2015;45(4):378–386. doi:10.1111/hepr.12359

19. Weiner AA, Olsen J, Ma D, et al. Stereotactic body radiotherapy for primary hepatic malignancies—report of a phase I/II institutional study. *Radiother Oncol*. 2016;121(1):79–85. doi:10.1016/j.radonc.2016.07.020

20. Velec M, Haddad CR, Craig T, et al. Predictors of liver toxicity following stereotactic body radiation therapy for hepatocellular carcinoma. *Int J Radiat Oncol Biol Phys*. 2017;97(5):939–946. doi:10.1016/j.ijrobp.2017.01.221

21. Barry A, Knox JJ, Wei AC, et al. Can stereotactic body radiotherapy effectively treat hepatocellular carcinoma? *J Clin Oncol*. 2016;34(5):404–408. doi:10.1200/JCO.2015.64.8097

22. Wahl DR, Stenmark MH, Tao Y, et al. Outcomes after stereotactic body radiotherapy or radiofrequency ablation for hepatocellular carcinoma. *J Clin Oncol*. 2016;34(5):452–459. doi:10.1200/JCO.2015.61.4925

23. Rajyaguru DJ, Borgert AJ, Smith AL, et al. Radiofrequency ablation versus stereotactic body radiotherapy for localized hepatocellular carcinoma in nonsurgically managed patients: analysis of the national cancer database. *J Clin Oncol*. 2018;36(6):600–608. doi:10.1200/JCO.2017.75.3228

24. Pollom EL, Lee K, Durkee BY, et al. Cost-effectiveness of stereotactic body radiation therapy versus radiofrequency ablation for hepatocellular carcinoma: a Markov modeling study. *Radiology.* 2017;283(2):460–468. doi:10.1148/radiol.2016161509

25. Klein J, Dawson LA, Jiang H, et al. Prospective longitudinal assessment of quality of life for liver cancer patients treated with stereotactic body radiation therapy. *Int J Radiat Oncol Biol Phys.* 2015;93(1):16–25. doi:10.1016/j.ijrobp.2015.04.016

26. Huo YR, Eslick GD. Transcatheter arterial chemoembolization plus radiotherapy compared with chemoembolization alone for hepatocellular carcinoma: a systematic review and meta-analysis. *JAMA Oncol.* 2015;1(6):756–765. doi:10.1001/jamaoncol.2015.2189

27. Zeng ZC, Seong J, Yoon SM, et al. Consensus on stereotactic body radiation therapy for small-sized hepatocellular carcinoma at the 7th Asia-Pacific Primary Liver Cancer Expert Meeting. *Liver Cancer.* 2017;6(4):264–274. doi:10.1159/000475768

28. Rim CH, Kim CY, Yang DS, et al. Comparison of radiation therapy modalities for hepatocellular carcinoma with portal vein thrombosis: a meta-analysis and systematic review. *Radiother Oncol.* 2018;129:112–122. doi:10.1016/j.radonc.2017.11.013

29. Nakayama H, Sugahara S, Tokita M, et al. Proton beam therapy for hepatocellular carcinoma: the University of Tsukuba experience. *Cancer.* 2009;115(23):5499–5506. doi:10.1002/cncr.24619

30. Fukumitsu N, Sugahara S, Nakayama H, et al. A prospective study of hypofractionated proton beam therapy for patients with hepatocellular carcinoma. *Int J Radiat Oncol Biol Phys.* 2009;74(3):831–836. doi:10.1016/j.ijrobp.2008.10.073

31. Bush DA, Kayali Z, Grove R, Slater JD. The safety and efficacy of high-dose proton beam radiotherapy for hepatocellular carcinoma: a phase 2 prospective trial. *Cancer.* 2011;117(13):3053–3059. doi:10.1002/cncr.25809

32. Bush DA, Smith JC, Slater JD, et al. Randomized clinical trial comparing proton beam radiation therapy with transarterial chemoembolization for hepatocellular carcinoma: results of an interim analysis. *Int J Radiat Oncol Biol Phys.* 2016;95(1):477–482. doi:10.1016/j.ijrobp.2016.02.027

33. Hong TS, Wo JY, Yeap BY, et al. Multi-institutional phase II study of high-dose hypofractionated proton beam therapy in patients with localized, unresectable hepatocellular carcinoma and intrahepatic cholangiocarcinoma. *J Clin Oncol.* 2016;34(5):460–468. doi:10.1200/JCO.2015.64.2710

34. Toramatsu C, Katoh N, Shimizu S, et al. What is the appropriate size criterion for proton radiotherapy for hepatocellular carcinoma? a dosimetric comparison of spot-scanning proton therapy versus intensity-modulated radiation therapy. *Radiat Oncol.* 2013;8:48. doi:10.1186/1748-717X-8-48

35. Gandhi SJ, Liang X, Ding X, et al. Clinical decision tool for optimal delivery of liver stereotactic body radiation therapy: photons versus protons. *Pract Radiat Oncol.* 2015;5(4):209–218. doi:10.1016/j.prro.2015.01.004

36. Qi WX, Fu S, Zhang Q, et al. Charged particle therapy versus photon therapy for patients with hepatocellular carcinoma: a systematic review and meta-analysis. *Radiother Oncol.* 2015;114(3):289–295. doi:10.1016/j.radonc.2014.11.033

37. Gomez DR, Poenisch F, Pinnix CC, et al. Malfunctions of implantable cardiac devices in patients receiving proton beam therapy: incidence and predictors. *Int J Radiat Oncol Biol Phys.* 2013;87(3):570–575. doi:10.1016/j.ijrobp.2013.07.010

38. Park HC, Yu JI, Cheng JC, et al. Consensus for radiotherapy in hepatocellular carcinoma from the 5th Asia-Pacific Primary Liver Cancer Expert Meeting (APPLE 2014): current practice and future clinical trials. *Liver Cancer.* 2016;5(3):162–174. doi:10.1159/000367766

How I Treat Advanced Hepatocellular Cancer With Multikinase Inhibitors and Other Targeted Therapies

Kabir Mody and Ghassan K. Abou-Alfa

INTRODUCTION

Liver cancers, worldwide, account for more than 850,000 new cancer cases annually, and approximately 90% of these are hepatocellular carcinoma (HCC) (1,2). HCC is a lethal malignancy arising from hepatocytes. In the United States, HCC-related deaths represent 3% and 6% of all cancer-related deaths in females and males, respectively (3). HCC is the second leading cause of cancer-related death globally, and there is a recognizable increase in the mortality rates from HCC in most countries, including the United States (4,5).

There are several well-defined risk factors for the disease including cirrhosis, hepatitis B virus (HBV) infection, hepatitis C virus (HCV) infection, alcohol abuse, and nonalcoholic steatohepatitis (NASH) (1) (Figure 34.1). Other well-known and characterized colluding factors for development of the disease include intake of aflatoxin B1, and certain metabolic disorders including hemochromatosis. Newer studies have suggested that infection with adeno-associated virus 2 (AAV2) may be a novel cause of the disease, particularly in individuals without cirrhosis (6).

HCC is often diagnosed at advanced stages for which highly effective therapy options have been limited, with a 5-year survival rate of just 3% (3). Sorafenib arose as the singular standard in 2007 and recently, we have witnessed the rise of a number of additional options for patients with advanced HCC, including the emergence of three other tyrosine kinase inhibitors (TKIs) and checkpoint inhibitors. We discuss herein recent literature highlighting recently emergent options for management of this disease, as relevant to the management of our patients as medical oncologists.

FIRST-LINE THERAPY

Angiogenesis, defined as the process by which tumors develop new blood vessels needed for tumor growth, is a key process in HCC. An excess of angiogenic factors coming from tumor cells, vascular endothelial cells, and also surrounding immune cells results in the activation and recruitment of endothelial cells and pericytes (7). In fact, plasma concentrations of angiogenic factors vascular endothelial growth factor (VEGF), angiopoietin-2 (Ang2), and platelet-derived growth factor (PDGF)-B have been shown to be significantly elevated in HCC patients, compared with patients with cirrhosis alone (8).

Given the critical role of angiogenesis in the disease, multiple agents seeking to disrupt the process have been studied in HCC and agents targeting this process currently play a central role in the management of this disease.

The first therapeutic to demonstrate efficacy and garner Food and Drug Administration (FDA) approval for treatment of HCC was sorafenib. This agent acts by inhibiting the serine–threonine kinases Raf-1 and B-Raf and the receptor tyrosine kinase activity of vascular endothelial growth factor receptors (VEGFRs) 1, 2, and 3 and platelet-derived growth factor receptor β (PDGFR-β) (9,10). In the phase III multicenter, double-blind, placebo-controlled SHARP trial, 602 patients with advanced HCC and no previous systemic treatment were randomly assigned to receive either sorafenib or placebo (11). Sorafenib demonstrated a significant improvement

---

A Clinical Vignette ("How I Treat") is included at the end of the chapter.

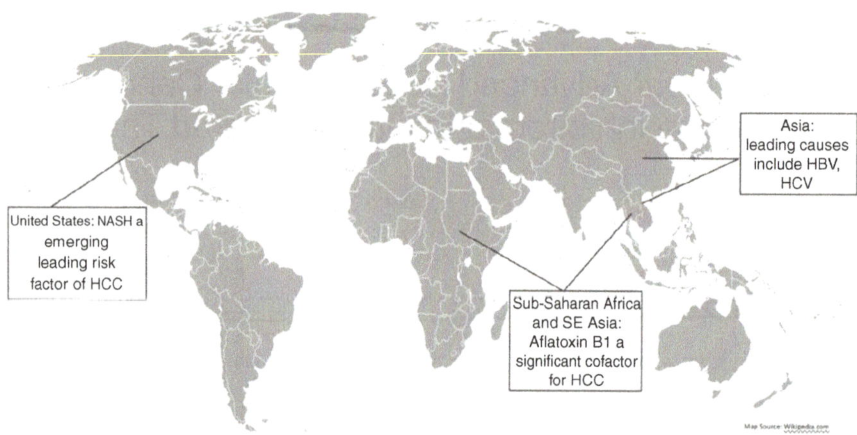

FIGURE 34.1   Global risk factors for HCC.

HBV, hepatitis B virus; HCC, hepatocellular carcinoma; HCV, hepatitis C virus; NASH, nonalcoholic steatohepatitis.

in median survival at 10.7 months, compared to 7.9 months for patients in the placebo group (hazard ratio [HR]: 0.69, $p < .001$) (11). Given the varied etiologies for patients' underlying liver disease and risk factors for HCC, the question of sorafenib's benefit in each of these different subgroups has been explored too. Subgroup analyses of phase II and III studies of sorafenib in HCC have shown greater benefit from the treatment in those with HCV-induced HCC versus other causes (12,13). An additional phase III trial of sorafenib versus placebo conducted in the Asia-Pacific region, involving patients mainly with HBV-induced disease, demonstrated a statistically significant survival advantage for sorafenib. However, this advantage was not to the same magnitude as that seen in the SHARP trial (6.5 vs. 4.2 months, $p = .014$) (14). Supportive of these results, a meta-analysis of phase III trial results demonstrated improved overall survival (OS) for sorafenib in patients who are both HBV negative and HCV positive (15). The differential activity of sorafenib in those with HCV-induced HCC, versus other etiologies of underlying liver disease, if real, may be secondary to high Raf kinase activity driven by the HCV core protein-1 in this subgroup (16). After almost a decade of suboptimal results of trials evaluating agents in the first-line setting in an effort to improve outcomes above and beyond sorafenib, recent data have offered a potential alternative, and data from ongoing trials to emerge in the coming months to years seek to raise the bar.

Lenvatinib, a molecule with a different and more varied target profile compared with sorafenib, is an inhibitor of VEGFRs 1–3, FGF receptors 1–4, PDGF receptor α, RET, and KIT and initially showed activity in a phase 2 study of patients with HCC (17). In a recently reported phase 3 open-label, multicenter noninferiority trial, OS was compared in patients treated with lenvatinib (12 mg/day for bodyweight ≥60 kg or 8 mg/day for bodyweight <60 kg) versus sorafenib as a first-line treatment for unresectable, systemic treatment-naïve HCC (18; Table 34.1). Over the course of about 2 years, 954 eligible patients were randomly assigned to lenvatinib or sorafenib. Median OS for lenvatinib was 13.6 months compared to sorafenib at 12.3 months (HR: 0.92, 95% confidence interval [CI]: 0.79–1.06), meeting the study primary criteria for noninferiority. Treatment was generally well tolerated. The most common any-grade adverse events were hypertension, diarrhea, decreased appetite, decreased weight, fatigue, nausea, palmar–plantar erythrodysesthesia, dysphonia, and proteinuria for lenvatinib. For sorafenib, the most common any-grade adverse events were alopecia, palmar–plantar erythrodysesthesia, diarrhea, hypertension, decreased appetite, and fatigue. The overall response rate, per mRECIST by independent reviewer, for patients on lenvatinib was 41% versus 12% for those in the sorafenib group. Disease control rates were 73% and 59%, respectively ($p < .0001$). The median duration on treatment was 5.7 months for patients on lenvatinib and 3.7 months for those on sorafenib. Subgroup analysis revealed no significant differences in OS among subgroups of patients receiving lenvatinib.

TABLE 34.1 First-Line Studies: Demographics and Outcomes

	Sorafenib (Llovet et al.) (11)	Sorafenib (Kudo et al.) (18)	Lenvatinib
Median Age	64.9	62	63
Male: Female (%)	87/13	84/16	85/15
Global region			
Western (Europe, North America, Australia)	97	33	33
Asia	0	67	67
Risk factor (%)			
Alcohol	26	4	8
Hepatitis B	19	48	53
Hepatitis C	29	26	19
Other/Unknown	25	21	21
ECOG performance status			
0	54	63	64
1	38	37	36
BCLC stage (%)			
B	18	19	22
C	82	81	78
Macroscopic vascular invasion, extrahepatic spread, or both	70	71	69
Macroscopic portal vein	36	23	19
Extrahepatic spread	53	61	62
Child–Pugh class (%)	95	99	99
Concomitant systemic antiviral therapy (%)	2	31	34
Previous anticancer procedures/surgery	63	72	68
Responses (RECIST: independent review) (%)			
CR	0	<1	<1
PR	2	6	18
SD	71	53	54
Disease control rate (%)	43	59	73
Median time to progression (Months)	5.5	3.7	7.4
Median PFS (Months)	NR	3.6	7.3
Median OS (Months)	10.7	12.3	13.6

BCLC, Barcelona Clinic Liver Cancer; CR, complete response; ECOG, Eastern Cooperative Oncology Group; NR, no response; OS, overall survival; PFS, progression-free survival; PR, partial response; SD, stable disease.

Case

The patient is treated with sorafenib 400 mg p.o. twice daily for 2 months. He tolerates the drug generally well experiencing mildly increased fatigue, though still with an Eastern Cooperative Oncology Group (ECOG) performance status of 0, and mild diarrhea controlled with as needed antidiarrheal medications. Repeat imaging after 2 months of therapy demonstrates stability of disease. After 4 months of therapy, abdominal MRI reveals that the mass involving the majority of the right hepatic lobe now measures approximately 11.1 × 5.8 × 9.6 cm with tumor thrombus throughout the right portal vein and extending into the left portal vein. The mass and tumor thrombus demonstrate arterial phase hyperenhancement, with washout on delayed images. The large porta hepatis lymph node now measures 7.6 × 5.2 × 5 cm. No ascites is seen. Osseous structures are unremarkable. CT chest now shows no new pulmonary nodules; however, the prior seen pulmonary nodules are still present now measuring, at largest, 3.0 cm.

Relevant labs include Hgb 10.8, white blood cell (WBC) 5.5, platelets 90, albumin 3.5, total bilirubin 1.0, alkaline phosphatase 140, aspartate aminotransferase (AST) 76, alanine aminotransferase (ALT) 77, and international normalized ratio (INR) 1.0. Alpha-fetoprotein (AFP) is now 11,393 ng/mL, Child–Pugh score is 6 (class A), and ECOG performance status is still 0.

SECOND-LINE THERAPY

In the second-line setting, a string of randomized phase 3 trials utilizing agents such as brivanib, ramucirumab, and everolimus in recent years has failed to show a benefit over placebo, though ramucirumab may have found a role in a particular subgroup of HCC patients. This impasse was broken the past year with the publication of both the RESORCE and CheckMate 040 trials, and the eventual FDA approval of both regorafenib and nivolumab (19,20).

The RESORCE trial was a randomized, double-blind, global phase 3 trial evaluating regorafenib (160 mg daily on days 1–21 of a 28-day cycle) versus placebo in adults with HCC who had tolerated sorafenib (≥400 mg/day for ≥20 of the last 28 days of treatment), progressed on sorafenib, and had Child–Pugh A liver function (19). Over a two-and-a-half-year period, 573 were randomized. Regorafenib demonstrated improved OS compared with placebo with an HR of 0.63 ($p < .0001$) and a median OS of 10.6 months versus 7.8 months, respectively. Median progression-free survival (PFS) was 3.1 months and 1.5 months, respectively. Adverse events were seen in all patients on regorafenib, with the most common clinically relevant grade 3 or 4 treatment-emergent events being similar to those seen in prior studies of regorafenib: hypertension, hand–foot skin reaction, fatigue, and diarrhea.

Yet another success with an agent targeting angiogenesis was reported upon recently, in the second-line setting. Ramucirumab, targeting VEGFR2, was evaluated in the REACH study in which 565 patients with advanced HCC were randomized to ramucirumab or placebo (21). Median OS for the ramucirumab group was 9.2 months versus 7.6 months for the placebo group (HR: 0.87, $p = .14$) (21). In a prespecified subgroup of patients with a baseline AFP concentration of ≥400 ng/mL, median OS was 7.8 versus 4.2 months, respectively (HR: 0.67, $p = .006$). On such basis, the follow-up REACH-2 study was launched for patients with advanced HCC with baseline AFP >400 ng/mL with progression during or after sorafenib. A press release reported this study was a positive one, and full results will be released soon (22).

Other than targeting angiogenesis and immune-related targets, other targets are demonstrating some value too and seek to establish their role in the management strategy in the coming years. One such target has been the cMET pathway, which has been a target of much interest in HCC in recent prior years, with strong preclinical support. Increased cMET activity can initiate, drive, or contribute to the development and progression of HCC. Aberrant cMET activity is associated with rapid tumor growth, aggressively invasive disease, and poor patient prognosis (23,24). cMET aberrations occur in approximately 50% of patients with HCC and can arise through gene mutation (4%), gene amplification (24%), increased mRNA expression (50%), and receptor overexpression (28%) (25–27). Unfortunately, here again we have seen a number of failed studies, until recently.

Tivantinib, an agent targeting the cMET kinase, was studied in a phase 3 METIV-HCC study, based on a prior phase 2 study. In the phase 2 study, cMET overexpression was noted to be associated with a more intriguing response rate to tivantinib. The subgroup of patients with MET overexpression showed an improvement in median OS from 3.8 to 7.2 months (HR: 0.38, $p = .01$) In the METIV-HCC study, 340 patients with cMET-high HCC, following treatment with sorafenib, were randomized to tivantinib or placebo. Median OS was 8.4 months in the tivantinib arm compared with 9.1 months in the placebo arm (HR: 0.97, p = .81). Median PFS was 2.1 months and 2 months, respectively (HR: 0.96, p = .81). The JET-HCC study in Japan also recently demonstrated no significant clinical benefit with very similar results in patients randomized to tivantinib versus placebo in the second-line setting (28). Median PFS was 2.8 versus 2.3 months (HR: 0.72, p = .065), respectively. Median OS was 9.9 versus 8.5 months (HR: 0.85). Other studies evaluating cMET targeting drugs such as foretinib and golvatinib have also failed.

In a counter argument about the necessity of cMET expression, another cMET inhibitor, cabozantinib, which targets cMET, in addition to RET, VEGFR2, AXL-1, and TIE-2, was studied in a phase 2 study in 41 patients, which demonstrated a response rate of 9% and an overall disease control rate of 71%, with a median OS of 15.1 months and a median PFS of 4.4 months (29). Based on these results, the phase 3 CELESTIAL randomized 707 patients with advanced HCC, who had received at least one prior systemic therapy to cabozantinib or placebo (30). The study demonstrated cabozantinib's efficacy compared with placebo with a median OS of 10.2 versus 8.0 months, respectively (HR: 0.76, p = .0049), and a median PFS of 5.2 versus 1.9 months (HR: 0.44, p < .001). The drug was generally well tolerated with the more common adverse effects being hand–foot skin reaction, hypertension, increased AST, fatigue, and diarrhea.

This lack of observed efficacy in many of the studies evaluating supposed cMET inhibitors has likely been secondary to a number of factors, including trial design, lack of patient selection according to tumor cMET status, and the prevalence of off-target activities of these agents, possibly indicating that their cMET inhibition is incomplete. On the other hand, selective cMET inhibitors such as tepotinib and capmatinib may be better poised to achieve complete inhibition of tumor cMET activity (31). Preliminary results suggest that selective cMET inhibitors have antitumor activity in HCC, with acceptable safety and tolerability in patients with Child–Pugh A liver function. Ongoing trials will keep cMET inhibition on the map as an area of continued promise in the management of HCC.

Of course, other options in the second-line setting also include immunotherapy agents. Prior preclinical data have demonstrated that several immunologic mechanisms play a role in HCC development and progression, and in thwarting effective patients' antitumor immune surveillance capabilities (32). This topic is dealt with in detail in Chapter 35, *How I Treat* Advanced Hepatocellular Cancer With Immunotherapy.

CONCLUSION

In the realm of management of advanced HCC, after 9 years of disappointment, sorafenib is no longer the sole kid on the block. Recent times have seen the FDA approval of two new agents, regorafenib and nivolumab. Additionally, two more agents, lenvatinib and cabozantinib, have demonstrated efficacy and await FDA review for possible approval (Figure 34.2). First-line

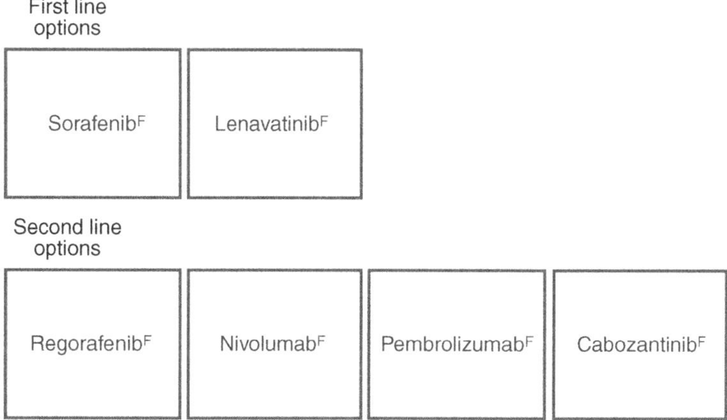

FIGURE 34.2 Current landscape of therapeutics for HCC.

[F]FDA approved for HCC.

FDA, Food and Drug Administration; HCC, hepatocellular carcinoma.

therapy options now number two, and with results of CheckMate-459 anxiously awaited, a game-changing third option may be on the horizon. Second-line options are also now plenty. While these agents provide a myriad of opportunities and options for our patients, many questions remain to be addressed. The most pressing challenge will be the optimal sequencing of first-line and second-line agents. Intense correlative efforts will be needed to elucidate predictive biomarkers and evidence-based sequencing pathways. Finally, the impact of these agents in various combinations in the advanced disease setting and also in earlier stages of disease and in combination with other treatment modalities is being explored and will undoubtedly introduce more options as well as questions.

Clinical Vignette 34.1

The patient is a 68-year-old man with a prior medical history of hyperlipidemia and hepatitis C for which he underwent successful antiviral treatment 3 years ago. He has neither a history of esophageal varices or gastrointestinal bleeding nor any history of ascites or symptoms of hepatic encephalopathy. He presented with complaints of upper abdominal pain and bloating intermittently, which was ongoing for 2 months. Physical exam is unremarkable. He has an ECOG performance status of 0. CT abdomen and pelvis is performed and demonstrates an ill-defined area in the lateral aspect measuring 6.4 cm in diameter of the right hepatic lobe with heterogeneous enhancement, with possible short segment focal filling defect in the right portal vein. Additionally there is a 4.5 centimeter mass in the porta hepatis region, likely a conglomerate lymph node. Initial laboratory studies reveal a complete blood count (CBC) within normal limits other than platelets of 95,000, chemistry panel within normal limits, and a liver panel revealing an albumin of 3.8, total bilirubin of 0.4, alkaline phosphatase 117, AST 74, ALT 54, and an INR of 1.1. Alpha-fetoprotein is elevated at 8,300 ng/mL. Child–Pugh class A (score: 5) MR Abd shows an infiltrative mass involving the majority of the right hepatic lobe measuring approximately 9.1 × 5.4 × 8.8 cm with tumor thrombus throughout the right portal vein and extending into left portal vein. The mass and tumor thrombus demonstrate arterial phase hyperenhancement, with washout on delayed images, features diagnostic of HCC. There is also a large porta hepatis lymph node measuring 6.6 × 5.6 × 4.4 cm. There is no ascites. Osseous structures are unremarkable. CT chest demonstrates five pulmonary nodules, two in the left lower lobe, two in the right lower lobe, and one in the right upper lobe, the largest measuring 1.5 cm. There is no lymphadenopathy within the axillae, lower cervical, mediastinal, or hilum regions. The heart is normal sized without pericardial effusion, nor any pleural effusions. Osseous structures demonstrate no concerning abnormality. Biopsy of a pulmonary nodule in the right upper lobe is performed with pathology consistent with moderately differentiated HCC.

REFERENCES

1. Llovet JM, Zucman-Rossi J, Pikarsky E, et al. Hepatocellular carcinoma. *Nat Rev Dis Primers*. 2016;2:16018. doi:10.1038/nrdp.2016.18
2. Torre LA, Bray F, Siegel RL, et al. Global cancer statistics, 2012. *CA Cancer J Clin*. 2015;65(2):87–108. doi:10.3322/caac.21262
3. Siegel R, Miller KD, Jemal A. Cancer Statistics, 2018. *CA Cancer J Clin*. 2018;68(1):7–30. doi:10.3322/caac.21442
4. Bertuccio P, Turati F, Carioli G, et al. Global trends and predictions in hepatocellular carcinoma mortality. *J Hepatol*. 2017;67(2);302–309. doi:10.1016/j.jhep.2017.03.011
5. GBD 2013 Mortality and Causes of Death Collaborators. (2015). Global, regional, and national age-sex specific all-cause and cause-specific mortality for 240 causes of death, 1990-2013: a systematic analysis for the Global Burden of Disease Study 2013. *Lancet*. 2015;385(9963), 117–171. doi:10.1016/S0140-6736(14)61682-2
6. Nault JC, Datta S, Imbeaud S, et al. Recurrent AAV2-related insertional mutagenesis in human hepatocellular carcinomas. *Nat Genet*. 2015;47(10):1187–1193. doi:10.1038/ng.3389

7. Zhu AX, Duda DG, Sahani DV, et al. HCC and angiogenesis: possible targets and future directions. *Nat Rev Clin Oncol*. 2011;8(5):292–301. doi:10.1038/nrclinonc.2011.30
8. Mas VR, Maluf DG, Archer KJ, et al. Angiogenesis soluble factors as hepatocellular carcinoma noninvasive markers for monitoring hepatitis C virus cirrhotic patients awaiting liver transplantation. *Transplantation*. 2007;84(10):1262–1271. doi:10.1097/01.tp.0000287596.91520.1a
9. Chang YS, Adnane J, Trail PA, et al. Sorafenib (BAY 43-9006) inhibits tumor growth and vascularization and induces tumor apoptosis and hypoxia in RCC xenograft models. *Cancer Chemother Pharmacol*. 2007;59(5):561–574. doi:10.1007/s00280-006-0393-4
10. Wilhelm SM, Carter C, Tang L, et al. BAY 43-9006 exhibits broad spectrum oral antitumor activity and targets the RAF/MEK/ERK pathway and receptor tyrosine kinases involved in tumor progression and angiogenesis. *Cancer Res*. 2004;64(19):7099–7109. doi:10.1158/0008-5472.CAN-04-1443
11. Llovet JM, Ricci S, Mazzaferro V, et al. Sorafenib in advanced hepatocellular carcinoma. *N Engl J Med*. 2008;359(4):378–390. doi:10.1056/NEJMoa0708857
12. Abou-Alfa GK. Selection of patients with hepatocellular carcinoma for sorafenib. *J Natl Compr Canc Netw*. 2009;7(4);397–403.
13. Abou-Alfa GK, Schwartz L, Ricci S, et al. Phase II study of sorafenib in patients with advanced hepatocellular carcinoma. *J Clin Oncol*. 2006;24(26);4293–4300. doi:10.1200/JCO.2005.01.3441
14. Cheng AL, Kang YK, Chen Z, et al. Efficacy and safety of sorafenib in patients in the Asia-Pacific region with advanced hepatocellular carcinoma: a phase III randomised, double-blind, placebo-controlled trial. *Lancet Oncol*. 2009;10(1):25–34. doi:10.1016/S1470-2045(08)70285-7
15. Jackson R, Psarelli EE, Berhane S, et al. Impact of viral status on survival in patients receiving sorafenib for advanced hepatocellular cancer: a meta-analysis of randomized phase III trials. *J Clin Oncol*. 2017;35(6):622–628. doi:10.1200/JCO.2016.69.5197
16. Giambartolomei S, Covone F, Levrero M, et al. Sustained activation of the Raf/MEK/Erk pathway in response to EGF in stable cell lines expressing the Hepatitis C Virus (HCV) core protein. *Oncogene*. 2001;20(20), 2606–2610. doi:10.1038/sj.onc.1204372
17. Ikeda K, Kudo M, Kawazoe S, et al. Phase 2 study of lenvatinib in patients with advanced hepatocellular carcinoma. *J Gastroenterol*. 2017;52(4):512–519. doi:10.1007/s00535-016-1263-4
18. Kudo M, Finn RS, Qin S, et al. Lenvatinib versus sorafenib in first-line treatment of patients with unresectable hepatocellular carcinoma: a randomised phase 3 non-inferiority trial. *Lancet*. 2018;391(10126):1163–1173. doi:10.1016/S0140-6736(18)30207-1
19. Bruix J, Qin S, Merle P, et al. Regorafenib for patients with hepatocellular carcinoma who progressed on sorafenib treatment (RESORCE): a randomised, double-blind, placebo-controlled, phase 3 trial. *Lancet*. 2017;389(10064):56–66. doi:10.1016/S0140-6736(16)32453-9
20. El-Khoueiry AB, Sangro B, Yau T, et al. Nivolumab in patients with advanced hepatocellular carcinoma (CheckMate 040): an open-label, non-comparative, phase 1/2 dose escalation and expansion trial. *Lancet*. 2017;389(10088):2492–2502. doi:10.1016/S0140-6736(17)31046-2
21. Zhu AX, Park JO, Ryoo BY, et al. Ramucirumab versus placebo as second-line treatment in patients with advanced hepatocellular carcinoma following first-line therapy with sorafenib (REACH): a randomised, double-blind, multicentre, phase 3 trial. *Lancet Oncol*. 2015;16(7):859–870. doi:10.1016/S1470-2045(15)00050-9
22. Lilly Announces CYRAMZA® (ramucirumab) Phase 3 REACH-2 Study in Second-Line Hepatocellular Carcinoma Patients Met Overall Survival Endpoint (2018). [Press release]
23. Boccaccio C, Comoglio PM. Invasive growth: a MET-driven genetic programme for cancer and stem cells. *Nat Rev Cancer*. 2006;6(8):637–645. doi:10.1038/nrc1912
24. Kim JH, Kim HS, Kim BJ, et al. Prognostic value of c-Met overexpression in hepatocellular carcinoma: a meta-analysis and review. *Oncotarget*. 2017;8(52):90351–90357. doi:10.18632/oncotarget.20087
25. Cecchi F, Rabe DC, Bottaro DP. Targeting the HGF/Met signaling pathway in cancer therapy. *Expert Opin Ther Targets*. 2012;16(6):553–572. doi:10.1517/14728222.2012.680957
26. Lee SJ, Lee J, Sohn I, et al. A survey of c-MET expression and amplification in 287 patients with hepatocellular carcinoma. *Anticancer Res*. 2013;33(11):5179–5186.
27. Xin Y, Jin D, Eppler S, et al. Population pharmacokinetic analysis from phase I and phase II studies of the humanized monovalent antibody, onartuzumab (MetMAb), in patients with advanced solid tumors. *J Clin Pharmacol*. 2013;53(11):1103–1111. doi:10.1002/jcph.148
28. Kobayashi S, Ueshima K, Moriguchi M, et al. *JET-HCC: A phase 3 randomized, double-blind, placebo-controlled study of tivantinib as a second-line therapy in patients with c-Met high hepatocellular carcinoma*. Paper presented at the ESMO 2017; 2017; Madrid, Spain.
29. Cohn A, Kelley RK, Yang T, et al. Activity of cabozantinib (XL184) in hepatocellular carcinoma patients (pts): results from a phase II randomized discontinuation trial (RDT). *J Clin Oncol*. 2012;30(4_suppl):261. doi:10.1200/jco.2012.30.4_suppl.261

30. Abou-Alfa G, Meyer T, Cheng A-L, et al. Cabozantinib (C) versus placebo (P) in patients (pts) with advanced hepatocellular carcinoma (HCC) who have received prior sorafenib: Results from the randomized phase III CELESTIAL trial. *J Clin Oncol.* 2018;36(4_suppl 4S):207. doi:10.1200/jco.2018.36.4_suppl.207
31. Bouattour M, Raymond E, Qin S, et al. Recent developments of c-Met as a therapeutic target in hepatocellular carcinoma. *Hepatology.* 2018;67(3):1132–1149. doi:10.1002/hep.29496
32. Harding JJ, El Dika I, Abou-Alfa GK. Immunotherapy in hepatocellular carcinoma: Primed to make a difference? *Cancer.* 2016;122(3):367–377. doi:10.1002/cncr.29769

How I Treat Advanced Hepatocellular Cancer With Immunotherapy

Olatunji B. Alese and Katerina Zakka

INTRODUCTION

Hepatocellular carcinoma (HCC) frequently presents in advanced stages, with limited curative treatment options (1). Early-stage HCC can be treated with locoregional therapies, surgical resection (1), or liver transplantation. However, systemic therapy is the mainstay in advanced or extrahepatic HCC. This has been mostly molecular targeted therapies, and the recent introduction of checkpoint inhibitors into clinical practice has expanded treatment options. The immune system is a key player in HCC as well as a therapeutic option in different cancers.

Patients have unique anti- or protumor responses during the development and progression of HCC. Immune changes reported in HCC include tumor-associated antigen (TAA)-specific CD8+ T-cell immune responses, T-cell infiltration after locoregional therapy, T-regulatory cell intratumoral accumulation, and myeloid-derived suppressor cell accumulation, all of which have been correlated with disease progression and poor survival (2). Under physiologic states, the liver induces immune tolerance by means of blocking the activation of effector T-cells in the liver microenvironment. This mechanism protects the liver from autoimmune damage due to ongoing immune stimulation from continuous antigen exposure. Although immune tolerance is advantageous in a healthy liver, it is detrimental in HCC since it prevents an adequate immune response against malignant cells. Furthermore, the intrahepatic immunosuppressive environment in HCC is worsened by the chronic inflammation underlying fibrosis and cirrhosis. This is characterized by the continued expression of different cytokines and recruitment of immune cells to the liver, contributing to the propagation of HCC by further activating immunosuppressive mechanisms. Ultimately, an inability to escalate an adequate antitumor response results in disease progression (2–4).

Immune responses occur in livers affected by HCC, and numerous clinical studies have demonstrated the efficacy of immunotherapy in the disease. The immune response is significantly suppressed in HCC, allowing malignant cells to escape the host immune system. In this context, immunotherapy restores the patient's immune status, playing an important antitumor role in eliminating micrometastatic residual disease and thus, reducing the risk of recurrence. Lymphocyte infiltration of the tumor and a high CD4+:CD8+ T-cell ratio have been associated with reduced risk of tumor recurrence following liver transplantation for HCC (5). This finding implies a key role of T-cells in regulating tumor progression and provides a strong justification for T-cell immunotherapy in HCC. This is further supported by the antitumor activity after treatment with immune checkpoint inhibitors in patients with advanced HCC (6,7).

IMMUNOTHERAPY AGENTS CURRENTLY IN CLINICAL PRACTICE

Immunotherapeutic approaches have demonstrated efficacy in several cancer types, including HCC. The ability of the immune system to detect and fight cancer was first demonstrated by the development of a killed bacterial vaccine for cancer in the late 1800s by William Coley (8). Activation of lymphocytes is regulated by a balance between costimulatory and coinhibitory molecules, namely "immune checkpoints," belonging to the B7/CD28 superfamily and the TNF/TNFR superfamily (9). The term "immune checkpoint inhibitor" was thus coined, referring to any compound inhibiting the function of an immune checkpoint, in the form of peptides,

---

A Clinical Vignette ("How I Treat") is included at the end of the chapter.

nucleic acid molecules, small molecules, and preferentially antibodies (10). Immune checkpoint inhibitors enhance the proliferation, migration, persistence, and/or cytotoxic activity of T-cells in a subject and in particular, the tumor infiltrating T-cells (9).

Two categories of immune checkpoint inhibitors have been adopted for cancer therapy in clinical practice: the anti-cytotoxic T-lymphocyte-associated protein 4 (CTLA-4) antibody and the anti-programmed cell death protein 1 pathway (PD-1/PD-L1) antibodies (11). Examples include anti-CTLA-4 antibodies (ipilimumab, tremelimumab), anti-PD-1 antibodies (nivolumab, pembrolizumab), and anti-PD-L1 antibodies (atezolizumab, avelumab, durvalumab). CTLA-4 is a protein receptor on the surface of T-cells. Anti-CTLA-4 antibodies block the binding of CTLA-4 and CD80/86 present on the surface of antigen presenting cells (APCs), resulting in antitumor immune responses mediated by T-cells (12,13). PD-1 is a cell surface receptor expressed on T-cells and pro-B cells. When bound to one of its ligands, PD-L1 or PD-L2, the receptor inhibits the activation of T-cells. Anti-PD-1 and anti-PD-L1 antibodies interfere with the binding of PD-1 and PD-L1/2, allowing T-cell proliferation and cytokine release for malignant cell destruction (14). Additionally, activated PD-L1 facilitates failure of T-cell responses to eradicate hepatitis C or B viral infections, and blockade of the PD-L1/PD-1 pathway may have implications for virus clearance. This is of particular importance given the unique tumor biology of HCC with recurrences due to tumor dissemination of the original tumor or de novo carcinogenesis due to field cancerization, multicentric carcinogenesis with persistent active hepatitis and hepatic fibrosis (15).

The efficacy of nivolumab was shown in CheckMate 040 (16) leading to its approval as second-line monotherapy in advanced HCC that had progressed on sorafenib (16–19). This phase 1/2, open-label, noncomparative, dose escalation and expansion trial of nivolumab was conducted in patients with histologically confirmed advanced HCC with or without hepatitis C or B infection. The trial excluded patients with active autoimmune disease, brain metastasis, a history of hepatic encephalopathy, clinically significant ascites, infection with HIV, or active coinfection with hepatitis B virus (HBV) and hepatitis C virus (HCV) or HBV and hepatitis D virus (HDV). Seventy-one percent (71%) of patients had extrahepatic spread, 29% had macrovascular invasion, and 37% had alfa-fetoprotein (AFP) levels ≥400 μg/L. With a primary end point of objective response rate, the dose expansion phase allowed only patients with Child–Pugh A and an Eastern Cooperative Oncology Group performance status of 1 or less. Nivolumab 3 mg/kg was given every 2 weeks to 214 enrolled patients in four cohorts: sorafenib untreated or intolerant without viral hepatitis (n = 56), patients without viral hepatitis following progression on sorafenib (n = 57), HCV infected (n = 50), and HBV infected (n = 51). The objective response rate was 20% (95% confidence interval [CI]: 15–26), including three complete responses (CRs) and 39 partial responses (PRs). Forty-five percent of the patients had stable disease, with disease stabilizations lasting at least 6 months in 57% of these cases. The disease control rate (DCR) was 64%. About 69% of the objective responses occurred before 3 months, with a median duration of response of 9.9 months (95% CI: 8.3 to not estimable [NE]). The 9-month overall survival ranged from 63% in the cohort of patients without viral hepatitis following progression on sorafenib to 89% in patients naïve or intolerant to sorafenib without viral hepatitis. The observed durable responses and significantly longer overall survival compared to the small molecule tyrosine kinase inhibitors (TKIs) are remarkable. The most common adverse reactions (≥20%) were fatigue (38%), musculoskeletal pain (36%), abdominal pain (34%), pruritus (27%), diarrhea (27%), rash (26%), cough (23%), and decreased appetite (22%). Treatment-emergent grade 3 or 4 aspartate aminotransferase (AST) elevation was in 18%, grade 3 or 4 alanine aminotransferase (ALT) elevation in 11%, and grade 3 or 4 increased bilirubin in 7% of the treated patients.

Similar treatment responses were seen in Keynote-224 trial of pembrolizumab in patients previously treated with sorafenib. This nonrandomized, multicenter, open-label, phase 2 trial enrolled patients with comparable eligibility criteria to those of CheckMate 040. The median age was 68 years (range 43–87). About 26% had HCV and 21% had HBV infection. Extrahepatic disease was present in 63.5%, 17% had vascular invasion, and 9% had both. Thirty-eight percent (38%) of patients had AFP levels ≥400 μg/L and 79.8% had progressed on sorafenib treatment. Twenty percent of the patients were unable to tolerate sorafenib but no patient received more than one prior systemic therapy (sorafenib). With an objective response of 17% (95% CI: 11–26), there were one (1%) complete and 17 (16%) PRs. Forty-six of the 104 patients (44%) had stable disease and 34 (33%) had progressive disease. The responses were similar across subgroups with different etiology. Ninety-four percent of responders were estimated to have a response duration greater than or equal to 6 months. Seventy-three percent of the patients had treatment-related adverse events, which were serious in 15% of the patients. Results of the first-line phase III CheckMate 459 trial (nivolumab vs. sorafenib in advanced HCC) were pending at the time of this publication (20). The phase III trial (pembrolizumab vs. placebo) in the second-line therapy of advanced HCC is ongoing.

INDICATIONS AND RISK ASSESSMENT FOR IMMUNOTHERAPY

Immune checkpoint inhibitors have unique risk–benefit ratios due to associated immune-related adverse events (irAEs). Baseline laboratory parameters are indicated before, during, and following cessation of immunotherapy in HCC patients. Relative and absolute contraindications include preexisting pulmonary disease, inflammatory bowel disease, hepatic or renal dysfunction, uncontrolled autoimmune or thyroid diseases, and prior allogeneic stem cell or solid organ transplant. Although clinical and laboratory biomarkers for optimal patient selection are yet to be developed in HCC immunotherapy, current trends appear to be different from other tumor types such as lung cancer where response correlates with the level of PD-L1 expression. Other nondiscriminatory factors include viral or alcohol cirrhosis etiology, prior sorafenib therapy, or level of serum AFP.

Nivolumab is currently approved in HCC patients who have been previously treated with, or intolerant to, sorafenib. It is administered as an intravenous (IV) infusion of 240 mg every 2 weeks or 480 mg every 4 weeks, over 30 minutes until disease progression or unacceptable toxicity. Pembrolizumab is similarly approved in patients following progression on sorafenib. The recommended dose is 200 mg administered as an IV infusion over 30 minutes every 3 weeks until disease progression, unacceptable toxicity, or up to 24 months in patients without disease progression.

COMMON ADVERSE EVENTS AND MANAGEMENT

irAEs from immune checkpoint inhibitors occur as a result of impaired self-tolerance from loss of T-cell inhibition (21). The disadvantage of an amplified immune response driven by T-cell activation is the potential autoimmune-related inflammation of normal tissue. They can involve any organ system but gastrointestinal, dermatologic, hepatic, and endocrine are frequently affected. These side effects are manageable with immune-modulatory medications (IMMs), but can be sometimes fatal. Spatial correlation and onset of the suspected irAE is important in its management. In a pooled analysis of patients treated with nivolumab, the median onset of skin irAEs was 5 weeks, gastrointestinal 7.3 weeks, hepatic 7.7 weeks, pulmonary 8.9 weeks, endocrine 10.4 weeks, and renal irAEs was 15.1 weeks (22). Pembrolizumab has a median onset of moderate to severe toxicity around 9 weeks, compared to 6 weeks with ipilimumab (23). Late-onset irAEs may also occur long after treatment has been completed (24,25). Steroids are the mainstay of moderate and severe irAEs. Other IMMs used in steroid-refractory cases include the anti-TNF-alpha antibody infliximab, the antimetabolite mycophenolate mofetil, and the calcineurin inhibitors tacrolimus and cyclosporine (21). T-cell depleting antibodies such as antithymocyte globulin have been necessary in rare cases (26).

Diarrhea is one of the most common irAEs, occurring at any grade in 8% to 30% of those treated with anti-PD1 antibodies. Management of diarrhea and colitis due to immune checkpoint inhibitors depends on the severity of the symptoms. In a patient with abdominal pain or if diarrhea exceeds six episodes per day, steroids should be immediately initiated and the immunotherapy agent should be withheld for moderate or grade 2 toxicity. Infliximab should be considered if there is no improvement after 48 to 72 hours. Other immunosuppressants such as tacrolimus or mycophenolate mofetil have been used in steroid- and infliximab-refractory cases (21). Immune-related hepatitis (increasing levels of ALT or AST with or without elevated bilirubin) typically occurs between 6 and 14 weeks after initiation of therapy (21). It occurs in 1% to 6% of patients treated with anti-PD1 agents. Management includes steroid therapy in patients with ALT or AST greater than 5 times the upper limit of normal. If hepatitis does not respond to steroids, mycophenolate mofetil should be added. Less frequent gastrointestinal irAEs include pancreatitis (21), inflammatory enteric neuropathy with constipation (27), and esophagitis (21). The recommended dose of steroids in moderate to severe irAEs is 1 to 2 mg/kg/day of prednisolone or IV equivalent.

Skin toxicity includes rash, pruritus, and vitiligo, often occurring within the first few weeks of treatment (22,28). Severe skin toxicity (grades 3 and 4) is rare, with the highest frequency in combination immunotherapy. Most cases improve with steroids, and resolution occurs in 2 to 6 weeks. Pneumonitis is an uncommon side effect of immune checkpoint inhibitors in HCC treatment. Usually asymptomatic, pneumonitis may be observed during treatment continuation. The development of symptoms often leads to discontinuation of immunotherapy and initiation of steroids. Renal injury can present as elevated creatinine, autoimmune nephritis, and interstitial nephritis, occurring in 0% to 4% of cases (23,29–34). Management includes steroids for creatinine levels more than 1.5 to 3 times the baseline value.

Thyroid dysfunction can occur as hypothyroidism, common with anti-PD1 antibodies (4%–10%), and is rarely severe (23,31,34). Hyperthyroidism is less common (1%–7%). Management of hypothyroidism is hormone replacement with levothyroxine. Tachycardia and tremors in hyperthyroidism can be managed with beta-blockers. Steroids should be started if the patient is symptomatic, and thyroid suppressive medications such as carbimazole should be used in syndromes resembling Graves disease. Other endocrine adverse events include adrenal crisis for which a stress dose of IV steroids must be given promptly (21).

Although rare and occurring in no more than 3% of patients (23,29–34), neurologic irAEs may include myasthenia gravis and Guillain–Barré syndrome. Nivolumab has been associated with polyneuropathy (33), facial and abducens nerve paresis, and demyelination (21). Posterior reversible leukoencephalopathy (35), radiculoneuropathy (36), Bell's palsy (24), and aseptic meningitis (37) are more common in anti-CTLA4 therapy. High-dose steroid therapy with oral prednisolone or IV equivalent should be instituted. In steroid-refractory cases, plasmapheresis or IVIG is required in myasthenic syndromes and in the primary management of Guillain–Barré syndrome (21). Rheumatological adverse events including myalgias and arthralgias occur in 2% to 12% of patients (23,29–34), especially with anti-PD1 antibodies. Mild symptoms can be managed with acetaminophen or nonsteroidal anti-inflammatory drugs (NSAIDs), while moderate to severe cases require steroids. Ocular toxicities include uveitis, conjunctivitis, iritis, and Graves ophthalmopathy. Management of mild to moderate symptoms that are not associated with visual change includes use of topical steroid eye drops. Prompt initiation of oral or IV steroids is mandatory with visual changes.

EMERGING AND NOVEL THERAPIES

Novel treatment strategies are needed in the treatment of HCC due to the current dismal outcomes. Despite the moderate preliminary activity of anti-CTLA-4 and anti-PD-1/PD-L1 monotherapy, combinational approaches may extend responses in HCC (38). Studies evaluating combination therapy with multiple immune checkpoints such as anti-PD-1 antibody plus anti CTLA-4 antibody (nivolumab and ipilimumab) in HCC are ongoing. The concurrent use of an anti-CTLA-4 antibody could augment the inhibition of the B7-CTLA-4 pathway, increasing CD8+ T-cell proliferation in the lymph nodes and their infiltration into tumor tissues with subsequent antitumor effects (39).

Combination therapies with immune checkpoint inhibitors and molecular targeted agents have also received considerable attention (40,41). The combination of atezolizumab and bevacizumab as a first-line therapy demonstrated promising results in a phase Ib study (NCT02715531) (42). The patients were treated with atezolizumab (1,200 mg) + bevacizumab (15 mg/kg) IV every 3 weeks until progression of disease or unacceptable toxicity. There were PRs in 13 of 21 patients (62%). This was regardless of HCC etiology, region (Asia or the United States), baseline AFP levels, or extrahepatic disease. There are also ongoing trials for the combination therapy of lenvatinib with pembrolizumab in a phase Ib study in Japan (JapicCTI-173494) and sorafenib with nivolumab as a first-line therapy in advanced HCC (NCT03439891).

Other treatment approaches for HCC include the combination of immune checkpoint inhibitors and conventional locoregional therapies (38). Radiotherapy, transarterial chemoembolization (TACE), and radiofrequency ablation (RFA) can stimulate the immune system and increase the effect of immunotherapy by inducing local inflammation and releasing neoantigens (39). In addition, hypoxia from embolization therapies modulates the expression of critical immunotherapy targets, including CD137, OX40, and PD-L1, in the tumor microenvironment (43,44). In this context, a recent clinical study reported the treatment efficacy of anti-CTLA-4 antibody combined with locoregional therapy in patients with advanced HCC (45). Thirty-two patients were given tremelimumab at two dose levels (3.5 and 10 mg/kg IV) every 4 weeks for six doses, and a subtotal RFA or chemoablation was done on day 36. This was followed by 3-monthly infusions till toxicity or progression of disease as per protocol. Median overall survival was 12.3 months, with median time to tumor progression of 7.4 months. There are ongoing trials evaluating the utility of Nivolumab as adjuvant therapy after resection or ablation (46,47). In addition to CTLA-4 and PD-1/PD-L1 blockade, preclinical data have indicated that other immune inhibitory checkpoints (e.g., LAG3 (48), TIM-3 (49), and KIR (50)) and agonists to stimulatory molecules (e.g., CD137 (51) and OX40 (52)) can be therapeutic in T-cell-mediated tumor killing.

Other immune targets used in clinical practice include immunomodulators (cytokines, interleukins [ILs], and chemokines). All three types of interferon (IFN-α, IFN-β, IFN-γ) have been shown to be effective in inhibiting HCC by inducing tumor cell apoptosis or autophagy (53–55). Preliminary clinical studies have evaluated the efficacy of IL-2 or IL-12 alone or in combination, with disappointing results (56,57). Several chemokine-associated signaling, including CXCR4/CXCL12 and CCR6/CCL20 axes, are also being explored for therapy options. Numerous approaches have been explored to create a tumor vaccine for HCC. AFP and glypican-3 (GPC3) are two frequently used tumor antigens in HCC peptide-based vaccines. Tumor vaccines using APCs to induce tumor antigen-specific cytotoxic T lymphocytes (CTLs) (58), activate natural killer (NK) cells, and inhibit Treg cells have also shown some activity in HCC patients. A study of pulsed APC vaccine was conducted with autologous tumor lysate in 31 patients with advanced HCC. The first 14 patients were treated with weekly therapy with five courses of dendritic cell vaccination while the remaining 17 patients had monthly boost vaccinations after the initial pulsed therapy. There were PRs in 12.9% while 54.8% had stable disease. The overall 1-year survival rate was about 40%.

Adoptive immunotherapy using chimeric antigen receptor (CAR) T-cells recognizes the cell surface antigens, irrespective of tumor variations in the expression of major histocompatibility complex (MHC) antigens considered a common mechanism of tumor immune escape (59,60). A preclinical study conducted by Gao et al. demonstrated that third-generation CAR T-cells targeting GPC3, expressed in HCC but not in normal liver tissue (61,62), could eradicate established GPC3-positive HCC xenografts in vivo (63). Thus, these cells might represent a promising treatment strategy for HCC patients. In addition, strategies such as dual-targeted CAR T-cells to reduce on-target, off-tumor toxicities are also being explored. The first target for stimulatory signaling is overexpressed in tumor tissues, but not in normal tissues. The second target for costimulatory signaling is tissue-specific proteins with high-level expression in the tumor tissues. An example is the asialoglycoprotein receptor 1 (ASGR1), a cell surface receptor expressed exclusively on hepatic parenchymal cells, which increases the antitumor activities of first-generation GPC3-targeted CAR T-cells against HCC cells expressing both ASGR1 and GPC3 (64).

CONCLUSION

Immunotherapy remains an attractive therapeutic option in HCC. Patients who respond favorably to immune checkpoint inhibitors in monotherapy or a combination of various agents show prolonged survival (65,66). The combinations of immune checkpoint inhibitors with molecular targeted agents, cytotoxic agents, radiation therapy, or locoregional therapy may bring a paradigm shift in HCC treatment. An array of translational research and clinical trials are being conducted to assess novel immunotherapies in HCC.

Clinical Vignette 35.1

Case 1: A 50-year-old female patient with liver cirrhosis secondary to chronic HCV and metastatic HCC presented after disease progression on first-line treatment with sorafenib. Her past medical history includes diet-controlled diabetes mellitus, hypertension, and hypercholesterolemia controlled with medications. She vaguely remembered being treated for inflammatory bowel disease as a teenager, but has not had any symptoms for more than two decades, prior to her diagnosis of cancer. She had been treated on a tolerated 120 mg daily dose of sorafenib, with disease control for 6 months. Restaging scans showed new lesions in both lungs, and increased left adrenal metastasis. She is interested in immunotherapy, but has heard that it is contraindicated in autoimmune disorders. How would you address her treatment preferences?

Case 2: A 68-year-old male with advanced unresectable HCC with portal vein tumor thrombosis was started on second-line nivolumab. Past medical history includes chronic obstructive pulmonary disease (COPD) bronchitis controlled on bronchodilator inhalers and a previous ICU admission for Clostridium difficile colitis 8 years ago that required experimental fecal transplant. He has not had a recurrence of C. diff diarrhea since that episode. Five weeks after starting nivolumab, he presented to the office with a fine macular rash over his trunk and upper extremities that improved with a steroid cream. Two weeks later, he developed frequent loose bowel motions (up to 8 times within 24 hours), abdominal pain, and bloody stool. He presented to the emergency room (ER), where intravenous fluid (IVF) was started and a sample for C. diff was taken and sent to the lab. As the oncologist on call, what would be your recommendations to the ER staff?

Answers
Case 1: A remote history of inflammatory bowel disease or other autoimmune conditions is not a contraindication to checkpoint inhibitors. She can be offered either nivolumab or pembrolizumab as second-line treatment for her metastatic HCC. She should be closely monitored for onset of irAEs, including diarrhea and counseled to immediately seek medical care.

Case 2: Discontinue immunotherapy and initiate high-dose steroids. His past medical history of severe Clostridium difficile colitis is significant but he should be treated for moderate immune-related colitis pending the result of his stool sample.

REFERENCES

1. Finn RS. Emerging targeted strategies in advanced hepatocellular carcinoma. *Semin Liver Dis.* 2013;33(Suppl 1):S11–S19. doi:10.1055/s-0033-1333632
2. Stauffer JK, Scarzello AJ, Jiang Q, et al. Chronic inflammation, immune escape, and oncogenesis in the liver: a unique neighborhood for novel intersections. *Hepatology.* 2012;56(4):1567–1574. doi:10.1002/hep.25674
3. Greten TF, Wang XW, Korangy F. Current concepts of immune based treatments for patients with HCC: from basic science to novel treatment approaches. *Gut.* 2015;64(5):842–848. doi:10.1136/gutjnl-2014-307990
4. Makarova-Rusher OV, Medina-Echeverz J, Duffy AG, et al. The yin and yang of evasion and immune activation in HCC. *J Hepatol.* 2015;62(6):1420–1429. doi:10.1016/j.jhep.2015.02.038
5. Unitt E, Marshall A, Gelson W, et al. Tumour lymphocytic infiltrate and recurrence of hepatocellular carcinoma following liver transplantation. *J Hepatol.* 2006;45(2):246–253. doi:10.1016/j.jhep.2005.12.027
6. Nishida N, Kudo M. Immune checkpoint blockade for the treatment of human hepatocellular carcinoma. *Hepatol Res.* 2018;48(8):622–634. doi:10.1111/hepr.13191
7. Sangro B, Gomez-Martin C, de la Mata M, et al. A clinical trial of CTLA-4 blockade with tremelimumab in patients with hepatocellular carcinoma and chronic hepatitis C. *J Hepatol.* 2013;59(1):81–88. doi:10.1016/j.jhep.2013.02.022
8. Hoption Cann SA, van Netten JP, van Netten C. Dr William Coley and tumour regression: a place in history or in the future. *Postgrad Med J.* 2003;79(938):672–680.
9. Chen L, Flies DB. Molecular mechanisms of T cell co-stimulation and co-inhibition. *Nat Rev Immunol.* 2013;13(4):227–242. doi:10.1038/nri3405
10. Pardoll DM. The blockade of immune checkpoints in cancer immunotherapy. *Nat Rev Cancer.* 2012;12(4):252–264. doi:10.1038/nrc3239
11. Daher S, Massarwa M, Benson AA, et al. Current and future treatment of hepatocellular carcinoma: an updated comprehensive review. *J Clin Transl Hepatol.* 2018;6(1):69–78. doi:10.14218/jcth.2017.00031

12. Grohmann U, Orabona C, Fallarino F, et al. CTLA-4-Ig regulates tryptophan catabolism in vivo. *Nat Immunol*. 2002;3(11):1097–1101. doi:10.1038/ni846

13. Schneider H, Downey J, Smith A, et al. Reversal of the TCR stop signal by CTLA-4. *Science*. 2006;313(5795):1972–1975. doi:10.1126/science.1131078

14. Okazaki T, Maeda A, Nishimura H, et al. PD-1 immunoreceptor inhibits B cell receptor-mediated signaling by recruiting src homology 2-domain-containing tyrosine phosphatase 2 to phosphoty-rosine. *Proc Natl Acad Sci U S A*. 2001;98(24):13866–13871. doi:10.1073/pnas.231486598

15. Gao Q, Wang XY, Qiu SJ, et al. Overexpression of PD-L1 significantly associates with tumor aggressiveness and postoperative recurrence in human hepatocellular carcinoma. *Clin Cancer Res*. 2009;15(3):971–979. doi:10.1158/1078-0432.Ccr-08-1608

16. El-Khoueiry AB, Sangro B, Yau T, et al. Nivolumab in patients with advanced hepatocellular carcinoma (CheckMate 040): an open-label, non-comparative, phase 1/2 dose escalation and expansion trial. *Lancet*. 2017;389(10088):2492–2502. doi:10.1016/s0140-6736(17)31046-2

17. Bruix J, Qin S, Merle P, et al. Regorafenib for patients with hepatocellular carcinoma who pro-gressed on sorafenib treatment (RESORCE): a randomised, double-blind, placebo-controlled, phase 3 trial. *Lancet*. 2017;389(10064):56–66. doi:10.1016/s0140-6736(16)32453-9

18. Kudo M, Finn RS, Qin S, et al. Lenvatinib versus sorafenib in first-line treatment of patients with unresectable hepatocellular carcinoma: a randomised phase 3 non-inferiority trial. *Lancet*. 2018;391(10126):1163–1173. doi:10.1016/s0140-6736(18)30207-1

19. Llovet JM, Ricci S, Mazzaferro V, et al. Sorafenib in advanced hepatocellular carcinoma. *N Engl J Med*. 2008;359(4):378–390. doi:10.1056/NEJMoa0708857

20. Vance S, Liu E, Zhao L, et al. Selective radiosensitization of p53 mutant pancreatic cancer cells by combined inhibition of Chk1 and PARP1. *Cell Cycle*. 2011;10(24):4321–4329. doi:10.4161/cc.10.24.18661

21. Spain L, Diem S, Larkin J. Management of toxicities of immune checkpoint inhibitors. *Cancer Treat Rev*. 2016;44:51–60. doi:10.1016/j.ctrv.2016.02.001

22. Weber JS, Hodi FS, Wolchok JD, et al. Safety profile of nivolumab monotherapy: a pooled analysis of patients with advanced melanoma. *J Clin Oncol*. 2017;35(7):785–792. doi:10.1200/jco.2015.66.1389

23. Robert C, Schachter J, Long GV, et al. Pembrolizumab versus ipilimumab in advanced mela-noma. *N Engl J Med*. 2015;372(26);2521–2532. doi:10.1056/NEJMoa1503093

24. Johnson DB, Friedman DL, Berry E, et al. Survivorship in immune therapy: assessing chronic immune toxicities, health outcomes, and functional status among long-term ipilimumab sur-vivors at a single referral center. *Cancer Immunol Res*. 2015;3(5):464–469. doi:10.1158/2326-6066.Cir-14-0217

25. Ryder M, Callahan M, Postow MA, et al. Endocrine-related adverse events following ipilimumab in patients with advanced melanoma: a comprehensive retrospective review from a single insti-tution. *Endocr Relat Cancer*. 2014;21(2):371–381. doi:10.1530/erc-13-0499

26. Chmiel KD, Suan D, Liddle C, et al. Resolution of severe ipilimumab-induced hepatitis after anti-thymocyte globulin therapy. *J Clin Oncol*. 2011;29(9):e237–e240. doi:10.1200/jco.2010.32.2206

27. Bhatia S, Huber BR, Upton MP, et al. Inflammatory enteric neuropathy with severe constipation after ipilimumab treatment for melanoma: a case report. *J Immunother*. 2009;32(2);203–205. doi:10.1097/CJI.0b013e318193a206

28. Weber JS, Kahler KC, Hauschild A. Management of immune-related adverse events and kinetics of response with ipilimumab. *J Clin Oncol*. 2012;30(21):2691–2697. doi:10.1200/jco.2012.41.6750

29. Brahmer J, Reckamp KL, Baas P, et al. Nivolumab versus docetaxel in advanced squamous-cell non-small-cell lung cancer. *N Engl J Med*. 2015;373(2):123–135. doi:10.1056/NEJMoa1504627

30. Garon EB, Rizvi NA, Hui R, et al. Pembrolizumab for the treatment of non-small-cell lung cancer. *N Engl J Med*. 2015;372(21):2018–2028. doi:10.1056/NEJMoa1501824

31. Larkin J, Hodi FS, Wolchok JD. Combined nivolumab and ipilimumab or monotherapy in untreated melanoma. *N Engl J Med*. 2015;373(13):1270–1271. doi:10.1056/NEJMc1509660

32. Motzer RJ, Rini BI, McDermott DF, et al. Nivolumab for metastatic renal cell carcinoma: results of a randomized phase II trial. *J Clin Oncol*. 2015;33(13):1430–1437. doi:10.1200/jco.2014.59.0703

33. Rizvi NA, Mazieres J, Planchard D, et al. Activity and safety of nivolumab, an anti-PD-1 immune checkpoint inhibitor, for patients with advanced, refractory squamous non-small-cell lung cancer (CheckMate 063): a phase 2, single-arm trial. *Lancet Oncol*. 2015;16(3):257–265. doi:10.1016/s1470-2045(15)70054-9

34. Weber JS, D'Angelo SP, Minor D, et al. Nivolumab versus chemotherapy in patients with advanced melanoma who progressed after anti-CTLA-4 treatment (CheckMate 037): a ran-domised, controlled, open-label, phase 3 trial. *Lancet Oncol*. 2015;16(4):375–384. doi:10.1016/s1470-2045(15)70076-8

35. Maur M, Tomasello C, Frassoldati A, et al. Posterior reversible encephalopathy syndrome during ipilimumab therapy for malignant melanoma. *J Clin Oncol.* 2012;30(6):e76–e78. doi:10.1200/jco.2011.38.7886

36. Manousakis G, Koch J, Sommerville RB, et al. Multifocal radiculoneuropathy during ipilimumab treatment of melanoma. *Muscle Nerve.* 2013;48(3):440–444. doi:10.1002/mus.23830

37. Voskens CJ, Goldinger SM, Loquai C, et al. The price of tumor control: an analysis of rare side effects of anti-CTLA-4 therapy in metastatic melanoma from the ipilimumab network. *PLoS One.* 2013;8(1):e53745. doi:10.1371/journal.pone.0053745

38. Harding JJ, El Dika I, Abou-Alfa GK. Immunotherapy in hepatocellular carcinoma: primed to make a difference? *Cancer.* 2016;122(3):367–377. doi:10.1002/cncr.29769

39. Kudo M. Immuno-oncology in hepatocellular carcinoma: 2017 update. *Oncology.* 2017;93(Suppl 1):147–159. doi:10.1159/000481245

40. Kudo M. Molecular targeted therapy for hepatocellular carcinoma: where are we now? *Liver Cancer.* 2015;4(3):i–vii. doi:10.1159/000367753

41. Zhang B, Finn RS. Personalized clinical trials in hepatocellular carcinoma based on biomarker selection. *Liver Cancer.* 2016;5(3):221–232. doi:10.1159/000367763

42. Stein S, Pishvaian MJ, Lee MS, et al. Safety and clinical activity of 1L atezolizumab + bevacizumab in a phase Ib study in hepatocellular carcinoma (HCC). *J Clin Oncol.* 2018;36(15_suppl):4074–4074. doi:10.1200/JCO.2018.36.15_suppl.4074

43. Labiano S, Palazon A, Melero I. Immune response regulation in the tumor microenvironment by hypoxia. *Semin Oncol.* 2015;42(3):378–386. doi:10.1053/j.seminoncol.2015.02.009

44. Palazon A, Martinez-Forero I, Teijeira A, et al. The HIF-1alpha hypoxia response in tumor-infiltrating T lymphocytes induces functional CD137 (4-1BB) for immunotherapy. *Cancer Discov.* 2012;2(7):608–623. doi:10.1158/2159-8290.Cd-11-0314

45. Duffy AG, Ulahannan SV, Makorova-Rusher O, et al. Tremelimumab in combination with ablation in patients with advanced hepatocellular carcinoma. *J Hepatol.* 2017;66(3):545–551. doi:10.1016/j.jhep.2016.10.029

46. Klempner SJ, Gershenhorn B, Tran P, et al. BRAFV600E mutations in high-grade colorectal neuroendocrine tumors may predict responsiveness to BRAF-MEK combination therapy. *Cancer Discov.* 2016;6(6):594–600. doi:10.1158/2159-8290.CD-15-1192

47. Kudo M, Izumi N, Sakamoto M, et al. Survival analysis over 28 years of 173,378 patients with hepatocellular carcinoma in Japan. *Liver Cancer.* 2016;5(3):190–197. doi:10.1159/000367775

48. Barathan M, Gopal K, Mohamed R, et al. Chronic hepatitis C virus infection triggers spontaneous differential expression of biosignatures associated with T cell exhaustion and apoptosis signaling in peripheral blood mononucleocytes. *Apoptosis.* 2015;20(4):466–480. doi:10.1007/s10495-014-1084-y

49. Li H, Wu K, Tao K, et al. Tim-3/galectin-9 signaling pathway mediates T-cell dysfunction and predicts poor prognosis in patients with hepatitis B virus-associated hepatocellular carcinoma. *Hepatology.* 2012;56(4):1342–1351. doi:10.1002/hep.25777

50. Cariani E, Missale G. KIR/HLA immunogenetic background influences the evolution of hepatocellular carcinoma. *Oncoimmunology.* 2013;2(12):e26622–e26622. doi:10.4161/onci.26622

51. Gauttier V, Judor JP, Le Guen V, et al. Agonistic anti-CD137 antibody treatment leads to antitumor response in mice with liver cancer. *Int J Cancer.* 2014;135(12):2857–2867. doi:10.1002/ijc.28943

52. Morales-Kastresana A, Sanmamed MF, Rodriguez I, et al. Combined immunostimulatory monoclonal antibodies extend survival in an aggressive transgenic hepatocellular carcinoma mouse model. *Clin Cancer Res.* 2013;19(22):6151–6162. doi:10.1158/1078-0432.Ccr-13-1189

53. Herzer K, Hofmann TG, Teufel A, et al. IFN-alpha-induced apoptosis in hepatocellular carcinoma involves promyelocytic leukemia protein and TRAIL independently of p53. *Cancer Res.* 2009;69(3):855–862. doi:10.1158/0008-5472.Can-08-2831

54. Li P, Du Q, Cao Z, et al. Interferon-gamma induces autophagy with growth inhibition and cell death in human hepatocellular carcinoma (HCC) cells through interferon-regulatory factor-1 (IRF-1). *Cancer Lett.* 2012;314(2):213–222. doi:10.1016/j.canlet.2011.09.031

55. Obora A, Shiratori Y, Okuno M, et al. Synergistic induction of apoptosis by acyclic retinoid and interferon-beta in human hepatocellular carcinoma cells. *Hepatology.* 2002;36(5):1115–1124. doi:10.1053/jhep.2002.36369

56. Lygidakis NJ, Kosmidis P, Ziras N, et al. Combined transarterial targeting locoregional immunotherapy-chemotherapy for patients with unresectable hepatocellular carcinoma: a new alternative for an old problem. *J Interferon Cytokine Res.* 1995;15(5):467–472. doi:10.1089/jir.1995.15.467

57. Sangro B, Mazzolini G, Ruiz J, et al. Phase I trial of intratumoral injection of an adenovirus encoding interleukin-12 for advanced digestive tumors. *J Clin Oncol.* 2004;22(8):1389–1397. doi:10.1200/jco.2004.04.059

58. Sun JC, Pan K, Chen MS, et al. Dendritic cells-mediated CTLs targeting hepatocellular carcinoma stem cells. *Cancer Biol Ther.* 2010;10(4):368–375.

59. Gilham DE, Debets R, Pule M, et al. CAR-T cells and solid tumors: tuning T cells to challenge an inveterate foe. *Trends Mol Med.* 2012;18(7):377–384. doi:10.1016/j.molmed.2012.04.009

60. Sadelain M, Brentjens R, Riviere I. The promise and potential pitfalls of chimeric antigen receptors. *Curr Opin Immunol.* 2009;21(2):215–223. doi:10.1016/j.coi.2009.02.009

61. Baumhoer D, Tornillo L, Stadlmann S, et al. Glypican 3 expression in human nonneoplastic, preneoplastic, and neoplastic tissues: a tissue microarray analysis of 4,387 tissue samples. *Am J Clin Pathol.* 2008;129(6):899–906. doi:10.1309/hcqwpwd50xhd2dw6

62. Hass HG, Jobst J, Scheurlen M, et al. Gene expression analysis for evaluation of potential biomarkers in hepatocellular carcinoma. *Anticancer Res.* 2015;35(4):2021–2028.

63. Gao H, Li K, Tu H, et al. Development of T cells redirected to glypican-3 for the treatment of hepatocellular carcinoma. *Clin Cancer Res.* 2014;20(24):6418–6428. doi:10.1158/1078-0432. Ccr-14-1170

64. Chen C, Li K, Jiang H, et al. Development of T cells carrying two complementary chimeric antigen receptors against glypican-3 and asialoglycoprotein receptor 1 for the treatment of hepatocellular carcinoma. *Cancer Immunol Immunother.* 2017;66(4):475–489. doi:10.1007/s00262-016-1949-8

65. Sharma P, Allison JP. The future of immune checkpoint therapy. *Science.* 2015;348(6230):56–61. doi:10.1126/science.aaa8172

66. Sharma P, Allison JP. Immune checkpoint targeting in cancer therapy: toward combination strategies with curative potential. *Cell.* 2015;161(2):205–214. doi:10.1016/j.cell.2015.03.030

IV

Gastric and Esophageal Cancer

Epidemiology of Gastric and Esophageal Cancer

Mohamad Bassam Sonbol and Daniel H. Ahn

INTRODUCTION

Gastric and esophageal cancers are a significant cause of mortality in the United States with an estimated annual incidence of 26,240 and 17,290 cases, and 10,800 and 15,800 yearly deaths for gastric and esophageal cancers, respectively (1). Worldwide, gastric and esophageal cancers are the second highest cause of cancer deaths after lung cancer with the highest incidence in Eastern Asia and Central and Eastern Europe (2). Such differences are partially attributed to several risk factors that include certain dietary patterns as well as infectious etiologies (3).

Esophageal cancer can be stratified into esophageal adenocarcinoma, esophageal squamous cell carcinoma (SCC), and gastroesophageal junction (GEJ) adenocarcinoma. Likewise, gastric cancer can be further divided into gastric adenocarcinoma, intestinal type and gastric adenocarcinoma, diffuse type (4).

Historically, esophageal SCC in the upper and middle esophagus used to be the most common type of esophageal cancer. Over the past several decades, the incidence of esophageal SCC has been decreasing in the United States and worldwide, overtaken by the dramatic increase of esophageal and GEJ adenocarcinoma (5). On the other hand, both the incidence and mortality rates of gastric cancers have rapidly declined. These changes are related to the risk factors associated with each subtype as described in the following.

The decline in incidence of gastric cancer is partially due to the recognition of certain risk factors such as *Helicobacter pylori* (*H. pylori*) infection, as well as an understanding of the importance of food refrigeration (6). *H. pylori* infection is known to be associated with an increased risk of gastritis and noncardia gastric adenocarcinoma. Worldwide, approximately half of the population is infected with higher rates in Asia and South America, while lower rates are observed in the Western population (7). Two previous meta-analyses composed primarily of Asian-based patient population studies showed *H. pylori* eradication resulted in lower rates of gastric cancer (7,8). This was supported by a subsequent nationwide, population-based Swedish study (9). Based on these findings, the current recommendation from the American College of Gastroenterology (ACG) is for H. pylori testing to be conducted in high-risk patient populations (10).

In addition to *H. pylori*, nutritional and environmental factors have been identified as risk factors for gastric adenocarcinoma. High-salt diet, nutritional deficiencies (vitamin A and C deficiency), smoked foods, and lack of refrigeration along with poor quality water are associated with a higher likelihood of gastric cancers (11). Other risk factors also include cigarette smoking, Epstein–Barr virus (EBV), and hereditary and genetic syndromes (Table 36.1).

Esophageal SCC is associated with carcinogen exposure, which includes cigarette smoking and excessive alcohol consumption (16,17). On the other hand, esophageal and GEJ adenocarcinomas are associated with obesity, smoking, and Barrett's metaplasia (18,19).

TABLE 36.1 Selected Hereditary Syndromes With High Frequency of Gastric Cancer

Syndrome	Gene	Other Association
HDGC (12)	*CDH1*	• Prostate cancer • Lobular breast cancer • Signet-ring colon cancer
Peutz–Jeghers syndrome (13)	*STK11*	• Colorectal • Pancreas • Breast cancer • Gynecological cancers • Testicular • Lung • Benign skin pigmentations
FAP (14)	*APC; MutYH*	• Colon cancer • Pancreatic cancer • Papillary thyroid
Juvenile polyposis (15)	*SMAD 4*	• Colon cancer • Small intestine cancer • Pancreas • Hereditary hemorrhagic telangiectasia

FAP, familial adenomatous polyposis; HDGC, hereditary diffuse gastric cancer.

REFERENCES

1. Siegel RL, Miller KD, Jemal A. Cancer statistics, 2018. *CA Cancer J Clin*. 2018;68(1):7–30. doi:10.3322/caac.21442
2. Torre LA, Siegel RL, Ward EM, et al. Global cancer incidence and mortality rates and trends—an update. *Cancer Epidemiol Biomarkers Prev*. 2016;25(1):16–27. doi:10.1158/1055-9965. EPI-15-0578
3. Torre LA, Bray F, Siegel RL, et al. Global cancer statistics, 2012. *CA Cancer J Clin*. 2015;65(2):87–108. doi:10.3322/caac.21262
4. Lauren P. The two histological main types of gastric carcinoma: diffuse and so-called intestinal-type carcinoma: an attempt at a histo-clinical classification. *Acta Pathol Microbiol Scand*. 1965;64:31–49. doi:10.1111/apm.1965.64.1.31
5. Lagergren J, Lagergren P. Recent developments in esophageal adenocarcinoma. *CA Cancer J Clin*. 2013;63(4):232–248. doi:10.3322/caac.21185
6. Haenszel W. Variation in incidence of and mortality from stomach cancer, with particular reference to the United States. *J Natl Cancer Inst*. 1958;21(2):213–262. doi:10.1093/jnci/21.2.213
7. Peleteiro B, Bastos A, Ferro A, et al. Prevalence of Helicobacter pylori infection worldwide: a systematic review of studies with national coverage. *Dig Dis Sci*. 2014;59(8):1698–1709. doi:10.1007/s10620-014-3063-0
8. Ford AC, Forman D, Hunt RH, et al. Helicobacter pylori eradication therapy to prevent gastric cancer in healthy asymptomatic infected individuals: systematic review and meta-analysis of randomised controlled trials. *BMJ*. 2014;348:g3174. doi:10.1136/bmj.g3174
9. Doorakkers E, Lagergren J, Engstrand L, et al. Helicobacter pylori eradication treatment and the risk of gastric adenocarcinoma in a Western population. *Gut*. 2018;67(12):2092–2096. doi:10.1136/gutjnl-2017-315363
10. Chey WD, Leontiadis GI, Howden CW, et al. ACG clinical guideline: treatment of Helicobacter pylori infection. *Am J Gastroenterol*. 2017;112(2):212–239. doi:10.1038/ajg.2016.563
11. Liu C, Russell RM. Nutrition and gastric cancer risk: an update. *Nutr Rev*. 2008;66(5):237–249. doi:10.1111/j.1753-4887.2008.00029.x
12. van der Post RS, Vogelaar IP, Carneiro F, et al. Hereditary diffuse gastric cancer: updated clinical guidelines with an emphasis on germline CDH1 mutation carriers. *J Med Genet*. 2015;52(6):361–374. doi:10.1136/jmedgenet-2015-103094
13. van Lier MG, Wagner A, Mathus-Vliegen EM, et al. High cancer risk in Peutz-Jeghers syndrome: a systematic review and surveillance recommendations. *Am J Gastroenterol*. 2010;105(6):1258–1264; author reply 65. doi:10.1038/ajg.2009.725

14. Syngal S, Brand RE, Church JM, et al. ACG clinical guideline: genetic testing and management of hereditary gastrointestinal cancer syndromes. *Am J Gastroenterol*. 2015;110(2):223–262; quiz 63. doi:10.1038/ajg.2014.435

15. Latchford AR, Neale K, Phillips RK, et al. Juvenile polyposis syndrome: a study of genotype, phenotype, and long-term outcome. *Dis Colon Rectum*. 2012;55(10):1038–1043. doi:10.1097/DCR.0b013e31826278b3

16. Freedman ND, Abnet CC, Caporaso NE, et al. Impact of changing US cigarette smoking patterns on incident cancer: risks of 20 smoking-related cancers among the women and men of the NIH-AARP cohort. *Int J Epidemiol*. 2016;45(3):846–856. doi:10.1093/ije/dyv175

17. Islami F, Fedirko V, Tramacere I, et al. Alcohol drinking and esophageal squamous cell carcinoma with focus on light-drinkers and never-smokers: a systematic review and meta-analysis. *Int J Cancer*. 2011;129(10):2473–2484. doi:10.1002/ijc.25885

18. Lauby-Secretan B, Scoccianti C, Loomis D, et al. Body fatness and cancer—viewpoint of the IARC working group. *N Engl J Med*. 2016;375(8):794–798. doi:10.1056/NEJMsr1606602

19. Thrift AP, Shaheen NJ, Gammon MD, et al. Obesity and risk of esophageal adenocarcinoma and Barrett's esophagus: a Mendelian randomization study. *J Natl Cancer Inst*. 2014;106(11):dju252. doi:10.1093/jnci/dju252

37

Diagnosis and Staging of Gastric and Esophageal Cancer

Mohamad Bassam Sonbol and Daniel H. Ahn

ESOPHAGEAL CANCER

The tumor, node, and metastasis (TNM) staging is the established method for staging esophageal and gastroesophageal junction (GEJ) cancers and is strongly associated with prognosis. At the time of presentation, an upper endoscopy is needed to obtain a tissue biopsy for diagnosis. Furthermore, in order to determine the tumor depth penetration (tumor stage, T) and mediastinal lymph node status (nodal stage, N), an endoscopic ultrasound (EUS) has become the de facto standard in the initial workup and evaluation of esophageal cancer (1). In a study of 117 patients with node negativity by PET/CT, EUS was positive (upstaging) for metastatic lymph node disease in 33% of the cases (2). The sensitivity and specificity of regional lymph node metastases on PET/CT were estimated to be at 57% and 85%, respectively (1). Thus, PET/CT should be used in combination with EUS to reliably stage the regional lymph node in esophageal and GEJ cancers as there is a significant difference in overall survival in patients with node-negative versus node-positive (N+) disease (2,3). To accurately stage patients with esophageal cancers above the carina with no evidence of distant metastatic disease (M0), bronchoscopy is recommended by the National Comprehensive Cancer Network (NCCN) guidelines (4). The benefit of PET/CT is primarily in the evaluation of the extent of the disease and for the detection of occult metastatic disease, especially before planned curative surgery.

GASTRIC CANCER

Gastric cancer is also most often diagnosed by upper endoscopy. As in esophageal cancer, the American Joint Committee on Cancer (AJCC) TNM staging is the most widely used method for staging gastric cancers (5). EUS is useful and recommended by the NCCN guidelines in evaluating early/locally advanced disease. CT scans with oral and intravenous (IV) contrast are useful to identify distant metastatic disease. However, CT scans are unreliable when it comes to evaluating peritoneal metastases as approximately 20% of CT-negative cases are found to have intraperitoneal disease by staging laparoscopy (6). Similarly, PET/CT scan is helpful in identifying occult distant metastases but also remains unreliable in ruling out peritoneal involvement. Furthermore, most diffuse-type gastric cancers are not fluorodeoxyglucose (FDG) avid (7). Therefore, staging laparoscopy with cytology evaluation is a useful tool to assess for intraperitoneal involvement. Patients whose tumors exhibit positive peritoneal cytology are at increased risk for disease recurrence and are associated with poorer outcomes (8,9). The NCCN guidelines recommend considering diagnostic laparoscopy with cytology in patients with T1b or higher (5). However, diagnostic laparoscopy is not indicated for patients planned for palliative resection.

REFERENCES

1. van Vliet EP, Heijenbrok-Kal MH, Hunink MG, et al. Staging investigations for oesophageal cancer: a meta-analysis. *Br J Cancer.* 2008;98(3):547–557. doi:10.1038/sj.bjc.6604200
2. Foley KG, Lewis WG, Fielding P, et al. N-staging of oesophageal and junctional carcinoma: is there still a role for EUS in patients staged N0 at PET/CT? *Clin Radiol.* 2014;69(9):959–964. doi:10.1016/j.crad.2014.04.023

3. Allum WH, Griffin SM, Watson A, et al. Guidelines for the management of oesophageal and gastric cancer. *Gut*. 2002;50(Suppl 5):v1–v23. doi:10.1136/gut.50.suppl_5.v1

4. NCCN. Esophageal and Esophagogastric Junction Cancers. Version 1.2019-March 14, 2019. https://www.nccn.org/professionals/physician_gls/pdf/esophageal.pdf

5. NCCN. Gastric Cancer. version1.2019-March14, 2019. https://www.nccn.org/professionals/physician_gls/pdf/gastric.pdf

6. Power DG, Schattner MA, Gerdes H, et al. Endoscopic ultrasound can improve the selection for laparoscopy in patients with localized gastric cancer. *J Am Coll Surg*. 2009;208(2):173–178. doi:10.1016/j.jamcollsurg.2008.10.022

7. Mukai K, Ishida Y, Okajima K, et al. Usefulness of preoperative FDG-PET for detection of gastric cancer. *Gastric Cancer*. 2006;9(3):192–196. doi:10.1007/s10120-006-0374-7

8. Bentrem D, Wilton A, Mazumdar M, et al. The value of peritoneal cytology as a preoperative predictor in patients with gastric carcinoma undergoing a curative resection. *Ann Surg Oncol*. 2005;12(5):347–353. doi:10.1245/ASO.2005.03.065

9. De Andrade JP, Mezhir JJ. The critical role of peritoneal cytology in the staging of gastric cancer: an evidence-based review. *J Surg Oncol*. 2014;110(3):291–297. doi:10.1002/jso.23632

38

Molecular Diagnostic Guidelines of Gastric and Esophageal Cancer

Mohamad Bassam Sonbol and Daniel H. Ahn

MOLECULAR DIAGNOSTIC GUIDELINES

After obtaining tumor tissue to confirm the diagnosis, further molecular testing is recommended to guide future therapies. Human epidermal growth factor receptor 2 (HER2) assessment is recommended in patients with gastric, esophageal, and gastroesophageal junction (GEJ) adenocarcinoma. HER2 is a member of the family of epidermal growth factor receptor (EGFR) extracellular receptors that is linked to tumor growth and apoptosis (1). HER2 assessment can be performed by immunohistochemistry (IHC), followed by fluorescence in situ hybridization (FISH) in cases that show equivocal (2+) expression by IHC. The rates of HER2 positivity vary based on tumor location and subtype. The incidence of HER2 overexpression is higher in GEJ cancers compared to the gastric cancers (32% vs. 21%) (2). Additionally, for gastric adenocarcinoma, the rates of HER2 positivity are higher in the intestinal histology (33%) compared to the diffuse histology (8%) (3,4). On the other hand, esophageal adenocarcinoma tends to be associated with higher rates of HER2 (15%–30%) than esophageal SCC (5%–13%) (5). In TOGA, an open-label, international, phase 3 randomized controlled clinical trial, the addition of trastuzumab, a monoclonal antibody that targets HER2, to fluoropyrimidine platinum based chemotherapy in patients with HER2 overexpressing advanced gastric or GEJ cancers led to improvement in overall survival from 11.1 to 13.8 months (6). Testing for microsatellite instability (MSI) and PD-L1 is also currently recommended for patients with metastatic gastric, esophageal, and GEJ adenocarcinoma who are candidates for treatment with PD-1 inhibitors with the recent approval of pembrolizumab (7). In KEYNOTE-059, an open-label single-arm phase 2 trial, patients with treatment-refractory PD-L1+ advanced gastric or GEJ cancer experienced a 15.5% objective response rate, which resulted in the Food and Drug Administration (FDA) approval in 2017 for pembrolizumab in patients whose tumors exhibited PD-L1 positivity (8).

Molecular Subtypes of Gastric Cancer

In 2014, The Cancer Genome Atlas (TCGA) defined four subtypes of gastric cancers (9): Epstein–Barr virus (EBV; 9%), MSI high (22%), genomically stable (GS; 20%), and chromosomal instability (CIN; 50%) subtypes (Table 38.1). The EBV-positive subtype comprises 9% of gastric cancers and mostly occurs in the gastric fundus or body with male predilection. These tumors display recurrent *PIK3CA* mutations, extreme DNA hypermethylation, recurrent *JAK2* and *ERBB2* amplifications, and amplification of PD-L1 and PD-L2. In addition, EBV-positive gastric cancers have more frequent tumor-infiltrating CD8+ and Foxp3+ cells. Together with the MSI-high subtype, EBV-positive gastric cancers represent an attractive target for checkpoint inhibitors that target immune cells in the microenvironment (10). MSI-high gastric cancers were also noted to have high rates of mutations in *PIK3CA*, *ERBB3*, *ERBB2*, and *EGFR*. However, while the association has been described in colon cancer, *BRAF* V600E mutations were absent in MSI-high gastric cancers. The CIN subtype has high rates of receptor tyrosine kinase oncogenes such as *FGFR2*, *EGFR*, *HER2*, and *MET*. The differences observed in these subtypes might provide further insight into the heterogeneity in treatment responses to various therapeutic approaches and help better refine patient selection in future clinical trials (11).

TABLE 38.1 Molecular Subtypes of Gastric Cancers

Gastric Cancer Subtype	Frequency	Molecular and Genetic Characteristics
CIN	50%	RTK-RAS activation; *TP53* mutation
GS	20%	*CDH1* and *RHOA* mutations
MSI	22%	Mutations in *PIK3CA, ERBB3, ERBB2, EGFR*; *MLH1* silencing
EBV	9%	DNA hypermethylation; *PIK3CA*; *PD-L1, PD-L2*; *JAK2*; *ERBB2* (amplification)

CIN, chromosomal instability; EBV, Epstein–Barr virus; GS, genomically stable; MSI, microsatellite instability.

REFERENCES

1. Gravalos C, Jimeno A. HER2 in gastric cancer: a new prognostic factor and a novel therapeutic target. *Ann Oncol*. 2008;19(9):1523–1529. doi:10.1093/annonc/mdn169
2. Van Cutsem E, Bang YJ, Feng-Yi F, et al. HER2 screening data from ToGA: targeting HER2 in gastric and gastroesophageal junction cancer. *Gastric Cancer*. 2015;18(3):476–484. doi:10.1007/s10120-014-0402-y
3. Kunz PL, Mojtahed A, Fisher GA, et al. HER2 expression in gastric and gastroesophageal junction adenocarcinoma in a US population: clinicopathologic analysis with proposed approach to HER2 assessment. *Appl Immunohistochem Mol Morphol*. 2012;20(1):13–24. doi:10.1097/PAI.0b013e31821c821c
4. Tanner M, Hollmen M, Junttila TT, et al. Amplification of HER-2 in gastric carcinoma: association with Topoisomerase IIalpha gene amplification, intestinal type, poor prognosis and sensitivity to trastuzumab. *Ann Oncol*. 2005;16(2):273–278. doi:10.1093/annonc/mdi064
5. Dreilich M, Wanders A, Brattstrom D, et al. HER-2 overexpression (3+) in patients with squamous cell esophageal carcinoma correlates with poorer survival. *Dis Esophagus*. 2006;19(4):224–231. doi:10.1111/j.1442-2050.2006.00570.x
6. Bang YJ, Van Cutsem E, Feyereislova A, et al. Trastuzumab in combination with chemotherapy versus chemotherapy alone for treatment of HER2-positive advanced gastric or gastro-oesophageal junction cancer (ToGA): a phase 3, open-label, randomised controlled trial. *Lancet*. 2010;376(9742):687–697. doi:10.1016/S0140-6736(10)61121-X
7. FDA. FDA grants accelerated approval to pembrolizumab for advanced gastric cancer. 2017.
8. Fuchs CS, Doi T, Jang RW, et al. Safety and efficacy of pembrolizumab monotherapy in patients with previously treated advanced gastric and gastroesophageal junction cancer: phase 2 clinical KEYNOTE-059 trial. *JAMA Oncol*. 2018;4(5):e180013. doi:10.1001/jamaoncol.2018.0013
9. Cancer Genome Atlas Research Network. Comprehensive molecular characterization of gastric adenocarcinoma. *Nature*. 2014;513(7517):202–209. doi:10.1038/nature13480
10. Ma J, Li J, Hao Y, et al. Differentiated tumor immune microenvironment of Epstein-Barr virus-associated and negative gastric cancer: implication in prognosis and immunotherapy. *Oncotarget*. 2017;8(40):67094–67103. doi:10.18632/oncotarget.17945
11. Ahn DH, Bekaii-Saab TS. Genetic Diversity and treatment implications in gastric and gastro-esophageal cancers: one size does not fit all. *J Oncol Pract*. 2018;14(4):227–228. doi:10.1200/JOP.18.00158

How I Treat Early-Stage Gastric and Esophageal Cancer With Neoadjuvant Therapy

William A. Stokes and Karyn A. Goodman

EVIDENCE

Surgery comprises the mainstay of treatment for esophageal, gastroesophageal junction (GEJ), and gastric cancers and should be offered to all patients who are operative candidates. However, for those patients with locally advanced disease, such as the patient in Clinical Vignette 39.1, combined-modality therapy (CMT) is indicated. Despite multiple studies evaluating the use of preoperative chemoradiation therapy (CRT) for esophageal cancer over the past three decades, only recent studies have established trimodality therapy as the preferred approach for locally advanced esophageal and GEJ cancers. For gastric cancer, perioperative chemotherapy has been established, and the role of adjuvant CRT remains controversial.

CRT was initially developed in the nonsurgical setting after the landmark trial Radiation Therapy Oncology Group (RTOG) 8501 demonstrated the benefit of CRT (50 Gy with cisplatin/5-fluorouracil [5-FU]) over radiation therapy (RT) alone (64 Gy) (1). Until recently, the role of neoadjuvant CRT prior to surgery remained a subject of controversy. Older trials were limited by methodological issues, nonstandard chemotherapy regimens and RT doses, outdated RT techniques, underrepresentation of adenocarcinoma histology, and small study populations. A more modern study, Cancer and Leukemia Group B (CALGB) 9781, randomized patients to either immediate surgery or neoadjuvant CRT consisting of 50.4 Gy and concurrent 5-FU and cisplatin followed by surgery. While this study closed due to poor accrual with only 56 patients enrolled out of an intended population of 500, the addition of CRT significantly prolonged overall survival (OS; median 54 vs. 21 months) and progression-free survival (PFS; median 42 vs. 12 months), and it did not increase postoperative mortality (2).

More recently, the seminal ChemoRadiotherapy for Oesophageal Cancer Followed by Surgery Study (CROSS) overcame the small sample size of CALGB 9781 and other limitations. This phase III trial conducted in the Netherlands enrolled patients with tumors of the esophagus or GEJ with clinical stages of T1N1M0 or T2-3N0-1M0. In total, 363 patients, of whom 75% had adenocarcinoma histology, were randomized to either neoadjuvant CRT followed by surgery or immediate surgery, with CRT consisting of 41.4 Gy in 23 fractions delivered concurrently with five weekly infusions of carboplatin and paclitaxel. The addition of CRT significantly improved surgical completion (R0 rates of 92% vs. 69%), PFS (median 38 vs. 16 months), and OS (median 49 vs. 24 months) (3,4).

An analysis of patterns of failure demonstrated that CRT patients experienced significant reductions in anastomotic, mediastinal, peritoneal, and hematogenous recurrences (5). Importantly, the incidence and distribution of postoperative complications did not meaningfully differ between arms, indicating that the oncologic benefits of CRT did not come at the cost of excess morbidity; nor was quality of life affected in the postoperative or long-term periods (4,6,7). Ultimately, the dramatic improvements in disease control and survival seen with CMT in the CROSS trial have established trimodality therapy with neoadjuvant CRT followed by surgery as the preferred approach to esophageal and GEJ cancers.

Perioperative or preoperative chemotherapy without RT has also been investigated in esophageal cancer in two large randomized trials. Intergroup 0113 and the Medical Research Council (MRC) OEO1 have yielded conflicting results (e.g., 8,9); however, a meta-analysis evaluating the addition of neoadjuvant chemotherapy to surgery that encompasses 10 trials and 2,062 patients (10) demonstrated a significant improvement in survival with chemotherapy

---

A Clinical Vignette ("How I Treat") is included at the end of the chapter.

(hazard ratio: 0.87, 95% confidence interval [CI]: 0.79–0.96) and provided justification for neoadjuvant chemotherapy prior to resection.

Thus, it makes intuitive sense to question the role of neoadjuvant CRT given the aforementioned improvement in outcomes following neoadjuvant chemotherapy alone. The results of the PreOperative therapy in Esophagogastric adenocarcinoma Trial (POET) from Germany are instructive in this regard. Despite an initial enrollment target of 354 patients, only 125 individuals with GEJ adenocarcinomas were eventually randomized to undergo either induction chemotherapy and surgery or the same approach with intervening CRT. Induction chemotherapy consisted of cisplatin and 5-FU, and CRT consisted of 30 Gy in 15 fractions with concurrent cisplatin and etoposide. Long-term results of this study indicated a trend toward improved OS and significant improvements in locoregional control and PFS with CRT (11). Therefore, despite being underpowered, the POET study suggests that chemotherapy alone is insufficient as neoadjuvant therapy and that RT constitutes an essential component of CMT.

Intensification of neoadjuvant systemic therapy via the addition of a human epidermal growth factor receptor 2 (HER2) directed agent is being evaluated in RTOG 1010. This trial randomized patients with HER2-overexpressing esophageal adenocarcinoma to either neoadjuvant CRT (50.4 Gy with carboplatin and paclitaxel) and surgery or to the same approach with trastuzumab added to CRT (NCT01196390). With accrual completed, the results of this trial are eagerly anticipated.

The optimal chemotherapeutic regimen has yet to be established, as a variety of doublets have been studied in neoadjuvant CRT, including 5-FU and cisplatin on CALGB 9781 (2), 5-FU and oxaliplatin on SWOG 0356 (12), carboplatin and paclitaxel on CROSS (4), and cisplatin and etoposide on POET (11). Unfortunately, high-quality comparative data are lacking to guide the selection of one regimen over others. At this time, therefore, the selection of chemotherapy should be individualized according to the specific patient's performance status, comorbidities, and preferences. However, it should be noted that the National Comprehensive Cancer Network (NCCN) considers only carboplatin and paclitaxel, 5-FU and oxaliplatin, and 5-FU and cisplatin as "category 1" regimens, with only the first two qualifying as "preferred" combinations (13).

As with chemotherapy, the appropriate RT approach in the neoadjuvant setting continues to be debated. CALGB employed a CRT dose of 50.4 Gy (2), while the CROSS trial utilized a lower CRT dose of 41.4 Gy. The significant improvement in outcomes with CRT observed in both of these trials justifies the use of 41.4 to 50.4 Gy in the neoadjuvant approach to esophageal cancer (13). Of note, the NEOSCOPE trial falls in between these values, featuring 45 Gy (14).

As patients with esophageal cancer are at high risk of systemic spread, there have been attempts to improve outcomes by intensifying chemotherapy with the addition of induction chemotherapy before CRT, thereby treating patients with a three-step approach analogous to the experimental arm of the POET trial (11). A phase II trial conducted at MD Anderson Cancer Center evaluated the addition of induction chemotherapy to preoperative CRT and surgery. Patients were randomized to CRT with 50.4 Gy of RT with 5-FU and oxaliplatin followed by surgery, with or without induction chemotherapy consisting of a more intensive regimen of the same agents. The primary end point of a significant difference in pathologic complete response (pCR) rate was not reached among 109 evaluable subjects; nevertheless, roughly twice as many patients receiving induction chemotherapy achieved a pCR as compared to those who did not (26% vs. 13%), a trend that approached statistical significance at $p = .09$ (15). Additional single-arm trials have demonstrated the feasibility of adding induction chemotherapy to preoperative CRT and surgery (16–19).

This three-step approach to esophageal cancer holds appeal in the era of personalized medicine. At present, the advantages of neoadjuvant CRT with respect to pCR, disease control, and survival do not extend to all patients who undergo CMT, and the identification of those patients at risk for suboptimal outcomes may allow a beneficial change in therapeutic strategy. The three-step approach allows clinicians to "test the biology" of tumors by assessing their response to induction chemotherapy, tailor the CRT regimen accordingly, and thereby optimize outcomes following surgery. Such an adaptive approach requires two essential features: (a) a suitable biomarker and (b) efficacious treatment alternatives.

PET utilizing ^{18}F has emerged as a predictive biomarker in esophageal cancer. Changes in metabolic activity as assessed by PET during neoadjuvant therapy strongly predict clinical outcomes (20–23). Some of the most robust evidence supporting the prognostic discrimination of PET and its application comes from investigators at the Technical University of Munich. Retrospectively analyzing their GEJ patients undergoing preoperative cisplatin-based chemotherapy, they identified and subsequently validated a ≥35% (vs. <35%) reduction in metabolic activity between baseline and day 14 of chemotherapy as a cutoff that accurately differentiates "responders" from "nonresponders" with respect to changes in radiographic tumor size, pathologic response, time to progression, and survival (24,25). These provocative results led the investigators to conduct the first Metabolic response evalUatioN for Individualization of neoadjuvant Chemotherapy in Oesophageal and oesophagogastric adeNocarcinoma (MUNICON I) study, a phase II trial that prospectively assigned all patients to a strategy consisting of upfront platinum-based chemotherapy for 2 weeks. Responders went on to receive platinum-based chemotherapy for 10 additional weeks prior to surgery, while nonresponders aborted chemotherapy and proceeded directly to surgery. Out of 104 patients receiving surgery, the 50 responders experienced improved OS (median not reached vs. 26 months) and event-free survival (median 30 vs. 14 months) (26).

MUNICON II, used the same 35% PET response cutoff to 14 days of cisplatin-based CT to identify responders and nonresponders. Responders again continued to receive chemotherapy for a total of 12 weeks; however, in an effort to improve outcomes among nonresponders, therapy was intensified with preoperative CRT prior to surgery, rather than immediate surgery as in MUNICON I. CRT consisted of 32 Gy delivered twice daily in 20 fractions with concurrent cisplatin. Among 56 patients, pathologic response and OS were numerically but not significantly better for responders; however, responders experienced significantly longer time to progression (median not reached vs. 15 months) (27). Together, the two MUNICON trials demonstrate the feasibility of using PET to identify nonresponders to upfront chemotherapy and then altering therapy in these patients with a goal of redirecting the patient to more effective therapy. The MUNICON approach is limited, however, by the nonuniform application of CRT prior to surgery, nonstandard RT fractionation schedule, and limited population size.

The randomized CALGB 80803 study built on the PET-directed therapy paradigm established by MUNICON. This trial randomized patients with T3–4 or node-positive adenocarcinoma of the esophagus or GEJ to one of two upfront induction chemotherapy regimens: 5-FU and oxaliplatin delivered for three 2-week cycles or two 3-week cycles of carboplatin and paclitaxel. Response was assessed at 36 to 42 days and defined as ≥35% reduction in metabolic activity from baseline. All patients then proceeded to CRT to a dose of 50.4 Gy, with responders continuing their assigned chemotherapy during CRT and nonresponders switching to the alternative chemotherapy regimen for CRT. Surgical resection was planned 6 weeks post-CRT. With 240 patients evaluable, of whom approximately 40% were nonresponders, the primary end point of improving pCR from 5% to 20% among nonresponders was met (28). At a median follow-up of 42 months, the median OS for PET responders was 47 months, compared with 29 months for nonresponders (29). The median survival in the nonresponders compares favorably with historical median OS rates among nonresponders that failed to exceed 18 months (26,27,30). The findings suggest that early PET response assessment may be used as both a prognostic and a predictive tool in patients with esophageal and GEJ adenocarcinomas and can help individualize therapy for these patients. While the study was not powered for a head-to-head comparison of the two induction regimens, the median survival of 50 months among responders receiving induction and concurrent 5-FU and oxaliplatin is encouraging and warrants further evaluation with a prospective study to compare chemotherapy regimens.

Representative outcomes from trials in esophageal and GEJ cancers are depicted in Table 39.1.

Our discussion to this point has been predicated on our patient having a tumor of the GEJ and would also apply to a patient with esophageal cancer. If, however, our patient described in Clinical Vignette 39.1 had a tumor that extended more than 5 cm into the gastric cardia (i.e., a Siewert III GEJ tumor) or was arising entirely from the stomach, we would recommend a gastric cancer treatment paradigm. Two distinct approaches have emerged. The first was established by the MRC Adjuvant Gastric Infusional Chemotherapy (MAGIC) trial, which randomized 503 patients with GEJ or gastric cancer to surgery with or without perioperative chemotherapy, consisting of epirubicin, cisplatin, and 5-FU delivered preoperatively for three cycles and postoperatively for three cycles. The addition of perioperative chemotherapy significantly prolonged both PFS and OS, while postoperative complications and mortality were comparable between arms (31). Notably, a recent CALGB trial demonstrated that the removal of epirubicin from perioperative chemotherapy did not compromise outcomes (32). The other accepted approach is based on the Intergroup 0116 trial, which randomized 559 patients with cancers of the GEJ or stomach to surgery with or without adjuvant CRT, consisting of 45 Gy delivered with 5-FU. CRT significantly improved both relapse-free and OS (33).

With the experimental arms of MAGIC and Intergroup 0116 both featuring chemotherapy, the additional benefit of RT, as utilized in the latter, remains controversial. The Adjuvant Chemoradiotherapy in Stomach Tumors (ARTIST) trial, conducted in South Korea, directly

TABLE 39.1 Pathologic and Survival Outcomes Following Neoadjuvant Therapy for Esophageal and GEJ Cancers in Selected Prospective Trials

Trial (Arm)	Neoadjuvant regimen	pCR %	Median OS Months	4-Year OS %
MUNICON I (nonresponders)	FOLFOX (no RT)	0	26	NR
CALGB 9781 (neoadjuvant)	Cis&5-FU-based CRT	40	54	~56
CROSS (neoadjuvant)	C&P-based CRT	23	42	45
POET (CRT)	Cis&5-FU → Cis&Etop-based CRT	14	31	~40
MUNICON II (nonresponders)	Cis&5-FU → Cis-/5-FU-based CRT	4	18	NR
NEOSCOPE ("winner")	CapOx → C&P-based CRT	29	NR	NR
CALGB 80803 (C&P nonresponders)	C&P → FOLFOX-based CRT	17	28	42
CALGB 80803 (C&P responders)	C&P → C&P-based CRT	13	40	45
CALGB 80803 (FOLFOX nonresponders)	FOLFOX → C&P-based CRT	19	31	38
CALGB 80803 (FOLFOX responders)	FOLFOX → FOLFOX-based CRT	38	50	53

5-FU, 5-fluorouracil; CapOx, capecitabine and oxaliplatin; Cis, cisplatin; C&P, carboplatin and paclitaxel; Etop, etoposide; FOLFOX, 5-FU and oxaliplatin; GEJ, gastroesophageal junction; NR, not reported; OS, overall survival; pCR, pathologic complete response.

assessed the addition of RT to adjuvant chemotherapy following resection of gastric cancer. This study randomized 458 resected patients to either chemotherapy, consisting of capecitabine and cisplatin for up to six cycles, or to CRT, consisting of the same chemotherapy delivered before, during, and after 45 Gy of RT. The addition of RT failed to significantly prolong OS or disease-free survival in the study population but did reduce locoregional relapse (34). Intriguingly, unplanned subgroup analyses suggested a benefit with CRT among patients with node-positive or intestinal-type cancers. The ARTIST 2 trial is specifically evaluating the benefit of adjuvant CRT in the setting of node-positive disease (NCT01761461). At this time, our institutional practice is to treat gastric cancer patients with perioperative chemotherapy, generally consisting of FOLFOX, as an extrapolation from the data using cisplatin and 5-FU from CALGB 80101 (32). We reserve adjuvant CRT primarily for cases of a positive margin after surgery with the goal of improving local control.

Clinical Vignette 39.1

A 60-year-old man presents with 3 months of progressive dysphagia, over which time he has lost 15 pounds. He endorses long-standing postprandial epigastric pain, and for the past month he has noted feeling more fatigued than usual but has not had to cut back from his full-time job as a technology consultant. His past medical history is remarkable for obesity and hypertension, for which he takes amlodipine; family and past surgical histories are noncontributory. Labwork is consistent with mild iron-deficiency anemia but indicates no metabolic disturbance or abnormalities in hepatic or renal function. He undergoes an upper gastrointestinal endoscopy, which demonstrates normal esophageal mucosa in the proximal and middle portions; however, the distal esophagus exhibits diffuse salmon-colored mucosa and an ulcerated mass, located 38 to 42 centimeters from the incisors, that encompasses two-thirds of the esophageal luminal circumference and extends into the gastric cardia. The remainder of the stomach and duodenum appear unremarkable. Biopsy of the mass yields adenocarcinoma, poorly differentiated, with negative staining for HER2. Endoscopic ultrasound demonstrates a distal hypoechoic GEJ mass penetrating through the muscularis propria into the surrounding adventitia, but not into surrounding structures; in addition, four round lymph nodes ranging from 1.0 to 1.4 centimeters in width are noted in the lower paraesophageal and perigastric regions. A PET/CT scan demonstrates soft-tissue thickening of the distal esophagus extending into the cardia with a maximum standardized uptake value (SUV) of 24.6, in addition to numerous avid paraesophageal and perigastric lymph nodes (Figure 39.1); no avid lesions are noted in the rest of the body. The patient is evaluated by a multidisciplinary team and based on staging exams, he is deemed to have a Siewert II GEJ cancer. Based on the location of the tumor, the options for this patient include treating him according to an esophageal paradigm with neoadjuvant CRT followed by surgery or according to a gastric cancer approach, which typically entails perioperative chemotherapy. Our institutional approach in Siewert II GEJ cancer is to offer a neoadjuvant approach with induction chemotherapy, CRT, and then planned surgical resection. As discussed earlier, for patients with PET-avid disease, based on the results now reported in abstract form from CALGB 80803 (29), we use induction FOLFOX. The benefit of initiating chemotherapy first is that there is generally significant improvement in patients' dysphagia, and patients who are able to eat tend to tolerate CRT better. After induction chemotherapy, we until recently switched to carboplatin and paclitaxel for CRT; however, with the recent update on survival outcomes, we now perform a PET scan if possible after the 2 months of chemotherapy to evaluate response, and we will then either continue with the 5-FU and oxaliplatin with RT for PET responders or switch to carboplatin and paclitaxel for nonresponders (Figure 39.2). We aim to deliver CRT to 50.4 Gy but consider lower doses (e.g., 41.4 Gy) in patients with compromised lung function. Patients undergo surgical resection at 6 to 8 weeks after completion of CRT. During treatment and prior to surgery, patients are offered to participate in a prehabilitation program including nutrition consultation and follow-up, implementation of protein supplements, intravenous fluids 2 to 3 times per week, distress screening, and a physical fitness program two times per week with the goal of maximizing fitness for surgery and reducing the risk of postoperative complications.

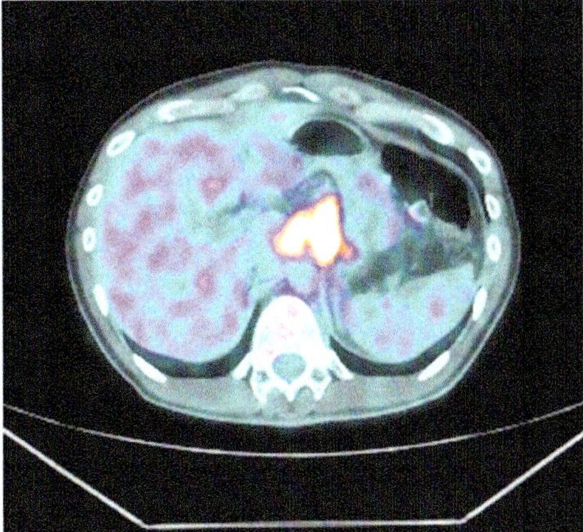

FIGURE 39.1   Representative axial slice of PET/CT depicting avidity associated with distal esophageal mass and adjacent paraesophageal lymph nodes.

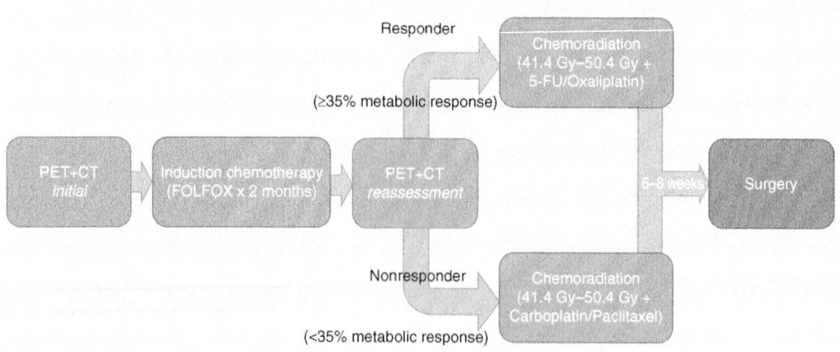

FIGURE 39.2   Treatment algorithm for PET-directed therapy in the neoadjuvant management of esophageal and GEJ cancer.

FOLFOX, 5-fluorouracil and oxaliplatin; GEJ, gastroesophageal junction.

REFERENCES

1   Herskovic A, Martz K, al Sarraf M, et al. Combined chemotherapy and radiotherapy compared with radiotherapy alone in patients with cancer of the esophagus. *N Engl J Med.* 1992;326(24):1593–1598. doi:10.1056/nejm199206113262403

2. Tepper J, Krasna MJ, Niedzwiecki D, et al. Phase III trial of trimodality therapy with cisplatin, fluorouracil, radiotherapy, and surgery compared with surgery alone for esophageal cancer: CALGB 9781. *J Clin Oncol.* 2008;26(7):1086–1092. doi:10.1200/jco.2007.12.9593

3. Shapiro J, van Lanschot JJB, Hulshof M, et al. Neoadjuvant chemoradiotherapy plus surgery versus surgery alone for oesophageal or junctional cancer (CROSS): long-term results of a randomised controlled trial. *Lancet Oncol.* 2015;16(9):1090–1098. doi:10.1016/s1470-2045(15)00040-6

4. van Hagen P, Hulshof MC, van Lanschot JJ, et al. Preoperative chemoradiotherapy for esophageal or junctional cancer. *N Engl J Med.* 2012;366(22):2074–2084. doi:10.1056/NEJMoa1112088

5. Oppedijk V, van der Gaast A, van Lanschot JJ, et al. Patterns of recurrence after surgery alone versus preoperative chemoradiotherapy and surgery in the CROSS trials. *J Clin Oncol.* 2014;32(5):385–391. doi:10.1200/jco.2013.51.2186

6. Noordman BJ, Verdam MGE, Lagarde SM, et al. Effect of neoadjuvant chemoradiotherapy on health-related quality of life in esophageal or junctional cancer: results from the randomized CROSS trial. *J Clin Oncol.* 2018;36(3):268–275. doi:10.1200/jco.2017.73.7718

7. Noordman BJ, Verdam MGE, Lagarde SM, et al. Impact of neoadjuvant chemoradiotherapy on health-related quality of life in long-term survivors of esophageal or junctional cancer: results from the randomized CROSS trial. *Ann Oncol.* 2018;29(2):445–451. doi:10.1093/annonc/mdx726

8. Kelsen DP, Ginsberg R, Pajak TF, et al. Chemotherapy followed by surgery compared with surgery alone for localized esophageal cancer. *N Engl J Med.* 1998;339(27):1979–1984. doi:10.1056/nejm199812313392704

9. MRC. Surgical resection with or without preoperative chemotherapy in oesophageal cancer: a randomised controlled trial. *Lancet.* 2002;359(9319):1727–1733. doi:10.1016/s0140-6736(02)08651-8

10. Sjoquist KM, Burmeister BH, Smithers BM, et al. Survival after neoadjuvant chemotherapy or chemoradiotherapy for resectable oesophageal carcinoma: an updated meta-analysis. *Lancet Oncol.* 2011;12(7):681–692. doi:10.1016/s1470-2045(11)70142-5

11. Stahl M, Walz MK, Riera-Knorrenschild J, et al. Preoperative chemotherapy versus chemoradiotherapy in locally advanced adenocarcinomas of the oesophagogastric junction (POET): long-term results of a controlled randomised trial. *Eur J Cancer.* 2017;81:183–190. doi:10.1016/j.ejca.2017.04.027

12. Leichman LP, Goldman BH, Bohanes PO, et al. S0356: a phase II clinical and prospective molecular trial with oxaliplatin, fluorouracil, and external-beam radiation therapy before surgery for patients with esophageal adenocarcinoma. *J Clin Oncol.* 2011;29(34):4555–4560. doi:10.1200/jco.2011.36.7490

13. Ajani JA, D'Amico TA, Baggstrom M, et al. NCCN Esophageal Cancer Guidelines (Version 2.2018); 2018. https://www.nccn.org/professionals/physician_gls/pdf/esophageal.pdf

14. Mukherjee S, Hurt CN, Gwynne S, et al. NEOSCOPE: a randomised phase II study of induction chemotherapy followed by oxaliplatin/capecitabine or carboplatin/paclitaxel based pre-operative chemoradiation for resectable oesophageal adenocarcinoma. *Eur J Cancer*. 2017;74:38–46. doi:10.1016/j.ejca.2016.11.031

15. Ajani JA, Xiao L, Roth JA, et al. A phase II randomized trial of induction chemotherapy versus no induction chemotherapy followed by preoperative chemoradiation in patients with esophageal cancer. *Ann Oncol*. 2013;24(11):2844–2849. doi:10.1093/annonc/mdt339

16. Henry LR, Goldberg M, Scott W, et al. Induction cisplatin and paclitaxel followed by combination chemoradiotherapy with 5-fluorouracil, cisplatin, and paclitaxel before resection in localized esophageal cancer: a phase II report. *Ann Surg Oncol*. 2006;13(2):214–220. doi:10.1245/aso.2006.01.001

17. Ilson DH, Minsky BD, Ku GY, et al. Phase 2 trial of induction and concurrent chemoradiotherapy with weekly irinotecan and cisplatin followed by surgery for esophageal cancer. *Cancer*. 2012;118(11):2820–2827. doi:10.1002/cncr.26591

18. Rivera F, Galan M, Tabernero J, et al. Phase II trial of preoperative irinotecan-cisplatin followed by concurrent irinotecan-cisplatin and radiotherapy for resectable locally advanced gastric and esophagogastric junction adenocarcinoma. *Int J Radiat Oncol Biol Phys*. 2009;75(5):1430–1436. doi:10.1016/j.ijrobp.2008.12.087

19. Ruhstaller T, Widmer L, Schuller JC, et al. Multicenter phase II trial of preoperative induction chemotherapy followed by chemoradiation with docetaxel and cisplatin for locally advanced esophageal carcinoma (SAKK 75/02). *Ann Oncol*. 2009;20(9):1522–1528. doi:10.1093/annonc/mdp045

20. Downey RJ, Akhurst T, Ilson D, et al. Whole body 18FDG-PET and the response of esophageal cancer to induction therapy: results of a prospective trial. *J Clin Oncol*. 2003;21(3):428–432. doi:10.1200/jco.2003.04.013

21. Duong CP, Hicks RJ, Weih L, et al. FDG-PET status following chemoradiotherapy provides high management impact and powerful prognostic stratification in oesophageal cancer. *Eur J Nucl Med Mol Imaging*. 2006;33(7):770–778. doi:10.1007/s00259-005-0040-z

22. Flamen P, Van Cutsem E, Lerut A, et al. Positron emission tomography for assessment of the response to induction radiochemotherapy in locally advanced oesophageal cancer. *Ann Oncol*. 2002;13(3):361–368.

23. Wieder HA, Brucher BL, Zimmermann F, et al. Time course of tumor metabolic activity during chemoradiotherapy of esophageal squamous cell carcinoma and response to treatment. *J Clin Oncol*. 2004;22(5):900–908. doi:10.1200/jco.2004.07.122

24. Ott K, Weber WA, Lordick F, et al. Metabolic imaging predicts response, survival, and recurrence in adenocarcinomas of the esophagogastric junction. *J Clin Oncol*. 2006;24(29):4692–4698. doi:10.1200/jco.2006.06.7801

25. Weber WA, Ott K, Becker K, et al. Prediction of response to preoperative chemotherapy in adenocarcinomas of the esophagogastric junction by metabolic imaging. *J Clin Oncol*. 2001;19(12):3058–3065. doi:10.1200/jco.2001.19.12.3058

26. Lordick F, Ott K, Krause BJ, et al. PET to assess early metabolic response and to guide treatment of adenocarcinoma of the oesophagogastric junction: the MUNICON phase II trial. *Lancet Oncol*. 2007;8(9):797–805. doi:10.1016/s1470-2045(07)70244-9

27. zum Buschenfelde CM, Herrmann K, Schuster T, et al. (18)F-FDG PET-guided salvage neoadjuvant radiochemotherapy of adenocarcinoma of the esophagogastric junction: the MUNICON II trial. *J Nucl Med*. 2011;52(8):1189–1196. doi:10.2967/jnumed.110.085803

28. Goodman KA, Niedzwiecki D, Hall N, et al. Initial results of CALGB 80803 (Alliance): a randomized phase II trial of PET scan-directed combined modality therapy for esophageal cancer. *J Clin Oncol*. 2017;35(4_suppl):1. doi:10.1200/jco.2017.35.4_suppl.1

29. Goodman KA, Hall N, Bekaii-Saab TS, et al. Survival outcomes from CALGB 80803 (Alliance): a randomized phase II trial of PET scan-directed combined modality therapy for esophageal cancer. *J Clin Oncol*. 2018;36(15_suppl):4012. doi:10.1200/jco.2018.36.15_suppl.4012

30. Ku GY, Kriplani A, Janjigian YY, et al. Change in chemotherapy during concurrent radiation followed by surgery after a suboptimal positron emission tomography response to induction chemotherapy improves outcomes for locally advanced esophageal adenocarcinoma. *Cancer*. 2016;122(13):2083–2090. doi:10.1002/cncr.30028

31. Cunningham D, Allum WH, Stenning SP, et al. Perioperative chemotherapy versus surgery alone for resectable gastroesophageal cancer. *N Engl J Med*. 2006;355(1):11–20. doi:10.1056/NEJMoa055531

32. Fuchs CS, Niedzwiecki D, Mamon HJ, et al. Adjuvant chemoradiotherapy with epirubicin, cisplatin, and fluorouracil compared with adjuvant chemoradiotherapy with fluorouracil and leucovorin after curative resection of gastric cancer: results from CALGB 80101 (Alliance). *J Clin Oncol*. 2017;35(32):3671–3677. doi:10.1200/jco.2017.74.2130

33. Smalley SR, Benedetti JK, Haller DG, et al. Updated analysis of SWOG-directed intergroup study 0116: a phase III trial of adjuvant radiochemotherapy versus observation after curative gastric cancer resection. *J Clin Oncol*. 2012;30(19):2327–2333. doi:10.1200/jco.2011.36.7136
34. Park SH, Sohn TS, Lee J, et al. Phase III trial to compare adjuvant chemotherapy with capecitabine and cisplatin versus concurrent chemoradiotherapy in gastric cancer: final report of the adjuvant chemoradiotherapy in stomach tumors trial, including survival and subset analyses. *J Clin Oncol*. 2015;33(28):3130–3136. doi:10.1200/jco.2014.58.3930

How I Treat Early-Stage Gastric and Esophageal Cancer With Surgery

Sajid A. Khan, Vadim Kurbatov, and Mitchell C. Posner

ESOPHAGEAL CANCER

Esophageal cancer is a global health problem accounting for 310,440 cases yearly and is the sixth most common cause for cancer deaths globally. In the United States, it will be diagnosed in 17,650 Americans in 2019, with 16,080 expected deaths from the disease. Only 18.8% of patients are alive 5 years after diagnosis (1). More than 60% of cases have an adenocarcinoma histology, most commonly arising in the distal esophagus. Common risk factors include Barrett's esophagus, obesity, and gastroesophageal reflux disease, and less common risk factors are achalasia, caustic injury, diverticula, esophageal web, and tylosis. Squamous cell carcinoma (SCC) accounts for a majority of the remaining cases, typically arising in the proximal and mid esophagus. These tumors are strongly associated with tobacco and alcohol use. While human papillomavirus (HPV) may be associated with SCC in high incidence areas in Asia and South Africa, there is growing evidence against the association between HPV and progression of Barrett's esophagus to adenocarcinoma (2,3).

Given the complexity of this disease, it is imperative that a new diagnosis of esophageal cancer prompt discussion between members of an experienced multidisciplinary team regarding the optimal coordinated treatment plan before deciding on a curative or palliative approach. Early cases are often diagnosed by surveillance endoscopy, most commonly for Barrett's esophagus. A careful clinical workup begins with a thorough history and physical, including assessment for symptoms of local invasion, which would preclude esophagectomy. Key symptoms to elicit are the presence of progressive dysphagia, weight loss, odynophagia, anorexia, and retrosternal pain. Symptoms of local invasion into the recurrent laryngeal nerve or paratracheal node involvement should be sought after and these include stridor, hoarse voice, and coughing. A history of aspiration pneumonia may suggest tracheoesophageal fistula. Finally, one should be aware of a high risk for second primary cancers of the head, neck, and lung. A patient's performance and nutritional status must be carefully judged, as the physiologic stress of esophagectomy is not trivial.

Clinical staging should include an esophagogastroduodenoscopy (EGD) to make a diagnosis, assess tumor epicenter, proximal and distal tumor extent relative to incisors, presence of concomitant Barrett's or dysplasia proximal to the tumor, extension into stomach, and degree of obstruction. The eight edition of the American Joint Committee on Cancer (AJCC) Staging Manual has moved away from Siewert classification for esophagogastric junction (EGJ) cancer staging. Instead, tumors with their epicenter located >2 cm away from the EGJ onto the proximal stomach are staged as gastric cancer. Cardia cancers not involving the EGJ are staged as stomach cancers. Tumors with their epicenter <2 cm from the EGJ onto the proximal stomach are staged as esophageal cancer (4). An endoscopic ultrasound (EUS) is required to determine the depth of invasion (T stage) and nodal status (N stage). We routinely obtain a CT chest/abdomen/pelvis with and without intravenous (IV) contrast and a PET–CT (5). For EGJ tumors, we frequently perform a staging laparoscopy with peritoneal washings since the presence of positive peritoneal cytology equates to M1 disease and is a relative contraindication to resection. Pulmonary function studies are useful in the assessment of a patient's ability to tolerate a major resection. If suspicion for airway invasion exists, an endobronchial ultrasound is indicated.

Patients with high-grade dysplasia and those with tumors limited to the mucosa (T1a) are best treated with endoscopic mucosal resection (EMR) and radiofrequency ablation (RFA)

Two Clinical Vignettes ("How I Treat") are included in the chapter.

because they have an exceedingly low risk for lymph node metastasis (6). In retrospective analyses, the rates of lymph node metastasis in patients with T1a SCC and adenocarcinoma were found to be 0% to 3% and 0% to 2%, respectively (7–10). These tumors may be treated with acceptable oncologic outcomes with EMR, potentially sparing patients from the morbidity and mortality of an esophagectomy. To this end, Ell et al. reported prospective outcomes from 100 consecutive patients treated with EMR for favorable T1a esophageal adenocarcinoma, showing a 5-year survival rate of 95% (11). T1b tumors that demonstrate favorable characteristics (well differentiated without lymphovascular invasion) can undergo endoscopic submucosal dissection (ESD) as the initial staging and therapeutic intervention. Lesions limited to the first submucosal layer (sm1) have been reported to have excellent outcomes, though the standard of care for these patients remains surgical resection in those with a good performance status (12). In general, tumors with invasion beyond the mucosa (≥T1b) without evidence of distant metastases require a more aggressive multimodal approach.

Patients with node-positive disease or tumors that are T2 or greater potentially benefit from neoadjuvant therapy, which can downstage disease, eradicate occult micrometastases, and increase the rate of resection with negative circumferential margins (R0 resection). Preoperative therapy can be administered as preoperative chemoradiotherapy (carboplatin and paclitaxel, 41.4 Gy) as supported by the Netherlands CROSS trial or as perioperative chemotherapy, most recently supported by the FLOT4-AIO trial (13,14). The CROSS trial demonstrated that addition of neoadjuvant therapy improved median overall survival (OS) from 24 to 48.6 months. Some equipoise remains, stemming from a randomized clinical trial (RCT) of 195 patients with early esophageal adenocarcinoma by Mariette et al., in which patients had excellent rates of R0 resection and similar survival outcomes irrespective of randomization (15). Burmeister et al. performed a 256-patient RCT, randomizing patients to surgery alone versus neoadjuvant chemoradiation followed by resection, and also found no survival benefit, but did note a 21% higher rate of R0 resection in the arm treated with neoadjuvant chemoradiation (16).

Tumor histology is an important consideration since the management of SCC and adenocarcinoma differs, though the prognosis is similar. Cervical or mid-esophageal cancers, which are primarily of squamous cell histology, are particularly radiosensitive and can be treated nonsurgically with definitive chemoradiotherapy. This results in lower rates of morbidity and mortality, potential for laryngeal preservation, and good rates of locoregional and distant control with comparable OS. Salvage surgery can be reserved for nonresponders to therapy (17).

After completion of neoadjuvant therapy, patients are restaged with a CT chest/abdomen/pelvis and PET–CT, and if there is no evidence of progression of disease, we plan for an esophagectomy. The choice of surgical approach, transthoracic versus transhiatal esophagectomy, continues to be debated with the aim to optimize cancer outcomes with minimal surgical morbidity and mortality. The transhiatal approach resects esophageal lesions through abdominal and cervical incisions, sparing formal thoracotomy that can lead to substantial pain and subsequent pulmonary complications and avoidance of an intrathoracic anastomotic leak, with progression to mediastinitis. The literature suggests oncologic equivalence of both approaches, with the transhiatal approach benefiting from a more favorable side-effect profile. Orringer et al. report on the largest single-institution experience of 1,525 patients treated with the transhiatal approach, finding overall 5-year survival to be 29%, with significantly improved stage-specific 5-year survival of 65% for stage I disease. Their results highlight the manageable nature of the most common surgical complications associated with the approach. Anastomotic leak (12%) was managed with cervical wound opening, turning the leak into a controlled fistula. Recurrent laryngeal nerve neurapraxia or injury (4.5%) was transient in 99% of cases (18).

Meta-analysis of studies to 1999, including data from three RCTs, suggests the transthoracic approach has a different distribution of operative complications, associated with higher intraoperative blood loss, higher risk of postoperative pulmonary complications, chyle leak, and wound infection (19–21). The impact of these complications on cancer-specific and mortality outcomes was minimal. The equivalence in long-term outcomes was confirmed by a study by Hulscher et al., which prospectively randomized 220 patients not undergoing chemotherapy or radiation therapy to either transhiatal esophagectomy or transthoracic esophagectomy with two-field lymph node dissection, and found 5-year survival of 34% and 36%, respectively (22). A 2008 review of Surveillance, Epidemiology, and End Results (SEER) data reached a similar conclusion, identifying an early survival benefit to transhiatal approach, which did not translate to improved 5-year survival (23). A 2011 meta-analysis of 5,905 patients similarly found patients undergoing a transthoracic approach to have a significantly higher 30-day mortality and higher rate of pulmonary complications.

We strongly believe that a surgeon should perform the operation via the surgical approach he or she is most comfortable with. We prefer the transhiatal approach as follows. After laparoscopy to rule out distant metastases, we proceed with a transhiatal esophagectomy through an upper midline incision. The right gastroepiploic pedicle is identified and carefully preserved throughout the operation. The short gastric arteries are divided, left gastric artery is ligated and divided, lesser omentum divided, wide Kocher maneuver performed, and a longitudinal pyloromyotomy performed to reduce gastric stasis in the future gastric conduit (24,25). We divide the phrenoesophageal membrane to provide wide exposure to the lower mediastinum to facilitate lymph node clearance and margin clearance. We place a needle jejunostomy catheter to complete the intra-abdominal portion of the surgery. We make a cervical incision along the anterior border of the sternocleidomastoid muscle, divide platysma and omohyoid muscle, and circumferentially come around the cervical esophagus, preserving the recurrent laryngeal nerve. The upper mediastinal dissection is completed by blunt dissection via the abdominal and cervical incisions. The cervical esophagus is divided and thoracic esophagus is delivered through the posterior mediastinum into the peritoneal cavity. A gastric tube is formed with multiple fires of a linear stapling device and after confirmation of negative surgical margins, we commence with the reconstruction (26). We perform an end-to-side cervical esophagogastrostomy with an EEA stapler. The cervical and abdominal incisions are approximated in layers in standard fashion.

Particular consideration needs to be paid to adequate lymph node dissection to achieve an appropriate oncologic resection. Options include a standard or extended (en bloc) approach. As per AJCC eight edition guidelines, we resect at least 15 lymph nodes to achieve adequate nodal staging (4). This practice is supported by data in patients who have not undergone neoadjuvant therapy, but data in patients who have undergone neoadjuvant therapy are lacking. More aggressive en bloc resection and nodal dissection has been evaluated in an attempt to achieve more durable disease-free and overall survival. Altorki et al. reviewed outcomes for 128 patients undergoing esophagectomy, 61% of which received extended lymphadenectomy. The groups had similar in-hospital mortality and major complication rates. Four-year survival was significantly improved in the extended resection group (27). However, given the retrospective and single-institutional nature of the study, this may be attributable to selection bias and stage migration. Lagergren et al. published recent prospective data from 606 patients and found no statistically significant association between extended lymphadenectomy and all-cause or disease-specific mortality (28).

Alternatively, a minimally invasive approach can be employed, with evidence suggesting no compromise in oncologic outcome. Luketich et al. report their experience at Pittsburgh with 1,011 patients treated with either three-incision minimally invasive esophagectomy (MIE) or Ivor Lewis MIE. The procedure was associated with a low median ICU stay of 2 days, low 30-day perioperative mortality of 1.7%, and high R0 resection rate of 98%. However, long-term follow-up data for this cohort are not available. The same group's outcomes for 80 consecutive patients treated with MIE for T1 lesions showed 5-year OS to be 62% and 3-year disease-free survival (DFS) to be 80% (29). Biere et al. performed the first, multicenter, randomized controlled trial, randomizing 56 patients to MIEs versus open esophagectomy. The MIE approach resulted in a short-term benefit of less postoperative pulmonary infections (30). The TIME multicenter RCT of 115 patients randomized to MIEs versus open esophagectomy found MIEs to be associated with a reduction in pulmonary complications and length of stay. Updated publication of 3-year follow up data suggests no differences in disease-free and overall 3-year survival for open and MI esophagectomy (31). Takeuchi et al. used the National Clinical Database (NCD) in Japan to retrospectively compare outcomes of 5,354 patients treated with MIE or open esophagectomy. They too found significantly longer operative time and less blood loss associated with the MIE approach. Additionally, MIE had a higher rate of anastomotic leakage and need for reoperation within 30 days. The study did not assess long-term outcomes for the procedure (32).

In order to further optimize outcomes, we recommend and implement several strategies. Risk reduction programs include cessation programs for drinking and smoking. Furthermore, we recommend that individuals seek out and are referred to high-volume facilities, as several lines of evidence support improved patient outcomes in the hands of high-volume surgeon specialists and centers of excellence. Reviewing Medicare data in 2003, Birkmeyer concluded that hospital volume and operative mortality are largely mediated by surgeon volume for complex cases and patients can improve their chances of survival substantially by selecting surgeons who perform the operations frequently. The survival difference was not trivial. Patients operated by a surgeon performing 2 esophagectomies a year at an institution performing less than 5 had an adjusted operative mortality of 21.7%, significantly higher than 8% in patients operated by surgeons performing >6 procedures yearly at a hospital with a yearly volume of >13 cases (33). Further rationale for centralizing the operation to high-volume surgeons was noted by Bilimoria et al., showing 5-year OS to be 30.4% and 20.7% for high- and low-volume surgeons, respectively (34).

Patients typically spend 2 days in the ICU with careful monitoring of hemodynamics. Jejunal tube feeds are started on postoperative day 1 and advanced toward the goal (35). After audible return of bowel function, we commence with a clear liquid diet, often between postoperative days 5 and 7, and as this is tolerated, then a postgastrectomy diet.

There are several postoperative complications that may occur. Careful examination for the cervical incision each day is important to monitor for an anastomotic leak at the esophagogastrostomy. If there is crepitance or erythema, the cervical incision should be opened since this heralds an anastomotic dehiscence. Local wound care is all that is necessary and will result in eventual healing in 100% of patients albeit with a higher incidence of stricture. Chylothorax is rare but if it does occur, it can be addressed by drainage and interventional duct embolization or an early minimally invasive surgery (MIS) thoracotomy with thoracic duct clips. Complications such as pneumonia and venous thromboembolism can be reduced by early ambulation and chemical prophylaxis. Long-term complications include anastomotic stricture, which requires upper endoscopic dilation (36). Postvagotomy diarrhea can be minimized by strict adherence to a postgastrectomy diet. Generally speaking, patients experience a very good quality of life postresection (37).

Clinical Vignette 40.1

Here, we discuss the details of surgical management of an otherwise healthy 51-year-old male with complaints of worsening dysphagia, odynophagia, epigastric pain, and 30 lb weight loss. He had a 25 pack-year history of cigarette smoking and alcohol intake for the past 15 years. This worrisome presentation prompted EGD, which showed an EGJ mass 36 to 39 cm from the incisors and biopsy proven invasive moderately to poorly differentiated adenocarcinoma (Figure 40.1). Staging EUS was performed, demonstrating a T3N1 lesion with abnormal distal paraesophageal and celiac lymph nodes. Staging laparoscopy with peritoneal washings was negative and neoadjuvant chemoradiation was initiated. Restaging with PET–CT and EGD revealed no progression of disease (Figure 40.2). He then underwent a transhiatal esophagectomy with gastric conduit, pyloromyotomy, and feeding jejunostomy. He was discharged on POD#7 after an unremarkable course and surgical pathology revealed ypT0N0 disease, with all 31 lymph nodes sampled negative for carcinoma and one node demonstrating histiocyte reaction consistent with treatment effect. He did not receive postoperative chemotherapy.

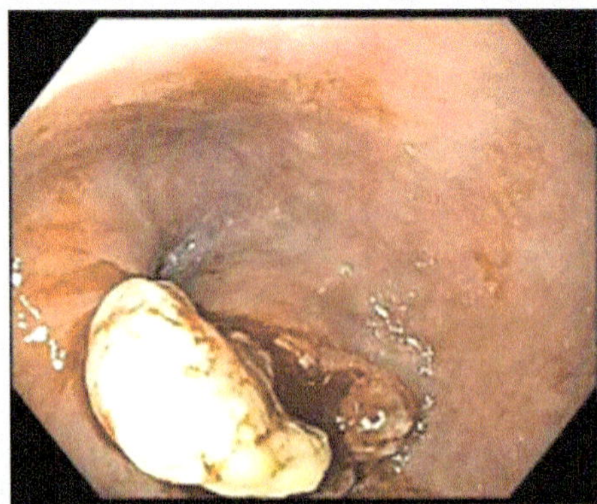

FIGURE 40.1   EGD showed erythematous ulcerated mass involving the gastroesophageal junction.

EGD, esophagogastroduodenoscopy.

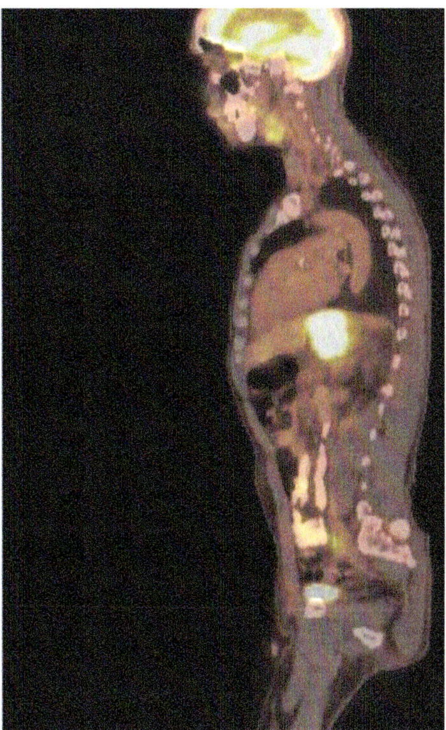

FIGURE 40.2   PET–CT showed no evidence of disease progression after neoadjuvant chemoradiation.

GASTRIC CANCER

Gastric cancer is estimated to be diagnosed in 27,510 Americans in 2019, accounting for 1.7% of all new cancer cases and 11,140 deaths (1). Overall, it has a better prognosis compared to esophageal cancer, with a 5-year OS of 31% (38). Despite an overall decreasing incidence over the past 40 years from 11.67 to 6.49 per 100,000 patients, in part due to changes in food preparation, diet, and the environment, there has been a steady rise in the incidence of tumors located in the cardia and gastroesophageal junction from 0.7 to 3.2 patients per 100,000, from 1976 to 1994 (38,39). The majority of gastric tumors are of adenocarcinoma histology, and the remainder of this chapter focuses on this variant.

Optimal cancer-related and surgical outcomes are predicated on the multidisciplinary team approach and it is imperative that an oncologic workup be complete prior to embarking on a treatment pathway. We routinely perform an EGD/EUS to obtain tissue confirmation and assess T stage including multivisceral extension and N stage. To confirm there is no evidence of distant metastases, CT of the abdomen and pelvis with and without IV contrast and CT chest without IV contrast are obtained. To complete the clinical staging workup, the patient should undergo a staging laparoscopy for $\geq$T2, or Nany tumors.

Optimal cancer treatment is initially based on T stage identified on EUS. For well-differentiated tumors that invade into lamina propria or muscularis mucosae (cT1a) and that are $\leq$2 cm in diameter, an EMR is performed with comparable 10-year OS and shorter hospital length of stays to gastrectomies (38,40). ESD is a technique that is increasingly being performed, primarily in Asia, for select patients with small early gastric cancers (41). This technique has the advantage of achieving en bloc resection of early lesions >2 cm in size, which is difficult to accomplish with EMR. Chung et al. describe their experience treating 1,000 patients with ESD, demonstrating complete en bloc resection was achieved in 87% of patients, and other groups have reported similar long-term survival to patients undergoing gastrectomy for early-stage gastric cancers (42).

Patients without distant metastases who have node-positive cancer (cN+) and/or invasion into or beyond the muscularis propria (cT2–4) should undergo a perioperative chemotherapy approach as this multimodality approach improves survival as demonstrated in the MAGIC and FLOT4-AIO randomized trials (14,43). If upfront gastrectomy is pursued, adjuvant chemoradiation can be administered based on data from several landmark studies. The Intergroup-116 trial, which randomized patients to R0 resection with and without adjuvant chemoradiotherapy, demonstrated relapse-free and OS benefit on long-term follow-up (44). The more recent CALGB 80101 trial demonstrated that adjuvant radiation after gastrectomy can be administered concurrently with FU-LV or ECF with similar 5-year OS (45). The ARTIST trial randomized 458 patients treated with curative resection and D2 lymphadenectomy to receiving adjuvant chemotherapy with capecitabine and cisplatin or adjuvant radiotherapy with capecitabine. The addition of radiation did not improve DFS with the exception of the subgroup with lymph node positive disease (46). The ARTIST II trial that is actively accruing patients is powered to determine if the addition of radiotherapy improves DFS in node-positive patients. Finally, the CLASSIC trial from investigators in South Korea have shown postoperative chemotherapy with capecitabine and oxaliplatin after D2 gastrectomy for stage II and III cancers improves 5-year OS from 69% to 78% compared to no adjuvant therapy (47).

We perform a D2 lymphadenectomy with en bloc with resection of the primary tumor as follows. For distal gastrectomy, we dissect station 4 and 6 perigastric lymph nodes along the greater curve and for total gastrectomy station 2 lymph nodes are taken with the primary tumor. All of the soft tissue along stations 1, 3, and 5 along the lesser curve is resected en bloc with the gastrectomy to complete resection of perigastric nodes. This dissection would complete a D1 lymphadenectomy; however, we prefer a D2 lymphadenectomy for the reasons described earlier. The soft tissue overlying the left gastric vein and artery is resected to address the station 7 nodes, followed by mobilization of the soft tissue at station 8 (hepatic artery), station 9 (celiac axis), and the splenic artery (station 11 lymph nodes). For tumors not involving the splenic hilum and which do not require a splenectomy, the station 10 lymph nodes are preserved.

Rate of lymph node metastasis in early gastric cancer was evaluated by Gotada et al. in a series of 5,265 patients with well-differentiated, nonulcerated tumors <3 cm. After treatment gastrectomy and lymph node dissection, none of the 1,230 patients with well-differentiated intramucosal tumors <3 cm were found to have lymph node metastases. However, the rate of nodal metastasis markedly grew with submucosal invasion and increasing tumor size (48). The incidence of lymph node metastasis in early gastric cancer is well illustrated by a study of a 1,577-patient U.S. cohort, revealing lymph node metastases existed in 60% of T2 lesions after R0 resections (49).

The extent of lymph node dissection has been one of the major areas of controversy in surgical oncology, particularly since current AJCC nodal staging requires ≥16 nodes be examined for presence of locoregional disease. The arguments in support of a more extensive lymphadenectomy are improved staging, improved OS, and prevention of locoregional recurrence. An RCT by Wu et al. demonstrated improved survival with a D3 lymphadenectomy compared to D1 lymphadenectomy (50). However, the debate regarding D2 over D1 lymphadenectomy is dominated by prospective data from the Dutch and MRC studies (51,52). Each study randomized patients to D2 versus D1 lymphadenectomy, with splenectomy and distal pancreatectomy routinely performed in the D2 dissection group. These studies concluded that the addition of a D2 lymphadenectomy did not equate to a better OS. Further, the more aggressive lymphadenectomy had the unintended consequence of increasing perioperative morbidity and mortality, in retrospect, believed to be due to concomitant pancreatectomy and splenectomy with a D2 dissection. However, 15-year follow-up of the Dutch trial demonstrated that D2 lymphadenectomy is associated with lower locoregional recurrence and less gastric cancer specific deaths than D1 lymphadenectomy (52). Several retrospective studies have concluded that more extensive lymphadenectomy equates to improved survival; however, stage migration from a more extensive lymphadenectomy makes it difficult to draw definitive conclusions from these studies. This includes the German Gastric Carcinoma Study Group of 1,654 patients showing that patients who underwent a D2 lymphadenectomy with retrieval of >25 lymph nodes had an improved survival rate compared to patients who had a standard lymph node dissection (6). On the other hand, several studies including an RCT from the Japanese Clinical Oncology Group-9501 (D2 vs. D2 plus para-aortic node dissection) have shown that performing a lymphadenectomy more aggressive than a D2 dissection does not appear to result in improved long-term survival (53–55).

A D2 lymphadenectomy should be spleen and pancreas sparing unless there is direct tumor involvement of these structures, which requires a distal pancreatectomy or splenectomy. The Italian Gastric Cancer Study Group RCT trial of 162 patients randomized D1 and D2 pancreas sparing lymphadenectomies showing no increased morbidity or mortality in the D2 group, with measures of technical and clinical success comparable to those reported in Japan (56). Further, subset analysis of the D2 group revealed improved disease-specific survival with node-positive disease or advanced T stage. This evidence drives our practice of performing a spleen and pancreas sparing D2 lymphadenectomy for staging and locoregional control when performing gastrectomy for early gastric cancer. However, if there is direct tumor involvement of the pancreas and spleen, one must be prepared for an en bloc multivisceral resection.

Multiple groups have evaluated the use of sentinel lymph node (SLN) biopsy using indocyanine green. Hiratsuka et al. concluded that SLN status can predict the lymph node involvement with a high degree of accuracy, with 100% sensitivity in 44 patients with T1 disease (57). However, a recent Japanese pilot study evaluating accuracy of SLN biopsy in T1 disease was stopped early due to a 46% rate of false-negative nodal status (58). Based on current evidence, we do not see SLN biopsy as an alternative to D2 lymphadenectomy.

Distal tumors are treated with a distal subtotal gastrectomy with the general principle to preserve stomach if it can be without compromising proximal margins of 5 cm. The oncologic equivalence of this approach was addressed by several European prospective RCTs comparing total gastrectomy to subtotal gastrectomy for distal gastric cancer. Each of these studies revealed a similar OS with equivalent surgical morbidity and mortality, thus supporting our approach of subtotal gastrectomy for distal-based tumors (59–61). If an adequate margin cannot be achieved or for tumors with a more proximal location, we perform a total gastrectomy. In rare circumstances such as in the very elderly or in those patients with substantial comorbid conditions that would preclude a total gastrectomy, we do consider a proximal subtotal gastrectomy and have not found the described complications of bile reflux to be a substantial issue.

The reconstruction option that we use for distal gastrectomy is a hand-sewn retrocolic Roux-en-Y retrocolic end-to-side gastrojejunostomy. A 2018 RCT, randomizing 162 patients to receive Billroth II (BII) or Roux-en-Y gastrojejunostomy (RYGJ) reconstruction after distal subtotal gastrectomy showed similar survival after 1-year follow-up, with similar quality-of-life measures (62). Long-term evidence showing superiority of one reconstruction option is lacking at this time. For total gastrectomy, we perform a retrocolic, end-to-side Roux-en-Y esophagojejunostomy with a stapled anastomosis with a 25 mm circular stapler. All patients who undergo total gastrectomy receive a concomitant needle catheter feeding jejunostomy. We do not perform a jejunal pouch reconstruction although Fein et al. showed improved quality of life for Roux-en-Y pouch reconstruction at 3-, 4-, and 5-year time points in 138 patients randomized for Roux-en-Y reconstruction with or without a pouch, and recommended a pouch for patients with a good prognosis (63). Recent meta-analysis reports that pouch formation is safe and portends improved quality of life through reduction of dumping syndrome and heartburn (64–66).

Radical gastrectomy can be performed through a traditional open upper midline incision. or with a minimally invasive approach as long as oncologic principles are not compromised. Long-term outcomes from a small RCT randomizing patients to laparoscopic versus open subtotal gastrectomy for distal gastric cancer provided early evidence for this practice. After 5 years of follow-up, overall morbidity and mortality were equivalent while 5-year OS and DFS did not differ. The authors concluded that laparoscopic subtotal gastrectomy is feasible and has similar short- and long-term outcomes as open surgery (67). Investigators from South Korea demonstrated in a large-scale case–control and case-matched study that a laparoscopic approach could provide equivalent oncologic outcomes with less postoperative opiate use and slightly shorter length of stay (68). They analyzed 2,976 patients treated with either laparoscopic or open gastrectomy and with a median follow-up of 70.8 months; there was no difference in survival, with the exception that for stage IA gastric cancer, laparoscopic gastrectomy had improved survival (95.3% 5-year survival) versus open gastrectomy (90.3% 5 year survival; $p < .001$), suggesting a rationale for utility particularly in cases of early gastric cancer. Recently, preliminary results from a large prospective RCT have been reported.

The KLASS-01 study prospectively randomized 1,416 patients with clinical stage I cancer to laparoscopic distal gastrectomy (n = 705) or open gastrectomy (n = 711), reporting equivalent lymph node retrieval and a lower wound complication rate in the laparoscopic group though major abdominal complications and perioperative mortality were the same. Five-year outcomes for the KLASS-01 study, and outcomes from JCOG0912, which randomizes 920 patients with early gastric cancer (stage IA or IB) to laparoscopic or open distal gastrectomy, will provide more conclusive evidence for noninferiority of the methodology and potentially validate currently noted advantages of the MIS gastrectomy (69–71). Robotically assisted laparoscopic gastrectomy has also been described, and in our experience there is not a clear advantage to this approach with the exception of better exposure during the D2 lymphadenectomy. Each surgeon should utilize the approach he or she is most comfortable with and which provides superior oncologic outcomes. Robotic surgery offers a potential advantage of more degrees of freedom of instrument and tremor filtration. Short-term outcomes suggest comparable morbidity and adequate lymphadenectomy. On the other hand, long-term outcomes data have demonstrated comparable 5-year survival outcomes between patients undergoing laparoscopic and open gastrectomy (72–74).

Routine postoperative care begins with early mobilization and pulmonary toilet the evening of surgery, patient-controlled anesthesia, and maintenance IV fluids. If a jejunostomy tube was placed, tube feeds are initiated within 24 hours of completion of surgery. Routine gastrografin swallow studies are not indicated and only utilized when suspicion for a leak exists, and we often perform a CT with enteral contrast to rule out problems other than a leak if clinical suspicion exists. Ice chips and hard candy are initiated on postoperative day 1, sips of water are initiated on postoperative day 2, and after audible return of bowel function a clear liquid diet is initiated followed by a postgastrectomy diet consisting of six small meals daily.

Clinical Vignette 40.2

We discuss the case of a 76-year-old man who presented with anemia and upper endoscopy, revealing a 6 cm fungating mass in the angularis, which was a biopsy confirmed moderately differentiated adenocarcinoma of intestinal type (Figure 40.3). EUS documented uT3N1 disease and CT chest/abdomen/pelvis did not reveal distant metastases (Figure 40.4). Staging laparoscopy with washings was performed, showing no evidence of occult metastasis. He completed four cycles of neoadjuvant chemotherapy (docetaxel, oxaliplatin, fluorouracil) with no evidence of disease progression on CT chest/abdomen/pelvis. We proceeded with distal subtotal gastrectomy and D2 lymphadenectomy.

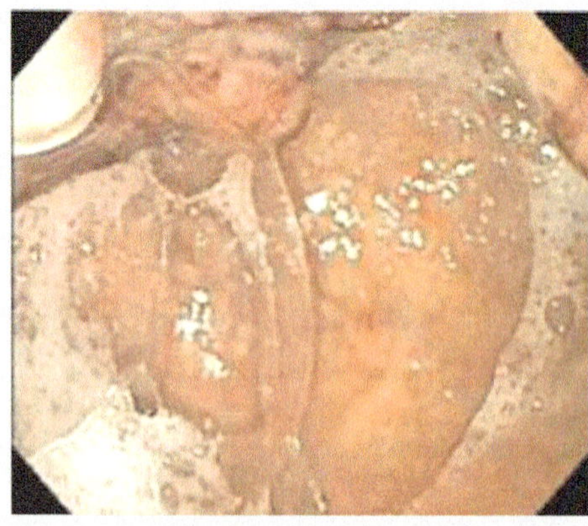

FIGURE 40.3   3 × 3 cm friable fungating mass in the angularis seen on endoscopy.

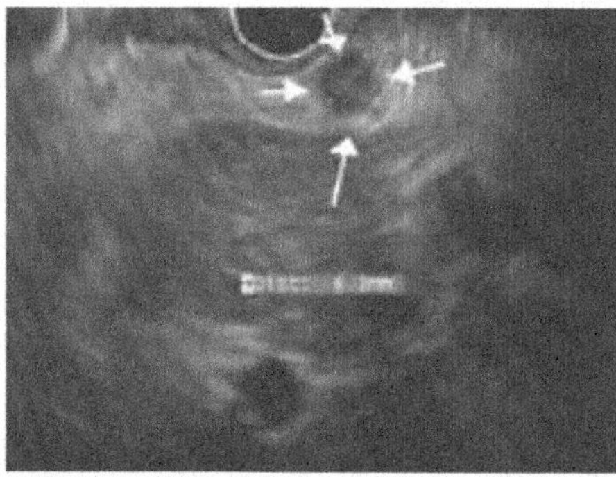

FIGURE 40.4　Abnormal lymph node on EUS upstaged to T3N1 disease.

EUS, endoscopic ultrasound.

REFERENCES

1. Siegel RL, Miller KD, Jemal A. Cancer statistics, 2019. *CA Cancer J Clin.* 2019;69(1):7–34. doi:10.3322/caac.21551
2. El-Serag HB, Hollier JM, Gravitt P, et al. Human papillomavirus and the risk of Barrett's esophagus. *Dis Esophagus.* 2013;26(5):517–521. doi:10.1111/j.1442-2050.2012.01392.x
3. Iyer A, Rajendran V, Adamson CS, et al. Human papillomavirus is detectable in Barrett's esophagus and esophageal carcinoma but is unlikely to be of any etiologic significance. *J Clin Virol.* 2011;50:205–208. doi:10.1016/j.jcv.2010.11.015
4. Amin MB, Edge SB, Greene FL, et al. *AJCC Cancer Staging Manual.* 8th ed. New York, NY: Springer Publishing; 2017.
5. Shimada H, Okazumi S. Japanese Gastric Cancer Association Task Force for Research Promotion : clinical utility of 18 F-fluoro-2-deoxyglucose positron emission tomography in gastric cancer. A systematic review of the literature. *Gastric Cancer.* 2011;14:13. doi:10.1007/s10120-011-0017-5
6. Merkow RP, Bilimoria KY, Keswani RN, et al. Treatment Trends, Risk of Lymph Node Metastasis, and Outcomes for Localized Esophageal Cancer. *J Natl Cancer Inst.* 2014;106(7):dju133. doi:10.1093/jnci/dju133
7. Araki K, Ohno S, Egashira A, et al. Pathologic features of superficial esophageal squamous cell carcinoma with lymph node and distal metastasis. *Cancer. 2002;*94:570–575. doi:10.1002/cncr.10190
8. Endo M, Yoshino K, Kawano T, et al. Clinicopathologic analysis of lymph node metastasis in surgically resected superficial cancer of the thoracic esophagus. *Dis Esophagus. 2000;*13:125–129. doi:10.1046/j.1442-2050.2000.00100.x
9. Westerterp M, Koppert LB, Buskens CJ, et al. Outcome of surgical treatment for early adenocarcinoma of the esophagus or gastro-esophageal junction. *Virchows Arch.* 2005;446:497–504. doi:10.1007/s00428-005-1243-1
10. Leers JM, DeMeester SR, Oezcelik A, et al. The prevalence of lymph node metastases in patients with T1 esophageal adenocarcinoma a retrospective review of esophagectomy specimens. *Ann Surg. 2011;*253:271–278. doi:10.1097/SLA.0b013e3181fbad42
11. Ell C, May A, Pech O, et al. Curative endoscopic resection of early esophageal adenocarcinomas (Barrett's cancer). *Gastrointest Endosc.* 2007;65:3–10. doi:10.1016/j.gie.2006.04.033
12. Manner H, Pech O, Heldmann Y, et al. Efficacy, safety, and long-term results of endoscopic treatment for early stage adenocarcinoma of the esophagus with low-risk sm1 invasion. *Clin Gastroenterol Hepatol.* 2013;11:630–635. doi:10.1016/j.cgh.2012.12.040
13. Shapiro J, Lanschot JB, Van Hulshof MCCM, et al. Neoadjuvant chemoradiotherapy plus surgery versus surgery alone for oesophageal or junctional cancer (CROSS): long-term results of a randomised controlled trial. *Lancet Oncology.* 2015;16(9):1090–1098. doi:10.1016/S1470-2045(15)00040-6

14. Al-Batran SE, Homann N, Schmalenberg H, et al. Perioperative chemotherapy with docetaxel, oxaliplatin, and fluorouracil/leucovorin (FLOT) versus epirubicin, cisplatin, and fluorouracil or capecitabine (ECF/ECX) for resectable gastric or gastroesophageal junction (GEJ) adenocarcinoma (FLOT4-AIO): a multicenter, randomized phase 3 trial. *J Clin Oncol.* 2017;35(15_suppl):4004. doi:10.1200/jco.2017.35.15_suppl.4004

15. Mariette C, Dahan L, Mornex F, et al. Surgery alone versus chemoradiotherapy followed by surgery for stage I and II esophageal cancer: final analysis of randomized controlled phase III trial FFCD 9901. *J Clin Oncol.* 2014;32(23), 2416–2422. doi:10.1200/JCO.2013.53.6532

16. Burmeister BH, Smithers BM, Gebski V, et al. Surgery alone versus chemoradiotherapy followed by surgery for resectable cancer of the oesophagus: a randomised controlled phase III trial. *Lancet Oncol.* 2005;6(9):659–668. doi:10.1016/S1470-2045(05)70288-6

17. Cao CN, Luo JW, Gao L, et al. Primary radiotherapy compared with primary surgery in cervical esophageal cancer. *JAMA Otolaryngol Head Neck Surg. 2014;*140(10):918–926. doi:10.1001/jamaoto.2014.2013

18. Orringer MB, Marshall B, Chang AC, et al. Two thousand transhiatal esophagectomies: changing trends, lessons learned. *Ann Surg.* 2007;246:363–372. doi:10.1097/SLA.0b013e31814697f2

19. Goldminc M, Maddern G, LePrise E, et al. Oesophagectomy by transhiatal approach or thoracotomy: a prospective randomized trial. *Br J Surg.* 1993;80:367–370. doi:10.1002/bjs.1800800335

20. Chu KM, Law SY, Fok M, et al. A prospective randomized comparison of transhiatal and transthoracic resection for lower-third esophageal carcinoma. *Am J Surg.* 1997;174:320–324. doi:10.1016/S0002-9610(97)00105-0

21. Jacobi CA, Zieren HU, Muller M, et al. Surgical therapy of esophageal carcinoma: the influence of surgical approach and esophageal resection on cardiopulmonary function. *Eur J Cardiothorac Surg.* 1997;11:32–37. doi:10.1016/S1010-7940(96)01106-2

22. Hulscher JB, Tijssen JG, Obertop H, et al. Transthoracic versus transhiatal resection for carcinoma of the esophagus: a meta-analysis. Ann Thorac Surg. 2001;72:306–313. doi:10.1016/S0003-4975(00)02570-4

23. Chang AC, Ji J, Birkmeyer NJ, et al. Outcomes after transhiatal and transthoracic esophagectomy for cancer. *Ann Thorac Surg.* 2008;85:424–429. doi:10.1016/j.athoracsur.2007.10.007

24. Fok M, Cheng SW, Wong J. Pyloroplasty versus no drainage in gastric replacement of the esophagus. *Am J Surg.* 1991;162:447–452. doi:10.1016/0002-9610(91)90258-F

25. Urschel JD, Blewett CJ, Young JE, et al. Pyloric drainage (pyloroplasty) or no drainage in gastric reconstruction after esophagectomy: a meta-analysis of randomized controlled trials. *Dig Surg.* 2002;19:160–164. doi:10.1159/000064206

26. Casson AG, Darnton SJ, Subramanian S, et al. What is the optimal distal resection margin for esophageal carcinoma? *Ann Thorac Surg.* 2000;69(1):205–209. doi:10.1016/S0003-4975(99)01262-X

27. Altorki NK, Girardi L, Skinner DB. En bloc esophagectomy improves survival for stage III esophageal cancer. *J Thorac Cardiovasc Surg.* 1997;114:948–955. doi:10.1016/S0022-5223(97)70009-6

28. Lagergren J, Mattsson F, Zylstra J, et al. Extent of lymphadenectomy and prognosis after esophageal cancer surgery. *JAMA Surg.* 2016;151(1):32–39. doi:10.1001/jamasurg.2015.2611

29. Luketich JD, Pennathur A, Awais O. Outcomes after minimally invasive esophagectomy: review of over 1000 patients. *Ann Surg.* 2012;256:95–103. doi:10.1097/SLA.0b013e3182590603

30. Biere SS, Van Berge Henegouwen MI, Maas KW, et al. Minimally invasive versus open oesophagectomy for patients with oesophageal cancer: a multicentre, open-label, randomised controlled trial. *Lancet.* 2012;379(9829):1887–1892. doi:10.1016/S0140-6736(12)60516-9

31. Straatman J, van der Wielen N, Cuesta MA, et al. Minimally invasive versus open esophageal resection: three-year follow-up of the previously reported randomized controlled trial: the TIME trial. *Ann Surg.* 2017;266(2):232–236. doi:10.1097/SLA.0000000000002171

32. Takeuchi H, Miyata H, Gotoh M, et al. A risk model for esophagectomy using data of 5354 patients included in a Japanese nationwide web-based database. *Ann Surg.* 2014;260(2):259–266. doi:10.1097/SLA.0000000000000644

33. Birkmeyer J, Therese S, Siewers A, et al. Surgeon volume and operative mortality in the united states. *N Engl J Med.* 2003;349:2117–2127. doi:10.1056/NEJMsa035205

34. Bilimoria KY, Bentrem, DJ, Feinglass JM, et al. Directing surgical quality improvement initiatives: comparison of perioperative mortality and long-term survival for cancer surgery. *J Clin Oncol.* 2008;26:4626–4633. doi:10.1200/JCO.2007.15.6356

35. Kobayashi K, Koyama Y, Kosugi S, et al. Is early enteral nutrition better for postoperative course in esophageal cancer patients? *Nutrients.* 2013;5(9):3461–3469. doi:10.3390/nu5093461

36. Park JY, Song H, Kim JH, et al. Benign anastomotic strictures after esophagectomy: long-term effectiveness of balloon dilation and factors affecting recurrence in 155 patients. *Am J Roentgenol.* 2012;198(5):1208–1213. doi:10.2214/AJR.11.7608

37. Greene CL, Demeester SR, Worrell SG, et al. Alimentary satisfaction, gastrointestinal symptoms, and quality of life 10 or more years after esophagectomy with gastric pull-up. *J Thorac Cardiovasc Surg*. 2003;147(3):909–914. doi:10.1016/j.jtcvs.2013.11.004

38. Devesa SS, Blot WJ, Fraumeni JF Jr. Changing patterns in the incidence of esophageal and gastric carcinoma in the United States. *Cancer*. 1998;83(10):2049–2053. doi:10.1002/(SICI)1097-0142(19981115)83:10<2049::AID-CNCR1>3.0.CO;2-2

39. Noone AM, Howlader N, Krapcho M, et al. eds. SEER Cancer Statistics Review, 1975-2015; 2017. National Cancer Institute: Bethesda, MD. https://seer.cancer.gov/csr/1975_2015

40. Meng FS, Zhang ZH, Wang YM, et al. Comparison of endoscopic resection and gastrectomy for the treatment of early gastric cancer: a meta-analysis. *Surg Endosc*. 2016;30(9):3673–3683. doi:10.1007/s00464-015-4681-0

41. Japanese Gastric Cancer Association. Japanese gastric cancer treatment guidelines 2010 (ver. 3). *Gastric Cancer*. 2011;14:113–123. doi:10.1007/s10120-011-0042-4

42. Chung IK, Lee JH, Lee SH, et al. Therapeutic outcomes in 1000 cases of endoscopic submucosal dissection for early gastric neoplasms: Korean ESD Study Group multicenter study. *Gastrointest Endosc*. 2009;69(7):1228–1235. doi:10.1016/j.gie.2008.09.027

43. Cunningham D, Allum, WH, Stenning SP, et al. Perioperative chemotherapy versus surgery alone for resectable gastroesophageal cancer. *N Engl J Med*. 2006;355(1):11–20. doi:10.1056/NEJMoa055531

44. Smalley SR, Benedetti JK, Haller DG, et al. Updated analysis of SWOG-directed intergroup study 0116: a phase III trial of adjuvant radiochemotherapy versus observation after curative gastric cancer resection. *J Clin Oncol*. 2012;30(19):2327–2333. doi:10.1200/JCO.2011.36.7136

45. Fuchs CS, Niedzwiecki D, Mamon HJ, et al. Adjuvant chemoradiotherapy with epirubicin, cisplatin, and fluorouracil compared with adjuvant chemoradiotherapy with fluorouracil and leucovorin after curative resection of gastric cancer: results from CALGB 80101 (Alliance). *J Clin Oncol*. 2017;35(32):3671–3677. doi:10.1200/JCO.2017.74.2130

46. Lee J, Lim DH, Kim S, et al. Phase III trial comparing capecitabine plus cisplatin versus capecitabine plus cisplatin with concurrent capecitabine radiotherapy in completely resected gastric cancer with D2 lymph node dissection: the ARTIST trial. *J Clin Oncol*. 2012;30(3):268–273. doi:10.1200/JCO.2011.39.1953

47. Noh SH, Park SR, Yang H-K, et al. on behalf of the CLASSIC trial investigators. Adjuvant capecitabine plus oxaliplatin for gastric cancer after D2 gastrectomy (CLASSIC): 5-year follow-up of an open-label, randomised phase 3 trial. *Lancet Oncol*. 2014;15(12):1389–1396. doi:10.1016/S1470-2045(14)70473-5

48. Gotoda T, Yanagisawa A, Sasako M, et al. Incidence of lymph node metastasis from early gastric cancer: estimation with a large number of cases at two large centers. *Gastric Cancer*. 2000;3(4):219–225. doi:10.1007/PL00011720

49. D'Angelica M, Gonen M, Brennan MF, et al. Patterns of initial recurrence in completely resected gastric adenocarcinoma. *Ann Surg*. 2004;240:808–816. doi:10.1097/01.sla.0000143245.28656.15

50. Wu CW, Hsiung CA, Lo SS, et al. Nodal dissection for patients with gastric cancer: a randomized controlled trial. *Lancet Oncol*. 2006;7:309–315. doi:10.1016/S1470-2045(06)70623-4

51. Cuschieri A, Weeden S, Fielding J, et al. Patient survival after D1 and D2 resections for gastric cancer: long-term results of the MRC randomized surgical trial. Surgical Co-operative Group. *Br J Cancer*. 1999;79:1522–1530. doi:10.1038/sj.bjc.6690243

52. Songun I, Putter H, Kranenbarg EM, et al. Surgical treatment of gastric cancer: 15-year follow-up results of the randomised nationwide Dutch D1D2 trial. *Lancet Oncol*. 2010;11:439–449. doi:10.1016/S1470-2045(10)70070-X

53. Sano T, Sasako M, Yamamoto S, et al. Gastric cancer surgery: morbidity and mortality results from a prospective randomized controlled trial comparing D2 and extended para-aortic lymphadenectomy—Japan Clinical Oncology Group study 9501. *J Clin Oncol*. 2004;22:2767–2773. doi:10.1200/JCO.2004.10.184

54. Sasako M, Sano T, Yamamoto S, et al. D2 lymphadenectomy alone or with para-aortic nodal dissection for gastric cancer. *N Engl J Med*. 2008;359:453–462. doi:10.1056/NEJMoa0707035

55. Yonemura Y, Wu CC, Fukushima N, et al. Randomized clinical trial of D2 and extended paraaortic lymphadenectomy in patients with gastric cancer. *Int J Clin Oncol*. 2008;13:132–137. doi:10.1007/s10147-007-0727-1

56. Degiuli M, Sasako M, Calgaro M, et al. Morbidity and mortality after D1 and D2 gastrectomy for cancer : interim analysis of the Italian Gastric Cancer Study Group (IGCSG) randomised surgical trial. *Euro J of Surg Onc*. 2004;30(3):303–308. doi:10.1016/j.ejso.2003.11.020

57. Hiratsuka M, Miyashiro I, Ishikawa O, et al. Application of sentinel node biopsy to gastric cancer surgery. *Surgery*. 2001;129(3):335–340. doi:10.1067/msy.2001.111699

58. Miyashiro I, Hiratsuka M, Sasako M, et al. High false-negative proportion of intraoperative histological examination as a serious problem for clinical application of sentinel node biopsy for early gastric cancer: final results of the Japan Clinical Oncology Group multicenter trial JCOG0302. *Gastric Cancer*. 2014;17:316–323. doi:10.1007/s10120-013-0285-3

59. Gouzi JL, Huguier M, Fagniez PL, et al. Total versus subtotal gastrectomy for adenocarcinoma of the gastric antrum. A French prospective controlled study. *Ann Surg*. 1989;209:162–166. doi:10.1097/00000658-198902000-00005

60. Robertson CS, Chung SC, Woods SD, et al. A prospective randomized trial comparing R1 subtotal gastrectomy with R3 total gastrectomy for antral cancer. *Ann Surg*. 1994;220:176–182. doi:10.1097/00000658-199408000-00009

61. Bozzetti F, Marubini E, Bonfanti G, et al. Subtotal versus total gastrectomy for gastric cancer: five-year survival rates in a multicenter randomized Italian trial. Italian Gastrointestinal Tumor Study Group. *Ann Surg*. 1999;230:170–178. doi:10.1097/00000658-199908000-00006

62. So JBY, Rao J, Wong ASY, et al. Roux-en-Y or Billroth II Reconstruction After Radical Distal Gastrectomy for Gastric Cancer: a Multicenter Randomized Controlled Trial. *Ann Surg*. 2018;267(2):236–242. doi:10.1097/sla.0000000000002229

63. Fein M, Fuchs KH, Thalheimer A, et al. Long-term benefits of Roux-en-Y pouch reconstruction after total gastrectomy: a randomized trial. *Ann Surg*. 2008;247(5):759–765. doi:10.1097/SLA.0b013e318167748c

64. Schomas DA, Quevedo JF, Donahue JM, et al. The prognostic importance of pathologically involved celiac node metastases in node-positive patients with carcinoma of the distal esophagus or gastroesophageal junction: a surgical series from the Mayo Clinic. *Dis Esophagus*. 2010;23(3):232–239. doi:10.1111/j.1442-2050.2009.00990.x

65. Lynch HT, Kaurah P, Wirtzfeld D, et al. Hereditary diffuse gastric cancer: diagnosis, genetic counseling, and prophylactic total gastrectomy. *Cancer*. 2008;112(12):2655–2663. doi:10.1002/cncr.23501

66. Strong VE, Gholami S, Shah MA, et al. Total Gastrectomy for hereditary diffuse gastric cancer at a single center: postsurgical outcomes in 41 patients. *Ann Surg*. 2017;266(6):1006–1012. doi:10.1097/SLA.0000000000002030

67. Huscher CGS, Mingoli A, Sgarzini G, et al. Laparoscopic versus open subtotal gastrectomy for distal gastric cancer: five-year results of a randomized prospective trial. *Ann Surg*. 2005;241(2):232–237. doi:10.1097/01.sla.0000151892.35922.f2

68. Kim H-H, Ahn SH. The current status and future perspectives of laparoscopic surgery for gastric cancer. *J Korean Surg Soc*. 2011;81(3):151–162. doi:10.4174/jkss.2011.81.3.151

69. Kim HH, Han SU, Kim MC, et al. Prospective randomized controlled trial (phase III) to comparing laparoscopic distal gastrectomy with open distal gastrectomy for gastric adenocarcinoma (KLASS 01). *J Korean Surg Soc*. 2013;84:123–130. doi:10.4174/jkss.2013.84.2.123

70. Nakamura K, Katai H, Mizusawa J, et al. A phase III study of laparoscopy-assisted versus open distal gastrectomy with nodal dissection for clinical stage IA/IB gastric cancer (JCOG0912). *Jpn J Clin Oncol*. 2013;43,3:324–327. doi:10.1093/jjco/hys220

71. Kim W, Kim HH, Han SU, et al. Decreased morbidity of laparoscopic distal gastrectomy compared with open distal gastrectomy for stage I gastric cancer: short-term outcomes from a multicenter randomized controlled trial (KLASS-01). *Ann Surg*. 2016;263(1):28–35. doi: 10.1097/SLA.0000000000001346

72. Marano A, Choi YY, Hyung WJ, et al. Robotic versus Laparoscopic versus open gastrectomy: a meta-analysis. *J Gastric Cancer*. 2013;13(3):136–148. doi:10.5230/jgc.2013.13.3.136

73. Kim MC, Heo GU, Jung GJ. Robotic gastrectomy for gastric cancer: surgical techniques and clinical merits. *Surg Endosc*. 2010;24(3):610–615. doi:10.1007/s00464-009-0618-9

74. Kim HH, Han SU, Kim MC, et al. Long-term results of laparoscopic gastrectomy for gastric cancer: a large-scale case-control and case-matched Korean multicenter study. *J Clin Oncol*. 2014;32(7):627–633. doi:10.1200/JCO.2013.48.8551

How I Treat Metastatic Gastric and Esophageal Cancer With Chemotherapy and Choice of Biologics

Mehmet Akce

INTRODUCTION

Approximately 45,160 esophagogastric cancer cases will be diagnosed in the United States in 2019 (1). More than one-third of esophagogastric cancers present with metastatic disease with a 5-year survival rate of 5% (1,2). The majority of gastric and esophageal cancers are adenocarcinoma. Systemic chemotherapy options are similar for both adenocarcinoma and squamous cell carcinoma. Systemic chemotherapy and/or targeted therapy have been shown to improve survival and palliate symptoms in both adenocarcinoma and squamous cell carcinoma histology (3–5). Approved targeted therapy options include trastuzumab for human epidermal growth factor receptor 2 (HER2) positive metastatic gastric and esophageal cancer in combination with chemotherapy in the first line and antiangiogenic ramucirumab for adenocarcinoma histology in the second line. Active systemic chemotherapy agents include fluorouracil, cisplatin, docetaxel, irinotecan, paclitaxel, epirubicin, and doxorubicin. Performance status, organ function, and patient preference should be taken into consideration in individualized treatment planning.

FIRST-LINE CHEMOTHERAPY REGIMENS FOR METASTATIC GASTRIC AND ESOPHAGEAL CANCER

In the first-line setting, several randomized clinical trials have shown survival benefit and improved overall response rates in metastatic gastric and esophageal cancers (see Table 41.1). Systemic chemotherapy provides approximately a 7-month survival benefit compared to best supportive care in metastatic gastric cancer (6). Compared to best supportive care, chemotherapy and/or targeted therapy improve survival in metastatic esophageal and gastroesophageal junction cancers without compromising quality of life (3). Combination chemotherapy is more effective than single-agent chemotherapy and provides a modest survival improvement compared to single-agent chemotherapy (6). Use of chemotherapy regimens varies globally, and current treatment guidelines recommend doublet or triplet platinum-based regimens alone or with trastuzumab in HER2-positive disease (7–10).

In the first-line setting of metastatic gastric and esophageal cancer, both two- and three-drug chemotherapy combinations improved overall survival (OS) and response rates in randomized clinical trials (see Table 41.1). More toxicities were encountered with three-drug regimens and later the survival benefit of the third cytotoxic drug, mainly docetaxel or epirubicin, was questioned. The V325 trial compared docetaxel/cisplatin/5-fluorouracil (5-FU; DCF) to cisplatin/5-FU (CF) in 457 advanced gastric cancer patients (97% metastatic). The triplet regimen resulted in improvement in response rate and a modest 0.6-month improvement in OS. Unfortunately, the triplet regimen did result in a significant increase in treatment-related toxicity (11) including grade 3 or 4 adverse events, 69% versus 59%, respectively. More grade 3 and 4 neutropenia, neutropenic infections, and infections were encountered in the DCF arm.

The randomized epirubicin, cisplatin and fluorouracil (ECF) for advanced and locally advanced esophagogastric cancer 2 (REAL-2) trial compared epirubicin/cisplatin plus 5-FU or capecitabine (ECX) versus epirubicin/oxaliplatin plus 5-FU or capecitabine (EOX) in two-by-two design (15). This trial established noninferiority of oxaliplatin compared to cisplatin, and the hazard ratio (HR) of the oxaliplatin-containing group was 0.92 (95% confidence interval

---

A Clinical Vignette ("How I Treat") is included at the end of the chapter.

TABLE 41.1 Established Chemotherapy Regimens in the First-Line Treatment of Metastatic Gastric and Esophageal Cancer

Chemotherapy Regimen	Phase	Response Rate (%)	Median PFS (Months)	Median OS (Months)
Docetaxel/cisplatin/5-FU (11)	II/III	37.0	-	9.2
5-FU/oxaliplatin/folinic acid (12)	III	34.8	5.8	10.7
5-FU/cisplatin/folinic acid (12)		24.5	3.9	8.8
Cisplatin/capecitabine (13)	III	46.0	5.6	10.5
Cisplatin/S1 (14)	III	54.0	6.0	13.0
Epirubicin/cisplatin/5-FU (15)	III	40.7	6.2	9.9
Epirubicin/cisplatin/capecitabine (15)		46.4	6.7	9.9
Epirubicin/oxaliplatin/5-FU (15)		42.4	6.5	9.3
Epirubicin/oxaliplatin/capecitabine (15)		47.9	7.0	11.2
Docetaxel/cisplatin/5-FU (11)	III	37.0	5.6	9.2
Trastuzumab plus cisplatin/capecitabine or 5-FU (16)	III	47.0	6.7	13.8
5-FU/irinotecan (17)	III	39.2	5.3	9.5

5-FU, 5-fluorouracil; OS, overall survival; PFS, progression-free survival.

[CI]: 0.80–1.10). Furthermore, less neutropenia, alopecia, thromboembolism, and kidney toxicity were reported in the oxaliplatin group, but a higher rate of diarrhea and neuropathy was reported in the same group as compared to the cisplatin-containing group. In essence, the oxaliplatin-containing regimen was noninferior and less toxic. In a separate randomized phase III trial, the 5-FU and cisplatin (FLP) regimen was compared with the 5-FU and oxaliplatin regimen (FLO) in metastatic esophagogastric adenocarcinoma and showed no difference in OS but a trend toward better progression-free survival (PFS) with FLO (12). Less renal toxicity, thromboembolism, anemia, nausea, alopecia, and fatigue were observed with the FLO regimen. The FLO regimen was associated with more peripheral neuropathy compared to FLP. Patients above the age of 65 derived better PFS (6.0 vs. 3.1 months, $p = .029$) and OS (13.9 vs. 7.2 months, $p = .83$) with FLO as compared to FLP in the same study.

In clinical practice, capecitabine could be substituted for 5-FU as supported by randomized clinical trials. The REAL-2 study proved that capecitabine was noninferior compared to 5-FU (HR: 0.86, 95% CI: 0.80–0.99) (13). In a separate study from Asia, 316 patients were randomized to 5-FU/cisplatin versus capecitabine/cisplatin, and noninferiority of capecitabine was proven (13). Furthermore, a meta-analysis of these two trials revealed superior OS with capecitabine-containing regimens compared to 5-FU combinations (18).

In patients who cannot tolerate or are ineligible for platinum compounds, 5-FU/irinotecan (FOLFIRI) combination could be a viable first-line therapy option (17,19). FOLFIRI was compared with the ECX regimen in 416 patients with advanced gastric and gastroesophageal cancer in a phase III randomized clinical trial, and better time to treatment failure was reported with FOLFIRI (5.1 vs. 4.2 months, $p = .008$). Median OS, PFS, and response rate were not different between the two arms, and FOLFIRI was better tolerated with less grade 3 or 4 toxicity (69% vs. 84%, $p < .001$). In the same trial, second-line therapy was predefined and patients were offered ECX if they progressed on FOLFIRI and vice versa. A considerable number or patients proceeded with second-line therapy (101 FOLFIRI and 81 ECX).

Utilization of triple combinations versus doublet combinations differs in clinical practice. In general, triple regimens could be offered to younger patients with good performance status and organ function due to concerns for higher treatment-related toxicity. Triple regimens were found to be associated with more adverse events as shown in the V325 trial. Increased toxicity with triple regimens is a particular concern for elderly patients. In a randomized phase II study, 143 patients ≥65 years of age with locally advanced and metastatic gastric and gastroesophageal junction cancer were treated with 5-FU/leucovorin/oxaliplatin/docetaxel (FLOT) chemotherapy regimen versus 5-FU/leucovorin/oxaliplatin (FLO) (20). More than two-thirds of the patients in the trial had metastatic disease. The FLOT regimen was related with significantly more grade 3 or 4 adverse events ($p < .001$) such as neutropenia (52.8% vs. 12.9%), leukopenia (29.2% vs. 5.7%), and nausea (20.8% vs. 7.3%). The FLOT regimen impacted quality of life negatively. Additionally, overall grade 3 or 4 adverse events were almost twice as high with the FLOT regimen (81.9% vs. 38.6%, $p < .001$). The response rates were not different between the two arms in patients ≥70 years old and metastatic disease although in the entire cohort and patients aged <70 FLOT was associated with higher response rates. In general, study population median OS did not differ between the two arms (FLO 14.5 months, FLOT 17.3 months, $p = .39$). In patients >75 years old, median PFS was not different between the two regimens (FLO 7.5 months vs. FLOT 7.6 months, $p = .65$).

The first-line chemotherapy choice differs globally and a recent network meta-analysis provides guidance on treatment selection. It incorporated 17 different chemotherapy regimens from prospective phase II and III randomized clinical trials with direct comparisons for OS in 50 studies with 10,249 patients and PFS in 34 studies with 7,795 patients (21). This study showed that fluoropyrimidine noncisplatin doublets (such as fluoropyrimidine plus oxaliplatin or irinotecan or taxane) were more effective compared to cisplatin doublets (cisplatin plus irinotecan or fluoropyrimidine or taxane). Additionally, anthracycline-containing triplet regimens were not superior to fluoropyrimidine doublets. This finding and other earlier trials questioned the benefit of anthracyclines (17).

S-1 is an oral fluoropyrimidine that is approved for advanced gastric cancer in East Asia and Europe but not in the United States (14,22). It was shown to be noninferior to 5-FU in Japanese patients in the first-line setting (23). The FLAGS trial compared cisplatin/S-1 versus cisplatin/5-FU in 1,053 non-Asian patients and did not show superiority (24). The median OS was 8.6 versus 7.9 months with no statistical significance, and less toxicity was seen in the S-1 arm. It should be noted that the S-1 arm included a lower dose of cisplatin (75 mg/m^2 vs. 100 mg/m^2). Herceptin plus S-1/cisplatin was studied in HER2-positive metastatic gastric cancer in a phase II study and reported improved median PFS and OS (16 and 7.8 months) (25).

INCORPORATION OF BIOLOGICS TO FIRST-LINE THERAPY

Trastuzumab and ramucirumab are currently approved biologics in the treatment of metastatic gastric and esophageal cancers (26). Clinically relevant key signaling pathways that have been targeted in clinical trials in gastric and esophageal cancer include HER2, vascular endothelial growth factor (VEGF), epidermal growth factor receptor (EGFR), cMET, and mTOR (27). Despite multiple clinical trials targeting these pathways, so far only targeting the HER2 pathway was shown to improve survival in the first-line setting and the VEGF pathway in the second-line setting. HER2 is a proto-oncogene and overexpressed in up to 40% of gastric and esophageal cancers (28). HER2 overexpression or amplification is checked in tumor tissue by immunohistochemistry (IHC) and gene amplification by using fluorescence in situ hybridization (FISH) methods as recommended by guidelines (see Table 41.2) (8,9,26,28). Trastuzumab is a humanized monoclonal antibody against the extracellular domain of HER2 receptor; it inhibits HER2-mediated cellular signaling and causes antibody-dependent cytotoxicity. Trastuzumab for Gastric Cancer (ToGA) trial compared chemotherapy (cisplatin/5-FU or cisplatin/capecitabine) versus chemotherapy plus trastuzumab in 594 HER2-overexpressed gastric and gastroesophageal cancer patients and reported significantly improved OS with trastuzumab combination (11.1 versus 13.8 months) (16). The vast majority of the patients in both arms were treated with capecitabine-containing regimens; 87% of patients were treated with cisplatin/capecitabine plus trastuzumab regimen versus 86% with the cisplatin/capecitabine regimen. Cardiac toxicity did not differ between the treatment groups (6% in each group). The clinical benefit was higher in patients with a high degree of HER2 overexpression (defined as IHC 3+ HER2 overexpression or IHC 2+ with positive FISH test).

If the HER2 status is determined after the chemotherapy regimen is already commenced, trastuzumab can still be added to the first-line chemotherapy. If the HER2-positive patients did not receive trastuzumab in the first-line setting, it could be added to the second-line chemotherapy regimen. This approach is supported by a phase II study from Japan, in which 47 patients with HER2-positive metastatic gastric cancer without prior trastuzumab exposure were treated with trastuzumab and paclitaxel combination and reported 37% response rate and 17.1 months OS (29). No new safety concerns were raised in this study compared to the first-line setting.

TABLE 41.2 Scoring Guidelines for Interpretation of HER2 Immunohistochemistry in Gastric and Esophageal Cancer

Surgical Specimen–Staining Pattern	Biopsy Specimen–Staining Pattern	Score	HER2 Expression Assessment
No reactivity or membranous reactivity in <10% of tumor cells	No reactivity or membranous reactivity in any tumor cells	0	Negative
Faint/barely perceptible membranous reactivity in ≥10% of tumor cells; cells are reactive only in part of their membrane	Tumor cell cluster* with a faint/barely perceptible membranous reactivity irrespective of percentage of tumor cells stained	1+	Negative
Weak to moderate, complete, basolateral, or lateral membranous reactivity in ≥10% of tumor cells	Tumor cell cluster* with a weak to moderate, complete, basolateral, or lateral membranous reactivity respective of percentage of tumor cells stained	2+	Equivocal
Strong, complete, basolateral, or lateral membranous reactivity in ≥10% of tumor cells stained	Tumor cell cluster* with a strong, complete, basolateral, or lateral membranous reactivity respective of percentage of tumor cells stained	3+	Positive

*Tumor cell cluster (>5 neoplastic cells).

Source: From Bartley AN, Washington MK, Colasacco C, et al. HER2 Testing and Clinical Decision Making in Gastroesophageal Adenocarcinoma: Guideline From the College of American Pathologists, American Society for Clinical Pathology, and the American Society of Clinical Oncology. *J Clin Oncol.* 2017;35:446–464. doi:10.1200/jco.2016.69.4836

Treatment beyond progression or maintenance therapy with trastuzumab is not an established approach. There are data mainly from retrospective studies suggesting potential benefit for treatment beyond progression with trastuzumab but data from randomized clinical trials is lacking (30–32). A prospective phase II study evaluating trastuzumab as a single agent beyond progression on platinum- or fluoropyrimidine-containing first-line regimen was terminated due to poor accrual (NCT020054484). A retrospective study from MD Anderson Cancer Center reported results of trastuzumab and chemotherapy backbone (predominantly 5-FU/irinotecan regimen) treatment beyond disease progression in 43 patients with HER2-positive metastatic gastric cancer who were initially treated with trastuzumab and chemotherapy (predominantly 5-FU/oxaliplatin regimen) (30). PFS and median OS were 5 and 11 months, respectively. A retrospective study form France reported results of treatment beyond progression with trastuzumab plus chemotherapy versus chemotherapy in 104 patients with HER2-positive metastatic gastric and gastroesophageal cancer. PFS was 4.4 versus 2.3 months ($p = .002$) and OS was 12.6 versus 6.1 months ($p = .001$) in favor of maintenance trastuzumab (31). In a multicenter prospective observational cohort study conducted in China, 32 patients with HER2-positive metastatic gastric and gastroesophageal cancer were treated with trastuzumab and a second-line chemotherapy agent versus 27 patients were treated with second-line chemotherapy agent alone (32). A longer PFS2 calculating from the time of second-line therapy was reported (3.1 versus 2 months, $p = .008$). However, no difference in median OS2 was shown. No new safety concerns were encountered. Despite potential benefit suggested by retrospective studies, a recent phase II study compared weekly paclitaxel plus trastuzumab versus weekly paclitaxel alone in 91 patients with HER2-positive gastric and gastroesophageal cancer who progressed during first-line trastuzumab plus chemotherapy and failed to show any improvement in PFS or OS (33). Currently, it is not the standard of care to continue trastuzumab beyond progression. Maintenance therapy in patients with no progression on initial chemotherapy and trastuzumab combination is being explored in the ongoing phase II PLATFORM trial (NCT02678182).

Combinations of trastuzumab and anthracycline-containing regimens are not recommended by the current clinical guidelines due to concerns of increased cardiotoxicity (8,9).

Other relevant molecular targets were also studied in randomized clinical trials. In the first-line setting, EXPAND and REAL-3 clinical trials with biologics targeting EGFR with cetuximab or panitumumab were negative (34,35). Dual tyrosine kinase inhibitor lapatinib targets EGFR and HER2. The LOGiC trial compared lapatinib plus capecitabine/oxaliplatin versus capecitabine/oxaliplatin in treatment-naïve HER2-positive metastatic gastric and esophageal cancer patients, and no survival benefit was found compared to standard treatment (36). The TyTAN trial compared lapatinib plus paclitaxel to paclitaxel in the second-line setting and reported no OS benefit in Asian patients (37). The GATSBY trial compared trastuzumab emtansine (TDM-1) to paclitaxel or docetaxel in the second-line setting and failed to show any OS benefit (38). The AVAGAST trial targeting VEGF-A with bevacizumab and capecitabine/cisplatin versus capecitabine/cisplatin combination did not improve OS in the first-line setting (39). The Granite-1 trial targeting mTOR pathway with everolimus plus capecitabine/cisplatin versus capecitabine/cisplatin combination also did not improve OS in the second- and third-line setting (40). Ramucirumab plus capecitabine/cisplatin was studied as a first-line treatment, but it did not improve OS although it improved PFS (41).

Fluoropyrimidine and platinum combination plus trastuzumab is the first-line systemic chemotherapy option for HER2-overexpressed metastatic gastric and esophageal cancers. Fluoropyrimidine and platinum combination is the most commonly utilized option in the HER2-negative setting although the standard is not established (7–9). In medically fit and young patients, a triplet regimen could be considered.

SECOND-LINE CHEMOTHERAPY REGIMENS AND BEYOND SECOND-LINE CHEMOTHERAPY

The treatment regimens after progression with first-line chemotherapy must be individualized and several different single-agent and combination chemotherapy regimens have been shown to be effective in the second-line setting (see Table 41.3). In patients with microsatellite instability high (MSI-H) gastric and esophageal adenocarcinoma, as a second-line therapy, and in patients with PD-L1 positive tumors, as a third-line therapy, immunotherapy with PD-1 inhibitor pembrolizumab is an option; the role of immunotherapy is reviewed in Chapter 42, *How I Treat Metastatic Gastric and Esophageal Cancer With Immunotherapy.*

In advanced gastric and esophageal cancer patients who progressed after a platinum- or fluoropyrimidine-based chemotherapy, the COUGAR-02 trial compared docetaxel versus best supportive care in 168 patients (44). Single-agent docetaxel improved median OS, 5.2 versus 3.6 months as well as achieved better symptom control with less pain, nausea, vomiting, and dysphagia. Docetaxel was associated with higher neutropenia and febrile neutropenia. In a similar patient population, single agent irinotecan was compared to best supportive care in a phase III randomized trial and, due to poor accrual, the study was terminated prematurely (45). A total of

TABLE 41.3 Established Chemotherapy Regimens in Second-Line Treatment and Beyond in Metastatic Gastric and Esophageal Cancer

Chemotherapy Regimen	Phase	Response Rate (%)	Median PFS (Months)	Median OS (Months)
Ramucirumab/paclitaxel* (42)	III	27.9	4.4	9.6
Ramucirumab* (43)	III	4.0	2.1	5.2
Docetaxel (44)	III	7.0	-	5.2
Irinotecan (45)	III	0	2.5	4.0
Paclitaxel (46) Irinotecan (46)	III	20.9 13.6	3.6 2.3	9.5 8.4
5-FU/irinotecan (17)	III	10.1[†]	-	-

*Adenocarcinoma only.

[†]Response rate in patients who received FOLFIRI as a second-line therapy per trial protocol after they progressed on ECX regimen in the trial.

5-FU, 5-fluorouracil; OS, overall survival; PFS, progression-free survival.

40 patients were enrolled and single agent irinotecan improved median OS (4 months) compared to best supportive care (2.4 months). Median PFS was calculated only for irinotecan and was reported to be 2.5 months. No objective responses were reported but disease stability at 6 weeks was achieved in 53% of patients, and 50% of patients reported improvement in their symptoms. The WJOG 4007 trial randomized 219 platinum and fluoropyrimidine combination resistant advanced gastric cancer patients to single agent paclitaxel or irinotecan. Both agents appeared to be suitable second-line agents in the trial (46). Similar median OS and PFS were noted, 9.5 versus 8.4 months and 3.6 versus 2.3 months, respectively. Overall response rates were 20.9% versus 13.6%. Similar grade 3 and 4 adverse events were encountered between the two groups.

INCORPORATION OF BIOLOGICS TO SECOND-LINE THERAPY AND BEYOND

The VEGF pathway plays a role in gastric and esophageal cancer development and has been studied in randomized clinical trials as a therapeutic target based on preclinical data. Following positive results of REGARD and RAINBOW randomized phase III trials, ramucirumab, a VEGFR-2 antagonist, as a single agent and in combination with paclitaxel, was established as standard second-line treatment options (42,43).

In the REGARD study, 355 patients with gastric and gastroesophageal adenocarcinoma who progressed on first-line fluoropyrimidines or platinum-containing chemotherapy were randomized to ramucirumab or placebo in a two-to-one ratio (43). Median OS was improved significantly with ramucirumab therapy compared to placebo, 5.2 versus 3.8 months. Other than a higher rate of hypertension in the ramucirumab arm, reported adverse events were similar.

In the RAINBOW study, 665 patients with therapy resistant gastric and gastroesophageal adenocarcinoma after progression with chemotherapy regimens including fluoropyrimidines, platinum, or an anthracycline agent were randomized to ramucirumab plus paclitaxel versus placebo plus paclitaxel in a one-to-one ratio (42). Median OS was significantly improved in the ramucirumab plus paclitaxel combination, 9.6 versus 7.4 months. Higher rates of grade 3 or higher adverse events were reported in the combination arm, including neutropenia, hypertension, fatigue, anemia, and abdominal pain.

More recently, apatinib, an oral VEGF-2, was studied in a phase III randomized trial in comparison with placebo in 267 patients with metastatic gastric and gastroesophageal cancer in the third-line setting in China and was shown to improve median OS compared to placebo (6.5 vs. 4.7 months) (47). Currently, apatinib is approved as a third-line therapy for metastatic gastric cancer only in China.

CASE STUDY

A 70-year-old man with a history of HER2-positive metastatic gastroesophageal adenocarcinoma progressed on FOLFOX and trastuzumab therapy. His complete blood count (CBC) and comprehensive metabolic panel (CMP) are acceptable. His Eastern Cooperative Oncology Group (ECOG) score is 1. He is interested in further systemic therapy. Which of the following options should not be offered to this patient?

A. FOLFIRI
B. Paclitaxel
C. Ramucirumab
D. Ramucirumab plus paclitaxel
E. Paclitaxel plus trastuzumab

Answer: A, B, C, or D could be offered as a second-line treatment option to the patient (see Table 41.2). However, E could not be offered as trastuzumab beyond progression is not the standard of care and a recent phase II trial failed to show any benefit of trastuzumab beyond progression.

SUMMARY

Systemic chemotherapy improves survival and quality of life in metastatic gastric and esophageal cancer. A fluoropyrimidine and platinum agent with trastuzumab can be utilized as

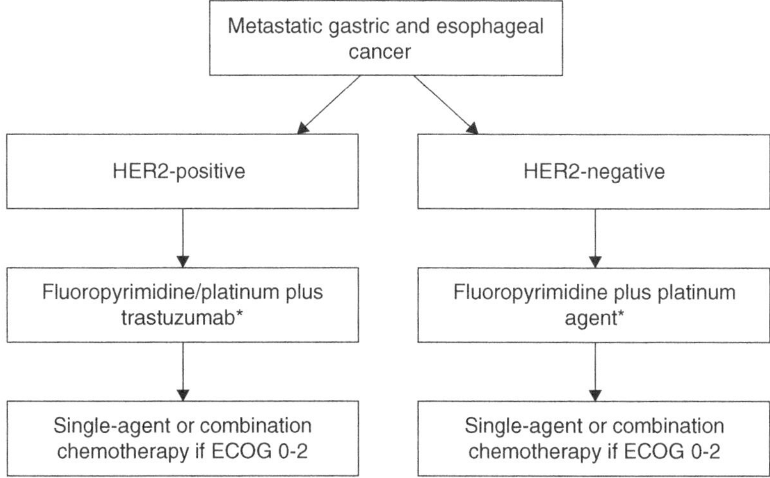

FIGURE 41.1   Chemotherapy and Biological Therapy Approach to Gastric and Esophageal Cancer ECOG, Eastern Cooperative Oncology Group.

standard first-line therapy in HER2-positive gastric and esophageal cancer (Figure 41.1). In HER2-negative disease, combination of fluoropyrimidines and platinum agent can be offered as first-line therapy. In younger patients with normal organ function and performance status, triple drug combinations could be an option. Ramucirumab single agent or ramucirumab plus paclitaxel is a standard option in metastatic gastric and esophageal adenocarcinoma patients with good performance status and organ function who progress on first-line chemotherapy. Several single agent and combination treatment regimens have reasonable clinical activity in the second-line setting and beyond if patients maintain reasonable performance status, organ function, and willingness to continue therapy. In the rapidly changing landscape of potential treatments and better understanding of the molecular pathogenesis of gastric and esophageal cancers, clinical trials should be offered as an option if available in all lines of therapy.

Clinical Vignette 41.1

A 69-year-old man with newly diagnosed metastatic gastric adenocarcinoma presented for further treatment. He has a past medical history of hypertension, hyperlipidemia, and gastroesophageal reflux disease (GERD). His social history is significant for smoking. He has no family history of cancer. He has normal organ function and ECOG score 1. Immunohistochemistry (IHC) exam of his tumor tissue revealed HER2 expression 3+. Which of the following should not be offered as a first-line treatment option to this patient?

A. 5-FU/oxaliplatin plus trastuzumab
B. Capecitabine/oxaliplatin plus trastuzumab
C. 5-FU/cisplatin plus trastuzumab
D. Capecitabine/cisplatin plus trastuzumab
E. Epirubicin/cisplatin/5-FU plus trastuzumab

Answer: Based on current treatment guidelines and randomized clinical trials (see Table 41.1), A, B, C, or D could be offered to this patient. However, due to increased risk of cardiotoxicity, trastuzumab and anthracycline combination is not recommended (E).

REFERENCES

1. Siegel RL, Miller KD, Jemal A. Cancer statistics, 2019. *CA Cancer J Clin*. 2019;69(1):7–34. doi:10.3322/caac.21551
2. Noone AM, Howlader N, Krapcho M, et al, eds. SEER Cancer Statistics Review, 1975–2015, National Cancer Institute. Bethesda, MD. https://seer.cancer.gov/csr/1975_2015/, based on November 2017 SEER data submission, posted to the SEER web site, April 2018.
3. Janmaat VT, Steyerberg EW, van der Gaast A, et al. Palliative chemotherapy and targeted therapies for esophageal and gastroesophageal junction cancer. *Cochrane Database Syst Rev*. 2017;11:Cd004063. doi:10.1002/14651858.CD004063.pub4
4. Glimelius B, Hoffman K, Haglund U, et al. Initial or delayed chemotherapy with best supportive care in advanced gastric cancer. *Ann Oncol*. 1994;5:189–190. doi:10.1093/oxfordjournals.annonc.a058778
5. Al-Batran SE, Ajani JA. Impact of chemotherapy on quality of life in patients with metastatic esophagogastric cancer. *Cancer*. 2010;116:2511–2518, doi:10.1002/cncr.25064
6. Wagner AD, Syn NLX, Moehler M, et al. Chemotherapy for advanced gastric cancer. *Cochrane Database Syst Rev*. 2017;8:Cd004064. doi:10.1002/14651858.CD004064.pub4
7. Waddell T, Verheij M, Allum W, et al. Gastric cancer: ESMO-ESSO-ESTRO clinical practice guidelines for diagnosis, treatment and follow-up. *Eur J Surg Oncol*. 2014;40:584–591. doi:10.1016/j.ejso.2013.09.020
8. NCCN Clinical Practice Guidelines in Oncology. *Gastric Cancer*. Version 2.2018-May 22, 2018.
9. NCCN Clinical Practice Guidelines in Oncology. *Esophageal and Esophagogastric Junction Cancers*. Version 2.2018-May 22, 2018.
10. Japanese Gastric Cancer Association. Japanese gastric cancer treatment guidelines 2014 (ver. 4). *Gastric Cancer*. 2017;20:1–19. doi:10.1007/s10120-016-0622-4
11. Van Cutsem E, Moiseyenko VM, Tjulandin S, et al. Phase III study of docetaxel and cisplatin plus fluorouracil compared with cisplatin and fluorouracil as first-line therapy for advanced gastric cancer: a report of the V325 Study Group. *J Clin Oncol*. 2006;24:4991–4997. doi:10.1200/jco.2006.06.8429
12. Al-Batran SE, Hartmann JT, Probst S, et al. Phase III trial in metastatic gastroesophageal adenocarcinoma with fluorouracil, leucovorin plus either oxaliplatin or cisplatin: a study of the Arbeitsgemeinschaft Internistische Onkologie. *J Clin Oncol*. 2008;26:1435–1442. doi:10.1200/jco.2007.13.9378
13. Kang YK, Kang WK, Shin DB, et al. Capecitabine/cisplatin versus 5-fluorouracil/cisplatin as first-line therapy in patients with advanced gastric cancer: a randomised phase III noninferiority trial. *Ann Oncol*. 2009;20:666–673. doi:10.1093/annonc/mdn717
14. Koizumi W, Narahara H, Hara T, et al. S-1 plus cisplatin versus S-1 alone for first-line treatment of advanced gastric cancer (SPIRITS trial): a phase III trial. *Lancet Oncol*. 2008;9:215–221. doi:10.1016/s1470-2045(08)70035-4
15. Cunningham D, Starling N, Rao S, et al. Capecitabine and oxaliplatin for advanced esophagogastric cancer. *N Engl J Med*. 2008;358:36–46. doi:10.1056/NEJMoa073149
16. Bang YJ, Van Cutsem E, Feyereislova A, et al. Trastuzumab in combination with chemotherapy versus chemotherapy alone for treatment of HER2-positive advanced gastric or gastro-oesophageal junction cancer (ToGA): a phase 3, open-label, randomised controlled trial. *Lancet*. 2010;376:687–697. doi:10.1016/s0140-6736(10)61121-x
17. Guimbaud R, Louvet C, Ries P, et al. Prospective, randomized, multicenter, phase III study of fluorouracil, leucovorin, and irinotecan versus epirubicin, cisplatin, and capecitabine in advanced gastric adenocarcinoma: a French intergroup (Federation Francophone de Cancerologie Digestive, Federation Nationale des Centres de Lutte Contre le Cancer, and Groupe Cooperateur Multidisciplinaire en Oncologie) study. *J Clin Oncol*. 2014;32:3520–3526. doi:10.1200/jco.2013.54.1011
18. Okines AF, Norman AR, McCloud P, et al. Meta-analysis of the REAL-2 and ML17032 trials: evaluating capecitabine-based combination chemotherapy and infused 5-fluorouracil-based combination chemotherapy for the treatment of advanced oesophago-gastric cancer. *Ann Oncol*. 2009;20:1529–1534. doi:10.1093/annonc/mdp047
19. Dank M, Zaluski J, Barone C, et al. Randomized phase III study comparing irinotecan combined with 5-fluorouracil and folinic acid to cisplatin combined with 5-fluorouracil in chemotherapy naive patients with advanced adenocarcinoma of the stomach or esophagogastric junction. *Ann Oncol*. 2008;19:1450–1457. doi:10.1093/annonc/mdn166
20. Al-Batran SE, Pauligk C, Homann N, et al. The feasibility of triple-drug chemotherapy combination in older adult patients with oesophagogastric cancer: a randomised trial of the Arbeitsgemeinschaft Internistische Onkologie (FLOT65+). *Eur J Cancer*. 2013;49:835–842. doi:10.1016/j.ejca.2012.09.025

21. Ter Veer E, Mohammad NH, van Valkenhoef G, et al. The efficacy and safety of first-line chemotherapy in advanced esophagogastric cancer: a network meta-analysis. *J Natl Cancer Inst.* 2016;108:djw166. doi:10.1093/jnci/djw166

22. Lordick F, Lorenzen S, Yamada Y, et al. Optimal chemotherapy for advanced gastric cancer: is there a global consensus? *Gastric Cancer.* 2014;17:213–225. doi:10.1007/s10120-013-0297-z

23. Boku N, Yamamoto S, Fukuda H, et al. Fluorouracil versus combination of irinotecan plus cisplatin versus S-1 in metastatic gastric cancer: a randomised phase 3 study. *Lancet Oncol.* 2009;10:1063–1069. doi:10.1016/s1470-2045(09)70259-1

24. Ajani JA, Rodriguez W, Bodoky G, et al. Multicenter phase III comparison of cisplatin/S-1 with cisplatin/infusional fluorouracil in advanced gastric or gastroesophageal adenocarcinoma study: the FLAGS trial. *J Clin Oncol.* 2010;28:1547–1553. doi:10.1200/jco.2009.25.4706

25. Kurokawa Y, Sugimoto N, Miwa H, et al. Phase II study of trastuzumab in combination with S-1 plus cisplatin in HER2-positive gastric cancer (HERBIS-1). *Br J Cancer.* 2014;110:1163–1168. doi:10.1038/bjc.2014.18

26. Wong N, Amary F, Butler R, et al. HER2 testing of gastro-oesophageal adenocarcinoma: a commentary and guidance document from the Association of Clinical Pathologists Molecular Pathology and Diagnostics Committee. *J Clin Pathol.* 2018;71:388–394. doi:10.1136/jclinpath-2017-204943

27. Kumar V, Soni P, Garg M, et al. Emerging therapies in the management of advanced-stage gastric cancer. *Front Pharmacol.* 2018;9:404. doi:10.3389/fphar.2018.00404

28. Bartley AN, Washington MK, Colasacco C, et al. HER2 testing and clinical decision making in gastroesophageal adenocarcinoma: guideline grom the College of American Pathologists, American Society for Clinical Pathology, and the American Society of Clinical Oncology. *J Clin Oncol.* 2017;35:446–464. doi:10.1200/jco.2016.69.4836

29. Nishikawa K, Takahashi T, Takaishi H, et al. Phase II study of the effectiveness and safety of trastuzumab and paclitaxel for taxane- and trastuzumab-naive patients with HER2-positive, previously treated, advanced, or recurrent gastric cancer (JFMC45-1102). *Int J Cancer.* 2017;140:188–196. doi:10.1002/ijc.30383

30. Al-Shamsi HO, Fahmawi Y, Dahbour I, et al. Continuation of trastuzumab beyond disease progression in HER2-positive metastatic gastric cancer: the MD Anderson experience. *J Gastrointest Oncol.* 2016;7:499–505. doi:10.21037/jgo.2016.06.16

31. Palle J, Tougeron D, Pozet A, et al. Trastuzumab beyond progression in patients with HER2-positive advanced gastric adenocarcinoma: a multicenter AGEO study. *J Clin Oncol.* 2017;35:94–94. doi:10.1200/JCO.2017.35.4_suppl.94

32. Li Q, Jiang H, Li H, et al. Efficacy of trastuzumab beyond progression in HER2 positive advanced gastric cancer: a multicenter prospective observational cohort study. *Oncotarget.* 2016;7:50656–50665. doi:10.18632/oncotarget.10456

33. Makiyama A, Sagara K, Kawada J, et al. A randomized phase II study of weekly paclitaxel ± trastuzumab in patients with HER2-positive advanced gastric or gastro-esophageal junction cancer refractory to trastuzumab combined with fluoropyrimidine and platinum: WJOG7112G (T-ACT). *J Clin Oncol.* 2018;36:4011–4011. doi:10.1200/JCO.2018.36.15_suppl.4011

34. Lordick F, Kang Y-K, Chung H-C, et al. Capecitabine and cisplatin with or without cetuximab for patients with previously untreated advanced gastric cancer (EXPAND): a randomised, open-label phase 3 trial. *Lancet Oncol.* 2013;14:490–499. doi:10.1016/s1470-2045(13)70102-5

35. Waddell T, Chau I, Cunningham D, et al. Epirubicin, oxaliplatin, and capecitabine with or without panitumumab for patients with previously untreated advanced oesophagogastric cancer (REAL3): a randomised, open-label phase 3 trial. *Lancet Oncol.* 2013;14:481–489. doi:10.1016/s1470-2045(13)70096-2

36. Hecht JR, Bang Y-J, Qin SK, et al. Lapatinib in combination with capecitabine plus oxaliplatin in human epidermal growth factor receptor 2-positive advanced or metastatic gastric, esophageal, or gastroesophageal adenocarcinoma: TRIO-013/LOGiC--a randomized phase III trial. *J Clin Oncol.* 2016;34:443–451. doi:10.1200/jco.2015.62.6598

37. Satoh T, Xu R-H, Chung HC, et al. Lapatinib plus paclitaxel versus paclitaxel alone in the second-line treatment of HER2-amplified advanced gastric cancer in Asian populations: TyTAN--a randomized, phase III study. *J Clin Oncol.* 2014;32:2039–2049. doi:10.1200/jco.2013.53.6136

38. Thuss-Patience PC, Shah TA, Ohtsu A, et al. Trastuzumab emtansine versus taxane use for previously treated HER2-positive locally advanced or metastatic gastric or gastro-oesophageal junction adenocarcinoma (GATSBY): an international randomised, open-label, adaptive, phase 2/3 study. *Lancet Oncol.* 2017;18:640–653. doi:10.1016/s1470-2045(17)30111-0

39. Van Cutsem E, de Haas S, Kang Y-K, et al. Bevacizumab in combination with chemotherapy as first-line therapy in advanced gastric cancer: a biomarker evaluation from the AVAGAST randomized phase III trial. *J Clin Oncol.* 2012;30:2119–2127. doi:10.1200/jco.2011.39.9824

40. Ohtsu A, Ajani JA, Bai Y-X, et al. Everolimus for previously treated advanced gastric cancer: results of the randomized, double-blind, phase III GRANITE-1 study. *J Clin Oncol.* 2013;31:3935–3943. doi:10.1200/jco.2012.48.3552

41. Fuchs CS, Tabernero J, Al-Batran S, et al. A randomized, double-blind, placebo-controlled phase III study of cisplatin plus a fluoropyrimidine with or without ramucirumab as first-line therapy in patients with metastatic gastric or gastroesophageal junction (GEJ) adenocarcinoma (RAINFALL, NCT02314117). *J Clin Oncol.* 2016;34:TPS178–TPS178, doi:10.1200/jco.2016.34.4_suppl.tps178

42. Wilke H, Muro K, Van Cutsem E, et al. Ramucirumab plus paclitaxel versus placebo plus paclitaxel in patients with previously treated advanced gastric or gastro-oesophageal junction adenocarcinoma (RAINBOW): a double-blind, randomised phase 3 trial. *Lancet Oncol.* 2014;15:1224–1235. doi:10.1016/s1470-2045(14)70420-6

43. Fuchs CS, Tomasek T, Yong CJ, et al. Ramucirumab monotherapy for previously treated advanced gastric or gastro-oesophageal junction adenocarcinoma (REGARD): an international, randomised, multicentre, placebo-controlled, phase 3 trial. *Lancet.* 2014;383:31–39. doi:10.1016/s0140-6736(13)61719-5

44. Ford HE, Marshall A, Bridgewater JA, et al. Docetaxel versus active symptom control for refractory oesophagogastric adenocarcinoma (COUGAR-02): an open-label, phase 3 randomised controlled trial. *Lancet Oncol.* 2014;15:78–86. doi:10.1016/s1470-2045(13)70549-7

45. Thuss-Patience PC, Kretzschmar A, Bichev D, et al. Survival advantage for irinotecan versus best supportive care as second-line chemotherapy in gastric cancer--a randomised phase III study of the Arbeitsgemeinschaft Internistische Onkologie (AIO). *Eur J Cancer.* 2011;47:2306–2314. doi:10.1016/j.ejca.2011.06.002

46. Hironaka S, Ueda S, Yasui H, et al. Randomized, open-label, phase III study comparing irinotecan with paclitaxel in patients with advanced gastric cancer without severe peritoneal metastasis after failure of prior combination chemotherapy using fluoropyrimidine plus platinum: WJOG 4007 trial. *J Clin Oncol.* 2013;31:4438–4444. doi:10.1200/jco.2012.48.5805

47. Li J, Qin S, Xu J, et al. Randomized, double-blind, placebo-controlled phase III trial of apatinib in patients with chemotherapy-refractory advanced or metastatic adenocarcinoma of the stomach or gastroesophageal junction. *J Clin Oncol.* 2016;34:1448–1454. doi:10.1200/jco.2015.63.5995

How I Treat Metastatic Gastric and Esophageal Cancer With Immunotherapy

Curtis R. Chong and Yelena Y. Janjigian

INTRODUCTION

In 2018 in the United States, an estimated 17,290 and 26,240 patients will be diagnosed with cancer of the esophagus and stomach, respectively, and of these 15,850 and 10,800 patients will die (1). Although improvements in sanitation and diet and *Helicobacter pylori* (*H. pylori*) eradication have decreased the incidence of new gastric cancer cases worldwide, the incidence of tumors of the gastric cardia and gastroesophageal junction (GEJ) has increased, possibly due to greater obesity and reflux disease (2). Notably, there is a rising incidence of the diffuse/infiltrative subtype of gastric cancer, which has a worse prognosis and affects younger patients compared to the intestinal subtype (3).

At the time of diagnosis, patients are often surgically incurable, highlighting the need for systemic therapy. Traditional treatment approaches to metastatic esophagogastric cancer include cytotoxic chemotherapy and monoclonal antibodies that target human epidermal growth factor receptor 2 (HER2) or vascular endothelial growth factor receptor 2 (VEGFR2) (4,5). Currently approved frontline therapies are associated with objective response rates (ORRs) in the frontline setting of approximately 30% to 50%, with few complete responses. Toxicity also limits the use of these regimens, with the incidence of grade 3 or 4 adverse events of up to 77% seen for platinum doublets, with a significant number of patients discontinuing treatment due to renal toxicity or neuropathy (6–8). Despite advances in treatment, the current prognosis for patients with esophageal and esophagogastric junction cancers is grim, with reported 5-year survival in 2016 of approximately 10% (9). In the United States and Europe, the median overall survival (OS) for metastatic esophagogastric cancer is approximately 8 to 11 months, highlighting the need for new treatments (7).

The recent approval by the U.S. Food and Drug Administration (FDA) of pembrolizumab in the treatment of refractory PD-L1 overexpressing (≥ 1%) gastric tumors and in microsatellite instability high (MSI-H) or mismatch repair (MMR) deficient solid tumors has ushered in the era of immunotherapy in the management of these cancers. In this review, we discuss the scientific rationale for the use of immunotherapy in esophagogastric cancer, interpret recently published clinical trial data, and summarize ongoing and future approaches to treatment.

MOLECULAR CLUES MAY EXPLAIN SUSCEPTIBILITY TO IMMUNOTHERAPY

Comprehensive genomic profiling has identified four molecular subtypes of gastric cancers that may predict differing susceptibility to immunotherapies (10). Epstein–Barr virus (EBV) positive tumors, which are strongly associated with *PIK3CA* mutations and PD-L1/2 overexpression, tend to occur in the gastric body/fundus. The diffuse histologic subtype of gastric cancer is enriched with tumors with genomically stable DNA, as defined by the degree of aneuploidy. Tumors characterized by chromosomal instability and by *p53* mutations/*EGFR* amplification tend to be found in the GEJ/cardia. A fourth subgroup, characterized by high MSI, tends to be diagnosed in older patients. Genomic profiling of esophageal cancers reveals that tumors with squamous histology are genetically similar to squamous cell carcinomas of other organs (11).

A Clinical Vignette ("How I Treat") is included at the end of the chapter.

In contrast, esophageal adenocarcinomas are similar to the chromosomally unstable variant of gastric adenocarcinoma. The high incidence of genomic alterations in esophagogastric cancers may render these tumors more susceptible to immunotherapies (12). In particular, esophageal cancers have been shown to have the fourth highest prevalence of somatic mutation, behind melanoma and lung and bladder cancers, which are known to be highly responsive to immunotherapy (13).

Chronic inflammation from acid reflux or toxins like alcohol or tobacco and exposure to pathogenic bacteria such as *H. pylori* contribute to the pathogenesis of esophagogastric cancer (14). One possible response to chronic inflammation is immune modulation that may allow for tumor growth and survival. Specifically, myeloid-derived suppressor cells, regulatory T-cells, and Th17 cells create an immunosuppressed environment, which helps tumor cells evade the immune system (14). Approximately 42% of gastric cancers express PD-L1 (15). Within the tumor microenvironment of esophagogastric cancer, high expression of the immune checkpoint receptors PD-L1 and CTLA-4 is associated with a poor prognosis (16–18). In contrast, the presence of tumor-infiltrating immune cells correlates with improved survival, suggesting the immune system plays a role in controlling tumor growth (19). There may also be differences in the tumor microenvironment between Asian and non-Asian populations. Gene expression profiling of 1,016 gastric cancers from a diverse patient population shows an enrichment of signatures related to T-cells, including CTLA-4 signaling and decreased inhibitor FOXP3 in non-Asian patients (20).

IMMUNOTHERAPY OF ESOPHAGOGASTRIC CANCER

Agents that target the PD1 checkpoint receptor have become the standard of care in the treatment of refractory esophagogastric cancer, with the approval of pembrolizumab for PD-L1 overexpressing (≥ 1%) gastric tumors, and pembrolizumab for MSI-H, MMR deficient esophagogastric tumors. PD-1 is a member of the CD28/CTLA-4 IgG superfamily of transmembrane receptors that, upon engagement of its ligands PD-L1 or PD-L2, negatively regulate T-cell receptor signaling (21). Pembrolizumab and nivolumab are FDA-approved humanized monoclonal antibodies that disrupt the interaction between PD-1 and PD-L1 or PD-L2. Atezolizumab, avelumab, and durvalumab are monoclonal antibodies directed against PD-L1 and are currently undergoing clinical testing in esophagogastric cancer.

The efficacy of anti-PD1 therapy in esophagogastric tumors with MMR deficiency and/or MSI-H was demonstrated in a phase II study of pembrolizumab that showed an ORR of 53% and a complete response rate of 21% (22,23). Of 32 tumor types tested for MMR deficiency, gastric adenocarcinoma had the second highest incidence of MMR deficiency, compared to esophageal/GEJ tumors, which ranked third from last (22). Analysis of 149 patients with MSI-H or MMR deficient tumors from five single-arm clinical trials of pembrolizumab, which included six patients with esophagogastric cancer, demonstrated a response rate of 39.6%, with 7% complete responses. Nivolumab was also found to be effective in patients with MMR deficient/MSI-H colorectal cancers and is FDA-approved in this patient population.

In September 2017, based on results of KEYNOTE-059, the FDA granted accelerated approval for pembrolizumab for the treatment of PD-L1 positive (≥1%) gastric/GEJ adenocarcinoma after progression on ≥2 lines of chemotherapy, including platinum and fluoropyrimidine. The results of this single-arm, phase II trial are presented in Table 42.1 (24).

The median time to objective response was 2.1 months (range: 1.7–6.6); the ORRs were 16.4% in patients receiving pembrolizumab in the 3rd line and 6.4% in the 4th+ line, in the overall population. Only 7 patients in the study were MSI-H, and 4 experienced an objective response, compared to 15 of 157 patients with MSI-low tumors. Treatment-related adverse events were typical for anti-PD1 therapy. Notably, median OS in the study population was 9.9 months for patients with an Eastern Cooperative Oncology Group (ECOG) status of 0 versus 3.8 months for an ECOG status of 1. In contrast to the results of this trial, KEYNOTE-061, a phase III trial comparing second-line pembrolizumab versus paclitaxel in PD-L1 ≥1% patients after progression on fluoropyrimidine and platinum failed to show a progression-free survival (PFS) or OS benefit.

A clinical trial of nivolumab in the 3rd+ line setting in Asian patients with GEJ cancer showed an OS of 5.3 months compared to 4.1 months with a 26% versus 11% 1-year OS and an 11% versus 0% response rate (25). The time to response was approximately 6 weeks, and the duration of response 9.5 months. There was no statistically significant difference in OS between placebo or nivolumab treatment when stratified by PD-L1 expression, and this may be because

TABLE 42.1 Results of Keynote-059: Pembrolizumab in Patients With Progression on ≥2 Lines of Chemotherapy

	Overall Population	PD-L1 ≥1%	PD-L1 Negative
Median overall survival	5.6 months	5.8 months	4.9 months
Objective response rate (third-line patients only)	11.6% (16.4%)	15.5% (22.7%)	6.4% (8.6%)
Complete response rate	2.3%	2%	2.8%
Median duration of response	8.4 months	16.3 months	6.9 months

tissue samples were only available for 40% of the patients in the study. Encouraging results have also been presented for durvalumab (26) and avelumab (27) in esophagogastric cancer.

Single-agent ipilimumab in the maintenance setting after first-line chemotherapy showed no improvement in OS, and only one of 18 patients with metastatic esophagogastric cancer benefited from tremelimumab (28). One potential way to increase the potency of immunotherapy is to combine an agent that targets PD1/PDL1 with an anti-CTLA-4 antibody. Indeed, the addition of ipilimumab to nivolumab in refractory esophagogastric cancer improved the response rate regardless of PDL1 status in the phase I/II Checkmate-032 study; however, an OS benefit was only seen in patients with PD-L1 ≥1% (Table 42.2) (29).

The response rate for N1 + I3 in PD-L1 ≥1% patients compares favorably with chemotherapy in the frontline setting, with potentially improved toxicity: the incidence of grade 3/4 adverse events was 45% for immunotherapy compared to 77% generally observed with combination chemotherapy. Currently, N1 + I3 is being compared to nivolumab + a fluoropyrimidine/platinum doublet in HER2-negative patients. The combination of chemotherapy with immunotherapy may prove synergistic through inducing tumor hypermutation or activating the immune system. For example, fluoropyrimidines increase T-cell activation, decrease tumor-associated myeloid-derived suppressor cells, and increase tumor-infiltrating lymphocytes. In preclinical models, cisplatin triggers release of antigens involved in immunogenic cell death.

Nivolumab was found to have efficacy in refractory squamous cell carcinoma of the esophagus, with a response rate of 17%, a disease control rate of 42%, a PFS of 1.5 months, and a median OS of 10.8 months, in a single-arm phase II trial conducted in Japan (30). Based on these findings, a phase III trial comparing nivolumab to taxane therapy in patients is under way (NCT02569242).

Trastuzumab plays a central role in the treatment of *HER2*-overexpressing esophagogastric cancers. The phase IB KNO14-PANACEA trial (NCT02129556) demonstrated that the combination of trastuzumab is safe. A phase II clinical trial exploring the addition of pembrolizumab to fluoropyrimidine, platinum, and trastuzumab is currently under way (NCT02901301). This study draws on a potential synergistic interaction between trastuzumab, which enhances NK cell cytotoxicity, and pembrolizumab, which activates the immune system.

Agents targeting PD1/PDL1 are also being studied in combination with chemotherapy + radiation in potentially curable esophagogastric cancer. For example, durvalumab, which targets PD-L1, is being tested in the neoadjuvant treatment of resectable esophageal/GEJ adenocarcinoma, combined with carboplatin + paclitaxel + RT followed by adjuvant durvalumab (NCT02962063). A similar study is being performed in patients with nivolumab in esophageal cancer (NCT03044613).

TABLE 42.2 Response Rates from Checkmate-032

	Nivolumab 3 mg/ kg q2wk (N1)	Nivolumab 1 mg/kg + Ipilimumab 3 mg/kg q3wk (N1 + I3)	Nivolumab 3 mg/kg + Ipilimumab 1 mg/kg q3wk (N3 + I1)
PD-L1 <1%	12%	24%	0
PD-L1 ≥1%	19%	40%	23%
18-Month Overall Survival PD-L1 ≥1%			
	13%	50%	15%

FUTURE DIRECTIONS

Despite the success of PD1 inhibitors and promising initial results from combination chemoimmunotherapy, treatment of metastatic esophagogastric cancer remains palliative.

Future immunotherapies against gastric adenocarcinoma may be directed against coinhibitory ligands like B7-H3/CD276, HHLA2, galectin 3 and 9, and B76, which are upregulated within the tumor microenvironment (31,32). Additional diagnostic tests such as T-cell receptor and whole-exome sequencing, cell surface markers, serum chemokines/cytokines, peripheral blood mononuclear cell phenotype, lymphocyte subsets, and gene/protein expression patterns may help predict which patients will respond to immunotherapy. Given the direct interaction of the stomach/esophagus with the outside environment, the microbiome may play an important role in determining the response to immunotherapy. CAR T-cells directed against esophagogastric tumors will hopefully increase the number of patients who are able to achieve remission. Our prediction is that within the next 5 years the treatment of esophagogastric cancer will involve combinations of immunotherapy, chemotherapy, and/or targeted agents in patients highly selected by tumor and immune markers.

Clinical Vignette 42.1

A 47-year-old man with a history of hyperlipidemia and diet-controlled diabetes presents with dysphagia, anemia, and guaiac positive stools. The patient reports no smoking history and very rare alcohol use. Endoscopy reveals a 4 cm ulcerated mass at the gastric cardia that on biopsy is an HER2-negative (IHC), poorly differentiated invasive adenocarcinoma. CT of the chest/abdomen/pelvis reveals a 5.8 × 4.9 cm mass along the lesser curvature of the gastric cardia/fundus, with a 1.3 cm regional lymph node. Diagnostic laparoscopy reveals a tumor on the serosal surface, and adenocarcinoma is found on biopsy of a retroperitoneal lymph node. The patient undergoes treatment with palliative FOLFOX with a partial response; oxaliplatin is stopped after 11 cycles due to neuropathy. After a further 13 cycles of 5-FU/leucovorin, disease progression occurs in the primary gastric tumor and in the retroperitoneal lymph nodes. The patient is further treated with 22 cycles of docetaxel + 5-FU with a partial response before progression occurs with the gastric mass invading the caudate lobe of the liver (Figure 42.1A). Comprehensive genomic profiling reveals *KRAS* G12D and *PIK3CA* T1052K mutations.

The patient was found to be positive for EBV RNA by fluorescence in situ hybridization (FISH), and the *PIK3CA* mutation seen in this patient is common in EBV+ tumors. In 2014, the patient was enrolled in a phase II clinical trial of nivolumab (3 mg/kg) +

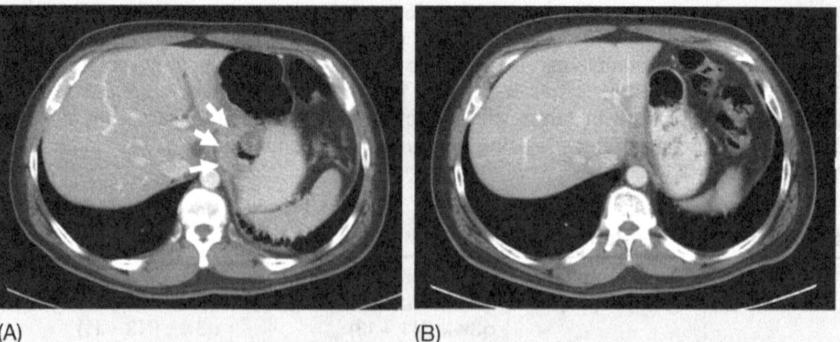

(A)   (B)

FIGURE 42.1   (A) Pretreatment CT scan demonstrates invasion of the liver by the primary gastric tumor (arrows). **(B)** Treatment effect of maintenance nivolumab demonstrates complete resolution of tumor invasion.

ipilimumab (1 mg/kg) × 4 cycles followed by nivolumab maintenance with resolution of the tumor invading the liver (Figure 42.1B). As of July 2018, the patient has stable disease in aortocaval lymph nodes and has tolerated 83 further cycles of maintenance nivolumab without toxicity.

REFERENCES

1. Siegel RL, Miller KD, Jemal A. Cancer statistics, 2018. *CA Cancer J Clin*. 2018;68(1):7–30. doi:10.33 22/caac.21442
2. Bertuccio P, Chatenoud L, Levi F, et al. Recent patterns in gastric cancer: a global overview. *Int J Cancer*. 2009;125(3):666–673 doi 10.1002/ijc.24290
3. Ikeda Y, Mori M, Kamakura T, et al. Improvements in diagnosis have changed the incidence of histological types in advanced gastric cancer. *Br J Cancer*. 1995;72(2):424–426. doi:10.1038/bjc.1995.349
4. Ajani JA, D'Amico TA, Almhanna K, et al. Esophageal and esophagogastric junction cancers, version 1.2015. *J Natl Compr Canc Netw*. 2015;13(2):194–227. doi:10.6004/jnccn.2015.0028
5. Ajani JA, D'Amico TA, Almhanna K, et al. Gastric Cancer, Version 3.2016, NCCN Clinical Practice Guidelines in Oncology. *J Natl Compr Canc Netw*. 2016;14(10):1286–1312. doi:10.6004/jnccn.2016.0137
6. Cunningham D, Starling N, Rao S, et al. Capecitabine and oxaliplatin for advanced esophago-gastric cancer. *N Engl J Med*. 2008;358(1):36–46. doi 10.1056/NEJMoa073149
7. Ohtsu A, Shah MA, Van Cutsem E, et al. Bevacizumab in combination with chemotherapy as first-line therapy in advanced gastric cancer: a randomized, double-blind, placebo-controlled phase III study. *J Clin Oncol*. 2011;29(30):3968–3976. doi:10.1200/JCO.2011.36.2236
8. Van Cutsem E, Moiseyenko VM, Tjulandin S, et al. Phase III study of docetaxel and cisplatin plus fluorouracil compared with cisplatin and fluorouracil as first-line therapy for advanced gastric cancer: a report of the V325 Study Group. *J Clin Oncol*. 2006;24(31):4991–4997. doi:10.1200/JCO.2006.06.8429
9. Rice TW, Ishwaran H, Hofstetter WL, et al. Recommendations for pathologic staging (pTNM) of cancer of the esophagus and esophagogastric junction for the 8th edition AJCC/UICC staging manuals. *Dis Esophagus*. 2016;29(8):897–905. doi:10.1111/dote.12533
10. Cancer Genome Atlas Research Network. Comprehensive molecular characterization of gastric adenocarcinoma. *Nature*. 2014;513(7517):202–209. doi:10.1038/nature13480
11. Cancer Genome Atlas Research Network, Analysis Working Group: Asian University, BC Cancer Agency, et al. Integrated genomic characterization of oesophageal carcinoma. *Nature*. 2017;541(7636):169–175. doi:10.1038/nature20805
12. Ajani JA, Lee J, Sano T, et al. Gastric adenocarcinoma. *Nat Rev Dis Primers*. 2017;3:17036. doi:10.1038/nrdp.2017.36
13. Alexandrov LB, Nik-Zainal S, Wedge DC, et al. Signatures of mutational processes in human cancer. *Nature*. 2013;500(7463):415–421. doi:10.1038/nature12477
14. Lin EW, Karakasheva TA, Hicks PD, et al. The tumor microenvironment in esophageal cancer. *Oncogene*. 2016;35(41):5337–5349. doi:10.1038/onc.2016.34
15. Wu C, Zhu Y, Jiang J, et al. Immunohistochemical localization of programmed death-1 ligand-1 (PD-L1) in gastric carcinoma and its clinical significance. *Acta Histochem*. 2006;108(1):19–24. doi:10.1016/j.acthis.2006.01.003
16. Ohigashi Y, Sho M, Yamada Y, et al. Clinical significance of programmed death-1 ligand-1 and programmed death-1 ligand-2 expression in human esophageal cancer. *Clin Cancer Res*. 2005;11(8):2947–2953. doi:10.1158/1078-0432.CCR-04-1469
17. Schlosser HA, Drebber U, Kloth M, et al. Immune checkpoints programmed death 1 ligand 1 and cytotoxic T lymphocyte associated molecule 4 in gastric adenocarcinoma. *Oncoimmunology*. 2016;5(5):e1100789. doi:10.1080/2162402X.2015.1100789
18. Wu P, Wu D, Li L, et al. PD-L1 and Survival in solid tumors: a meta-analysis. *PLoS One*. 2015;10(6):e0131403. doi:10.1371/journal.pone.0131403
19. Jiang W, Liu K, Guo Q, et al. Tumor-infiltrating immune cells and prognosis in gastric cancer: a systematic review and meta-analysis. *Oncotarget*. 2017;8(37):62312–62329. doi:10.18632/oncotarget.17602
20. Lin SJ, Gagnon-Bartsch JA, Tan IB, et al. Signatures of tumour immunity distinguish Asian and non-Asian gastric adenocarcinomas. *Gut*. 2015;64(11):1721–1731. doi:10.1136/gutjnl-2014-308252

21. Freeman GJ, Long AJ, Iwai Y, et al. Engagement of the PD-1 immunoinhibitory receptor by a novel B7 family member leads to negative regulation of lymphocyte activation. *J Exp Med*. 2000;192(7):1027–1034. doi:10.1084/jem.192.7.1027

22. Le DT, Durham JN, Smith KN, et al. Mismatch repair deficiency predicts response of solid tumors to PD-1 blockade. *Science*. 2017;357(6349):409–413. doi:10.1126/science.aan6733

23. Le DT, Uram JN, Wang H, et al. PD-1 blockade in tumors with mismatch-repair deficiency. *N Engl J Med*. 2015;372(26):2509–2520. doi:10.1056/NEJMoa1500596

24. Fuchs CS, Doi T, Jang RW, et al. Safety and efficacy of pembrolizumab monotherapy in patients with previously treated advanced gastric and gastroesophageal junction cancer: phase 2 clinical KEYNOTE-059 trial. *JAMA Oncol*. 2018;4(5):e180013. doi:10.1001/jamaoncol.2018.0013

25. Kang YK, Boku N, Satoh T, et al. Nivolumab in patients with advanced gastric or gastro-oesophageal junction cancer refractory to, or intolerant of, at least two previous chemotherapy regimens (ONO-4538-12, ATTRACTION-2): a randomised, double-blind, placebo-controlled, phase 3 trial. *Lancet*. 2017;390(10111):2461–2471. doi:10.1016/S0140-6736(17)31827-5

26. Segal NH, Hamid O, Hwu W, et al. A Phase I multi-arm dose-expansion study of the anti-programmed cell death-ligand-1 (PD-L1) antibody medi4736: preliminary data. *Ann Oncol*. 2014;25(suppl_4):iv365.

27. Chung HC, Arkenau H-T, Wyrwicz L, et al. Safran Safety, PD-L1 expression, and clinical activity of avelumab (MSB0010718C), an anti-PD-L1 antibody, in patients with advanced gastric or gastroesophageal junction cancer. *J Clin Oncol*. 2016;34(4_suppl):167. doi:10.1200/jco.2016.34.4_suppl.167

28. Ralph C, Elkord E, Burt DJ, et al. Modulation of lymphocyte regulation for cancer therapy: a phase II trial of tremelimumab in advanced gastric and esophageal adenocarcinoma. *Clin Cancer Res*. 2010;16(5):1662–1672. doi:10.1158/1078-0432.CCR-09-2870

29. Janjigian YY, Ott PA, Calvo E, et al. Nivolumab ± ipilimumab in pts with advanced (adv)/metastatic chemotherapy-refractory (CTx-R) gastric (G), esophageal (E), or gastroesophageal junction (GEJ) cancer: CheckMate 032 study. *J Clin Oncol*. 2017;35(15_suppl):4014. doi:10.1200/jco.2017.35.15_suppl.4014

30. Kudo T, Hamamoto Y, Kato K, et al. Nivolumab treatment for oesophageal squamous-cell carcinoma: an open-label, multicentre, phase 2 trial. *Lancet Oncol*. 2017;18(5):631–639. doi:10.1016/S1470-2045(17)30181-X

31. Janakiram M, Chinai JM, Fineberg S, et al. Expression, clinical significance, and receptor identification of the newest B7 family member HHLA2 protein. *Clin Cancer Res*. 2015;21(10):2359–2366. doi:10.1158/1078-0432.CCR-14-1495

32. Kouo T, Huang L, Pucsek AB, et al. Galectin-3 shapes antitumor immune responses by suppressing CD8+ T Cells via LAG-3 and inhibiting expansion of plasmacytoid dendritic cells. *Cancer Immunol Res*. 2015;3(4):412–423. doi:10.1158/2326-6066.CIR-14-0150

V

Rare Gastrointestinal Cancers

Molecular Diagnostic Guidelines of Cancers of the Bile Ducts and Gallbladder

Talal Hilal and Mitesh J. Borad

EPIDEMIOLOGY

Cancers of the bile ducts encompass a heterogeneous group of epithelial malignancies broadly divided into cholangiocarcinoma (CC) and gallbladder cancer (GBC). CC is the second most common primary hepatic neoplasm, after hepatocellular carcinoma, and is classified anatomically as intrahepatic cholangiocarcinoma (IHCCA) and extrahepatic cholangiocarcinoma (EHCCA). Historically, the majority of CCs were derived from EHCCA in the perihilar (50%) and distal (40%) region of the biliary tree (1). Although IHCCA constituted the minority of all cases, the incidence of IHCCA has been increasing over the past three decades while the incidence of EHCCA has remained stable (2). The peak age at diagnosis for CC is between ages 55 and 75 years. Unlike hepatocellular carcinoma, which is 5 to 6 times more prevalent in men, CC appears to have only a slight male predominance with female:male incidence rate ratios of 0.80 (95% confidence interval [CI]: 0.75–0.84) for IHCCA and 0.64 (95% CI: 0.61–0.68) for EHCCA (3). Worldwide, the highest prevalence is seen in Southeast Asia (4).

GBC is the most common biliary tract malignancy (5,6). The U.S. incidence rates of GBC are 0.9 and 0.5 per 100,000 females and males, respectively (7). Furthermore, there appear to be racial differences in incidence with American Indians/Alaskan natives, Asian/ Pacific Islanders, Blacks, and Hispanics having a higher incidence compared with non-Hispanic Whites (8). The mean age at diagnosis is 65 years with a female predominance (5).

RISK FACTORS

Chronic biliary tract inflammation is an established risk factor for both CC (9) and GBC (5). Some specific risk factors for CC include primary sclerosing cholangitis (PSC), intrahepatic lithiasis, and parasite infections such as *Clonorchis sinensis* and *Opisthorchis viverrini*. Chronic hepatitis B viral infection, hepatitis C viral infection, obesity, diabetes mellitus, and alcohol have also been described as risk factors specific for IHCCA (9). Most GBCs are adenocarcinomas arising from the gallbladder mucosa. Some specific risk factors include gallstones, gallbladder polyps, and porcelain gallbladder (5).

DIAGNOSIS

Tumor Markers

Carbohydrate antigen 19-9 (CA 19-9) is the most popular circulating marker for biliary and pancreatic malignancy. A raised CA 19-9 concentration has been shown to have a sensitivity of 77% and specificity of 87% for CC (10). However, there are drawbacks to this tumor marker. First, expression of CA 19-9 depends on the Lewis phenotype, and 7% of the population is negative for Lewis antigen (11). Second, CA 19-9 is elevated in pancreatic cancer, gastric cancer, cholangitis, or cholestasis (12). In these clinical scenarios, the specificity of the test is markedly reduced. Third, CA 19-9 is not of great utility in differentiating between benign strictures and CC in patients with PSC (13).

Carcinoembryonic antigen (CEA) has poor sensitivity and specificity (14). Serum cytokeratin 19 fragments measured using the CYFRA 21-1 assay have been shown to be elevated in CC with a sensitivity of 74% and specificity of 92% in a small case series (15). Further data evaluating CYFRA 21-1 and CA 19-9 have shown that a CYFRA 21-1 cutoff ≥1.5 ng/mL has a sensitivity of 56%, while a cut-off >3.0 ng/mL has a sensitivity of 30%. The specificity is high, however, at 88% and 97%, respectively. The combination of CYFRA 21-1 (>1.5 ng/mL) and CA 19-9 (>37 U/mL) resulted in a sensitivity and specificity of 45% and 96%, respectively (16). CYFRA 21-1 appears to be a better marker of prognosis rather than diagnosis, though it may be reasonable to use it as part of a diagnostic panel (including CA 19-9) given the high specificity.

Immunohistochemistry and In Situ Hybridization

Histopathologic differences between IHCCA and metastatic adenocarcinoma to the liver are subtle. A keratin profile of CK7+, CK19+, and CK20– is typical, but is common in other metastatic adenocarcinomas making IHC nonspecific.

Albumin was identified as the potential marker of IHCCA given its abundant and highly specific RNA expression in cells of hepatocyte origin. A branched-DNA platform for albumin RNA in situ hybridization was evaluated as a diagnostic modality to distinguish IHCCA from metastatic adenocarcinoma to the liver. Ferrone et al. reported a sensitivity of 99% for IHCCA and 100% for HCC. Perihilar and distal CC as well as metastatic carcinomas tested negative for albumin. Importantly, 22% of intrahepatic tumors previously diagnosed as carcinomas of undetermined primary tested positive for albumin and were reclassified as IHCCA (17).

Biliary Strictures and Molecular Markers

The distinction between a benign biliary stricture and a malignant one, which may represent a perihilar and distal CC (EHCCA), can be difficult. In patients with PSC, benign strictures are common, but the incidence of CC is significantly higher compared to the general population. Other nonmalignant causes such as choledocholithiasis, ischemia, and pancreatitis need to be considered. Routine cytology and intraductal forceps biopsy are often required to make a diagnosis of malignancy. However, the sensitivity of this modality is between 20% and 65% (18–20).

Aneuploid/aneusomic cells are markers of malignancy, but can be seen in premalignant lesions (e.g., colonic adenomas). In the biliary ducts, inflammation and cellular proliferation are rarely associated with aneuploidy/aneusomy. Therefore, molecular markers, such as digital image analysis (DIA) and fluorescence in situ hybridization (FISH), have been evaluated as methods for improving the accuracy of nonsurgical diagnosis of biliary strictures by detecting and quantifying abnormalities of nuclear DNA and loss or gain of chromosomes, respectively (21). Approximately 80% of biliary cancers exhibit aneuploidy (22). Based on these data, when routine cytology is negative, the addition of DIA and FISH serves as additional methods of detecting chromosomal instability (23).

In the study by Levy et al., the sensitivity of DIA was comparable to routine cytology for patients with PSC and higher than routine cytology for patients without PSC. In the overall population (PSC and non-PSC), FISH provided the greatest sensitivity when considering trisomy 7 as a marker of benign disease (45%). The specificity values for DIA and FISH were 95% and 100%, respectively. The composite DIA/FISH result increased diagnostic sensitivity one- to fivefold over routine cytology. Importantly, the negative predictive value of DIA, FISH, and composite DIA/FISH ranged from 56% to 70% (21).

Fritcher et al. have shown in another large clinical study that FISH was more sensitive than routine cytology for detecting biliary tract cancer. FISH was able to detect 49/227 (22%) cases of cancers that routine cytology interpreted as nonmalignant without compromising specificity. Specificity decreases substantially if trisomy 7 is included as a criterion for malignancy because only 50% of patients with trisomy 7 subsequently develop cancer on follow-up (24).

KRAS gene alterations have been identified in CC specimens (20%–100%) (14). In an effort to further improve the diagnostic accuracy using advanced molecular markers, testing for KRAS alterations was evaluated by Kipp et al. (25) who compared the performance of KRAS mutation analysis to cytology and FISH. The most common KRAS mutations are in codons 12 and 13, and less frequently, codon 61 (26). The study included patients with pancreatic adenocarcinoma and CC. Within the CC cohort, the sensitivity for KRAS mutation testing was 30% and improved to 54% with the combination of KRAS/FISH (only polysomic FISH results). The specificity of KRAS testing was 96% and combination KRAS/FISH was 96% (25).

Molecular Characteristics on Comprehensive Genomic Profiling
A large number of genetic alterations have been described in biliary tract cancers. Some of these alterations are relevant therapeutic targets that are currently under evaluation in clinical trials (27). However, they may also serve as an adjunct in diagnosis in some cases.

Isocitrate dehydrogenase (IDH) mutations (e.g., IDH1, IDH2) are more frequently observed in IHCCA (10%–28%) compared to EHCCA (28,29). Mutations in IDH1 or IDH2 were associated with longer overall survival and were independently associated with a longer time to recurrence after resection of IHCCA (30). Fibroblast growth factor receptor 2 (FGFR2) alterations are found in 13% to 20% of IHCCA cases and are typically fusions. They appear to confer less aggressive disease biology and are associated with improved overall survival (31). FGFR gene fusion positive cancers have shown to enhance susceptibility to FGFR inhibitors. KRAS mutations downstream of epidermal growth factor receptor (EGFR) are frequently seen in IHCCA (8%–54%) (32). KRAS mutations are associated with poor overall survival in all patients with IHCCA (33). Overexpression of p53 is less frequent in IHCCA (18%) compared to EHCCA (38%) or GBC (61%) (34). However, inactivating mutations are common in IHCCA (21%–37%) (34,35).

CONCLUSIONS

Molecular testing has proven to be of diagnostic and potential therapeutic utility in multiple clinical scenarios, in biliary tract cancers, such as correctly diagnosing carcinomas of unknown primary as IHCCA using albumin RNA in-situ hybridization, detecting chromosomal instability and diagnosing perihilar and distal CCs using FISH on cells from biliary strictures, and exploiting alterations via investigational agents on clinical trials using comprehensive genomic profiling for identification

REFERENCES

1. DeOliveira ML, Cunningham SC, Cameron JL, et al. Cholangiocarcinoma: thirty-one-year experience with 564 patients at a single institution. *Ann Surg.* 2007;245(5):755–762. doi:10.1097/01.sla.0000251366.62632.d3
2. Rizvi S, Gores GJ. Pathogenesis, diagnosis, and management of cholangiocarcinoma. *Gastroenterology.* 2013;145(6):1215–1229. doi:10.1053/j.gastro.2013.10.013
3. Saha SK, Zhu AX, Fuchs CS, et al. Forty-year trends in cholangiocarcinoma incidence in the U.S.: intrahepatic disease on the rise. *Oncologist.* 2016;21(5):594–599. doi:10.1634/theoncologist.2015-0446
4. Weindel M, Zulfiqar M, Bhalla A, et al. Molecular diagnostics in the neoplasms of the pancreas, liver, gall bladder, and extrahepatic biliary tract. *Clin Lab Med.* 2013;33(4):875–880. doi:10.1016/j.cll.2013.08.002
5. Wernberg JA, Lucarelli DD. Gallbladder cancer. *Surg Clin North Am.* 2014;94(2):343–360. doi:10.1016/j.suc.2014.01.009
6. Wistuba, II, Gazdar AF. Gallbladder cancer: lessons from a rare tumour. *Nat Rev Cancer.* 2004;4(9):695–706. doi:10.1038/nrc1429
7. Randi G, Malvezzi M, Levi F, et al. Epidemiology of biliary tract cancers: an update. *Ann Oncol.* 2009;20(1):146–159. doi:10.1093/annonc/mdn533
8. Castro FA, Koshiol J, Hsing AW, et al. Biliary tract cancer incidence in the United States-demographic and temporal variations by anatomic site. *Int J Cancer.* 2013;133(7):1664–1671. doi:10.1002/ijc.28161
9. Krasinskas AM. Cholangiocarcinoma. *Surg Pathol Clin.* 2018;11(2):403–429. doi:10.1016/j.path.2018.02.005
10. Kim HJ, Kim MH, Myung SJ, et al. A new strategy for the application of CA19-9 in the differentiation of pancreaticobiliary cancer: analysis using a receiver operating characteristic curve. *Am J Gastroenterol.* 1999;94(7):1941–1946. doi:10.1111/j.1572-0241.1999.01234.x
11. Locker GY, Hamilton S, Harris J, et al. ASCO 2006 update of recommendations for the use of tumor markers in gastrointestinal cancer. *J Clin Oncol.* 2006;24(33):5313–5327. doi:10.1200/JCO.2006.08.2644
12. Bonney GK, Craven RA, Prasad R, et al. Circulating markers of biliary malignancy: opportunities in proteomics? *Lancet Oncol.* 2008;9(2):149–158. doi:10.1016/S1470-2045(08)70027-5
13. Marrelli D, Caruso S, Pedrazzani C, et al. CA19-9 serum levels in obstructive jaundice: clinical value in benign and malignant conditions. *Am J Surg.* 2009;198(3):333–339. doi:10.1016/j.amjsurg.2008.12.031

14. Nehls O, Gregor M, Klump B. Serum and bile markers for cholangiocarcinoma. *Semin Liver Dis.* 2004;24(2):139–154. doi:10.1055/s-2004-828891
15. Kashihara T, Ohki A, Kobayashi T, et al. Intrahepatic cholangiocarcinoma with increased serum CYFRA 21-1 level. *J Gastroenterol.* 1998;33(3):447–453. doi:10.1007/s005350050112
16. Chapman MH, Sandanayake NS, Andreola F, et al. Circulating CYFRA 21-1 is a specific diagnostic and prognostic biomarker in biliary tract cancer. *J Clin Exp Hepatol.* 2011;1(1):6–12. doi:10.1016/S0973-6883(11)60110-2
17. Ferrone CR, Ting DT, Shahid M, et al. The ability to diagnose intrahepatic cholangiocarcinoma definitively using novel branched DNA-enhanced albumin RNA in situ hybridization technology. *Ann Surg Oncol.* 2016;23(1):290–296. doi:10.1245/s10434-014-4247-8
18. Pugliese V, Conio M, Nicolo G, et al. Endoscopic retrograde forceps biopsy and brush cytology of biliary strictures: a prospective study. *Gastrointest Endosc.* 1995;42(6):520–526. doi:10.1016/S0016-5107(95)70004-8
19. de Bellis M, Sherman S, Fogel EL, et al. Tissue sampling at ERCP in suspected malignant biliary strictures (Part 1). *Gastrointest Endosc.* 2002;56(4):552–561. doi:10.1016/S0016-5107(02)70442-2
20. de Bellis M, Sherman S, Fogel EL, et al. Tissue sampling at ERCP in suspected malignant biliary strictures (Part 2). *Gastrointest Endosc.* 2002;56(5):720–730. doi:10.1016/S0016-5107(02)70123-5
21. Levy MJ, Baron TH, Clayton AC, et al. Prospective evaluation of advanced molecular markers and imaging techniques in patients with indeterminate bile duct strictures. *Am J Gastroenterol.* 2008;103(5):1263–1273. doi:10.1111/j.1572-0241.2007.01776.x
22. Bergquist A, Tribukait B, Glaumann H, et al. Can DNA cytometry be used for evaluation of malignancy and premalignancy in bile duct strictures in primary sclerosing cholangitis? *J Hepatol.* 2000;33(6):873–877. doi:10.1016/S0168-8278(00)80117-8
23. Moreno Luna LE, Kipp B, Halling KC, et al. Advanced cytologic techniques for the detection of malignant pancreatobiliary strictures. *Gastroenterology.* 2006;131(4):1064–1072. doi:10.1053/j.gastro.2006.08.021
24. Fritcher EG, Kipp BR, Halling KC, et al. A multivariable model using advanced cytologic methods for the evaluation of indeterminate pancreatobiliary strictures. *Gastroenterology.* 2009;136(7):2180–2186. doi:10.1053/j.gastro.2009.02.040
25. Kipp BR, Fritcher EG, Clayton AC, et al. Comparison of KRAS mutation analysis and FISH for detecting pancreatobiliary tract cancer in cytology specimens collected during endoscopic retrograde cholangiopancreatography. *J Mol Diagn.* 2010;12(6):780–786. doi:10.2353/jmoldx.2010.100016
26. Kamisawa T, Tsuruta K, Okamoto A, et al. Frequent and significant K-ras mutation in the pancreas, the bile duct, and the gallbladder in autoimmune pancreatitis. *Pancreas.* 2009;38(8):890–895. doi:10.1097/MPA.0b013e3181b65a1c
27. DeLeon TT, Ahn DH, Bogenberger JM, et al. Novel targeted therapy strategies for biliary tract cancers and hepatocellular carcinoma. *Future Oncol.* 2018;14(6):553–566. doi:10.2217/fon-2017-0451
28. Kipp BR, Voss JS, Kerr SE, et al. Isocitrate dehydrogenase 1 and 2 mutations in cholangiocarcinoma. *Hum Pathol.* 2012;43(10):1552–1558. doi:10.1016/j.humpath.2011.12.007
29. Farshidfar F, Zheng S, Gingras MC, et al. Integrative genomic analysis of cholangiocarcinoma identifies distinct IDH-mutant molecular profiles. *Cell Rep.* 2017;19(13):2878–2880. doi:10.1016/j.celrep.2017.06.008
30. Sia D, Tovar V, Moeini A, et al. Intrahepatic cholangiocarcinoma: pathogenesis and rationale for molecular therapies. *Oncogene.* 2013;32(41):4861–4870. doi:10.1038/onc.2012.617
31. Graham RP, Barr Fritcher EG, Pestova E, et al. Fibroblast growth factor receptor 2 translocations in intrahepatic cholangiocarcinoma. *Hum Pathol.* 2014;45(8):1630–1638. doi:10.1016/j.humpath.2014.03.014
32. Isa T, Tomita S, Nakachi A, et al. Analysis of microsatellite instability, K-ras gene mutation and p53 protein overexpression in intrahepatic cholangiocarcinoma. *Hepatogastroenterology.* 2002;49(45):604–608.
33. Jang S, Chun SM, Hong SM, et al. High throughput molecular profiling reveals differential mutation patterns in intrahepatic cholangiocarcinomas arising in chronic advanced liver diseases. *Mod Pathol.* 2014;27(5):731–739. doi:10.1038/modpathol.2013.194
34. Hsu M, Sasaki M, Igarashi S, et al. KRAS and GNAS mutations and p53 overexpression in biliary intraepithelial neoplasia and intrahepatic cholangiocarcinomas. *Cancer.* 2013;119(9):1669–1674. doi:10.1002/cncr.27955
35. Khan SA, Thomas HC, Toledano MB, et al. p53 Mutations in human cholangiocarcinoma: a review. *Liver Int.* 2005;25(4):704–716. doi:10.1111/j.1478-3231.2005.01106.x

Surgery for Early-Stage Cancers of the Bile Ducts and Gallbladder

Jordan Cloyd, Charlie Kimbrough, and Timothy M. Pawlik

INTRODUCTION

Biliary tract cancers (BTCs) are a relatively uncommon but heterogeneous group of neoplasms arising from the biliary epithelium, further classified as cholangiocarcinoma or gallbladder cancer (GBC). Cholangiocarcinomas can be further distinguished as intrahepatic cholangiocarcinoma (IHCCA), arising from the secondary bile ducts or beyond; perihilar extrahepatic cholangiocarcinoma (pCCA), occurring at the confluence of the left and right hepatic ducts; distal extrahepatic cholangiocarcinoma (dCCA), typically arising inferior to the cyst duct. While all occur relatively infrequently in the United States, GBC represents the most commonly diagnosed BTC, followed by pCCA, dCCA, and IHCCA in decreasing order (1). Although often grouped together as BTCs, each subtype of cholangiocarcinoma has distinct anatomic, genetic, molecular, and clinical features with important prognostic and therapeutic implications (2).

Despite these differences, in general, the prognosis of patients with BTCs is poor. Most patients present with advanced-stage disease with only a minority (~35%) having early-stage disease amenable to surgical resection. This has profound prognostic implications since margin-negative resection is a requisite for long-term survival (3,4). In fact, the 5-year overall survival (OS) rates of patients with any type of BTC who are unable to undergo resection are less than 5% (5). While the development of more efficacious systemic and targeted therapies will be necessary to improve the dismal survival rates for BTCs, surgical resection with or without adjuvant therapy is the preferred treatment for all patients with localized BTC when appropriate. Given their distinct anatomic and clinical features, this chapter focuses on the salient surgical considerations relevant to optimizing the outcomes of patients with early-stage GBC, IHCCA, pCCA, and dCCA.

PREOPERATIVE CONSIDERATIONS

Diagnosis

Given their heterogeneity, the clinical presentation, diagnostic evaluation, and staging of patients with BTCs vary considerably. While not always necessary to perform prior to proceeding with surgery, a preoperative histopathologic diagnosis is preferred. IHCCA most commonly presents with an intrahepatic mass, either as an incidental finding on cross-sectional imaging, as part of screening for patients with cirrhosis, or less commonly due to symptoms of pain. An arterially enhancing lesion on MRI or CT with elevation of cancer antigen 19-9 is characteristic of IHCCA; percutaneous biopsy confirms the diagnosis. Particular attention should be given to the macroscopic histologic subtype: mass-forming, infiltrative, or intraductal (Figure 44.1).

The evaluation of patients with extrahepatic cholangiocarcinoma remains a diagnostic challenge. These patients most commonly present with jaundice due to either a biliary stricture or a soft-tissue mass at the hepatic confluence. Imaging studies may include magnetic resonance cholangiopancreatography (MRCP) to delineate the degree of biliary involvement or CT, which is helpful for evaluating proximity to vascular structures. Endoscopic retrograde cholangiopancreatography (ERCP) is an alternative option for evaluating biliary tract involvement but also enables cytologic diagnosis and placement of biliary stents. Recent advances

---

A Clinical Vignette is included at the end of the chapter.

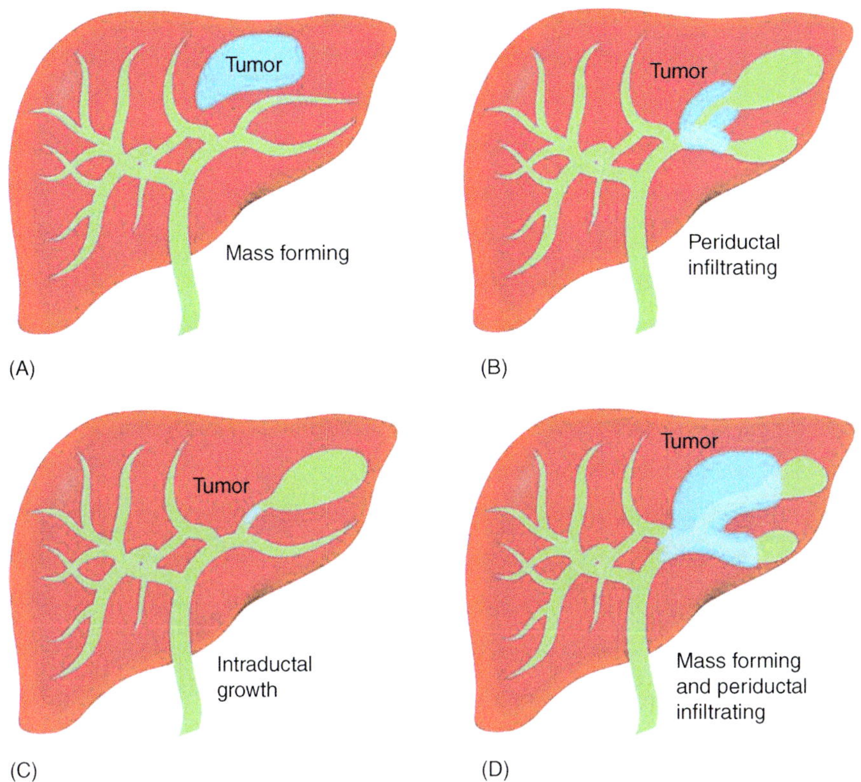

FIGURE 44.1   Macroscopic histology subtypes of intrahepatic cholangiocarcinoma.

Source: Used with permission from Brown KM, Geller DA. Surgical Management of Intra-Hepatic Cholangiocarcinoma. In: Herman J, Pawlik T, Thomas T, eds. *Biliary Tract and Gallbladder Cancer*. Medical Radiology. Springer, Berlin, Heidelberg; 2014:241–252. doi:10.1007/978-3-642-40558-7_15

in cell-based assays and molecular diagnostics have improved the diagnostic yield of biliary brushings (2). While endoscopic ultrasound (EUS) may play a role in evaluating hilar masses and/or adjacent lymph nodes, concern exists for peritoneal dissemination with EUS-guided fine-needle aspiration (FNA) (6). Finally, direct cholangioscopy, performed via ERCP, permits intraluminal evaluation and direct tissue acquisition.

GBC is a distinct entity from other BTCs and requires specialized diagnostic evaluation. The most common manifestation of GBC is an incidental finding on postoperative pathology following routine cholecystectomy. In other situations, a GBC may be incidentally encountered intraoperatively at the time of cholecystectomy. Finally, the onset of pain, vague abdominal symptoms, or even jaundice may lead to the identification of a gallbladder mass on cross-sectional imaging. In these situations, percutaneous, endoscopic, or surgical biopsies may be appropriate. In addition to MRI and CT, PET may be particularly helpful in identifying occult metastatic disease.

Staging

The American Joint Committee on Cancer (AJCC), eight edition, is used to stage BTC (Table 44.1). Staging provides important prognostic information but relies on meticulous surgical technique, stringent histopathologic review, and close long-term follow-up. Several changes have been made to the eight edition for hepatobiliary cancers (7), and early analyses suggest that the eight edition provides improved, though still imperfect, prognostication for at least some BTCs (8).

TABLE 44.1 TNM Staging of BTCs According to AJCC, Eight Edition

	Stage	IHCCA	pCCA	dCCA	GBC
T Stage	T1	Solitary tumor without vascular invasion	Confined to bile duct	Invades bile duct wall with depth <5 mm	Invades lamina propria or muscular layer
	T1a	≤5 cm	–	–	Invades lamina propria
	T1b	>5 cm	–	–	Invades muscular layer
	T2	• Solitary tumor with vascular invasion • Multifocal tumor	Invasion beyond bile duct	Invades bile duct wall with depth 5–12 mm	Invades perimuscular connective tissue
	T2a	–	To surrounding adipose tissue	–	Peritoneal side without invasion of serosa
	T2b	–	To adjacent liver parenchyma	–	Hepatic side without extension into liver
	T3	Perforates visceral peritoneum	Invades unilateral branches of PV or HA	Invades bile duct wall with depth >12 mm	• Perforates serosa • Invades liver and/or an adjacent organ/structure
	T4	Invades extrahepatic structures	• Invades main PV or bilateral branches • Invades unilateral second-order biliary radicals with contralateral PV or HA	Invades celiac axis, SMA, or HA	• Invades the main PV or HA • Invades ≥2 extrahepatic organs/structures
N Stage	N1	Left: inferior phrenic, hilar, gastrohepatic Right: hilar, periduodenal, peripancreatic	1–3 regional nodes: hilar or posterior pancreatoduodenal	1–3 regional nodes: hilar, anterior/posterior pancreatoduodenal, right lateral SMA	1–3 regional hilar nodes
	N2	–	≥4 regional nodes	≥4 regional nodes	≥4 regional nodes

(continued)

TABLE 44.1 TNM Staging of BTCs According to AJCC, Eight Edition (*continued*)

	Stage	IHCCA	pCCA	dCCA	GBC
M Stage	M1				
TNM Staging		*(see below)*	*(see below)*	*(see below)*	*(see below)*

IHCCA

T	N	M	Stage
1a	0	0	IA
1b	0	0	IB
2	0	0	II
3	0	0	IIIA
4	0	0	IIIB
Any	1	0	IIIB
Any	any	1	IV

pCCA

T	N	M	Stage
1	0	0	I
2	0	0	II
3	0	0	IIIA
4	0	0	IIIB
Any	1	0	IIIC
Any	2	0	IV
Any	any	1	IV

dCCA

T	N	M	Stage
1	0	0	I
1	1	0	IIA
1	2	0	IIIA
2	0	0	IIA
2	1	0	IIB
2	2	0	IIIA
3	0–1	0	IIB
3	2	0	IIIA
4	0–2	0	IIIB
Any	Any	1	IV

GBC

T	N	M	Stage
1	0	0	I
2a	0	0	IIA
2b	0	0	IIB
3	0	0	IIIA
1–3	1	0	IIIB
4	0–1	0	IVA
Any	2	0	IVB
Any	Any	1	IVB

AJCC, American Joint Committee on Cancer; BTC, biliary tract cancer; dCCA, distal extrahepatic cholangiocarcinoma; GBC, gallbladder cancer; HA, hepatic artery; IHCCA, intrahepatic cholangiocarcinoma; pCCA, perihilar extrahepatic cholangiocarcinoma; PV, portal vein; SMA, superior mesenteric artery; TNM, tumor, node, and metastasis.

Resectability

Although surgical resection of BTCs represents the best opportunity for long-term survival, assessing a patient's resectability is one of the important preoperative considerations a surgeon undertakes. In general, patient selection for major hepatopancreatobiliary surgery should be conducted along three domains: physiologic, oncologic, and technical. Physiologic resectability refers to the patient's capacity to safely tolerate major abdominal surgery. Severe comorbidities, poor functional status, inadequate nutrition, or underlying liver disease may indicate that a patient will not tolerate a major resection. Oncologic resectability refers to the indications for resection based on the underlying tumor biology. This may be impacted by the presence of extrahepatic disease, specific histopathologic features, degree of tumor marker elevation, response to previous therapies (if applicable), and, increasingly, the molecular features of the tumor. Finally, technical resectability is based on high-quality cross-sectional imaging and refers to the ability to achieve microscopically negative margins, while maintaining vascular inflow/outflow, biliary-enteric drainage, and an adequate future liver remnant (FLR) if liver resection is required.

If major liver resection is anticipated, accurate preoperative assessment of the FLR is critically important in order to minimize the risk of postoperative hepatic insufficiency (PHI) and mortality. Since FLR volume correlates with function and the risk of PHI, a systematic analysis of liver volumetry is imperative in patients undergoing extended hepatectomies or those with compromised liver function. Previous studies have identified FLR size thresholds at which the risk of PHI is prohibitively high: <20% in chemotherapy-naïve patients, <30% in chemotherapy-treated patients, and <40% to 50% in patients with cirrhosis (9). For those patients with inadequate FLR by volumetric analysis, preoperative portal vein embolization (PVE), which diverts portal blood flow and its inherent growth factors preferentially to the FLR, can be considered and typically results in 30% to 40% hypertrophic response for most patients (10).

Preoperative Biliary Decompression

The routine use of preoperative biliary decompression among patients with cholangiocarcinoma remains controversial. Patients with pCCA, who almost always present with hyperbilirubinemia, present the biggest challenge. Since jaundice impairs hepatic function, many prefer routine preoperative biliary decompression, especially among patients with low FLR volume, preoperative malnutrition, or cholangitis. Biliary obstruction also impairs the liver's response to PVE; so biliary decompression of the FLR, with a decrease in the bilirubin to at least a level of <5 mg/dL, is recommended prior to performing PVE (11). The optimal route of preoperative biliary drainage remains controversial. While endoscopic drainage with an internal stent may be more convenient for patients, there is a higher risk of cholangitis, occlusion, and procedural related complications compared to percutaneous drainage (12). While not typically performed in Western centers, some Japanese surgeons routinely use endoscopic nasobiliary drainage (13).

Jaundice in the setting of locally advanced GBC is a poor prognosis and a relative contraindication to surgical resection (14). These patients should undergo biliary decompression and neoadjuvant therapy, with surgical resection reserved for those patients with excellent performance status and favorable tumor biology. Biliary obstruction in the setting of IHCCA is relatively unusual and the decision to proceed with biliary drainage is made on a case-by-case basis. The evidence for preoperative biliary stenting among patients with dCCA and jaundice is typically extrapolated from studies of pancreatic ductal adenocarcinoma (PDAC). Randomized controlled trials in these populations do not support the routine use of preoperative biliary stent (15), but the individual decision should be made as part of a comprehensive multidisciplinary treatment plan.

Neoadjuvant Therapy

BTCs frequently present as locally advanced unresectable disease. While the routine use of neoadjuvant therapy in resectable BTCs has not been established, neoadjuvant therapy with an attempt to downstage patients with locally advanced disease is often employed. In reality, however, a minority of patients are successfully downstaged such that their cancers become resectable (16,17). This is likely a reflection of the relative lack of response to currently available systemic therapies. When indicated, most multidisciplinary teams have treated patients with combination gemcitabine and platinum based on the results of randomized controlled trials in the metastatic setting (18). Some have also had experience using locoregional therapies, including transarterial chemoembolization (TACE), radioembolization, or hepatic artery infusion therapy with implanted pump, to downstage patients with locally BTCs (19).

RESECTION FOR CURATIVE INTENT

Intrahepatic Cholangiocarcinoma

Curative intent surgery for IHCCA requires resection with negative margins and adequate lymphadenectomy. The need for major hepatectomy (typically defined as ≥ 3 Couinaud segments) should be anticipated based on the preoperative size, location, subtype, and number of tumors. Intraoperative ultrasound is used to define the borders of the tumor, identify satellite nodules, and localize important biliovascular structures. There is insufficient evidence to support anatomic versus nonanatomic resections. IHCCA tends to portray a locally aggressive phenotype and frequently involves major vascular structures. Similar long-term outcomes have been observed among patients undergoing major vascular resection as long as negative margins can be achieved (20).

Minimally invasive approaches are increasingly being used in the management of benign and malignant liver lesions with apparent improvements in postoperative pain control, length of hospital stay, and overall recovery (21). While randomized controlled trials have not been performed, the use of minimally invasive surgery in well-selected patients appears to be associated with similar oncologic outcomes compared to open surgery. In addition, the use of preoperative laparoscopy has been touted by some as a means of identifying occult metastatic disease and reducing the incidence of unnecessary laparotomy. However, with improvements in cross-sectional imaging, the efficacy and cost-effectiveness of routine laparoscopy has been called into question (22).

Due to a high rate of unresectability, there has been considerable interest in orthotopic liver transplantation (OLT) for IHCCA. Despite strong initial enthusiasm based on favorable outcomes from a single-institution series (23), subsequent experience with OLT for IHCCA has demonstrated high tumor recurrence rates (24,25). Currently, OLT is not recommended for IHCCA except as part of a clinical trial protocol at specialized centers (26).

Perihilar Cholangiocarcinoma

Although margin-negative resection is the most important intervention for patients with pCCA, their location at the hepatic duct confluence and proximity to adjacent vascular structures (Figure 44.2) makes complete tumor extirpation a significant challenge. Classification

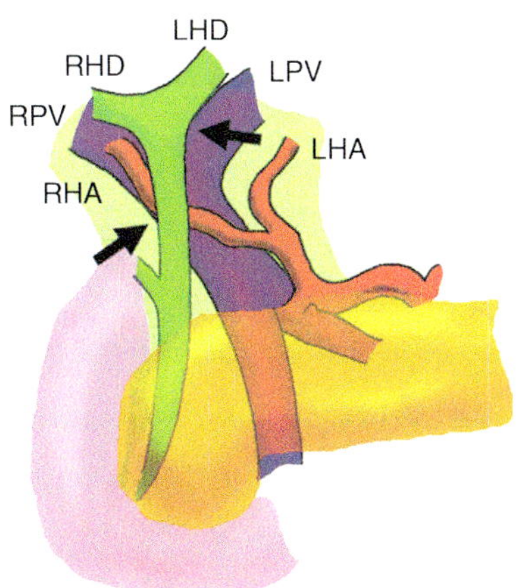

FIGURE 44.2 Vascular anatomy at the hepatic hilum.

LHA, left hepatic artery; LHD, left hepatic duct; LPV, left portal vein; RHA, right hepatic artery; RHD, right hepatic duct; RPV, right portal vein.

Source: Used with permission Shindoh J, Zimmitti G, Vauthey J-N. Surgical techniques for extrahepatic biliary tract cancers. In: Herman J, Pawlik T, Thomas T, eds. *Biliary Tract and Gallbladder Cancer*. Medical Radiology. Springer, Berlin, Heidelberg; 2014:253–263. doi:10.1007/978-3-642-40558-7_16

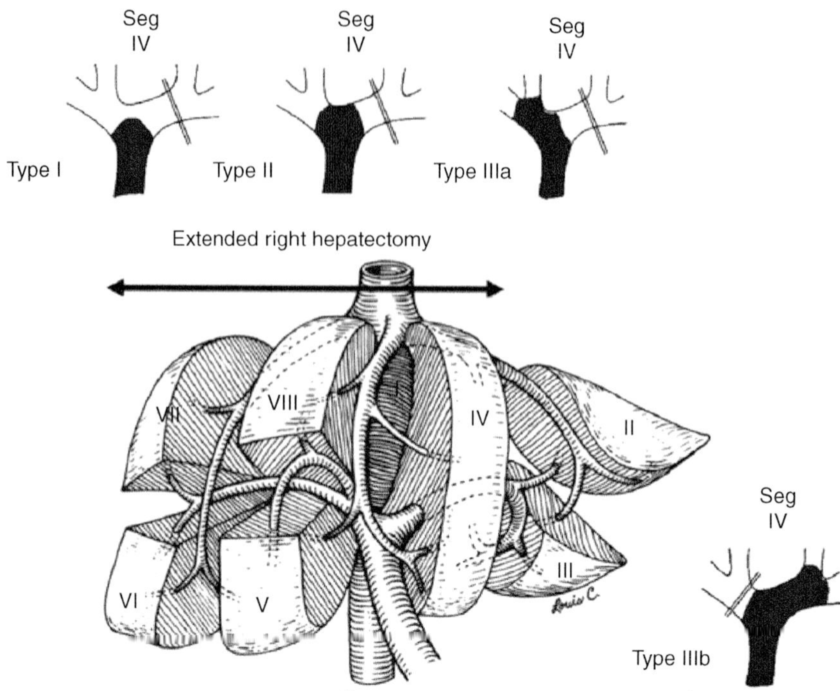

FIGURE 44.3   Extent of hepatic resection according to Bismuth–Corlette classification.

Source: Used with permission Shindoh J, Zimmitti G, Vauthey J-N. Surgical techniques for extrahepatic biliary tract cancers. In: Herman J, Pawlik T, Thomas T, eds. *Biliary Tract and Gallbladder Cancer*. Medical Radiology. Springer, Berlin, Heidelberg; 2014:253–263. doi:10.1007/978-3-642-40558-7_16

according to the Bismuth–Corlette system aids in surgical planning (Figure 44.3). For example, for types I, II, and IIIa, an extended right hepatectomy is recommended while for type IIIb, an extended left hepatectomy is recommended. In either case, segment IV must be completely or partially resected as pCCA frequently extends to the base of the quadrate lobe. Isolated bile duct resections or central hepatectomies have been described but, in general, are not recommended. While most institutions consider type IV tumors unresectable, some high-volume centers perform extended hepatectomy with arterial and venous reconstruction with or without combined pancreatoduodenectomy in an attempt to resect these challenging tumors (27,28). Careful attention to preoperative liver volumetry and function will determine the need for PVE prior to extended right hepatectomy.

Because the caudate lobe drains into the hepatic duct confluence, routine caudate lobectomy is generally recommended during resection for pCCA. Previous studies have demonstrated a high rate of caudate lobe (or its biliary branches) involvement in hilar cholangiocarcinoma (29) and that caudate lobectomy has been associated with both improved margin-negative resection rates (30) and OS (31). Since the Spiegel lobe drains into the left hepatic duct 90% of the time, some authors have suggested that partial preservation of the caudate lobe is acceptable in type IIIa tumors undergoing extended right hepatectomy.

pCCA frequently involves vascular structures, and the role of vascular resection remains controversial. While vascular involvement has historically been a contraindication to resection of pCCA, improvements in surgical technique have led to the increased use of vascular resection over the past few decades. In one series of 305 patients, major liver resection combined with portal vein resection was performed in 15% of resections for pCCA. While there was increased perioperative mortality with PVR compared to hepatectomy alone, long-term outcomes between the two groups were similar (32). A recent multi-institutional review of 201 patients with pCCA also found equivalent long-term survival outcomes in the subset of patients who underwent vascular resection, including hepatic artery reconstruction (33). Nevertheless, vascular resection is reserved for a highly selected group of patients and only when performed by experienced teams of surgeons (34).

Given its tendency to invade vascular structures, bilateral distal biliary radicals, or extrahepatic structures, pCCA is frequently deemed unresectable. OLT represents a viable option for these patients, though strict criteria must be met for eligibility. Patients should have unresectable disease (based on previously listed criteria) but with tumors <3 cm in size, have no evidence of distant or lymph node metastases, be medically appropriate to undergo liver transplantation, be able to receive full-dose neoadjuvant chemoradiation therapy, and have not previously undergone surgical exploration or transperitoneal biopsy. In these highly selected patients, the use of OLT according to the Mayo protocol in unresectable pCCA has resulted in excellent outcomes (Figure 44.4) (35). In fact, given the promising results observed with transplantation, some have recently questioned whether OLT should be utilized even in patients with resectable disease (36).

Distal Extrahepatic Cholangiocarcinoma

Pancreatoduodenectomy is the standard operation for dCCA, as it is necessary in order to sufficiently remove the entire distal bile duct tract. Indeed, only 10% of dCCAs are amenable

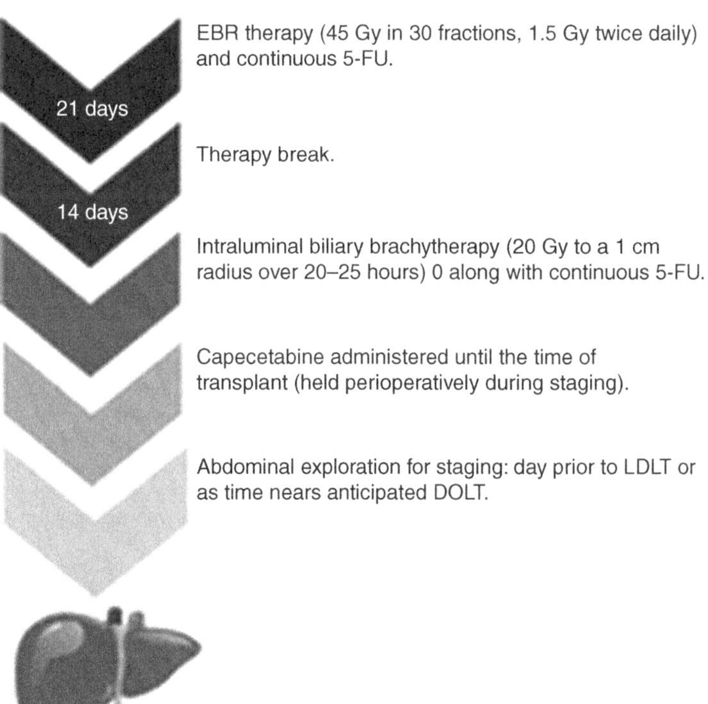

FIGURE 44.4 Description of Mayo protocol for treatment of unresectable perihilar cholangiocarcinoma.

Source: Used with permission Jadlowiec CC, Rosen CB. Transplantation for hilar cholangiocarcinoma. In: Pawlik T, Weber S, Gamblin T, eds. *Case-Based Lessons in the Management of Complex Hepato-Pancreato-Biliary Surgery*. Springer, Cham; 2017:259–273. doi:10.1007/978-3-319-50868-9_20

to common bile duct resection alone without pancreatoduodenectomy (37,38). Intraoperative frozen section analysis of the proximal hepatic duct margin should be evaluated. Rarely, combined hepatopancreatoduodenectomy would be required to obtain negative margins and caution should be given before committing to this procedure, which is associated with high morbidity and mortality rates.

Gallbladder Cancer

The surgical management of GBC depends on its initial presentation and pathologic T stage. For T1a GBC, diagnosed following initial cholecystectomy, no additional surgery or adjuvant therapy is typically recommended. For T1b and greater disease, additional operative intervention is indicated in patients healthy enough to undergo major surgery (39). The operative approach in these patients includes segment 4b/5 liver resection and porta hepatis lymphadenectomy. Reexcision of the cystic duct should be performed if this margin was positive for microscopic disease during the initial cholecystectomy; occasionally, resection of the common bile duct will be required in the setting of persistent microscopically positive disease. In addition, multiple reports have demonstrated the safety and feasibility of performing radical cholecystectomy in a minimally invasive fashion (40).

Both the incidence of residual disease and the long-term survival outcomes directly correlate with T stage (41). For this reason, many consider patients with T2 GBC to represent the cohort most likely to benefit from additional intervention. The management of T3/T4 GBC is slightly more controversial. Small series of well-selected patients suggest that extended radical resections of locally advanced tumors can result in long-term survival in some patients. While these patients have a high rate of lymph node positive and occult metastatic disease, aggressive operations, if margin-negative resection can be achieved, should be considered in well-selected patients (42).

Early reports following initial laparoscopic cholecystectomy for GBC noted a high incidence of recurrent disease at port sites, especially if gallbladder perforation or bile spillage occurred. This led surgeons to perform routine port site resections at the time of radical cholecystectomy. However, more recent evidence suggests that the incidence of port site disease is less common than initially thought and tends to serve as a marker of diffuse peritoneal involvement (43). In the absence of radiographic evidence of disease, routine port site resection is no longer encouraged. As in IHCCA, diagnostic laparoscopy can be used to complement high-quality CT, MRI, and/or PET to rule out metastatic disease or signs of unresectability.

ROLE OF LYMPHADENECTOMY

Intrahepatic Cholangiocarcinoma

Studies have consistently demonstrated the prognostic importance of lymph node positivity among patients with IHCCA (44). In addition, lymph node status is frequently used to guide decisions regarding adjuvant therapy. Therefore, lymphadenectomy at the time of surgical resection of IHCCA is routinely recommended. In fact, the National Comprehensive Cancer Network (NCCN) recommends sampling of at least six lymph nodes to ensure an adequate lymphadenectomy. On the other hand, only a minority of patients meet this criterion (45). This highlights the challenges of performing a complete porta hepatis lymphadenectomy and calls to attention the need for improved training in this area.

The divergent draining patterns of the right and left hemiliver should also be recognized (Figure 44.5). Left-sided tumors tend to drain to the gastrohepatic ligament and lesser curvature or cardia of the stomach while tumors of the right liver tend to drain to the hepatoduodenal ligament (58). Nevertheless, "crossover" does occur and, in general, a complete systematic lymphadenectomy for all IHCCA is recommended (46). Finally, the radiographic presence of suspicious lymph nodes on preoperative imaging portends a worse prognosis, and may represent an indication for systemic therapy, but does not currently represent an absolute contraindication to resection.

Extrahepatic Cholangiocarcinoma

Routine porta hepatis lymphadenectomy is recommended at the time of resection for pCCA as it provides important prognostic information (Figure 44.6). Patients with lymph

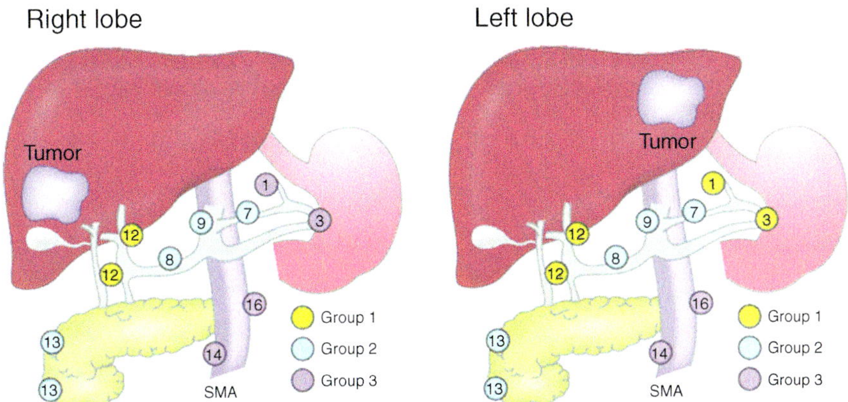

FIGURE 44.5 Divergent patterns of lymphatic spread for right and left intrahepatic cholangiocarcinomas.

SMA, superior mesenteric artery.

Source: Used with permission Brown KM, Geller DA. Surgical management of intra-hepatic cholangiocarcinoma. In: Herman J, Pawlik T, Thomas T, eds. *Biliary Tract and Gallbladder Cancer*. Medical Radiology. Springer, Berlin, Heidelberg; 2014:241–252. doi:10.1007/978-3-642-40558-7_15

node involvement beyond the hepatoduodenal ligament behave similar to stage IV patients, with a dismal 5-year survival of 0% to 12% (47). For this reason, metastatic lymph nodes outside the hepatoduodenal ligament along the celiac axis or in the aortocaval space are

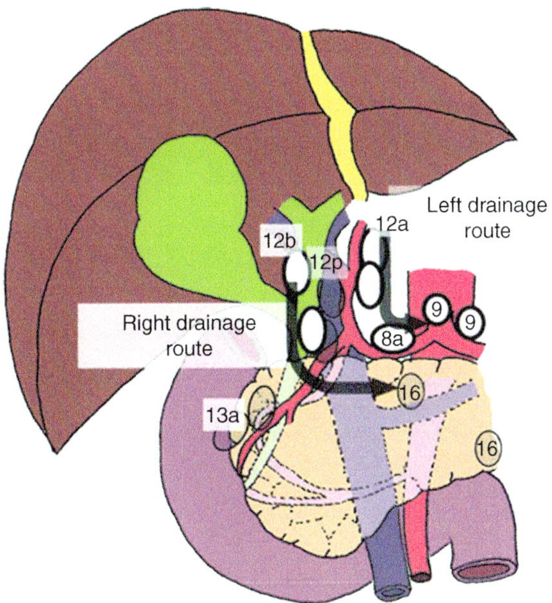

FIGURE 44.6 Lymphatic drainage of the extrahepatic biliary system.

Source: Used with permission Shindoh J, Zimmitti G, Vauthey J-N. Surgical techniques for extrahepatic biliary tract cancers. In: Herman J, Pawlik T, Thomas T, eds. *Biliary Tract and Gallbladder Cancer*. Medical Radiology. Springer, Berlin, Heidelberg; 2014:253–263. doi:10.1007/978-3-642-40558-7_16

usually considered contraindications to resection. A lymphadenectomy specimen with at least seven nodes is needed for adequate staging (48). Regional lymphadenectomy should be included at the time of surgery for dCCA as well. In general, this is easily obtained during pancreatoduodenectomy. For those rare cases, when isolated extrahepatic bile duct resection with negative margins is possible, porta hepatis lymphadenectomy should still be pursued. Previous studies have suggested at least 10 lymph nodes should be retrieved for optimal staging (49).

Gallbladder Cancer

GBC has a strong propensity for lymph node involvement, and this represents one of the most important determinants of long-term outcomes. Lymph node status correlates directly with T stage with positivity rates ranging from 20% to 40% in T2 GBCs (50). The lymphatic drainage pattern of GBCs has previously been described: cystic and pericholedochal stations are first involved, followed by portal vein, hepatic artery, and posterosuperior pancreatoduodenal stations (51). Given this pattern of spread and the locally advanced nature of many GBCs, the rate of combined pancreatoduodenectomy in some surgical series is quite high. However, morbidity and mortality rates of pancreatoduodenectomy, especially when combined with hemihepatectomy, are considerable and, in general, should be reserved for those patients with superb performance status. The routine lymphadenectomy for patients with clinically negative lymph nodes should include resection of the cystic, pericholedochal, hepatic artery, portocaval, and probably posterosuperior pancreatoduodenal lymph nodes. Some authors have recommended the routine excision of the common bile duct to facilitate a more complete lymphadenectomy though this has not been shown to reliably improve outcomes but does contribute to increased morbidity (52).

OUTCOMES

Perioperative morbidity and mortality following major resections for BTCs can be substantial. Fortunately, with improvements in patient selection and optimization, meticulous surgical technique, and enhanced perioperative care, postoperative mortality rates have decreased significantly over time (53). Major morbidity typically results from biliary fistula, PHI, infectious complications, venous thromboembolic events, and cardiopulmonary complications. Significant variability in outcomes are observed among low- and high-volume centers (54).

Despite best efforts, locoregional and distant recurrence remains a significant challenge for all BTCs and can reliably be predicted based on margin status, lymph node status, and histopathologic features. The use of adjuvant therapy strategies, in certain circumstances, may help mitigate the risk of recurrence. Distant recurrence should be treated with systemic chemotherapy while locoregional recurrences should be managed in a multidisciplinary fashion that may include systemic chemotherapy, transarterial therapies, radiation therapy and, rarely, repeat surgical resection (2).

CONCLUSIONS

The surgical management of BTC remains a significant challenge. BTCs represent a heterogeneous group of neoplasms that frequently present at advanced stages. High-quality cross-sectional imaging is imperative for evaluating the local extent of disease and planning the optimal surgical approach. Particular attention to preoperative nutritional status, FLR volume and function, and the need for preoperative biliary decompression must be emphasized. While the surgical considerations differ for each type of BTC, the aim of any operation is margin-negative resection with regional lymphadenectomy, which can increasingly be performed in a minimally invasive fashion. Although recent evidence has demonstrated the genetic, molecular, and clinical heterogeneity among BTCs, additional research is needed in order to translate these findings into personalized neoadjuvant and adjuvant treatment strategies. In the meantime, the delivery of safe and effective surgery with meticulous technique and sound oncologic principles remains the most important factor in achieving optimal outcomes.

Clinical Vignette 44.1

A 54-year-old man presented to his primary physician with abdominal pain, acholic stools, and new onset jaundice. Laboratory evaluation was remarkable for elevated liver function tests, including a total bilirubin of 7.5 mg/dL. CT of the abdomen/pelvis showed both intra- and extrahepatic biliary ductal dilation with no discrete mass. He was referred for endoscopic retrograde cholangiopancreatography (ERCP), which demonstrated a 1.5 cm stricture of the mid-distal common bile duct. Initial brushings were benign, but repeat ERCP with cholangioscopy and direct biopsy proved adenocarcinoma. Further evaluation with magnetic resonance cholangiopancreatography (MRCP) demonstrated an abnormally enhancing distal bile duct associated with a stricture (Figure 44.7), with no signs of lymphadenopathy or distant disease.

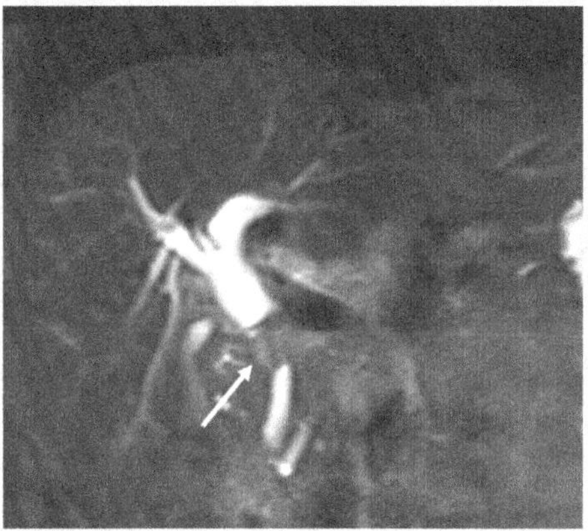

FIGURE 44.7   Representative image from MRCP for a patient with biliary stricture (arrow) secondary to extrahepatic distal cholangiocarcinoma.

MRCP, magnetic resonance cholangiopancreatography.

The patient was diagnosed with a distal extrahepatic cholangiocarcinoma and offered pancreatoduodenectomy. During surgery, the tumor was densely adherent to the portal vein and required a segmental vein resection with primary reanastomosis. Pathology confirmed a 1.8 cm, moderately differentiated adenocarcinoma with local infiltration into the portal vein. Final margins were negative and 8/28 lymph nodes were positive resulting in a pathologic stage of pT2N2M0. Following an uneventful recovery from surgery, adjuvant chemotherapy with capecitabine was initiated.

REFERENCES

1. Khan SA, Davidson BR, Goldin RD, et al. Guidelines for the diagnosis and treatment of cholangiocarcinoma: an update. *Gut.* 2012;61(12):1657–1669. doi:10.1136/gutjnl-2011-301748
2. Rizvi S, Khan SA, Hallemeier CL, et al. Cholangiocarcinoma - evolving concepts and therapeutic strategies. *Nat Rev Clin Oncol.* 2018;15(2):95–111. doi:10.1038/nrclinonc.2017.157
3. Endo I, Gonen M, Yopp AC, et al. Intrahepatic cholangiocarcinoma: rising frequency, improved survival, and determinants of outcome after resection. *Ann Surg.* 2008;248(1):84–96. doi:10.1097/SLA.0b013e318176c4d3
4. Nguyen KT, Steel J, Vanounou T, et al. Initial presentation and management of hilar and peripheral cholangiocarcinoma: is a node-positive status or potential margin-positive result a contraindication to resection? *Ann Surg Oncol.* 2009;16(12):3308–3315. doi:10.1245/s10434-009-0701-4
5. Siegel RL, Miller KD, Jemal A. Cancer statistics, 2017. *CA Cancer J Clin.* 2017;67(1):7–30. doi:10.3322/caac.21387

6. Heimbach JK, Sanchez W, Rosen CB, et al. Trans-peritoneal fine needle aspiration biopsy of hilar cholangiocarcinoma is associated with disease dissemination. *HPB*. 2011;13(5):356–360. doi:10.1111/j.1477-2574.2011.00298.x

7. Chun YS, Pawlik TM, Vauthey J-N. 8th Edition of the AJCC Cancer Staging Manual: Pancreas and Hepatobiliary Cancers. *Ann Surg Oncol*. 2018;25(4):845–847. doi:10.1245/s10434-017-6025-x

8. Spolverato G, Bagante F, Weiss M, et al. Comparative performances of the 7th and the 8th editions of the American Joint Committee on Cancer staging systems for intrahepatic cholangiocarcinoma. *J Surg Oncol*. 2017;115(6):696–703. doi:10.1002/jso.24569

9. Zorzi D, Laurent A, Pawlik TM, et al. Chemotherapy-associated hepatotoxicity and surgery for colorectal liver metastases. *Br J Surg*. 2007;94(3):274–286. doi:10.1002/bjs.5719

10. Makuuchi M, Thai BL, Takayasu K, et al. Preoperative portal embolization to increase safety of major hepatectomy for hilar bile duct carcinoma: a preliminary report. *Surgery*. 1990;107(5): 521–527.

11. Kennedy TJ, Yopp A, Qin Y, et al. Role of preoperative biliary drainage of liver remnant prior to extended liver resection for hilar cholangiocarcinoma. *HPB*. 2009;11(5):445–451. doi:10.1111/j.1477-2574.2009.00090.x

12. Al Mahjoub A, Menahem B, Fohlen A, et al. Preoperative biliary drainage in patients with resectable perihilar cholangiocarcinoma: is percutaneous transhepatic biliary drainage safer and more effective than endoscopic biliary drainage? a meta-analysis. *J Vasc Interv Radiol JVIR*. 2017;28(4):576–582. doi:10.1016/j.jvir.2016.12.1218

13. Kawashima H, Itoh A, Ohno E, et al. Preoperative endoscopic nasobiliary drainage in 164 consecutive patients with suspected perihilar cholangiocarcinoma: a retrospective study of efficacy and risk factors related to complications. *Ann Surg*. 2013;257(1):121–127. doi:10.1097/SLA.0b013e318262b2e9

14. Hawkins WG, DeMatteo RP, Jarnagin WR, et al. Jaundice predicts advanced disease and early mortality in patients with gallbladder cancer. *Ann Surg Oncol*. 2004;11(3):310–315. doi:10.1245/aso.2004.03.011

15. van der Gaag NA, Rauws EAJ, van Eijck CHJ, et al. Preoperative biliary drainage for cancer of the head of the pancreas. *N Engl J Med*. 2010;362(2):129–137. doi:10.1056/NEJMoa0903230

16. Grendar J, Grendarova P, Sinha R, et al. Neoadjuvant therapy for downstaging of locally advanced hilar cholangiocarcinoma: a systematic review. *HPB*. 2014;16(4):297–303. doi:10.1111/hpb.12150

17. Kato A, Shimizu H, Ohtsuka M, et al. Surgical resection after downsizing chemotherapy for initially unresectable locally advanced biliary tract cancer: a retrospective single-center study. *Ann Surg Oncol*. 2013;20(1):318–324. doi:10.1245/s10434-012-2312-8

18. Valle JW, Wasan H, Johnson P, et al. Gemcitabine alone or in combination with cisplatin in patients with advanced or metastatic cholangiocarcinomas or other biliary tract tumours: a multicentre randomised phase II study – The UK ABC-01 Study. *Br J Cancer*. 2009;101(4):621–627. doi:10.1038/sj.bjc.6605211

19. Sommer CM, Kauczor HU, Pereira PL. Locoregional therapies of cholangiocarcinoma. *Visc Med*. 2016;32(6):414–420. doi:10.1159/000453010

20. Ali SM, Clark CJ, Zaydfudim VM, et al. Role of major vascular resection in patients with intrahepatic cholangiocarcinoma. *Ann Surg Oncol*. 2013;20(6):2023–2028. doi:10.1245/s10434-012-2808-2

21. Ciria R, Cherqui D, Geller DA, et al. Comparative short-term benefits of laparoscopic liver resection: 9000 cases and climbing. *Ann Surg*. 2016;263(4):761–777. doi:10.1097/SLA.000 0000000001413

22. Gaujoux S, Allen PJ. Role of staging laparoscopy in peri-pancreatic and hepatobiliary malignancy. *World J Gastrointest Surg*. 2010;2(9):283–290. doi:10.4240/wjgs.v2.i9.283

23. Iwatsuki S, Starzl TE, Sheahan DG, et al. Hepatic resection versus transplantation for hepatocellular carcinoma. *Ann Surg*. 1991;214(3):221–228; discussion 228–229. doi:10.1097/000 00658-199109000-00005

24. Ghali P, Marotta PJ, Yoshida EM, et al. Liver transplantation for incidental cholangiocarcinoma: analysis of the Canadian experience. *Liver Transplant Off Publ Am Assoc Study Liver Dis Int Liver Transplant Soc*. 2005;11(11):1412–1416. doi:10.1002/lt.20512

25. Becker NS, Rodriguez JA, Barshes NR, et al. Outcomes analysis for 280 patients with cholangiocarcinoma treated with liver transplantation over an 18-year period. *J Gastrointest Surg Off J Soc Surg Aliment Tract*. 2008;12(1):117–122. doi:10.1007/s11605-007-0335-4

26. Lunsford KE, Javle M, Heyne K, et al. Liver transplantation for locally advanced intrahepatic cholangiocarcinoma treated with neoadjuvant therapy: a prospective case-series. *Lancet Gastroenterol Hepatol*. 2018;3(5):337–348. doi:10.1016/S2468-1253(18)30045-1

27. Nagino M, Nimura Y, Nishio H, et al. Hepatectomy with simultaneous resection of the portal vein and hepatic artery for advanced perihilar cholangiocarcinoma: an audit of 50 consecutive cases. *Ann Surg*. 2010;252(1):115–123. doi:10.1097/SLA.0b013e3181e463a7

28. Ebata T, Yokoyama Y, Igami T, et al. Hepatopancreatoduodenectomy for cholangiocarcinoma: a single-center review of 85 consecutive patients. *Ann Surg.* 2012;256(2):297–305. doi:10.1097/SLA.0b013e31826029ca

29. Mizumoto R, Kawarada Y, Suzuki H. Surgical treatment of hilar carcinoma of the bile duct. *Surg Gynecol Obstet.* 1986;162(2):153–158.

30. Bhutiani N, Scoggins CR, McMasters KM, et al. The impact of caudate lobe resection on margin status and outcomes in patients with hilar cholangiocarcinoma: a multi-institutional analysis from the US Extrahepatic Biliary Malignancy Consortium. *Surgery.* 2018;163(4):726–731. doi:10.1016/j.surg.2017.10.028

31. Sugiura Y, Nakamura S, Iida S, et al. Extensive resection of the bile ducts combined with liver resection for cancer of the main hepatic duct junction: a cooperative study of the Keio Bile Duct Cancer Study Group. *Surgery.* 1994;115(4):445–451.

32. de Jong MC, Marques H, Clary BM, et al. The impact of portal vein resection on outcomes for hilar cholangiocarcinoma: a multi-institutional analysis of 305 cases. *Cancer.* 2012;118(19):4737–4747. doi:10.1002/cncr.27492

33. Schimizzi GV, Jin LX, Davidson JT, et al. Outcomes after vascular resection during curative-intent resection for hilar cholangiocarcinoma: a multi-institution study from the US extrahepatic biliary malignancy consortium. *HPB.* 2018;20(4):332–339. doi:10.1016/j.hpb.2017.10.003

34. Abbas S, Sandroussi C. Systematic review and meta-analysis of the role of vascular resection in the treatment of hilar cholangiocarcinoma. *HPB.* 2013;15(7):492–503. doi:10.1111/j.1477-2574.2012.00616.x

35. Darwish Murad S, Kim WR, Harnois DM, et al. Efficacy of neoadjuvant chemoradiation, followed by liver transplantation, for perihilar cholangiocarcinoma at 12 US centers. *Gastroenterology.* 2012;143(1):88–98.e3; quiz e14. doi:10.1053/j.gastro.2012.04.008

36. Ethun CG, Lopez-Aguiar AG, Anderson DJ, et al. Transplantation versus resection for hilar cholangiocarcinoma: an argument for shifting treatment paradigms for resectable disease. *Ann Surg.* 2018;267(5):797–805. doi:10.1097/SLA.0000000000002574

37. Fong Y, Blumgart LH, Lin E, et al. Outcome of treatment for distal bile duct cancer. *Br J Surg.* 1996;83(12):1712–1715. doi:10.1002/bjs.1800831217

38. Wade TP, Prasad CN, Virgo KS, et al. Experience with distal bile duct cancers in U.S. Veterans Affairs hospitals: 1987–1991. *J Surg Oncol.* 1997;64(3):242–245. doi:10.1002/(sici)1096-9098(199703)64:3<242::aid-jso12>3.0.co;2-6

39. Hari Danielle M., Harrison HJ, Leung AM, et al. A 21-year analysis of stage I gallbladder carcinoma: is cholecystectomy alone adequate? *HPB.* 2012;15(1):40–48. doi:10.1111/j.1477-2574.2012.00559.x

40. Zimmitti G, Manzoni A, Guerini F, et al. Current role of minimally invasive radical cholecystectomy for gallbladder cancer. *Gastroenterol Res Pract.* 2016;2016:7684915. doi:10.1155/2016/7684915

41. Ishihara S, Horiguchi A, Miyakawa S, et al. Biliary tract cancer registry in Japan from 2008 to 2013. *J Hepato-Biliary-Pancreat Sci.* 2016;23(3):149–157. doi:10.1002/jhbp.314

42. Onoyama H, Yamamoto M, Tseng A, et al. Extended cholecystectomy for carcinoma of the gallbladder. *World J Surg.* 1995;19(5):758–763. doi:10.1007/bf00295925

43. Maker AV, Butte JM, Oxenberg J, et al. Is port site resection necessary in the surgical management of gallbladder cancer? *Ann Surg Oncol.* 2012;19(2):409–417. doi:10.1245/s10434-011-1850-9

44. de Jong MC, Nathan H, Sotiropoulos GC, et al. Intrahepatic cholangiocarcinoma: an international multi-institutional analysis of prognostic factors and lymph node assessment. *J Clin Oncol Off J Am Soc Clin Oncol.* 2011;29(23):3140–3145. doi:10.1200/JCO.2011.35.6519

45. Zhang X-F, Chen Q, Kimbrough CW, et al. Lymphadenectomy for Intrahepatic Cholangiocarcinoma: Has Nodal Evaluation Been Increasingly Adopted by Surgeons over Time? A National Database Analysis. *J Gastrointest Surg Off J Soc Surg Aliment Tract.* 2018;22(4):668–675. doi:10.1007/s11605-017-3652-2

46. Okami J, Dono K, Sakon M, et al. Patterns of regional lymph node involvement in intrahepatic cholangiocarcinoma of the left lobe. *J Gastrointest Surg Off J Soc Surg Aliment Tract.* 2003;7(7):850–856. doi:10.1016/s1091-255x(03)00140-9

47. Ramos E. Principles of surgical resection in hilar cholangiocarcinoma. *World J Gastrointest Oncol.* 2013;5(7):139–146. doi:10.4251/wjgo.v5.i7.139

48. Ito K, Ito H, Allen PJ, et al. Adequate lymph node assessment for extrahepatic bile duct adenocarcinoma. *Ann Surg.* 2010;251(4):675–681. doi:10.1097/SLA.0b013e3181d3d2b2

49. Schwarz RE, Smith DD. Lymph node dissection impact on staging and survival of extrahepatic cholangiocarcinomas, based on U.S. population data. *J Gastrointest Surg Off J Soc Surg Aliment Tract.* 2007;11(2):158–165. doi:10.1007/s11605-006-0018-6

50. Pugalenthi A, Fong Y. Surgical management of gallbladder cancer. In: Herman J, Pawlik T, & Thomas T. (Eds.), *Biliary Tract and Gallbladder Cancer.* Medical Radiology. Springer, Berlin, Heidelberg; 2014:265–274. doi:10.1007/978-3-642-40558-7_17

51. Shirai Y, Sakata J, Wakai T, et al. "Extended" radical cholecystectomy for gallbladder cancer: long-term outcomes, indications and limitations. *World J Gastroenterol*. 2012;18(34):4736–4743. doi:10.3748/wjg.v18.i34.4736

52. Gani F, Buettner S, Margonis GA, et al. Assessing the impact of common bile duct resection in the surgical management of gallbladder cancer. *J Surg Oncol*. 2016;114(2):176–180. doi:10.1002/jso.24283

53. Kingham TP, Correa-Gallego C, D'Angelica MI, et al. Hepatic parenchymal preservation surgery: decreasing morbidity and mortality rates in 4,152 resections for malignancy. *J Am Coll Surg*. 2015;220(4):471–479. doi:10.1016/j.jamcollsurg.2014.12.026

54. Buettner S, Gani F, Amini N, et al. The relative effect of hospital and surgeon volume on failure to rescue among patients undergoing liver resection for cancer. *Surgery*. 2016;159(4):1004–1012. doi:10.1016/j.surg.2015.10.025

55. Brown KM, Geller DA. Surgical Management of intra-hepatic cholangiocarcinoma. In: Herman J, Pawlik T, Thomas T, eds. *Biliary Tract and Gallbladder Cancer*. Medical Radiology. Berlin, Heidelberg: Springer Publishing; 2014:241–252. doi:10.1007/978-3-642-40558-7_15

56. Shindoh J, Zimmitti G, Vauthey J-N. Surgical techniques for extrahepatic biliary tract cancers. In: Herman J, Pawlik T, Thomas T, eds. *Biliary Tract and Gallbladder Cancer*. Medical Radiology. Berlin, Heidelberg: Springer Publishing; 2014:253–263. doi:10.1007/978-3-642-40558-7_16

57. Jadlowiec CC, Rosen CB. Transplantation for hilar cholangiocarcinoma. In: Pawlik T, Weber S, Gamblin T, eds. *Case-Based Lessons in the Management of Complex Hepato-Pancreato-Biliary Surgery*. Cham: Springer Publishing; 2017:259–273. doi:10.1007/978-3-319-50868-9_20

58. Shirabe K, Shimada M, Harimoto N, et al. Intrahepatic cholangiocarcinoma: its mode of spreading and therapeutic modalities. *Surgery*. 2002;131(1 Suppl):S159-164.

Adjuvant Therapy for Early-Stage Cancers of the Bile Ducts and Gallbladder

Flavio G. Rocha

INTRODUCTION

Biliary tract cancers (BTC) represent a heterogeneous group of tumors that arise anywhere from the liver down to the pancreas including intrahepatic, gallbladder cancer, perihilar, and distal cholangiocarcinoma (Figure 45.1). Although they represent malignant transformation of epithelium with cholangiocyte differentiation, they have proven to be incredibly diverse from a genetic standpoint (1). In addition, their etiology, clinical presentation, biologic behavior, and oncologic management can vary dramatically depending on the stage of disease and site of origin. Complete surgical resection with negative margins remains the only potentially curative treatment strategy (2). However, it is the minority of patients who are (a) fit for surgery, (b) present without locally advanced or metastatic disease, and (c) have favorable anatomy amenable to resection. Furthermore, complications from extensive multivisceral operations that include the liver and pancreas can be challenging to manage and can make recovery difficult at times leaving patients debilitated.

Over the past few years, improved patient selection, operative techniques, and perioperative care have benefited patients with these tumors; however, recurrence rates remain high and survival poor. Therefore adjuvant therapy has been proposed as a therapeutic option to improve outcomes. Given the rarity of these tumors, there has been a relative paucity of level 1 evidence to support any pre- or postoperative treatment for BTC. Most of the published literature is composed of single-institution retrospective series, population database studies, or expert consensus guidelines. The purpose of this chapter is to review the historical rationale for adjuvant therapy in BTC, highlight the recent prospective clinical trial data, and discuss the future directions for the multidisciplinary management of these aggressive cancers.

HISTORICAL PERSPECTIVE

Since the vast majority of patients with BTC present in advanced stages, much of the oncologic care has been directed at the treatment of systemic disease. However, until recently there was no consensus regarding the optimal chemotherapy regimen. Early, small phase II trials applied gemcitabine-based regimens that yielded response rates between 10% and 30% with mostly single-digit survival in months (3). Eckel et al. summarized these results in a pooled analysis of 104 trials with 2,810 patients from 1985 to 2006 of which only three were randomized, two were phase II, and one was phase III (4). The data suggested that gemcitabine combined with a platinum agent such as oxaliplatin or cisplatin increased the response rate and tumor control rate in advanced cholangiocarcinoma and gallbladder cancer compared to 5-fluorouracil (5-FU), irinotecan, anthracyclines, or taxanes. A subgroup analysis demonstrated that although gallbladder cancer patients had a higher response rate than cholangiocarcinoma patients (34% vs. 20%), the survival was longer in the latter (7.2 months vs. 9.3 months). It was not until the Advanced Biliary Cancer (ABC)-02 trial compared gemcitabine to the combination of gemcitabine and cisplatin in patients with recurrent or metastatic BTCs that an improved survival in the gemcitabine–cisplatin group (11.7 months vs. 8.1 months, $p < .001$) was confirmed in a prospective, randomized controlled fashion (5).

In the adjuvant space, there have been limited trials due to the relatively small volume of resected patients who are also eligible for additional treatment. Despite these limitations, several institutional and registry series have attempted to study the effect of adjuvant therapy

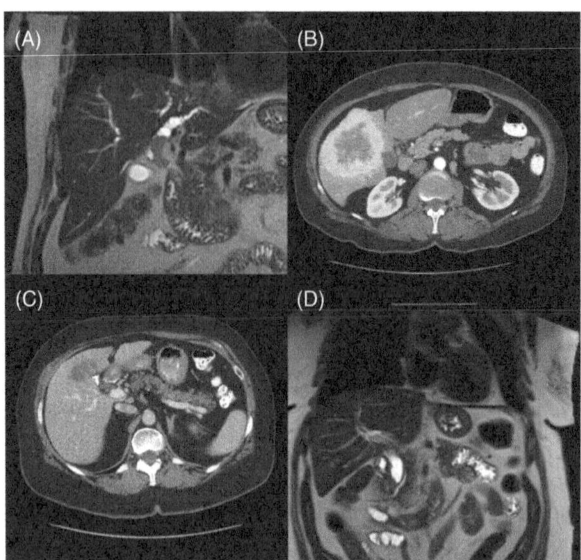

FIGURE 45.1 Radiographic images of different BTC tumor types. (A) hilar cholangiocarcinoma; (B) intrahepatic cholangiocarcinoma; (C) gallbladder cancer; (D) distal cholangiocarcinoma

BTC, biliary tract cancer.

in BTC. A large series from Japan encompassing 127 patients with cholangiocarcinoma (21 intrahepatic, 50 hilar, and 56 distal) suggested an improved 5-year survival from 36% to 47% in those patients who received adjuvant therapy with gemcitabine and S1 (6). This benefit particularly applied to those patients with negative margins and was not different among cholangiocarcinoma groups. An Italian study focused on 72 patients with resected intrahepatic cholangiocarcinoma of whom 25 received adjuvant therapy predominantly with gemcitabine also reported a more favorable 5-year survival of 65% compared to 40% in patients who underwent surgery alone (7). However, a contemporary retrospective study of 157 patients with gallbladder cancer and cholangiocarcinoma from MD Anderson Cancer Center did not find a survival benefit with neoadjuvant of adjuvant therapy if patients were resected with negative margins (8).

More recent population database studies with larger numbers of patients have demonstrated improved outcomes for adjuvant therapy in select cohorts of BTC. Two separate but overlapping analyses of the National Cancer Database (NCDB) focused on patients with gallbladder cancer showed that adjuvant therapy in the form of chemotherapy alone (9) or chemoradiation (10) was associated with longer survival only in patients with positive lymph nodes. In another study using the NCDB with propensity score matching, Miura and colleagues also only found a benefit of adjuvant chemotherapy in 2,751 patients with intrahepatic cholangiocarcinoma who had high-risk features such as higher T stage and positive lymph nodes or margins (11). Overall survival (OS) in the adjuvant therapy group was 19.8 months versus 10.7 months in N1 patients while it was 29.4 months versus 29 months in the N0 group. A similar result was found when examining the NCDB for patients with hilar cholangiocarcinoma again with propensity score matching. In this study of 1,846 patients, adjuvant chemotherapy was associated with a survival benefit of 29.5 months versus 23.6 months (12). The effect was even more pronounced in those patients with positive margins and the addition of radiation only marginally affected the outcomes.

In order to facilitate the interpretation of the existing data, a systematic review and meta-analysis of 83 comparative studies were performed of which 20 were selected for a pooled analysis (13). On unsupervised analysis, there was a nonsignificant improvement in survival with the addition of any adjuvant therapy (odds ratio [OR]: 0.74, 95% confidence interval [CI]: 0.55–1.01, $p > .06$). This trend held true for both gallbladder cancer and bile duct cancer groups. On sensitivity analysis, the protective effect of adjuvant therapy was preserved with chemotherapy and chemoradiation but not with radiation alone. A significant benefit of adjuvant therapy was also seen in node- and margin-positive resection patients. While the vast majority of N1 patients received chemotherapy alone, two-thirds of R1 patients had radiation alone where there was a suggestion of benefit in the adjuvant setting.

PROSPECTIVE CLINICAL TRIALS

One of the first phase III, prospective trials examining the role of adjuvant therapy for resected pancreaticobiliary cancers was published in 2002. This Japanese study randomized 508 patients (173 pancreas, 139 bile duct, 140 gallbladder, 50 ampullary) to surgery alone or surgery followed by mitomycin C and 5-FU (14). In the per-protocol analysis, there was a statistically significant benefit in the 5-year OS for the gallbladder cancer group only (26% vs. 14%, $p < .0367$); however, this difference disappeared when all patients were compared on an intention-to-treat basis.

In the ESPAC-3 trial, 428 patients with periampullary cancers (including 96 with bile duct cancer) were randomized to surgery alone versus surgery plus adjuvant 5-FU or gemcitabine (15). There was no difference in survival between the two chemotherapy regimens; however, patients treated with adjuvant therapy had a nonsignificant longer survival than those who were assigned to observation only (43.1 vs. 35.2 months, $p > .25$). This effect was most pronounced in the ampullary cancer patients as in the small subgroup of biliary cancers, 31 patients in the observation arm had an OS of 27.2 months while 31 patients in the 5-FU arm had an OS of 18.3 months, and 34 patients in the gemcitabine arm had an OS of 19.5 months.

More recently, four important trials in BTCs were completed and reported: SWOG (Southwest Oncology Group) S0809, BCAT (Biliary Cancer Adjuvant Trial), PRODIGE 12–ACCORD 18 trial (Gemcitabine Hydrochloride and Oxaliplatin or Observation in Treating Patients With Biliary Tract Cancer That Has Been Removed by Surgery), and BILCAP (Capecitabine or Observation After Surgery in Treating Patients With Biliary Tract Cancer) (Table 45.1).

SWOG S0809

The SWOG S0809 was a single-arm, phase II trial of adjuvant chemotherapy and chemoradiotherapy in patients following resection of gallbladder cancer or extrahepatic cholangiocarcinoma (perihilar and distal) (16). Patients received gemcitabine and capecitabine followed by capecitabine and radiotherapy. Adjuvant therapy was relatively well tolerated in this challenging population with 86% of patients completing therapy. The 2-year survival rate was 65% with a median OS of 35 months. Most notably, patients with positive margins (R1) had a similar OS as the patients with margin-negative resection (R0; 34 months vs. 35 months), suggesting efficacy of the treatment. Consistent with the expected disease biology, the patients with gallbladder cancer had a higher rate of distant recurrence (52%) compared to either the distal cholangiocarcinoma (42%) or perihilar cholangiocarcinoma (23%) groups. The lack of a control arm limits the impact of the findings (21). However, the feasibility of delivery and tolerability of the therapy coupled with the overall favorable survival results compared with historic cohorts support further consideration of this regimen in gallbladder cancer and extrahepatic cholangiocarcinoma.

BCAT

BCAT was a randomized, multicenter phase III trial in Japan that compared the administration of gemcitabine versus observation in resected extrahepatic cholangiocarcinoma (perihilar and distal) (17). Although initially conceived for 300 patients, it was composed of 225 patients who underwent either hepatobiliary resection or pancreaticoduodenectomy but also included isolated bile duct resections and hepatopancreaticoduodenectomies for tumors extending from the hepatic hilus to the pancreatic head. After a determination of futility on interim analysis, there was no statistical difference in OS (the primary end point) between the groups receiving adjuvant gemcitabine versus observation (62.3 months vs. 63.8 months). In addition, relapse-free survival was also similar between groups (36 months vs. 39.6 months), respectively. The authors also performed subgroup analyses including stratifying by node and margin positivity, but again there was no difference in outcomes although the study was not powered for these comparisons.

TABLE 45.1 Summary of Prospective Adjuvant Therapy Trials on Biliary Tract and Gallbladder Cancers

	SWOG S0809 (United States)	BCAT (Japan)	PRODIGE 12 (France)	BILCAP (UK)
Design	Single-arm phase 2	Randomized phase 3	Randomized phase 3	Randomized phase 3
Treatment	Gemcitabine/ Capecitabine + Capecitabine/XRT	Gemcitabine versus observation	Gemcitabine/ Oxaliplatin versus observation	Capecitabine versus observation
Number	79	225	196	440
BTC type	Gallbladder 32% Perihilar 48% Intrahepatic 0% Distal 20%	Gallbladder 0% Perihilar 48% Intrahepatic 0% Distal 52%	Gallbladder 19% Perihilar 8% Intrahepatic 45% Distal 28%	Gallbladder 18% Perihilar 28% Intrahepatic 19% Distal 35%
+Margin (%)	32	11	15	38
+Lymph nodes (%)	N/A	35	37	54
End point and summary	• 2-year OS 65% • Treatment well tolerated • R0/R1 OS similar at 35 and 34 months	• OS and RFS similar between treatment and control groups • No difference when stratified by resection margin and lymph nodes	• RFS similar between treatment and control groups • Treatment well tolerated based on QOL	• ITT median OS 51 versus 36 months (p = .097) • Per-protocol analysis median OS 53 versus 36 months (p = .028)

BCAT, Biliary Cancer Adjuvant Trial; BTC, biliary tract cancer; ITT, intention to treat; OS, overall survival; QOL, quality of life; RFS, recurrence-free survival; SWOG, Southwest Oncology Group.

PRODIGE 12–ACCORD 18

The PRODIGE 12–ACCORD 18 trial was a phase III randomized, multicenter trial evaluating adjuvant gemcitabine and oxaliplatin (GemOx) versus observation alone in resected BTC (18). The study randomized 196 patients at 33 French centers over a 5-year period and examined the recurrence-free survival (RFS) and quality of life (QOL). Unfortunately, the trial results were negative with no difference in RFS between study arms. The QOL was not different between the two arms, indicating that treatment was tolerated; however, only 33% of patients in the GemOx arm received all six cycles of planned treatment. Subgroup analysis by tumor type did not demonstrate any favorable trends (21).

BILCAP

The BILCAP trial was a phase III randomized, multicenter trial that evaluated adjuvant capecitabine (eight cycles) versus observation alone in patients with resected BTC (19). This trial accrued over an 8-year period at 44 sites in the UK. This study randomized 447 patients, and its primary end point was OS. In the intention-to-treat analysis, the median OS was 51 months for the capecitabine group as compared to 36 months for control (hazard ratio [HR]: 0.80, 95% CI: 0.63–1.04; p = .097); however, in the per-protocol analysis, median OS was 53 months in the capecitabine group as compared to 36 months in the control arm (HR: 0.75, 95% CI: 0.58–0.97; p = .028). Based on these findings, the investigators recommended adjuvant capecitabine as the standard of care in resected BTC.

FUTURE DIRECTIONS

Based on the recently reported trials of adjuvant therapy in resected BTC, adjuvant capecitabine is considered to be the new standard for all patients. In patients with gallbladder cancer or extrahepatic cholangiocarcinoma with a positive resection margin, there may be benefit to consideration of adding chemoradiation; however, additional investigation is warranted.

There are currently two additional clinical trials currently undergoing accrual that may provide answers to some of these questions. The Japanese Clinical Oncology Group is conducting the ASCOT, trial which is comparing the effect of adjuvant S-1 compared to observation in resected BTC in 440 patients. Meanwhile in Europe, the ACTICCA-1 investigators are randomizing BTC patients to receive combination gemcitabine cisplatin following surgery or capecitabine based on the encouraging results of the ABC-02 trial in the advanced setting. Because of the differential prognosis and pattern of recurrence of gallbladder cancer and cholangiocarcinoma, these patient cohorts will be analyzed separately.

This is an important distinction as all BTC adjuvant trials have failed to test the effectiveness of cytotoxic therapy across tumor types and locations. It is the hope that the inclusion of multinational collaborations particularly with Asian and South American centers that have a much higher incidence of BTC may help distinguish the individual contribution of adjuvant therapy in extra- and intrahepatic cholangiocarcinoma and gallbladder cancer. The role of adjuvant radiation in BTC also remains to be investigated and may yield further benefit in certain tumors with adverse features or in those patients with margin- and node-positive tumors. However, its role is still debated in resected pancreatic adenocarcinoma with conflicting trials between the United States and Europe.

The rapid availability of genomic sequencing particularly for advanced tumors has provided a new landscape for therapeutic targeting. Although BTCs share several oncologic pathways, there are signatures unique to certain histologic subtypes. For example, the isocitrate dehydrogenase (IDH) mutations and fibroblast growth factor (FGF) fusion rearrangements have been already identified as actionable targets for experimental drugs with promising initial results (20). Meanwhile, HER2 overexpression has been identified in up to one-fifth of advanced gallbladder cancer patients. While targeted monotherapy has yielded disappointing results, it is possible that combination treatment with active cytotoxic therapy may improve survival. Last, the recent explosion of immunotherapy has yet to be studied thoroughly in BTC. Pembrolizumab was recently approved as treatment for any mismatch repair (MMR) deficient tumor regardless of the tissue of origin. Although the fraction of BTC patients with MMR deficiency outside of Lynch syndrome who qualify for PD-1 therapy may be small, anecdotal reports have produced dramatic results with limited toxicity compared to traditional chemotherapy even in refractory or relapsed patients. Ongoing phase II trials in the metastatic setting may provide additional information that can be applied to patients with localized disease.

Given the aggressive nature of these malignancies and the relatively poor outcomes, even in anatomically resectable tumors, a neoadjuvant strategy may be the best approach to further understand the tumor biology and chemoresponsiveness of BTC. It is likely that most patients with BTC have micrometastatic disease at presentation, and neoadjuvant therapy may allow selection of patients most likely to benefit from surgical intervention and allow for evaluation of efficacy of specific therapy regimens either through objective response (tumor marker levels, morphologic changes) and/or metabolic response (21). It is also possible that the delivery of effective therapy prior to a complicated operation may be the optimal approach since patients may have difficulty tolerating more active agents postoperatively. If found to be promising, it may encourage hepatobiliary surgeons to perform more extensive resections and offer curative therapy to more patients with this devastating disease.

REFERENCES

1. Javle M, Bekaii-Saab T, Jain A, et al. Biliary cancer: utility of next-generation sequencing for clinical management. *Cancer*. 2016;122(24):3838–3847. doi:10.1002/cncr.30254
2. National Comprehensive Cancer Network. Hepatobiliary Cancers Version 1.2016. Vol 2016: National Comprehensive Cancer Network.
3. Prabhu R, Hwang J. Adjuvant therapy in biliary tract and gallbladder carcinomas: a review. *J Gastrointest Oncol*. 2017;8(2):302–313. doi:10.21037/jgo.2017.01.17
4. Eckel F, Schmid RM. Chemotherapy in advanced biliary carcinoma: a pooled analysis of clinical trials. *Br J Cancer*. 2007;96(6):896–902. doi:10.1038/sj.bjc.6603648
5. Valle J, Wasan H, Palmer DH, et al. Cisplatin plus gemcitabine versus gemcitabine for biliary tract cancer. *N Engl J Med*. 2010;362(14):1273–1281. doi:10.1056/NEJMoa0908721

6. Murakami Y, Uemura K, Sudo T, et al. Prognostic factors after surgical resection for intrahepatic, hilar, and distal cholangiocarcinoma. *Ann Surg Oncol*. 2011;18(3):651–658. doi:10.1245/s10434-010-1325-4

7. Ercolani G, Vetrone G, Grazi GL, et al. Intrahepatic cholangiocarcinoma: primary liver resection and aggressive multimodal treatment of recurrence significantly prolong survival. *Ann Surg*. 2010;252(1):107–114. doi:10.1097/SLA.0b013e3181e462e6

8. Glazer ES, Liu P, Abdalla EK, et al. Neither neoadjuvant nor adjuvant therapy increases survival after biliary tract cancer resection with wide negative margins. *J Gastrointest Surg*. 2012;16(9):1666–1671. doi:10.1007/s11605-012-1935-1

9. Bergquist JR, Shah HN, Habermann EB, et al. Adjuvant systemic therapy after resection of node positive gallbladder cancer: time for a well-designed trial? (Results of a US-national retrospective cohort study). *Int J Surg*. 2018;52:171–179. doi:10.1016/j.ijsu.2018.02.052

10. Hoehn RS, Wima K, Ertel AE, et al. Adjuvant therapy for gallbladder cancer: an analysis of the national cancer data base. *J Gastrointest Surg*. 2015;19(10):1794–1801. doi:10.1007/s11605-015-2922-0

11. Miura JT, Johnston FM, Tsai S, et al. Chemotherapy for surgically resected intrahepatic cholangiocarcinoma. *Ann Surg Oncol*. 2015;22(11):3716–3723. doi:10.1245/s10434-015-4501-8

12. Nassour I, Mokdad AA, Porembka MR, et al. Adjuvant therapy is associated with improved survival in resected perihilar cholangiocarcinoma: a propensity matched study. *Ann Surg Oncol*. 2018;25(5):1193–1201. doi:10.1245/s10434-018-6388-7

13. Horgan A, Amir E, Walter T, et al. Adjuvant therapy in the treatment of biliary tract cancer: a systematic review and meta-analysis. *J Clin Oncol*. 2012;30(16):1934–1940. doi:10.1200/JCO.2011.40.5381

14. Takada T, Amano H, Yasuda H, et al. Is postoperative adjuvant chemotherapy useful for gallbladder carcinoma? a phase III multicenter prospective randomized controlled trial in patients with resected pancreaticobiliary carcinoma. *Cancer*. 2002;95(8):1685–1695. doi:10.1002/cncr.10831

15. Neoptolemos JP, Moore MJ, Cox TF, et al. Effect of adjuvant chemotherapy with fluorouracil plus folinic acid or gemcitabine vs observation on survival in patients with resected periampullary adenocarcinoma: the ESPAC-3 periampullary cancer randomized trial. *JAMA*. 2012;308(2):147–156. doi:10.1001/jama.2012.7352

16. Ben-Josef E, Guthrie KA, El-Khoueiry AB, et al. SWOG S0809: a phase II intergroup trial of adjuvant capecitabine and gemcitabine followed by radiotherapy and concurrent capecitabine in extrahepatic cholangiocarcinoma and gallbladder carcinoma. *J Clin Oncol*. 2015;33(24):2617–2622. doi:10.1200/JCO.2014.60.2219

17. Ebata T, Hirano S, Konishi M, et al. Randomized clinical trial of adjuvant gemcitabine chemotherapy versus observation in resected bile duct cancer. *Br J Surg*. 2018;105(3):192–202. doi:10.1002/bjs.10776

18. Edeline J, Bonnetain F, Phelip JM, et al. Gemox versus surveillance following surgery of localized biliary tract cancer: results of the PRODIGE 12-ACCORD 18 (UNICANCER GI) phase III trial [abstract]. *J Clin Oncol*. 2017;35(4 Suppl):225. doi:10.1200/JCO.2017.35.4_suppl.225

19. Primrose JN, Fox R, Palmer DH, et al. Adjuvant capecitabine for biliary tract cancer: the BILCAP randomized study [abstract]. *J Clin Oncol*. 2017;35(15 Suppl):4006. doi:10.1200/JCO.2017.35.15_suppl.4006

20. Valle JW, Lamarca A, Goyal L, et al. New horizons for precision medicine in biliary tract cancers. *Cancer Discov*. 2017;7(9):943–962. doi:10.1158/2159-8290.CD-17-0245

21. Smoot RL, Rocha FG, Boughey JC. Adjuvant Therapies for Biliary Tract Cancers. *Bulletin of the American College of Surgeons*. 2018. http://bulletin.facs.org/2018/04/adjuvant-therapies-for-biliary-tract-cancers

Chemotherapy for Advanced Cancers of the Bile Ducts and Gallbladder

Jonathan Whisenant

INTRODUCTION

The overwhelming majority of patients with cholangiocarcinoma (CC) or gallbladder cancer (GBC) will present with locally advanced or metastatic disease or will experience relapse after a potentially curative resection (1–3). However, cancers of the bile duct and gallbladder comprise a widely heterogeneous group of diseases with a range of metastatic patterns and tremendous variability in disease course. For example, intrahepatic cholangiocarcinoma generally metastasizes to other sites in the liver, the peritoneal cavity, or potentially the lungs or pleura; perihilar cholangiocarcinomas (Klatskin tumors) will also frequently metastasize to the liver or peritoneal cavity but can spread to unusual sites including the brain and bones; GBCs frequently invade locally to the porta hepatis and liver, metastasize to regional lymph nodes, or metastasize to the liver, peritoneal cavity, or lungs. Additionally, while the median survival of patients with advanced cancers of the bile duct and gallbladder is approximately 1 year, many patients will progress and die rapidly while others may experience a very indolent course, living with metastatic disease for many years.

FIRST-LINE CHEMOTHERAPY

Prior to the publication of the UK ABC-02 trial in 2010 (4), decisions about treatment for patients with metastatic CC or GBC were based on case series and small nonrandomized trials. Several studies suggested clinical benefit in patients treated with 5-fluoropyrimidine or gemcitabine with an objective response rate (ORR) in the range of 15% to 35% and a median overall survival (OS) of less than 12 months. In the late 1990s, emerging data suggested encouraging efficacy with acceptable toxicity when patients are treated with combination chemotherapy including gemcitabine and cisplatin, demonstrating reproducible benefits with an ORR of approximately 20% to 40% and median OS of 1 year or greater (5,6).

The first large randomized phase 3 trial evaluating two different chemotherapy regimens was conducted in the United Kingdom from 2002 to 2008 (4). In the ABC-02 trial, 410 patients with locally advanced or metastatic CC (n = 241), GBC (n = 152), or ampullary cancer (n = 20) were randomized to receive either cisplatin 25 mg/m^2 followed by gemcitabine 1,000 mg/m^2 administered on days 1 and 8 every 21 days or gemcitabine alone 1,000 mg/m^2 on days 1, 8, and 15 every 28 days. Combination therapy with cisplatin and gemcitabine was associated with a significant improvement in OS (11.7 months vs. 8.1 months), progression-free survival (PFS, 8 months vs. 5 months), and rate of tumor control (81.4% vs. 71.8%). Treatment was well-tolerated with a modest increase in rates of neutropenia and anemia. This trial established combination chemotherapy with cisplatin and gemcitabine as a strong standard option as frontline treatment in patients with metastatic or locally advanced, unresectable CC or GBC (Figure 46.1).

Smaller phase 2 trials have suggested similar benefits when combining gemcitabine with oxaliplatin (GEMOX), possibly with a more favorable toxicity profile (7,8), with additional data supporting the use of combination therapy with gemcitabine and capecitabine (GEMCAP) as well (9,10). In general, these gemcitabine-based combination regimens appear to exhibit similar efficacy; if there is any difference in efficacy it is likely modest. However, in the absence of a randomized clinical trial demonstrating equivalent or superior efficacy of these regimens relative to treatment with cisplatin and gemcitabine, neither should be considered a standard option in the first-line setting. We favor combination therapy with gemcitabine and cisplatin in the front line

---

A Clinical Vignette is included at the end of the chapter.

as described in the aforementioned ABC-02 trial. Other regimens mentioned, however, should be considered reasonable alternatives especially in patients with potential contraindications to treatment with cisplatin (e.g., patients with renal insufficiency, hearing loss, neuropathy).

The optimal duration of frontline treatment is not well defined. Patients in the ABC-02 trial were treated for 6 months (eight cycles) and then observed (4); this practice is common in Europe. Although there are no clear data suggesting a benefit for treatment until evidence of disease progression compared to treatment for a defined period of time, many physicians will continue treatment beyond 6 months if patients are tolerating treatment well and have no evidence of disease progression. To improve tolerability, one approach frequently utilized is to stop cisplatin and continue treatment with gemcitabine alone if there is no evidence of disease progression after 6 months of treatment with combination therapy. Given the lack of data suggesting a clear benefit with ongoing treatment beyond 6 months, we maintain a low threshold to stop or modify treatment if there is significant toxicity or if it is felt that treatment is significantly impacting quality of life.

Of note, patients with intrahepatic CC generally experience lower response rates with chemotherapy than patients with extrahepatic CC and GBC. For example, in the ABC-02 trial, the ORR for GBC was 37.7% compared to an ORR of 18% in patients with bile duct cancers. This finding has been seen in other trials and is seen in our clinical practice as well.

When treating patients who present with locally advanced, unresectable disease, consideration can be given to radiotherapy as "consolidative" treatment. Limited clinical data support this approach, and the role of radiotherapy remains controversial. Many physicians will consider radiation after receiving systemic chemotherapy for some duration of time as long as there is no evidence of systemic metastatic disease. Retrospective reviews do suggest an improvement in survival in patients who receive chemoradiotherapy compared to patients receiving chemotherapy alone including a recent report suggesting a more convincing benefit with higher radiation dosing (11,12). This approach may also allow patients a "chemotherapy holiday," which may be considered a desirable goal in patients with a limited life expectancy. Given the possible survival benefit and the option of a chemotherapy holiday, consolidating therapy with radiation may be considered in select patients. Experienced radiation therapists approach this setting thoughtfully with important considerations including toxicity to healthy liver and nearby structures (including large and small bowel) as well as patterns of recurrence outside of the radiation field.

CHEMOTHERAPY OPTIONS IN THE SECOND LINE AND BEYOND

Optimal treatment in the salvage setting is poorly defined with no randomized prospective trials performed among this patient population. As patients are generally treated with a gemcitabine-based regimen in the first-line setting, most trials have evaluated fluoropyrimidine-based treatment in the salvage/second-line setting. Patients eligible for treatment generally have well-preserved performance status and many have had a favorable response to first-line treatment, suggesting a likely selection bias, but reported data suggest an apparent clinical benefit with fluoropyrimidine-based therapy, including treatment with 5-fluorouracil (5-FU), capecitabine, FOLFOX, and CAPOX (Figure 46.1). Response rates are generally low and duration of response is usually short with most reports suggesting an ORR of 5% to 20% and PFS of 2 to 3 months (13,14). However, patients who receive second-line chemotherapy do tend to live longer when compared to historical controls, but this may reflect a strong selection bias as many patients will not be candidates for second-line chemotherapy. Regardless, it is reasonable to consider second-line chemotherapy in select patients who retain a good performance status with interest in pursuing further systemic chemotherapy after a meaningful discussion about the pros and cons with a goal to establish realistic expectations.

OTHER THERAPEUTIC CONSIDERATIONS

The role of adding targeted agents to chemotherapy remains very unclear with several studies evaluating the addition of anti–vascular endothelial growth factor (VEGF) antibodies (bevacizumab, ramucirumab) or anti–epidermal growth factor receptor (EGFR) agents (cetuximab, panitumumab, erlotinib) to various chemotherapy backbones. Published data of small trials make it difficult to ascertain the additive benefit of these targeted agents but there does appear to be an emerging signal of efficacy, particularly with erlotinib, as trials suggest a modest

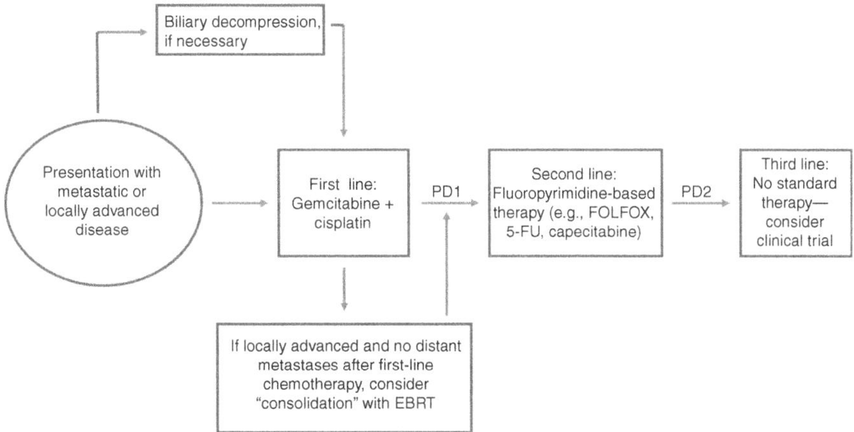

FIGURE 46.1   Treatment algorithm for patients with locally advanced or unresectable bile duct or gallbladder cancer.

EBRT, external body radiation therapy; PD1, first progression; PD2, second progression.

therapeutic benefit in patients receiving erlotinib either as a single agent (15) or when added to a chemotherapy backbone (16). However, given a lack of evidence demonstrating a clear survival benefit, we do not routinely add erlotinib to frontline chemotherapy but might consider a trial with erlotinib in the salvage setting in select patients. On the other hand, there is much more enthusiasm with several newer agents such as those targeting activating isocitrate dehydrogenase 1 (IDH1) mutations or fibroblast growth factor receptor 2 (FGFR2) fusions as well as immunotherapy options, which are being evaluated in ongoing clinical trials with promising early results. These treatments are addressed in Chapter 47, Emerging Therapies for Advanced Cancers of the Bile Ducts and Gallbladder.

SPECIAL CIRCUMSTANCES

Because of the pattern of progression and metastases, patients with unresectable or metastatic bile duct and gallbladder cancer frequently present unique challenges, largely related to biliary obstruction and/or liver dysfunction (17). These clinical problems must be kept in mind in making treatment decisions and when evaluating patients throughout their treatment course.

Patients with GBC or perihilar CC will frequently present with biliary obstruction as do patients with intrahepatic cholangiocarcinoma depending on the location of the primary tumor and the pattern of spread. When not candidates for curative resection, the immediate need is to alleviate the obstruction with biliary decompression, generally either endoscopically or percutaneously. In addition to effects on liver function, these patients will frequently require stent placement or percutaneous biliary drainage, both options placing them at ongoing risk for developing cholangitis. Treating physicians should review this risk with patients as life-threatening sepsis can set in rapidly. In general, physicians must maintain a low threshold to consider empiric antibiotics and evaluate the need to interrogate stent and/or catheter patency and possible need for exchange.

Similarly, biliary obstruction must be considered as a possible etiology of liver dysfunction at any time in the course of the disease, especially when manifesting primarily as hyperbilirubinemia. This can be a particular challenge in patients with diffuse liver involvement as it is often unclear whether an increasing bilirubin is due to biliary obstruction (which may be amenable to biliary duct decompression) or due to disease progression throughout the liver parenchyma resulting in generalized liver dysfunction. Evaluation requires a multidisciplinary approach involving expert radiology and gastroenterology evaluation, often requiring upper endoscopy with endoscopic retrograde cholangiopancreatography (ERCP) and/or magnetic resonance cholangiopancreatography (MRCP). This evaluation can be critical as patients who develop severe biliary obstruction may not be candidates for palliative therapy if the obstruction remains undetected, whereas biliary decompression can significantly improve symptoms and survival.

Patients presenting with abnormal liver function not relieved by biliary decompression present another clinical challenge given liver metabolism of chemotherapy. It is recommended that patients with mild to moderate hyperbilirubinemia receive a dose reduction of gemcitabine with close monitoring for toxicity; however, small trials suggest no dose adjustment is necessary even in the setting of bilirubin up to 10 × upper limit of normal (ULN) (18). Given these concerns, the experience of administering FOLFOX in the setting of severe liver dysfunction, and an unclear benefit with gemcitabine-based therapy over FOLFOX, many physicians will offer FOLFOX as first-line therapy in the setting of severe liver dysfunction.

Additionally, patients with metastatic CC and GBC exhibit a high risk of venous thromboembolism (VTE) (19). In addition to pulmonary embolism and extremity thrombosis, splanchnic thromboses are frequently discovered including thrombosis of portal, hepatic, splenic and mesenteric veins. As in other cancers, VTE in the setting of a metastatic CC or GBC is associated with a poorer survival when compared to patients without VTE. A high degree of suspicion is required when patients present with symptoms potentially attributable to VTE with prompt initiation of appropriate therapy.

SUMMARY

Most patients with bile duct and gallbladder cancers present unique clinical challenges and will eventually succumb to their disease. As with other cancers, physicians must consider the extent of disease, patient performance status, comorbidities, and personal goals as we address the role of palliative chemotherapy, including a thorough discussion of risks and expected benefits. Standard first-line chemotherapy with gemcitabine and cisplatin is well-tolerated and has been shown to improve survival. Other options for first-line treatment to be considered depending on clinical circumstances include GEMOX, GEMCAP, FOLFOX, or single-agent treatment with gemcitabine or a fluoropyrimidine. Treatment in the second-line setting is associated with modest benefits with consideration of a fluoropyrimidine-based regimen (e.g., FOLFOX, 5-FU, capecitabine) in patients initially treated with gemcitabine. There is very little data to support chemotherapy beyond the second-line setting for most patients, but emerging data evaluating the role of novel targeted agents appear promising. Given the paucity of data in this patient population, clinical trial participation is highly encouraged.

Clinical Vignette 46.1

A 57-year-old woman presents to the emergency room with right upper quadrant pain in April 2016. CT imaging demonstrates a large liver mass in the dome of the liver, a second smaller lesion anterolaterally, and malignant portal and para-aortic lymphadenopathy (Figure 46.2). CT-guided biopsy is obtained demonstrating a poorly differentiated adenocarcinoma with an immunohistochemical profile consistent with a hepatobiliary primary. Carbohydrate antigen 19-9 (CA 19-9) was elevated (373 U/mL) with a mildly elevated total bilirubin (1.4 mg/dL), mildly elevated alkaline phosphatase (141 U/L), and normal aspartate aminotransferase (AST) and alanine aminotransferase (ALT).

The patient begins treatment with palliative chemotherapy with gemcitabine and cisplatin. Treatment is well-tolerated with minimal change in CA 19-9 and improvement in liver function abnormalities. Follow-up imaging demonstrates overall stable disease. After 6 months of first-line chemotherapy, CA 19-9 is increasing (now 824 U/mL) (Figure 46.3) and imaging suggests disease progression with an increase in the size and number of liver lesions, increasing adenopathy, and new lung lesions (Figure 46.4).

The patient began treatment with mFOLFOX6. She experienced a drop in CA 19-9 after two cycles of treatment but ultimately had a clear increase in CA 19-9, worsening liver function testing, and clear radiographic progression after 3 months of treatment with mFOLFOX6 (Figures 46.5 and 46.6). At this time, she opted for hospice care. She passed away in April 2017, 11 months after her initial diagnosis.

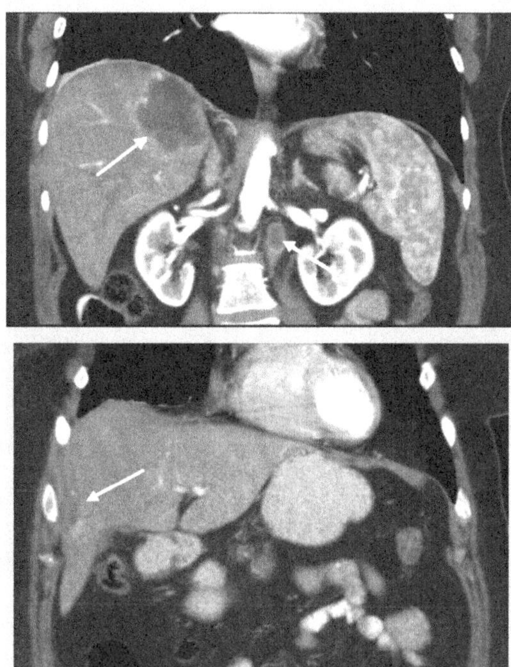

FIGURE 46.2   Imaging revealing multifocal liver disease and para-aortic adenopathy.

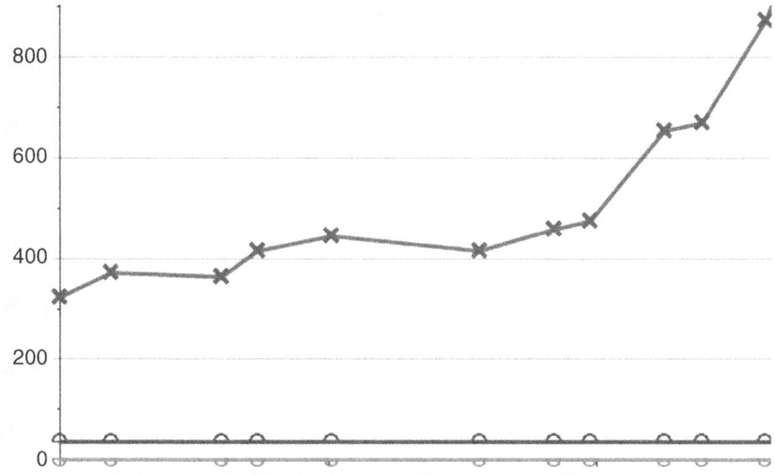

FIGURE 46.3   CA 19-9: June 2016–November 2016.

CA 19-9, carbohydrate antigen 19-9.

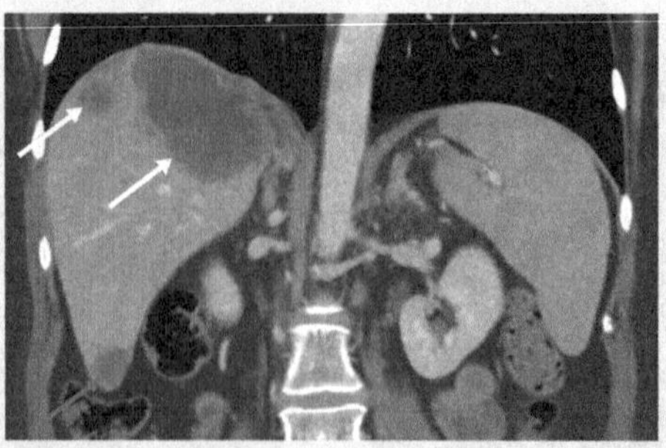

FIGURE 46.4   Imaging findings reveal increase in size of dominant liver mass with new lesions consistent with disease progression.

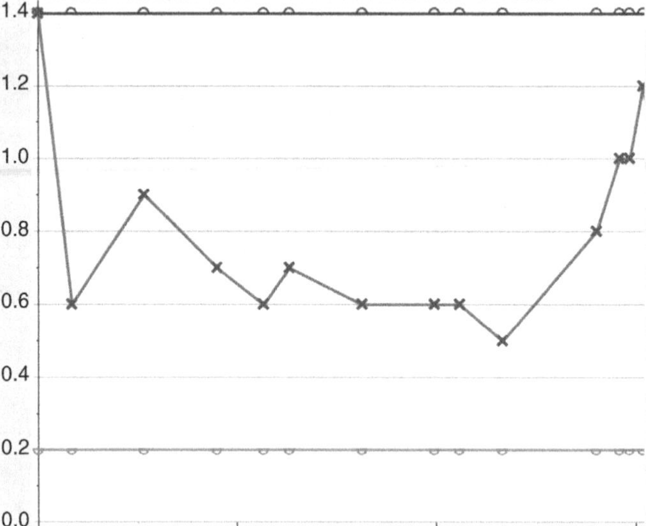

FIGURE 46.5   Bilirubin: June 2016–November 2016.

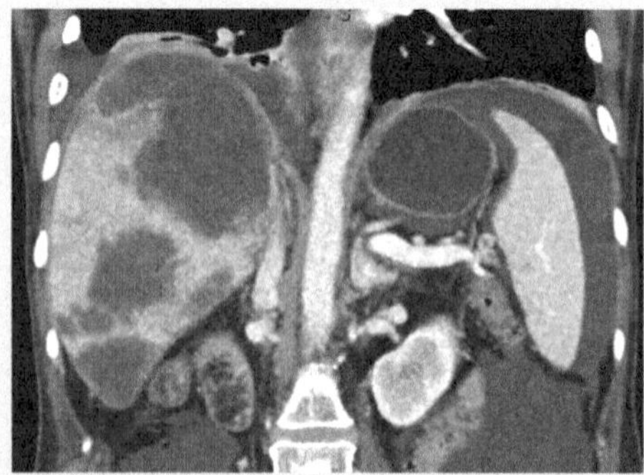

FIGURE 46.6   Imaging demonstrating marked disease progression after six cycles of mFOLFOX6 chemotherapy.

REFERENCES

1. Saha SK, Zhu AX, Fuchs CS, et al. Forty-year trends in cholangiocarcinoma incidence in the U.S.: intrahepatic disease on the rise. *Oncologist*. 2016;21(5):594–599. doi:10.1634/theoncologist.2015-0446

2. Fong Y, Blumgart LH, Lin E, et al. Outcome of treatment for distal bile duct cancer. *Br J Surg*. 1996;83(12):1712–1715. doi:10.1002/bjs.1800831217

3. Klempnauer J, Ridder GJ, von Wasielewski R, et al. Resectional surgery of hilar cholangiocarcinoma: a multivariate analysis of prognostic factors. *J Clin Oncol*. 1997;15(3):947–954. doi:10.1200/JCO.1997.15.3.947

4. Valle J, Wasan H, Palmer DH, et al. Cisplatin plus gemcitabine versus gemcitabine for biliary tract cancer. *N Engl J Med*. 2010;362(14):1273–1281. doi:10.1056/NEJMoa0908721

5. Thongprasert S, Napapan S, Charoentum C, et al. Phase II study of gemcitabine and cisplatin as first-line chemotherapy in inoperable biliary tract carcinoma. *Ann Oncol*. 2005;16(2):279–281. doi:10.1093/annonc/mdi046

6. Giuliani F, Gebbia V, Maiello E, et al. Gemcitabine and cisplatin for inoperable and/or metastatic biliary tree carcinomas: a multicenter phase II study of the Gruppo Oncologico dell'Italia Meridionale (GOIM). *Ann Oncol*. 2006;17(Suppl 7):vii73–vii77. doi:10.1093/annonc/mdl956

7. André T, Tournigand C, Rosmorduc O, et al. Gemcitabine combined with oxaliplatin (GEMOX) in advanced biliary tract adenocarcinoma: a GERCOR study. *Ann Oncol*. 2004;15(9):1339–1343. doi:10.1093/annonc/mdh351

8. Harder J, Riecken B, Kummer O, et al. Outpatient chemotherapy with gemcitabine and oxaliplatin in patients with biliary tract cancer. *Br J Cancer*. 2006;95(7):848–852. doi:10.1038/sj.bjc.6603334

9. Knox JJ, Hedley D, Oza A, et al. Combining gemcitabine and capecitabine in patients with advanced biliary cancer: a phase II trial. *J Clin Oncol*. 2005;23(10):2332–2338. doi:10.1200/JCO.2005.51.008

10. Cho JY, Paik YH, Chang YS, et al. Capecitabine combined with gemcitabine (CapGem) as first-line treatment in patients with advanced/metastatic biliary tract carcinoma. *Cancer*. 2005;104(12):2753–2758. doi:10.1002/cncr.21591

11. Kim YI, Park JW, Kim BH, et al. Outcomes of concurrent chemoradiotherapy versus chemotherapy alone for advanced-stage unresectable intrahepatic cholangiocarcinoma. *Radiat Oncol*. 2013;8:292. doi:10.1186/1748-717X-8-292

12. Tao R, Krishnan S, Bhosale PR, et al. Ablative radiotherapy doses lead to a substantial prolongation of survival in patients with inoperable intrahepatic cholangiocarcinoma: a retrospective dose response analysis. *J Clin Oncol*. 2016;34(3):219–226. doi:10.1200/JCO.2015.61.3778

13. Fornaro L, Vivaldi C, Cereda S, et al. Second-line chemotherapy in advanced biliary cancer progressed to first-line platinum-gemcitabine combination: a multicenter survey and pooled analysis with published data. *J Exp Clin Cancer Res*. 2015;34:156. doi:10.1186/s13046-015-0267-x

14. Lowery MA, Goff LW, Jordan E, et al. Second-line chemotherapy outcomes in advanced biliary cancers: a retrospective multicenter analysis. *J Clin Oncol*. 2016;34:437. doi:10.1200/jco.2016.34.4_suppl.437

15. Philip A, Mahoney MR, Allmer C, et al. Phase II study of erlotinib in patients with advanced biliary cancer. *J Clin Oncol*. 2006;24(19): 3069–3074. doi:10.1200/JCO.2005.05.3579

16. Lee J, Park SH, Chang HM, et al. Gemcitabine and oxaliplatin with or without erlotinib in advanced biliary-tract cancer: a multicenter, open-label, randomized, phase 3 study. *Lancet Oncol*. 2012;13(2):e49. doi:10.1016/S1470-2045(11)70301-1

17. Jarnagin WR, Ruo L, Little SA, et al. Patterns of Initial disease recurrence after resection of gallbladder carcinoma and hilar cholangiocarcinoma. *Cancer*. 2003;98(8):1689–1700. doi:10.1002/cncr.11699

18. Shibata T, Ebata T, Fujita K, et al. Optimal dose of gemcitabine for the treatment of biliary tract or pancreatic cancer in patients with liver dysfunction. *Cancer Sci*. 2016;107(2):168–172. doi:10.1111/cas.12851

19. Jeon HK, Kim DU, Baek DH, et al. Venous thromboembolism in patients with cholangiocarcinoma: focus on risk factors and impact on survival. *Eur J Gastroenterol Hepatol*. 2012;24(4):444–449. doi:10.1097/MEGI0b013e328350f93c

Emerging Therapies for Advanced Cancers of the Bile Ducts and Gallbladder

Madappa Kundranda and Milind Javle

INTRODUCTION

Biliary tract cancers (BTCs) are heterogeneous and highly lethal malignancies arising from the epithelial cells lining the biliary tree and include intrahepatic cholangiocarcinoma (IHCCA), extrahepatic cholangiocarcinoma (EHCCA), and gallbladder cancer (GBC). Epidemiological risk factors for BTC vary by region and include chronic inflammation (due to biliary and gallbladder stones, hepatobiliary flukes, primary sclerosing cholangitis, and viral hepatitis), developmental abnormalities such as cysts and Caroli's disease, and other environmental or metabolic factors such as diabetes and smoking (1). These tumors represent 10% to 20% of hepatobiliary neoplasms. IHCCA is the second most common primary liver cancer worldwide. The Global Burden of Disease study estimated 139,500 deaths from BTC in 2013, a 22% increase from the estimated 115,400 deaths in 1990, and this figure is increasing. This equates to age-standardized death rates from 2.3 to 3.4 per 100,000 per year, over this time period (2).

In the United States, gallbladder carcinoma is the most common, accounting for 60% of cases. The remaining 40% are cholangiocarcinomas and these are anatomically subclassified as intrahepatic when they arise from intrahepatic ducts or extrahepatic, when occurring at or below the confluence of the main left and right hepatic ducts (3). Regardless of the subtype, most BTCs present at an advanced disease stage where molecular classification may be of greater clinical relevance (4). In the minority of patients who are amenable to curative therapy, surgical resection with negative margins or liver transplantation offers the potential for cure. In the majority of patients with BTC who present with locally advanced or metastatic disease, there are limited effective therapeutic options (5). Systemic chemotherapy has been the mainstay of therapy for unresectable disease. A randomized phase 3 study was conducted in 410 patients with locally advanced or metastatic cholangiocarcinoma, GBC, and ampullary cancer with cisplatin (25 mg/m^2) followed by gemcitabine (1,000 mg/m^2) on days 1 and 8 every 21 days or gemcitabine (1,000 mg/m^2) on days 1, 8, and 15 every 28 days. The median overall survival (OS) was 11.7 months in the combination arm versus 8.1 months in the gemcitabine arm (hazard ratio [HR]: 0.64, 95% confidence interval [CI]: 0.52–0.80, $p < .001$) leading to the establishment of gemcitabine and cisplatin as the standard first-line therapy for biliary cancer. A significant benefit in both response rate and progression-free survival (PFS) was seen favoring the gemcitabine/cisplatin arm, with no clinically relevant increase in adverse events for the combination arm when compared with the single agent gemcitabine (6). A smaller phase 3 Japanese study of 84 patients with an identical design demonstrated similar results with an OS of cisplatin and gemcitabine at 11.2 months versus 7.7 months in the gemcitabine only arm (7). The gemcitabine plus cisplatin combination has not been directly compared with other gemcitabine combinations in phase 3 trials. After disease progression, no established alternatives are available, and the potential benefit of second-line chemotherapy is currently under investigation in the randomized phase III ABC-06 trial, comparing FOLFOX to best supportive care (NCT01926236). In addition, there are ongoing phase 2 trials in the second-line setting; gemcitabine, nab-paclitaxel, cisplatin, oxaliplatin, fluoropyrimidines, or a combination is used in BTCs. Even in small subsets of surgically resectable patients, the long-term outcomes are poor (about 30% 5-year survival) and in advanced disease, the results are dismal with the median survival being less than 1 year (8).

With BTCs increasing in incidence globally, there is an urgent need to develop more effective and tolerable treatments. A better understanding of the genomic landscape of this tumor type with respect to differences among the three anatomical subtypes (intrahepatic, extrahepatic, and gallbladder) may lead to more effective tailored therapies in these patients.

MOLECULAR SUBTYPES IN BTCS

The cascade of events leading to tumorigenesis from dysplasia to cancer is influenced by risk factors including: (a) chronic inflammation secondary to biliary lithiasis, hepatobiliary flukes, primary sclerosing cholangitis, and viral hepatitis; (b) developmental anomalies and choledochal cysts; and (c) environmental or metabolic factors such as obesity, smoking, and diabetes (9). These etiological differences may account for varied geographic distribution in cancer incidence with the highest incidence occurring in East and South Asia and certain regions of South America.

Earlier molecular studies by Miller et al. (10) evaluating 34 BTC surgical specimens by gene expression and comparative genomic hybridization (CGH) analysis reported that unsupervised hierarchical clustering analysis revealed that the three cancer subtypes (IHCCA, EHCCA, and GBC) did not cluster separately, implying that there was no difference in the global gene expression patterns between the subgroups. However, there was unique altered expression of 1633, 80, and 790 genes in IHCCA, EHCCA, and GBC, respectively. They also identified vascular invasion was associated with mutated expression of genes involved with electron transport and cellular metabolism. CGH analysis revealed that short segments of chromosomes 1p, 3p, 6q, 8p, 9p, and 14q were commonly deleted across all cancer subtypes while commonly amplified regions included segments of 1q, 3q, 5p, 7p, 7q, 8q, and 20q. This implication of using molecular signatures for both prognostic and therapeutic along with advances in whole genomic tumor profiling has led to the identification of a wide range of mutations, amplifications, and deletions that could potentially be targetable.

Important driver mutations including the epidermal growth factor (EGF) pathway with EGF receptor (EGFR), *KRAS*, and *BRAF* mutations or overexpression, as well as alteration in the mitogen-activated protein kinase and PI3K/mammalian target of rapamycin pathways, as well as TP53 have been identified. In addition, mutations in chromatin-remodeling genes *BAP1* (encoding a nuclear deubiquitinase), *ARID1A* (encoding a subunit of the SWI/SNF chromatin-remodeling complexes), and *PBRM1* (encoding a subunit of the ATP-dependent SWI/SNF chromatin-remodeling complexes) have been reported in frequencies of 10% to 25%. Also, mutations in the metabolic pathway involving isocitrate dehydrogenase 1 (IDH1) and isocitrate dehydrogenase 2 (IDH2) have also been observed. Furthermore, amplifications in cMET, FGF 19 (fibroblast growth factor 19), cyclin-dependent kinase 6, and cyclin d1, as well as deletions in cyclin-dependent kinase inhibitors 2A and 2B have been reported (11,12).

As we expand our understanding of the molecular pathways involved in BTCs, it is important to correlate it with the anatomical location of the tumor to identify new therapeutic targeted therapies. We have previously described that there exists a difference in the mutational profile based on the anatomical location of the tumor (11). Nakamura et al. (12) identified five molecular signatures, with alterations varying according to the anatomical location. They described potentially targetable genetic alterations in 38.9% of BTC cases (93/239). These potential targets included kinases (FGFR1, FGFR2, FGFR3, PIK3CA, ALK, EGFR, ERBB2, BRAF, and AKT3), oncogenes *(IDH1, IDH2, CCND1, CCND3,* and *MDM2)*, and tumor suppressor genes *(BRCA1* and *BRCA2)*. Importantly, they identified four molecular subgroups of gene expression, which clustered with clinical prognosis.

We have previously reported that targeted treatments would be most likely to improve outcomes in appropriately selected patients (13). Our study demonstrated a similar spread of genetic changes in a large cohort of 321 patients consistent with what has been previously reported. In the subset of patients with IHCCA receiving experimental targeted therapies, we observed a numerically better outcome than those on standard therapy (241 vs. 186 weeks, *p* = .07). In addition, patients identified to have a fibroblast growth factor receptor (FGFR) aberrant expression treated with an appropriate targeted therapy had an OS that exceeded those receiving non–FGFR-targeted therapy (25 vs. 80 months, *p* = .006).

KEY MOLECULAR PATHWAYS AND POTENTIAL EMERGING THERAPIES

EGFR Signaling Pathways

The EGFR family comprises four tyrosine kinase receptors (ERBB1–4) that regulate a multitude of cellular functions including cell proliferation, survival, angiogenesis, and invasion through ligand binding and subsequent activation of signal transduction cascades involving the MAPK pathway (Ras–Raf–MEK–ERK) and the PI3K/AKT pathway (14). Aberrant activation of the EGFR pathway in BTCs is common and has been associated with a poor clinical outcome (15). In BTCs, the most common pathways that are altered are the EGFR (ERBB1) and HER2/neu (ERBB2). Overexpression of EGFR occurs in 11% to 27% of IHCCA (16), 5% to 19% of EHCCA (16), and 12% in GBCs (17), whereas activating EGFR mutations are preferentially seen in GBC (4%–18%) but rarely in CCAs (12,18). Variable EGFR expression (10%–38%) was reported in the literature, depending upon the methodologies used. Whether this varies according to the geographic location or BTC type is unknown at this time (19,20).

A large phase III study evaluating the efficacy of gemcitabine and oxaliplatin with the addition of erlotinib was conducted among unselected/nonenriched patients with newly diagnosed metastatic BTC. Two hundred sixty-eight patients were randomized to receive either first-line treatment with chemotherapy alone (gemcitabine 1,000 mg/m^2 on day 1 and oxaliplatin 100 mg/m^2 on day 2) or chemotherapy plus erlotinib (100 mg daily). Although significantly more patients had an objective response in the chemotherapy plus erlotinib group than in the chemotherapy alone group (40 patients vs. 21 patients; p = .005), median OS was the same in both groups (9.5 months [95% CI: 7.5–11.5] in the chemotherapy alone group and 9.5 months [7.6–11.4] in the chemotherapy plus erlotinib group; HR: 0.93, 0.69–1.25; p = .611) (21). There have been other failed phase 2 trials with erlotinib, cetuximab, and panitumumab (Table 47.1). EGFR targeting in BTC has not been a promising strategy when combined with chemotherapy based on the aforementioned trials. However, these studies enrolled patients irrespective of their EGFR status or mutational profile. Single agents like erlotinib have been shown to have efficacy and this may be a very promising strategy in patients with EGFR mutation or amplification.

HER2/neu Amplification

HER2/neu (ERBB2), a key driver of tumorigenesis, mediates its signaling via the activation of downstream mitogen-activated protein kinase (MAPK)/ERK and phosphatidylinositol 3-kinase (PI3K)/PTEN/AKT pathways. Its overexpression as a result of gene amplification has been noted in several tumors including breast, non–small-cell lung cancer, and colorectal cancer. We have previously reported on HER2/neu protein expression in 187 cases of GBC using

TABLE 47.1 Completed Clinical Trials With Targeted Therapies in Biliary Cancers

Study	Phase	Patients (n)	Response Rate (%)	OS (Months)
Gemcitabine plus cetuximab (22)	II	44	20.4	13.5
GEMOX plus cetuximab (23)	II	30	63	15.2
GEMCAP plus cetuximab (24)	II	34	17.6	15.7
GEMOX plus panitumumab (25)	II	31	45	20.3
GEMOX-CAP plus panitumumab (26)	II	46	33	10
GEM-IRI plus panitumumab (27)	II	35	39	12.9
GEM-CIS-panitumumab vs. GEM-CIS (28)	II	93	45 vs. 39	12.8 vs. 21.4
Erlotinib (29)	II	42	8	7.5
GEMOX-erlotinib vs. GEMOX (21)	III	268	30 vs. 16	9.5 vs. 9.5

OS, overall survival.

the accepted College of American Pathologists (CAP)/American Society of Clinical Oncology (ASCO) criteria. Our study noted a 13% HER2/neu overexpression rate 3+ by immunohisto-chemistry (30). The incidence of HER2/neu overexpression in IHCCA has been reported at 0.9% (15) and EHCCA at 8% similar to other reports (19). The prognostic implication of HER2/neu amplification in BTC is unclear with several contradictory reports of a better or worse prognosis (13). Multiple phase 2 studies of single agent lapatinib (dual inhibitor of EGFR and HER2/neu) have not demonstrated any meaningful clinical benefit in BTCs (31,32). Preliminary results from an ongoing study combining pertuzumab + trastuzumab have demonstrated activity in HER2 amplified/overexpressed/mutated metastatic biliary tumors (33).

BRAF Mutation

BRAF is involved in the RAS/RAF/MEK/ERK molecular signaling pathway, and mutations occur in approximately 5% of patients with IHCCA (11). Given the significant survival advantage that was noted in the melanoma setting, a *BRAF V600* mutated IHCCA patient was evaluated with a combination of dabrafenib (BRAF inhibitor) and trametinib (MEK1 and MEK2 inhibitor) with a sustained partial response (34). Similar responses have been observed in our experience as well (Figure 47.1). Multiple trials are being conducted in the current setting (35).

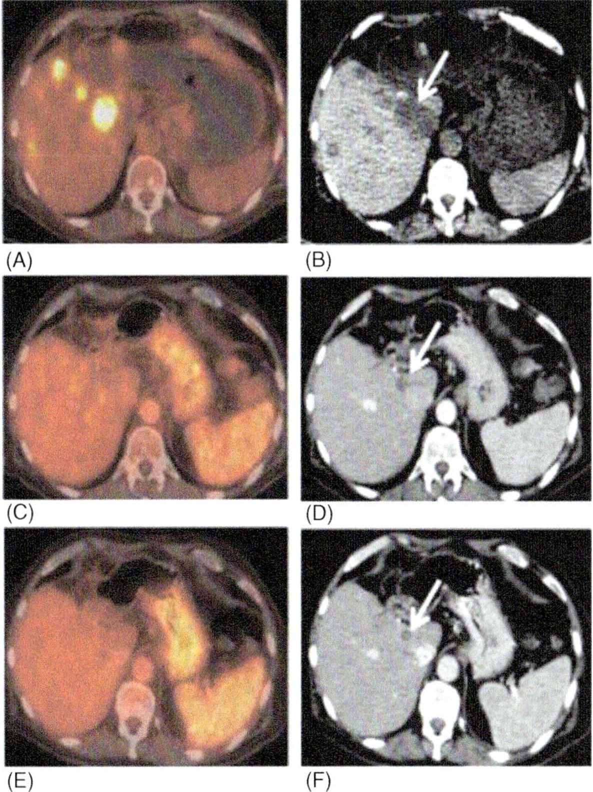

FIGURE 47.1   IHCCA with *BRAF* V600E mutation responds to RAF kinase inhibition.
Metastatic intrahepatic cholangiocarcinoma with BRAF V600E treated with a RAF kinase inhibitor. Axial (A) fused PET–CT and (B) unenhanced CT images from a PET scan demonstrate FDG avidity of multiple liver metastases. After 8 weeks of therapy, axial (C) fused PET–CT and (D) contrast-enhanced CT images demonstrate lack of FDG avidity and decreased size of liver metastases. After 16 weeks of therapy, axial (E) fused PET–CT and (F) contrast-enhanced CT images demonstrate continued lack of FDG avidity and further decreased size of liver metastases. The dominant lesion (arrow) decreased from 3.7 to 1.3 cm.

FDG, fluorodeoxyglucose; IHCCA, intrahepatic cholangiocarcinoma.

FGFR Signaling Pathway

The FGF pathway and *FGFR* genes are involved in multiple biologic processes, ranging from cell transformation, angiogenesis, and tissue repair to embryonic development (36). The FGFR family consists of four transmembrane receptors (FGFR 1–4), 22 FGFR ligands, and a heparan sulfate proteoglycan (HSPG) that stabilizes and sequesters the FGFs (37). The major downstream signaling pathways for FGFR are mediated through the Ras–Raf–MAPK, PI3K pathways, and the protein serine/threonine kinase AKT. Dysregulation of the FGFR pathway can occur through *FGFR* mutations, translocations, amplification, overexpression, and alteration of regulatory influences such as by FGF ligand amplification.

Although *FGFR* amplifications are rare in BTC, IHCCAs demonstrate a relative high incidence of *FGF* mutations and fusions (approximately 16%), which makes this a potentially attractive target for therapeutic interventions. Preclinical studies have demonstrated that only cells harboring the *FGFR* gene fusions were sensitive to FGFR inhibitors (38,39). FGF pathway antagonists include small molecule tyrosine kinase inhibitors that act at the receptor level to suppress oncogenic signaling (40). As a prognosticator, our data suggest that patients with an FGF2 GA including fusions portend to a more indolent natural course of the disease (16).

Clinical efficacy of FGFR2 inhibitors is being investigated in biomarker-driven clinical trials aimed at patients harboring FGFR2 pathway alterations. The pan-FGFR inhibitor BGJ398 has potent activity against FGFR1–3 and is under evaluation in advanced CCAs with FGFR genetic alterations. In a phase II study of 61 patients with FGFR genetic alterations (FGFR2 fusion = 48, mutation = 8, or amplification = 3), the overall response rate (ORR) was 14.8% (18.8% FGFR2 fusions only), disease control rate was 75.4% (83.3% FGFR2 fusions only), and estimated median PFS was 5.8 months (95% CI: 4.3–7.6 months). Figure 47.2 depicts the waterfall plot demonstrating the best radiological responses in these patients from baseline. The most common adverse events included hyperphosphatemia (72.1%), fatigue (36.1%), stomatitis (29.5%), and alopecia (26.2%) (41). Another example of a refractory patient with an *FGFR2–KCTD1* fusion treated with BGJ398 is illustrated in Figure 47.3. Currently, there are several phase II studies with various compounds including TAS-120 (NCT02052778), ponatinib (NCT 02272998), INCB054828 (NCT 02924376), erdafitinib (NCT02699606), and ARQ087 (NCT01752920).

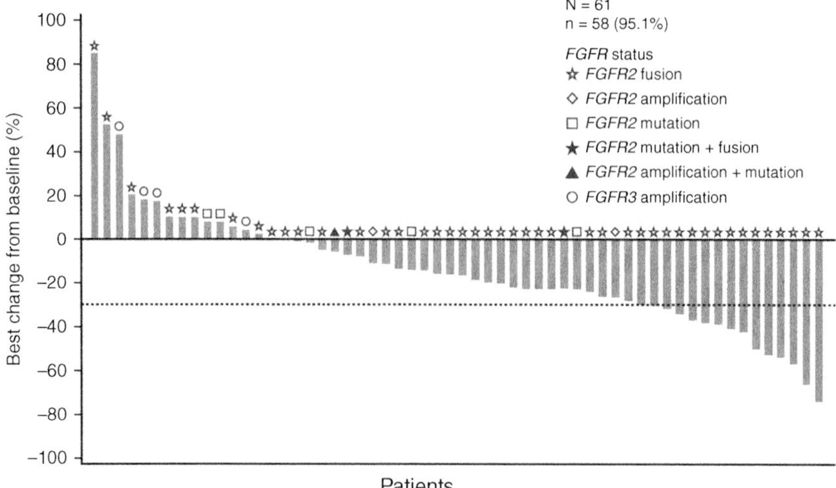

FIGURE 47.2   Waterfall plot of radiological responses in patients treated with BGJ398. Best percentage change in sum of longest tumor diameters from baseline. Only patients with baseline and at least one postbaseline assessment are included.

FGFR, fibroblast growth factor receptor; N, number of patients who received at least one study treatment; n, number of patients with baseline and at least one postbaseline assessment.

Source: From Javle M, Lowery M, Shroff RT, et al. Phase II study of BGJ398 in patients with FGFR-altered advanced cholangiocarcinoma. *J Clin Oncol.* 2018;36(3):276–282. doi:10.1200/JCO.2017.75.5009. Reprinted with permission. Copyright © 2017 American Society of Clinical Oncology. All rights reserved.

Before   After

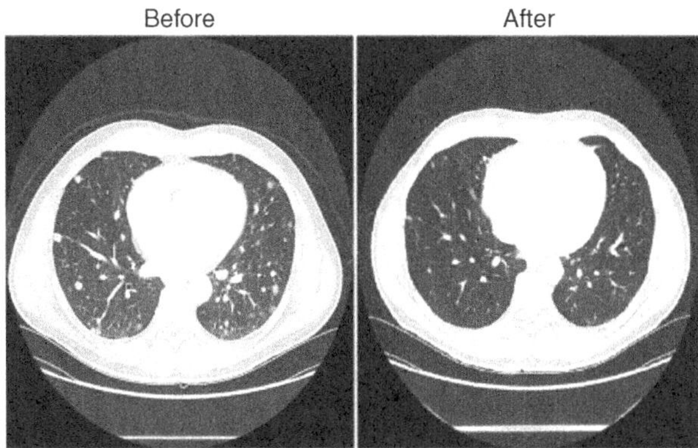

FIGURE 47.3   IHCCA with *FGFR2-KCTD1* fusion responds to BGJ398. Metastatic intrahepatic cholangiocarcinoma with *FGFR2-KCTD1* fusion treated with BGJ398. Axial CT images depict the before and after images of a patient with symptomatic pulmonary metastasis treatment with BGJ398. The patient sustained a partial response lasting over 7 months.

IHCCA, intrahepatic cholangiocarcinoma.

IDH1 and *IDH2* Mutations

The IDH family comprises three isozymes (IDH1, IDH2, and IDH3) that convert isocitrate to αKG via oxidative decarboxylation. IDH2 and IDH3 are located in the mitochondria, whereas IDH1 is located in the cytosol and peroxisome. IDH1 and IDH2 are obligate homodimers and utilize nicotinamide adenine dinucleotide phosphate (NADP$^+$) as a cofactor. The nicotinamide adenine dinucleotide (NAD$^+$)-dependent IDH3 isozyme exists as a heterotetramer consisting of two alpha, one beta, and one gamma subunit and plays a central role in the tricarboxylic acid (TCA) cycle, the final major metabolic pathway of cellular aerobic respiration. The utilization of NAD$^+$ by IDH3 is important in generating NADH for energy production. IDH thus plays an important role in exchanging key metabolites and shuttling electrons between the mitochondria and the cytosol (42).

The role of IDH mutations in tumorigenesis is that it may conjoin with other mutations to initiate and drive oncogenesis in multiple hematologic and solid tumors. High levels of 2-HG have been shown to inhibit αKG-dependent dioxygenases including histone and DNA demethylases, proteins that regulate cellular epigenetic status (43). In addition, IHD mutations with 2-HG promotes tumorigenesis via an effect on chromatin structure and tumors harboring IDH mutations display a CpG island methylator phenotype. Furthermore, Lu C et al. and others have demonstrated that overexpression of mutant IDH enzymes can induce histone and DNA hypermethylation, as well as block cellular differentiation (44). Interestingly this can be reversed by small molecule inhibition of the mutant enzymes (45). Together, these data suggest that cancer-associated IDH mutations can induce a block in cellular differentiation through epigenetic modifications, which contributes to tumor initiation and progression, thus building a solid clinical rationale to support the clinical evaluation of agents targeted at mutant IDH.

Mutations in *IDH1* and *IDH2* have been identified in BTCs. In IHCCA, an estimated 20% have IDH1, whereas 5% have IDH2 mutations. These mutations are typically not seen in EHCCA or GBC (16). The first molecule to enter clinical trials in late 2013 was enasidenib (AG-221), a selective, small molecule inhibitor of mutant IDH2 that was evaluated in patients with advanced myeloid malignancies. This was generally well-tolerated and induced hematologic responses in patients for whom prior acute myeloid leukemia therapy had failed with an ORR of 40.3%, and mOS of 9.3 months. Ivosidenib (AG-120) is a selective, small molecule inhibitor of mutant IDH1 and was evaluated in solid tumors including BTCs. In the cholangiocarcinoma dose escalation and expansion cohorts, 73 patients were evaluated. Among the 72 evaluable, 6% (n = 4) had a partial response and 56% (n = 40) experienced stable disease. The PFS rate at 6 months was 40%, and eight patients have been treated with AG-120 for $\geq$1 year (46). Following this, "ClarIDHy: A phase 3, multicenter, randomized, double-blind study of AG-120 vs placebo in patients with an advanced cholangiocarcinoma with an IDH1 mutation" is ongoing (47). In addition, several other trials of IDH inhibitors including AG-881 (NCT02481154) and IDH305 (NCT02381886) are under development.

DNA Repair Mutations

DNA mismatch repair (MMR) is a highly conserved biological pathway that plays a key role in maintaining genomic stability. MMR deficiency leading to microsatellite instability (MSI) has been recognized as a distinct oncogenic pathway. Lynch syndrome, defined by deleterious germline mutation in one of the four major MMR genes (*MLH1, MSH2, MSH6,* and *PMS2*) or the *EPCAM* gene, represents the hereditary prototype of MMR deficiency leading to tumor formation. Although MSI most commonly occurs in colorectal and endometrial cancers, a wide variety of other tumor types have been shown to exhibit MSI as well (13).

In BTCs there is a differential expression of the DNA repair mutations in the different cancer subtypes, and these may also vary depending upon disease etiology (48). Results of MSI may also vary depending upon the methodology used for analysis and reporting. A study by Liengswangwong and colleagues (49) using the National Cancer Institute (NCI) criteria (50) reported that none of their 37 intrahepatic cholangiocarcinomas exhibited microsatellite instability high (MSI-H). This group of patients was further evaluated by MMR IHCCA in a subsequent study and 5/29 tumors showed either MLH1 or MSH2 loss, for a total rate of MMR deficiency of 17% (51). This discrepancy further substantiates inconsistencies between the various methods used. MSI-H status was evaluated in 38 EHCCAs using seven microsatellite markers, and the investigators noted five (13%) showing instability at 1 or 2 loci, none involving mononucleotide markers and none fulfilling the MSI-H criterion that requires 40% or more of the tested loci being instable (52). Another study noted that 2/28 (7%) tumors showed MSI-H defined as instability at 40% of the six tested markers, both with mononucleotide instability (53).

Therefore, accurate and consistent evaluation of MMR deficiency in BTC has been very challenging as this was mostly measured by polymerase chain reaction (PCR) based MSI testing and/or utilizing MMR protein immunohistochemistry (IHC). In addition, small sample size, varied study populations, different microsatellite markers, different definitions for MSI, different antibody panels, and interpretational variations for MMR IHC have contributed adversely to this effort. In the current era of next-generation sequencing (NGS), it can be anticipated that large-scale genomic analysis will allow a more integrated view of the molecular alterations of the various biliary tumors. In our series of 321 BTC patients who underwent mutational profiling, DNA repair mutations (*MSH6, BRCA1, BRCA2, ATM, MLH1,* or *MSH2* gene) occurred in 13% of IHCCA, 26% of EHCCA, and 6% of GBC cases (13). Despite the variation in the incidence of MSI-H and MMR deficiency in BTC described in the aforementioned studies, current molecular profiling studies estimate a very low frequency (1%–2%) based on NGS. Immune therapy with checkpoint inhibitors is approved for the treatment of MSI-H BTC patients. It is also important to note that non-MSI-H patients harboring other DNA repair mutations including *BRCA1/2, ATM, ATR, RAD51, POLe,* and *FANC* family genes could potentially benefit from specific therapies targeting these pathways including poly(ADP-ribose) polymerase (PARP) inhibitors and/or immunotherapy.

Immunotherapy

There is evidence to suggest that at the earliest stages of tumor development, the host immune system is capable of both detecting and controlling the disease. However, over time this generates evolutionary pressure that favors the proliferation of cancer cells that are less immunogenic or otherwise capable of suppressing the host immune response (54,55). Interestingly, there often persists a small cohort of immune cells that remain able to identify and invade the tumor. The characteristics of this immune infiltrate may be of prognostic value in a variety of malignancies, including BTC (56).

The utilization of delicate interplay of the innate and the adaptive immune system is one of the founding principles of developing immune-based therapy in solid malignancies including BTCs. The innate immune system, consisting of the complement cascade, natural killer (NK) cells, granulocytes, and phagocytes, mounts an initial nonspecific defense against a multitude of pathogens and malignancy. The rate of tumor infiltration by the cellular components of the body's innate immune system is highly variable in solid tumors. In biliary tumors, less than half are penetrated by NK cells or mast cells (57,58), while macrophages are observed in the majority of them (57). Furthermore, infiltration of BTC by the innate immune system appears to be of limited clinical significance. Neither presence of mast cells nor NK cells correlated with outcome (58). However, the density of tumor-infiltrating macrophages is observed to increase as there is progression from premalignant precursors to invasive cancer and further ahead to metastatic disease (57). Although the exact mechanism is unclear, this is hypothesized to be secondary to activated macrophages releasing proinflammatory and proangiogenic cytokines including tumor necrosis factor-α, vascular endothelial growth factor A, and granulocyte macrophage colony-stimulating factor, which facilitates tumor growth (59).

The adaptive immune response starts with engulfing of foreign material (including cancer cells) by antigen presenting cells (APCs), most often dendritic cells. The antigen is then processed for presentation subsequently followed by the migration of dendritic cells to lymph nodes. In the lymph nodes, they stimulate the proliferation of antigen-specific lymphocytes and recruit CD4+ T-helper cells. The activated CD4+ cells release cytokines, which cause the differentiation of B-lymphocytes into antibody releasing plasma cells or activate cytotoxic CD8+ T-lymphocytes (CTL). After the antigen has been destroyed, both CD4+ and CD8+ T-cells can differentiate into memory T-cells. This leads to an expedited secondary immune response the next time there is an encounter with the offending antigen.

Like the innate immune system, there is considerable variability in the frequency of tumor infiltration by cells of the adaptive immune system. Although the exact percentage of BTC that contains dendritic cells is not clear, approximately 30% to 50% of BTC are infiltrated with CD4+ or CD8+ T-lymphocytes (57). In addition, tumor infiltration by the cellular mediators of the adaptive immune response is generally correlated with improved outcomes in BTC. The presence of dendritic cells, CD4+ T-cells, CD8+ T-cells, or plasma cells, within a biliary tumor is predictive of improved OS (57,60). This trend toward a more favorable prognosis is consistent with findings in other solid tumors and builds a strong preclinical scientific rationale for more effective therapies in BTCs.

There are several approaches to modulate the immune system including (a) peptide-based vaccines and personalized peptide vaccination, (b) dendritic cell–based vaccines, (c) adoptive immunotherapy, (d) immunostimulating cytokines, and (e) checkpoint inhibitors. The most promising techniques as pertaining to BTCs are discussed in the following.

Peptide-Based Vaccines
Peptide-based vaccines typically contain one or more antigens that are heavily expressed by malignant cells and often emulsified in Freund's adjuvant to increase immunogenicity. The main goal of immunization is to facilitate mass production of memory lymphocytes that can generate a strong secondary immune response against cancer cells that possess a particular antigen. Due to the heterogeneity of BTCs, the efficacy of any single peptide-based vaccine is intrinsically limited. At least two tumor-related antigens have been identified with moderate to high expression in biliary cancers—Wilms tumor 1 (WT1) and mucin 1 (MUC1) (61). In a phase I study of 25 patients, anti-WT1 vaccination and gemcitabine were administered to patients with unresectable BTCs and pancreatic adenocarcinoma. The disease control rate at 2 months was 50% and the median OS was 288 days for BTCs. Although objective clinical efficacy was not apparent, the safety of WT1 vaccine and GEM combination therapy was confirmed in that study (62). In another phase I trial of nine patients with advanced cholangiocarcinoma or pancreatic adenocarcinoma, monotherapy with peptide-based vaccines against MUC1 produced a single response of stable disease (54). The prospect of combination therapy with multiple peptide-based vaccines has been explored with a triple peptide vaccination against cell division cycle associated protein 1 (NUF2), cadherin 3 (CDH3), and kinesin family member 20A in patients with advanced BTCs. In a phase I study of nine patients, the median PFS and OS were 3.4 and 9.7 months, respectively, with minimal toxicities. In addition, peptide-specific T-cell responses were noted in all the patients (63).

Dendritic Cell–Based Vaccines
Dendritic cell–based vaccines expose the immune system to an antigen with the goal of generating memory lymphocytes, which will then likely produce a strong secondary immune response similar to peptide-based vaccines. However, rather than simply introducing a peptide that requires subsequent processing and presentation to the adaptive immune system, these vaccines contain dendritic cells that are already loaded with antigen. Although theoretically this can produce a greater antitumor response, it may also carry a risk of autoimmunity.

In a phase I/II proof-of-concept study, 12 patients with BTC and pancreatic adenocarcinomas received an anti-MUC1 dendritic cell–based vaccine in the adjuvant setting. A median OS of 26 months was observed, with 33% of patients surviving longer than 50 months. This was a limited study and not designed to differentiate between durable responses that occur due to vaccination and those that arise from complete surgical resection (64).

Both therapies could potentially have significant promise in the future. However, refining both the degree of immune response and distribution of the antigens needs to be optimized.

Adoptive Immunotherapy

The technique of adoptive immunotherapy is both exciting and very intriguing wherein the patient's own tumor-infiltrating lymphocytes are extracted, modified, and induced to clonally proliferate ex vivo. When these tumor-specific immune cells are reintroduced, they migrate back to the tumor and cause tumor-specific cell death. This concept was investigated in a study of 36 patients with IHCCA who were randomized to surgery alone versus surgery followed by combination adoptive immunotherapy with tumor lysate pulsed dendritic cells and transfer of activated T-cells (65). Of the 36 patients treated, the combination arm had a median PFS and OS of 18.3 and 31.9, respectively, versus 7.7 and 17.4 months with surgery alone. Interestingly, the 16 patients who produced the largest injection site reaction had a median OS of 95.5 months. Adoptive immunotherapy is both complex and in its infancy with BTCs but carries tremendous potential. Similar dramatic responses have been noted in case studies and studies are ongoing (66).

Checkpoint Inhibition

The activation of the T-cell is an important step in T-cell-mediated tumor cell death. T-cell activation depends on the interaction between the T-cell receptor (TCR) and a peptide, presented by APCs such as dendritic cells via major histocompatibility complex (MHC) class I or II molecules in the case of CD8 or CD4 T-cells, respectively. However, T-cell activation also requires an appropriate cytokine environment and a "second signal" in order to be effective. During T-cell activation, inhibitory receptors such as CTLA-4, PD-1, Lag-3, Tim-3, Tigit, and Viota are also induced to limit overstimulation of the immune system after antigen encounter, resulting in return to a resting state and to prevent an autoimmune process. The following new class of drugs inhibits these receptors to increase immune-mediated tumor-specific cell death.

PD-1 (programmed cell death ligand 1 or CD279) is a member of the immunoglobulin superfamily. It can be detected on activated T-cells, B-cells, and NK cells. PD-1 binds programmed death ligand 1 and 2, while PD-L1 also interacts with CD80 and PD-L2 interacts with repulsive guidance molecule B (RGMb) (67). PD-L1 is expressed by tumor cells and immune cells, while PD-L2 is only expressed on dendritic cells in normal tissue. All these interactions transmit an inhibitory signal. After binding, PD-1 becomes clustered with TCRs and recruits phosphatase SHP2 (Src homology 2 domain-containing tyrosine phosphatase 2) via its immunoreceptor tyrosine-based switch motif, which induces dephosphorylation of the proximal TCR signaling molecules and suppression of T-cell activation (68).

To evaluate the role of checkpoint inhibitors in BTCs, a trial of pembrolizumab in advanced biliary tract patients was conducted. In KEYNOTE-028, 89 patients with BTC were screened for PD-L1 expression, and 37 (42%) had PD-L1-positive tumors. In the reported interim analysis, ORR (confirmed and unconfirmed) was 17% (95% CI: 5%–39%). Eight patients (34%) had response or stable disease lasting 40+ weeks (69). Currently, a number of immunotherapy studies are ongoing including with nivolumab (NCT02829918), ipilimumab plus nivolumab (NCT02923934), and ramucirumab plus pembrolizumab (NCT02443324) in BTCs. Furthermore, immune therapy with checkpoint inhibitors is approved for the treatment of MSI-H BTC patients.

CONCLUSION

BTCs represent a heterogeneous and complex disease with a very grim prognosis. Historically, these cancers have been studied as a single entity with certain subsets having a better outcome than others. With the advent of newer technologies, comprehensive genomic profiling has revealed several distinct subsets such as IHCCAs, which have a high number of actionable mutations. These selected subsets have been successfully treated using therapies including immunotherapy and targeted therapy based on their molecular signatures. In addition, these biomarker-driven therapies have the potential to transform the prognosis of these cancers especially if they can be used earlier in the disease process and/or in conjunction with other modalities including surgery and radiation.

REFERENCES

1. Jemal A, Bray F, Center MM, et al. Global cancer statistics. *CA Cancer J Clin*. 2011;61(2):69–90. doi:10.3322/caac.20107
2. GBD 2013 Mortality and Causes of Death Collaborators. Global, regional, and national age-sex specific all-cause and cause-specific mortality for 240 causes of death, 1990-2013: a systematic analysis for the Global Burden of Disease Study 2013. *Lancet*. 2015;385(9963):117–171. doi:10.1016/S0140-6736(14)61682-2
3. Miller G, Jarnagin WR. Gallbladder carcinoma. *Eur J Surg Oncol*. 2008;34(3):306–312. doi:10.1016/j.ejso.2007.07.206
4. Jarnagin WR, Ruo L, Little SA, et al. Patterns of initial disease recurrence after resection of gallbladder carcinoma and hilar cholangiocarcinoma: implications for adjuvant therapeutic strategies. *Cancer*. 2003;98(8):1689–1700. doi:10.1002/cncr.11699
5. Hezel AF, Deshpande V, Zhu AX. Genetics of biliary tract cancers and emerging targeted therapies. *J Clin Oncol*. 2010;28(21):3531–3540. doi:10.1200/jco.2009.27.4787
6. Valle J, Wasan H, Palmer DH, et al. Cisplatin plus gemcitabine versus gemcitabine for biliary tract cancer. *N Engl J Med*. 2010;362(14):1273–1281. doi:10.1056/NEJMoa0908721
7. Okusaka T, Nakachi K, Fukutomi A, et al. Gemcitabine alone or in combination with cisplatin in patients with biliary tract cancer: a comparative multicentre study in Japan. *Br J Cancer*. 2010;103(4):469–474. doi:10.1038/sj.bjc.6605779
8. Siebenhuner AR, Seifert H, Bachmann H, et al. Adjuvant treatment of resectable biliary tract cancer with cisplatin plus gemcitabine: a prospective single center phase II study. *BMC Cancer*. 2018;18(1):72. doi:10.1186/s12885-017-3967-0
9. Rustagi T, Dasanu CA. Risk factors for gallbladder cancer and cholangiocarcinoma: similarities, differences and updates. *J Gastrointest Cancer*. 2012;43(2):137–147. doi:10.1007/s12029-011-9284-y
10. Miller G, Socci ND, Dhall D, et al. Genome wide analysis and clinical correlation of chromosomal and transcriptional mutations in cancers of the biliary tract. *J Exp Clin Cancer Res*. 2009;28:62. doi:10.1186/1756-9966-28-62
11. Jain A, Javle M. Molecular profiling of biliary tract cancer: a target rich disease. *J Gastrointest Oncol*. 2016;7(5):797–803. doi:10.21037/jgo.2016.09.01
12. Nakamura H, Arai Y, Totoki Y, et al. Genomic spectra of biliary tract cancer. *Nat Genet*. 2015;47(9):1003–1010. doi:10.1038/ng.3375
13. Javle M, Bekaii-Saab T, Jain A, et al. Biliary cancer: utility of next-generation sequencing for clinical management. *Cancer*. 2016;122(24):3838–3847. doi:10.1002/cncr.30254
14. Scaltriti M, Baselga J. The epidermal growth factor receptor pathway: a model for targeted therapy. *Clin Cancer Res*. 2006;12(18):5268–5272. doi:10.1158/1078-0432.CCR-05-1554
15. Yoshikawa D, Ojima H, Iwasaki M, et al. Clinicopathological and prognostic significance of EGFR, VEGF, and HER2 expression in cholangiocarcinoma. *Br J Cancer*. 2008;98(2):418–425. doi:10.1038/sj.bjc.6604129
16. Churi CR, Shroff R, Wang Y, et al. Mutation profiling in cholangiocarcinoma: prognostic and therapeutic implications. *PLoS One*. 2014;9(12):e115383. doi:10.1371/journal.pone.0115383
17. Javle M, Rashid A, Churi C, et al. Molecular characterization of gallbladder cancer using somatic mutation profiling. *Hum Pathol*. 2014;45(4):701–708. doi:10.1016/j.humpath.2013.11.001
18. Li M, Zhang Z, Li X, et al. Whole-exome and targeted gene sequencing of gallbladder carcinoma identifies recurrent mutations in the ErbB pathway. *Nat Genet*. 2014;46(8):872–876. doi:10.1038/ng.3030
19. Javle M, Churi C, Kang HC, et al. HER2/neu-directed therapy for biliary tract cancer. *J Hematol Oncol*. 2015;8:58. doi:10.1186/s13045-015-0155-z
20. Pignochino Y, Sarotto I, Peraldo-Neia C, et al. Targeting EGFR/HER2 pathways enhances the antiproliferative effect of gemcitabine in biliary tract and gallbladder carcinomas. *BMC Cancer*. 2010;10:631. doi:10.1186/1471-2407-10-631
21. Lee J, Park SH, Chang HM, et al. Gemcitabine and oxaliplatin with or without erlotinib in advanced biliary-tract cancer: a multicentre, open-label, randomised, phase 3 study. *Lancet Oncol*. 2012;13(2):181–188. doi:10.1016/S1470-2045(11)70301-1
22. Borbath I, Ceratti A, Verslype C, et al. Combination of gemcitabine and cetuximab in patients with advanced cholangiocarcinoma: a phase II study of the Belgian Group of Digestive Oncology. *Ann Oncol*. 2013;24(11):2824–2829. doi:10.1093/annonc/mdt337
23. Gruenberger B, Schueller J, Heubrandtner U, et al. Cetuximab, gemcitabine, and oxaliplatin in patients with unresectable advanced or metastatic biliary tract cancer: a phase 2 study. *Lancet Oncol*. 2010;11(12):1142–1148. doi:10.1016/S1470-2045(10)70247-3

24. Rubovszky G, Lang I, Ganofszky E, et al. Cetuximab, gemcitabine and capecitabine in patients with inoperable biliary tract cancer: a phase 2 study. *Eur J Cancer*. 2013;49(18):3806–3812. doi:10.1016/j.ejca.2013.07.143

25. Hezel AF, Noel MS, Allen JN, et al. Phase II study of gemcitabine, oxaliplatin in combination with panitumumab in KRAS wild-type unresectable or metastatic biliary tract and gallbladder cancer. *Br J Cancer*. 2014;111(3):430–436. doi:10.1038/bjc.2014.343

26. Jensen LH, Lindebjerg J, Ploen J, et al. Phase II marker-driven trial of panitumumab and chemotherapy in KRAS wild-type biliary tract cancer. *Ann Oncol*. 2012;23(9):2341–2346. doi:10.1093/annonc/mds008

27. Sohal DP, Mykulowycz K, Uehara T, et al. A phase II trial of gemcitabine, irinotecan and panitumumab in advanced cholangiocarcinoma. *Ann Oncol*. 2013;24(12):3061–3065. doi:10.1093/annonc/mdt416

28. Vogel A, Kasper S, Weichert W, et al. Panitumumab in combination with gemcitabine/cisplatin (GemCis) for patients with advanced kRAS WT biliary tract cancer: a randomized phase II trial of the Arbeitsgemeinschaft Internistische Onkologie (AIO). *J Clin Oncol*. 2015;33(15_suppl):4082–4082. doi:10.1200/jco.2015.33.15_suppl.4082

29. Philip PA, Mahoney MR, Allmer C, et al. Phase II study of erlotinib in patients with advanced biliary cancer. *J Clin Oncol*. 2006;24(19):3069–3074. doi:10.1200/JCO.2005.05.3579

30. Roa I, de Toro G, Schalper K, et al. Overexpression of the HER2/neu gene: a new therapeutic possibility for patients with advanced gallbladder cancer. *Gastrointest Cancer Res*. 2014;7(2):42–48.

31. Peck J, Wei L, Zalupski M, et al. HER2/neu may not be an interesting target in biliary cancers: results of an early phase II study with lapatinib. *Oncology*. 2012;82(3):175–179. doi:10.1159/000336488

32. Ramanathan RK, Belani CP, Singh DA, et al. A phase II study of lapatinib in patients with advanced biliary tree and hepatocellular cancer. *Cancer Chemother Pharmacol*. 2009;64(4):777–783. doi:10.1007/s00280-009-0927-7

33. Javle MM, Hainsworth JD, Swanton C, et al. Pertuzumab + trastuzumab for HER2-positive metastatic biliary cancer: preliminary data from MyPathway. *J Clin Oncol*. 2017;35(4_suppl):402–402. doi:10.1200/JCO.2017.35.4_suppl.402

34. Loaiza-Bonilla A, Clayton E, Furth E, et al. Dramatic response to dabrafenib and trametinib combination in a BRAF V600E-mutated cholangiocarcinoma: implementation of a molecular tumour board and next-generation sequencing for personalized medicine. *Ecancermedicalscience*. 2014;8:479. doi:10.3332/ecancer.2014.479

35. Goldstein D, Lemech C, Valle J. New molecular and immunotherapeutic approaches in biliary cancer. *ESMO Open*. 2017;2(Suppl 1):e000152. doi:10.1136/esmoopen-2016-000152

36. Chan E, Berlin J. Biliary tract cancers: understudied and poorly understood. *J Clin Oncol*. 2015;33(16):1845–1848. doi:10.1200/JCO.2014.59.7591

37. Beenken A, Mohammadi M. The FGF family: biology, pathophysiology and therapy. *Nat Rev Drug Discov*. 2009;8(3):235–253. doi:10.1038/nrd2792

38. Ross JS, Wang K, Gay L, et al. New routes to targeted therapy of intrahepatic cholangiocarcinomas revealed by next-generation sequencing. *Oncologist*. 2014;19(3):235–242. doi:10.1634/theoncologist.2013-0352

39. Wu YM, Su F, Kalyana-Sundaram S, et al. Identification of targetable FGFR gene fusions in diverse cancers. *Cancer Discov*. 2013;3(6):636–647. doi:10.1158/2159-8290.CD-13-0050

40. Arai Y, Totoki Y, Hosoda F, et al. Fibroblast growth factor receptor 2 tyrosine kinase fusions define a unique molecular subtype of cholangiocarcinoma. *Hepatology*. 2014;59(4):1427–1434. doi:10.1002/hep.26890

41. Javle M, Lowery M, Shroff RT, et al. Phase II study of BGJ398 in patients with FGFR-altered advanced cholangiocarcinoma. *J Clin Oncol*. 2018;36(3):276–282. doi:10.1200/JCO.2017.75.5009

42. Cohen AL, Holmen SL, Colman H. IDH1 and IDH2 mutations in gliomas. *Curr Neurol Neurosci Rep*. 2013;13(5):345. doi:10.1007/s11910-013-0345-4

43. Dang L, Yen K, Attar EC. IDH mutations in cancer and progress toward development of targeted therapeutics. *Ann Oncol*. 2016;27(4):599–608. doi:10.1093/annonc/mdw013

44. Lu C, Ward PS, Kapoor GS, et al. IDH mutation impairs histone demethylation and results in a block to cell differentiation. *Nature*. 2012;483(7390):474–478. doi:10.1038/nature10860

45. Kernytsky A, Wang F, Hansen E, et al. IDH2 mutation-induced histone and DNA hypermethylation is progressively reversed by small-molecule inhibition. *Blood*. 2015;125(2):296–303. doi:10.1182/blood-2013-10-533604

46. Lowery MA, Abou-Alfa GK, Burris HA, et al. Phase I study of AG-120, an IDH1 mutant enzyme inhibitor: results from the cholangiocarcinoma dose escalation and expansion cohorts. *J Clin Oncol*. 2017;35(15_suppl):4015–4015. doi:10.1200/JCO.2017.35.15_suppl.4015

47. Lowery MA, Abou-Alfa GK, Valle JW, et al. ClarIDHy: a phase 3, multicenter, randomized, double-blind study of AG-120 vs placebo in patients with an advanced cholangiocarcinoma with an IDH1 mutation. *J Clin Oncol.* 2017;35(15_suppl):TPS4142–TPS4142. doi:10.1200/JCO.2017.35.15_suppl.TPS4142

48. Hughes T, O'Connor T, Techasen A, et al. Opisthorchiasis and cholangiocarcinoma in Southeast Asia: an unresolved problem. *Int J Gen Med.* 2017;10:227–237. doi:10.2147/IJGM.S133292

49. Liengswangwong U, Nitta T, Kashiwagi H, et al. Infrequent microsatellite instability in liver fluke infection-associated intrahepatic cholangiocarcinomas from Thailand. *Int J Cancer.* 2003;107(3):375–380. doi:10.1002/ijc.11380

50. Boland CR, Thibodeau SN, Hamilton SR, et al. A National Cancer Institute Workshop on Microsatellite Instability for cancer detection and familial predisposition: development of international criteria for the determination of microsatellite instability in colorectal cancer. *Cancer Res.* 1998;58(22):5248–5257.

51. Liengswangwong U, Karalak A, Morishita Y, et al. Immunohistochemical expression of mismatch repair genes: a screening tool for predicting mutator phenotype in liver fluke infection-associated intrahepatic cholangiocarcinoma. *World J Gastroenterol.* 2006;12(23):3740–3745. doi:10.3748/wjg.v12.i23.3740

52. Suto T, Habano W, Sugai T, et al. Infrequent microsatellite instability in biliary tract cancer. *J Surg Oncol.* 2001;76(2):121–126. doi:10.1002/1096-9098(200102)76:2<121::aid-jso1022>3.0.co;2-7

53. Kim SG, Chan AO, Wu TT, et al. Epigenetic and genetic alterations in duodenal carcinomas are distinct from biliary and ampullary carcinomas. *Gastroenterology.* 2003;124(5):1300–1310. doi:10.1016/s0016-5085(03)00278-6

54. Gubin MM, Zhang X, Schuster H, et al. Checkpoint blockade cancer immunotherapy targets tumour-specific mutant antigens. *Nature.* 2014;515(7528):577–581. doi:10.1038/nature13988

55. Tumeh PC, Harview CL, Yearley JH, et al. PD-1 blockade induces responses by inhibiting adaptive immune resistance. *Nature.* 2014;515(7528):568–571. doi:10.1038/nature13954

56. Takahashi R, Yoshitomi M, Yutani S, et al. Current status of immunotherapy for the treatment of biliary tract cancer. *Hum Vaccin Immunother.* 2013;9(5):1069–1072. doi:10.4161/hv.23844

57. Goeppert B, Frauenschuh L, Zucknick M, et al. Prognostic impact of tumour-infiltrating immune cells on biliary tract cancer. *Br J Cancer.* 2013;109(10):2665–2674. doi:10.1038/bjc.2013.610

58. Nakakubo Y, Miyamoto M, Cho Y, et al. Clinical significance of immune cell infiltration within gallbladder cancer. *Br J Cancer.* 2003;89(9):1736–1742. doi:10.1038/sj.bjc.6601331

59. Pollard JW. Tumour-educated macrophages promote tumour progression and metastasis. *Nat Rev Cancer.* 2004;4(1):71–78. doi:10.1038/nrc1256

60. Oshikiri T, Miyamoto M, Shichinohe T, et al. Prognostic value of intratumoral CD8+ T lymphocyte in extrahepatic bile duct carcinoma as essential immune response. *J Surg Oncol.* 2003;84(4):224–228. doi:10.1002/jso.10321

61. Pauff JM, Goff LW. Current progress in immunotherapy for the treatment of biliary cancers. *J Gastrointest Cancer.* 2016;47(4):351–357. doi:10.1007/s12029-016-9867-8

62. Kaida M, Morita-Hoshi Y, Soeda A, et al. Phase 1 trial of Wilms tumor 1 (WT1) peptide vaccine and gemcitabine combination therapy in patients with advanced pancreatic or biliary tract cancer. *J Immunother.* 2011;34(1):92–99. doi:10.1097/CJI.0b013e3181fb65b9

63. Aruga A, Takeshita N, Kotera Y, et al. Phase I clinical trial of multiple-peptide vaccination for patients with advanced biliary tract cancer. *J Transl Med.* 2014;12:61. doi:10.1186/1479-5876-12-61

64. Lepisto AJ, Moser AJ, Zeh H, et al. A phase I/II study of a MUC1 peptide pulsed autologous dendritic cell vaccine as adjuvant therapy in patients with resected pancreatic and biliary tumors. *Cancer Ther.* 2008;6(B):955–964.

65. Shimizu K, Kotera Y, Aruga A, et al. Clinical utilization of postoperative dendritic cell vaccine plus activated T-cell transfer in patients with intrahepatic cholangiocarcinoma. *J Hepatobiliary Pancreat Sci.* 2012;19(2):171–178. doi:10.1007/s00534-011-0437-y

66. Marks EI, Yee NS. Immunotherapeutic approaches in biliary tract carcinoma: current status and emerging strategies. *World J Gastrointest Oncol.* 2015;7(11):338–346. doi:10.4251/wjgo.v7.i11.338

67. Xiao Y, Yu S, Zhu B, et al. RGMb is a novel binding partner for PD-L2 and its engagement with PD-L2 promotes respiratory tolerance. *J Exp Med.* 2014;211(5):943–959. doi:10.1084/jem.20130790

68. Yokosuka T, Takamatsu M, Kobayashi-Imanishi W, et al. Programmed cell death 1 forms negative costimulatory microclusters that directly inhibit T cell receptor signaling by recruiting phosphatase SHP2. *J Exp Med.* 2012;209(6):1201–1217. doi:10.1084/jem.20112741

69. Bang YJ, Doi T, Braud FD, et al. 525 Safety and efficacy of pembrolizumab (MK-3475) in patients (pts) with advanced biliary tract cancer: interim results of KEYNOTE-028. *Eur J Cancer.* 2015;51:S112. doi:10.1016/S0959-8049(16)30326-4

Neuroendocrine Tumors

Jonathan Strosberg

INTRODUCTION

Gastroenteropancreatic neuroendocrine tumors (GEP-NETs) include NETs of the gastrointestinal tract (also known as carcinoid tumors) and pancreatic neuroendocrine tumors. They are characterized by the ability to synthesize and secrete a variety of hormones and other vasoactive substances. The incidence of GEP-NETs has increased significantly in recent years, at least partly due to increases in imaging and endoscopy, which lead to incidental diagnoses of NETs (1). A traditional classification of GEP-NETs is based on embryonic derivation, distinguishing between foregut (gastroduodenal and pancreatic), midgut (jejunal, ileal, and cecal), and hindgut (distal colic and rectal) tumors (2). In general, midgut NETs are associated with the classical carcinoid syndrome (flushing and diarrhea) whereas hindgut tumors tend to be hormonally inactive.

Tumor grade and differentiation are important prognostic factors. Differentiation refers to the resemblance between the morphology of the tumor and tissue of origin, whereas tumor grade is quantified through markers of cell proliferation such as the Ki-67 index and mitotic rate. Low-grade tumors are defined as having a mitotic rate of 0 to 1 per 10 high-power fields (HPFs) or a Ki-67 index of 0% to 2%, intermediate-grade tumors having a mitotic rate of 2 to 20 or a Ki-67 index of 3% to 20%, and high-grade tumors having a mitotic rate or Ki-67 index >20% (3). Virtually all poorly differentiated tumors are high grade, typically with Ki-67 indexes >50%. Some high-grade tumors, particularly pancreatic NETs with Ki-67 in the 20% to 50% range, are relatively well differentiated (4). It is important to note that there can be significant heterogeneity in proliferative activity between different tumors within the same patient and changes in grade over the course of disease (5).

SMALL-INTESTINAL (MIDGUT) NETs

Most small intestinal NETs originate in the distal ileum (6). Approximately 25% of patients have multifocal tumors. Although generally slow-growing, midgut NETs have a particularly high malignant potential with lymph node or distant metastases observed in nearly all cases regardless of the tumor size. Metastases to the root of the mesentery are common and can cause desmoplastic fibrosis, resulting in bowel obstruction or ischemia (7).

Most advanced midgut NETs produce serotonin, among other hormonal substances, which causes carcinoid syndrome (8). Diarrhea is directly triggered by serotonin, whereas flushing is attributable to prostaglandins and tachykinins among other vasoactive substances (9–11). Carcinoid heart disease (CHD) typically occurs in patients with high levels of circulating serotonin, which causes fibrosis of right-sided cardiac valves leading to tricuspid regurgitation and pulmonary valve stenosis (12).

Nearly all midgut NETs are well differentiated with low proliferative activity. Despite their high propensity to metastasize, midgut NETs are associated with a relatively favorable long-term prognosis, even among patients with stage IV disease. Patients with metastatic tumors have 5-year survival rates exceeding 70% in large institutional databases (13).

GASTRIC NETs

Three types of gastric NETs have unique pathophysiologies and distinct treatment approaches.

Type 1 tumors are the most common subtype and arise in patients with chronic atrophic gastritis (14–16). In this condition, chronic absence of gastric acid causes antral G cells to secrete excess serum gastrin. Hypergastrinemia stimulates gastric neuroendocrine cell hyperplasia and development of multifocal NETs. These tumors generally behave in a benign fashion, and aggressive treatment is rarely appropriate. Most guidelines recommend endoscopic surveillance every 6 to 12 months with snare polypectomy of tumors (17,18). Diagnostic workup begins with conformation of elevated serum gastrin. Other findings supportive of the diagnosis include evidence of atrophic gastritis on biopsy of gastric tissue, and high gastric pH.

Type 2 gastric NETs are caused by hypergastrinemia in the setting of an underlying gastrinoma (19). As is the case with type 1 disease, tumors tend to be multifocal and relatively unaggressive. There is usually clinical or radiographic evidence of a gastrinoma and serum gastrin is elevated. Of note, proton pump inhibitors (PPIs) cause elevations of gastrin, so accurate gastrin measurement requires discontinuation of PPI therapy.

Type 3 gastric NETs are sporadic and are not associated with elevated gastrin levels. These tumors are more aggressive than type 1 or type 2 tumors. Oncological surgery (usually radical gastrectomy) is recommended in most cases; however small, superficial type 3 tumors can sometimes be managed with surgical wedge or even endoscopic resections (20).

APPENDICEAL NETs

NETs of the appendix are found in approximately 1 in 300 appendectomy specimens, nearly always incidentally (21,22). Tumor size is the most important prognostic factor for development of metastases. In one large series of patients, no metastases were observed in 127 cases in which tumors were smaller than 2 cm in diameter (21). Consequently, simple appendectomy was considered appropriate for patients with tumors <2 cm, whereas completion right hemicolectomy was recommended for larger tumors. In recent years, there have been reports of patients with tumors 1 to 2 cm in diameter who developed locoregional or distant metastases (23). Negative prognostic features for tumors in this size range include location in the base of the appendix (as opposed to tip), lymphovascular invasion, or extensive invasion into the mesoappendix (24).

COLORECTAL NETs

Most rectal NETs are detected incidentally during lower endoscopy, and are often small and submucosal in location (25). They are seldom associated with hormonal syndromes. Low-grade rectal NETs <1 cm rarely metastasize and can usually be resected endoscopically or transanally, whereas tumors >2 cm tend to be malignant (26,27). The metastatic potential of intermediate size tumors correlates with the depth of invasion.

Colonic NETs distal to the cecum can often be quite aggressive and many are poorly differentiated (28). Once metastatic, NETs of the colon and rectum tend to behave more aggressively than midgut NETs (29).

PANCREATIC NETs

Pancreatic NETs are heterogeneous neoplasms that can secrete a variety of peptide hormones including insulin, gastrin, glucagon, and vasoactive intestinal peptide (VIP). More than 75% of tumors are hormonally nonfunctioning (30,31). Insulinomas are the most common subtype of functional pancreatic NET with an annual incidence of roughly 0.5 per 100,000 (32). The large majority of insulinomas are <2 cm and considered relatively benign, although recurrences can occur after surgery (33). Patients typically present with symptoms of hypoglycemia including confusion, dizziness, diplopia, and diaphoresis, relieved with food or glucose administration (33).

Gastrinomas originate in the pancreas or duodenum (34–36). The Zollinger–Ellison syndrome (ZES), characterized by peptic ulceration, heartburn, and diarrhea (37), is caused by secretion of gastrin, which stimulates production of excess gastric acid. Diarrhea may occur due to the passage of excess gastric acid into the small intestine (38). ZES symptoms can be effectively palliated with PPIs, often at high doses (39). VIPomas secrete VIP, which stimulates intestinal secretion and inhibits electrolyte and water absorption. The resulting syndrome is characterized by profuse watery diarrhea and electrolyte abnormalities, including hypokalemia (40–42). Glucagonomas cause hyperglycemia, weight loss, venous thromboses, and an unusual rash called necrolytic migratory erythema (NME) (43,44).

Unlike hormone-producing tumors, which are often diagnosed as a result of the hormonal syndrome, nonfunctioning tumors are diagnosed as a result of tumor growth related symptoms or incidentally.

TUMOR BIOLOGY AND GENETIC SYNDROMES

Several hereditary syndromes are associated with GEP-NETs, particularly of pancreatic origin. Multiple endocrine neoplasia type 1 (MEN1) is an autosomal dominant syndrome, caused by mutations in chromosome 11q13, and characterized by neuroendocrine neoplasms of the anterior pituitary, parathyroid glands, and pancreas (45). *MEN1* encodes for menin, a nuclear protein that regulates gene transcription through chromatin remodeling (46). Pancreatic NETs in MEN1 are typically multifocal. Consequently, surgical resection is usually only recommended for tumors that are symptomatic or >2 cm in size (47,48).

Von Hippel–Lindau syndrome (VHL) is an autosomal dominant syndrome caused by mutations in the *VHL* gene located on chromosome 3p25 (49). VHL syndrome is linked to several different neoplasms including renal cell carcinomas, hemangioblastomas, pheochromocytomas, and pancreatic NETs, the last developing in only 10% of cases (50).

Most sporadic well-differentiated NETs contain a low burden of somatic mutations. Several recurrent somatic mutations have been identified in sporadic pancreatic NETs including mutations of the *MEN1* gene, mutations in *DAXX* or *ATRX* (genes encoding subunits of a chromatin remodeling complex), and mutations in mTOR pathway genes (51,52). The genetic landscape of midgut NETs is more poorly understood, and mutations are very infrequent (53). Epigenetic changes are thought to contribute significantly to NET pathogenesis (54).

DIAGNOSTIC PROCEDURES

Pathologic diagnosis of NETs is aided by immunohistochemical staining for the neuroendocrine markers synaptophysin and chromogranin A (CgA). Well-differentiated GEP-NETs tend to stain strongly for both synaptophysin and CgA whereas poorly differentiated tumors often maintain synaptophysin expression while losing CgA expression. Measurement of tumor proliferation via mitotic rate and Ki-67 index is an important component of pathological workup, and should be measured in the most mitotically active areas of the tumor (55). Patients who present with chronic diarrhea and/or flushing should undergo measurement of 5-hydroxyindoleacetic acid (5-HIAA), a metabolite of serotonin (56). Patients presenting with other suspected hormonal syndromes should undergo testing for the corresponding hormone level. If elevated, these hormone levels can be followed over time and used to help determine progression or response. CgA is a nonhormonal circulating tumor marker of modest utility in NETs. False elevations of CgA with PPI use are common. Other causes of false-positive tests include renal insufficiency, and inflammatory bowel disease. Other tumor markers include neuron-specific enolase (NSE), pancreatic polypeptide, and pancreastatin; however, their role in routine assessment of patients remains controversial (57). In a phase 3 study, elevations in both CgA and NSE were prognostic for progression-free and overall survival, and reductions in both serum biomarkers were predictive for radiographic response (58). At this time, there are insufficient data from large studies to select one particular tumor marker as the gold standard.

DIAGNOSTIC IMAGING

Radiographic evaluation of GEP-NETs relies on cross-sectional imaging using CT and MRI scans, as well as functional imaging studies, which are primarily based on somatostatin receptor (SSTR) expression. For optimal evaluation of liver metastases, guidelines recommend three-phase CT scans that include noncontrast images, arterial phase sequences (approximately

20 seconds after contrast injection), and portal venous phase sequences (approximately 70 seconds after contrast injection) (59). Multiphase CT scans are also useful for the identification of small pancreatic tumors (60). The presence of a mesenteric mass with surrounding desmoplastic fibrosis typically indicates a small intestinal primary.

MRI scans, particularly using gadoxetate contrast, are associated with an even higher sensitivity for detection of small liver metastases (61,62).

Most well-differentiated NETs express high levels of SSTRs. SSTR-based imaging was historically performed using indium-111 (^{111}In) somatostatin receptor scintigraphy (SRS; OctreoScan). In recent years, gallium-68 (^{68}Ga)-Dotatate PET scan has become the preferred modality for SSTR imaging due to its substantially improved sensitivity, reduced radiation exposure, and improved convenience to patients (one time versus multiday scanning). In one study of patients with known or suspected NET, a ^{68}Ga-Dotatate PET–CT detected 95% of lesions, compared to 45% with cross-sectional imaging and 31% with SRS (63). ^{68}Ga-Dotatate PET–CT imaging is useful for baseline whole-body staging, detection of small lymph node or bone metastases, identification of primary site (in cases of occult primary), and characterization of SSTR expression. High levels of SSTR expression are predictive of response to peptide receptor radiotherapy (PRRT) (64).

TREATMENT OF LOCALIZED TUMORS

Surgical therapy is usually offered to patients with local or locoregional tumors. However, there are exceptions. The correct approach to management of small (<2 cm), low-grade, incidentally detected pancreatic NETs is controversial: some advocate resection for all surgically fit patients based on possible risk of malignant behavior, whereas others advocate surveillance given the small likelihood of progression over time and excellent outcomes with a "watch and wait" approach (65). Pancreatic NETs >2 cm or those that are intermediate to high grade should be surgically resected in nearly all cases.

Virtually all midgut NETs exhibit malignant behavior despite their relatively slow growth rate, and should be surgically resected using appropriate oncologic techniques and resection of associated intestinal mesentery (24). Given the high incidence of multifocal tumors (approximately 25% of cases), the entire bowel should be palpated to rule out additional primary tumors.

NETs of the appendix are biologically unique. They are nearly always discovered incidentally during appendectomy for unrelated reasons and typically located at the tip of the appendix. A landmark analysis of 150 appendiceal NETs with long-term follow-up demonstrated no evidence of recurrence when tumors were <2 cm in diameter; therefore, completion right hemicolectomy has been traditionally recommended only for tumors >2 cm (21). In recent years, there have been several case reports of lymph node involvement in tumors 1 to 2 cm in size. Based on this data, right hemicolectomy can be recommended in some patients with tumors 1 to 2 cm in size along with other high-risk features such as location in the appendiceal base or extensive mesoappendiceal invasion (23). Low-grade tumors <1 cm almost never recur after simple appendectomy.

Most rectal NETs are small, submucosal tumors that are discovered incidentally. T1 rectal NETs smaller than 1 cm are often managed with endoscopic resection (29). In several studies, no recurrences were detected after endoscopic or transanal resection of T1 tumors (66,67).

Larger or more invasive rectal NETs, particularly >2 cm, are usually treated with formal oncologic surgery such as a low-anterior resection (LAR) with lymph node sampling (29,68,69).

The management of gastric NETs is complex. Type 1 gastric NETs are typically of low malignant potential and are usually managed with endoscopic surveillance rather than surgically. Antrectomy to remove the gastrin stimulus can be considered for patients with multifocal tumors that are enlarging or proliferating relatively rapidly. Type 3 (sporadic) gastric NETs are usually treated with partial gastrectomy and regional lymphadenectomy, although endoscopic resection may be considered for select patients with small, low-grade, T1 tumors (20).

SYSTEMIC THERAPY

Somatostatin Analogs (SSAs)

Analogs of the human hormone somatostatin were initially found to palliate hormonal symptoms associated with NETs. Both octreotide and lanreotide are synthetic octapeptides, which share similar SSTR affinities, binding avidly to SSTR subtype 2 (70). The first clinical trial of octreotide evaluated the drug in 25 patients with carcinoid syndrome, demonstrating significant improvements in flushing and diarrhea in more than 70% of cases (71). Subsequent studies showed high levels of activity in hormonal syndromes associated with pancreatic NETs, particularly VIPomas and glucagonomas (72).

Long-acting formulations of octreotide and lanreotide are now available, enabling dosing every 4 weeks (73). Both octreotide and lanreotide are well-tolerated with generally mild side effects including bloating and steatorrhea, as well as long-term cholelithiasis. Administration of SSAs at above-label dose or frequency can sometimes result in improved palliation of hormonal symptoms that are suboptimally controlled (74).

During the past decade, two phase 3 trials have revealed that SSAs significantly inhibit radiographic progression of NETs despite low objective response rates of roughly 1%. The first trial to demonstrate this antiproliferative effect was the PROMID study, which randomized patients with metastatic midgut NETs to receive octreotide LAR 30 mg every 4 weeks versus placebo (75). The time to tumor progression increased from 6 months in the placebo arm to 14.3 months in the octreotide LAR arm (p = .000072). Subsequently, the CLARINET trial compared lanreotide 120 mg every 4 weeks to placebo in patients with nonfunctioning, SSTR expressing enteropancreatic NETs (76). The study met its primary end point with a 53% improvement in progression-free survival (PFS; p = .0002). Based on these studies, SSAs are typically used as first-line drugs both for control of hormonal syndrome and control of tumor growth. Both drugs are generally considered to be equivalent therapeutically (18).

Everolimus

The mTOR pathway is frequently upregulated in NETs and discrete mutations in mTOR pathway genes are observed in approximately 15% of pancreatic NETs (52,77). The oral mTOR inhibitor everolimus has been evaluated in three phase 3 studies investigating distinct NET populations. In the RADIANT 2 study, 429 patients with hormonally functional (predominantly midgut) NETs were randomized to receive treatment with everolimus 10 mg plus octreotide versus placebo plus octreotide with crossover allowed from placebo at time of progression (78). Median PFS increased from 11.3 months on the placebo arm to 16.4 months on the everolimus arm (hazard ratio [HR]: 0.77, p = .026). This result fell short of the prespecified p value < .0246. There was no signal of overall survival (OS) improvement in the everolimus arm (79).

The RADIANT 3 trial randomly assigned 410 patients with low- and intermediate-grade pancreatic NETs to treatment with everolimus 10 mg versus placebo (80). This study demonstrated a clinically and statistically significant improvement in PFS with median PFS improving from 4.6 months on the placebo arm to 11 months on the everolimus arm (HR: 0.35, p < .001). There was also a trend toward improvement in OS (81).

The RADIANT 4 study compared everolimus versus placebo in 302 nonfunctioning NETs of the gastrointestinal tract and lungs (82). In this study, concurrent octreotide was prohibited. Median PFS improved from 3.9 on the placebo arm to 11.0 months on the everolimus arm (HR: 0.48, p < .000001), and there was a strong trend toward OS improvement on preliminary analysis.

It is noteworthy that the smallest benefit with everolimus was observed in the RADIANT 2 study, which enrolled predominantly patients with slow-growing midgut NETs. It is possible to infer that the risk/benefit profile of everolimus does not justify its use in patients with slowly progressive midgut NETs. In general, everolimus should be considered in patients with clinically significant disease progression, regardless of hormonal output.

Side effects of everolimus include rash, pneumonitis, diarrhea, hyperglycemia, aphthous oral ulcers, cytopenias, and atypical infections. While many toxicities are mild, chronic side effects may adversely impact patient quality of life. Objective response rates are lower than 10%.

Sunitinib

NETs are highly vascular, and increased levels of circulating vascular endothelial growth factor (VEGF) have been associated with tumor progression (83). The tyrosine kinase inhibitor (TKI) sunitinib targets VEGF receptors 1, 2, and 3. Based on relatively promising results in pancreatic NETs from a phase 2 study (84), a phase 3 trial randomized patients with low- and intermediate-grade pancreatic NETs to sunitinib 37.5 mg daily versus placebo. The study demonstrated a statistically significant improvement in median PFS from 5.5 months on the placebo arm to 11.1 months on the sunitinib arm (HR: 0.42; $p < .001$) (85). The objective response rate associated with sunitinib was 9%. Side effects of sunitinib included nausea, diarrhea, fatigue, cytopenias, palmar–plantar erythrodysesthesia, and hypertension. At this time, there are no phase 3 studies demonstrating benefit with a VEGF-inhibiting drug in nonpancreatic NETs.

Chemotherapy

Cytotoxic drugs are the cornerstone of therapy for patients with poorly differentiated neuroendocrine carcinomas. These aggressive malignancies are generally treated with platinum- and etoposide-based regimens, as used in small cell lung cancer. Several small studies evaluating cisplatin and etoposide in poorly differentiated gastrointestinal neuroendocrine carcinomas have shown objective response ranging from 42% to 67% (86,87). A large retrospective study in this population demonstrated that carboplatin has equivalent efficacy to cisplatin with lower rates of toxicity (88). Despite early responses, relapses generally occur within about 8 months of treatment, and median OS remains below 2 years. There are few known effective second-line therapies, with small studies suggesting some activity associated with 5-fluorouracil (5-FU) based regimens such as FOLFIRI or FOLFIRINOX (89,90).

Among well-differentiated NETs, pancreatic NETs appear to be particularly sensitive to temozolomide- or streptozocin-based regimens, typically combined with fluoropyrimidines such as 5-FU or capecitabine. A large retrospective study investigating the combination of streptozocin, 5-FU, and doxorubicin in 84 pancreatic NETs reported a response rate of 39% (91).

More recently, temozolomide-based studies have demonstrated objective response rates ranging from 33% to 70% in patients with pancreatic NETs (92–96). The highest response rates have been observed in studies combining temozolomide with capecitabine. A randomized phase 2 trial comparing temozolomide versus capecitabine plus temozolomide has completed accrual.

Nonpancreatic NETs are less sensitive, on average, to cytotoxic chemotherapy (92,93,97). However, there is likely some heterogeneity in chemosensitivity, with midgut NETs demonstrating lowest rates of response. Lung NETs may have higher response rates, but data are limited (98). It is unclear whether other clinical and biological factors such as tumor grade or expression of the DNA repair enzyme methylguanine methyltransferase (MGMT) are predictive for response (96,99,100).

Radiolabeled SSAs

Most well-differentiated NETs express high levels of somatostatin receptors and can therefore be treated in a targeted fashion with radiolabeled SSAs, a form of treatment also known as peptide receptor radiotherapy. Radiolabeled SSAs consist of a radionuclide, an SSA, and a chelator that binds them.

Most clinical trials of radiolabeled SSAs have evaluated either yttrium-90 (^{90}Y), a β-emitting isotope with a long particle range, or lutetium-177 (^{177}Lu), a β and γ particle emitter with intermediate particle range. Objective response rates have varied quite significantly in studies of ^{90}Y-based PRRT, possibly due to heterogeneity in the patient population as well as response criteria (101). Toxicities associated with ^{90}Y include renal insufficiency, which can occur even in patients who receive prophylactic amino acid infusions, which reduce glomerular uptake of radiolabeled peptides (102). ^{177}Lu-based PRRT treatments have been associated with similar or higher objective response rates, and substantially lower risk of nephrotoxicity. In a large prospective institutional database, objective response rates ranged from 31% in midgut NETs to 55% in pancreatic NETs, with intermediate response rates observed in colorectal and gastroduodenal NETs (103). Clinically significant nephrotoxicity occurred only in 0.3% of cases.

Bone marrow toxicity occurs with all forms of PRRT. Rates of grade 3 or 4 neutropenia and thrombocytopenia are approximately 2% to 5%. Lymphopenia is observed more commonly but is virtually never clinically significant. Long-term bone marrow toxicity, in the form of myelodysplastic syndrome (MDS) or acute leukemia, occurs in roughly 2% to 3% of cases, and is the most significant toxicity associated with this therapy (103,104).

The NETTER-1 trial was the first randomized, prospective phase 3 study to evaluate a radiolabeled SSA. Two hundred twenty-nine patients with somatostatin receptor positive midgut NETs, progressing on standard dose octreotide, were randomized to receive ^{177}Lu-dotatate every 8 weeks for four cycles plus octreotide 30 mg every 4 weeks versus high-dose octreotide (60 mg every 4 weeks) (105). The study revealed a 79% improvement in PFS with

[177]Lu-dotatate ($p < .00001$). Median PFS was 8 months on the control arm of the study and not reached with ^{177}Lu-dotatate at the time of primary analysis. There was a strong early signal for OS improvement with an HR of 0.4 ($p = .004$). Objective response was 18% on the investigational arm of the study versus 3% on the control arm. Grade 3 or 4 neutropenia and thrombocytopenia occurred in only 1% and 2% of patients treated with ^{177}Lu-dotatate, respectively. Results of the NETTER-1 study combined with single-arm study data resulted in the approval of ^{177}Lu-dotatate for the treatment of advanced GEP-NETs with evidence of SSTR expression on imaging studies. Patients must receive concurrent amino acid infusions to reduce the risk of nephrotoxicity: those containing arginine–lysine only are more tolerable than commercial amino acid solutions, which contain roughly 20 amino acids.

A standard course of treatment with ^{177}Lu-dotatate consists of four cycles administered every 8 weeks. There is evidence that patients who benefit but subsequently progress can be retreated, up to a lifetime maximum of about eight cycles (106).

Telotristat

Telotristat is an oral inhibitor of tryptophan hydroxylase, an enzyme involved in the conversion of tryptophan to serotonin. By reducing circulating levels of serotonin, telotristat has been shown to reduce diarrhea related to carcinoid syndrome. In the phase 3 TELESTAR trial, two doses of telotristat, 250 mg and 500 mg given three times a day, were compared to placebo in patients with history of carcinoid syndrome and at least four daily bowel movements despite SSA therapy (107). SSA treatment continued during the trial combined with telotristat. The primary end point was reduction in daily bowel movements, averaged over a 12-week period. There was an estimated daily reduction in bowel movements of –0.81 for the 250 mg dose and –0.69 for the 500 mg dose ($p < .01$). There were significant reductions in urine 5-HIAA levels (>30%) in 78% of patients receiving the 250 mg dose and 87% of patients receiving the 500 mg dose. The safety profile of telotristat was favorable.

Based on the TELESTAR trial, telotristat, at a dose of 250 mg three times daily, was approved for the treatment of refractory diarrhea associated with carcinoid syndrome. When evaluating candidates for telotristat, it is important to note that diarrhea in NET patients can be multifactorial with possible contributing factors including bile malabsorption, short gut syndrome, and pancreatic exocrine insufficiency caused by SSAs. The treatment should, ideally, target the underlying pathophysiology.

There is no clear evidence that telotristat impacts flushing, which is thought to be caused by vasoactive substances other than serotonin. In theory, telotristat should inhibit development or progression of CHD; however, there is yet no compelling clinical data demonstrating this effect.

Liver-Directed Treatment

Because the liver is the dominant site of metastases in GEP-NETs, liver-directed treatments are often used to reduce tumor bulk, control growth, and palliate symptoms. Treatment options include cytoreductive liver surgery in patients with resectable disease, liver embolization in patients with unresectable tumors, and liver transplant in highly selected patients with unresectable disease confined to the liver. Nearly all studies investigating liver-targeted therapies are retrospective, and there are no randomized data confirming benefit.

Cytoreductive (debulking) surgery is often recommended if at least 90% of disease can be resected (108,109). Ablative procedures are also commonly performed, either operatively or percutaneously (110,111). Long-term survival durations associated with surgery compare favorably with other treatments, although it is uncertain to what extent the outcomes are related to patient selection versus the surgical intervention.

Transarterial liver embolization procedures are often highly effective in NETs, partly due to their high vascularity. Embolization is typically performed in patients with clinically- or radiologically-progressive unresectable liver metastases. Two or three staged lobar embolizations are often required to treat the entire liver (112,113). Postembolization syndrome consists of abdominal pain, nausea, fevers, and fatigue. Embolizations consisting only of occlusive particles (bland embolization) or combined with chemotherapy (chemoembolization) are commonly performed, with no clear indication that one treatment modality is superior. The majority of institutional series report objective response rates averaging approximately 50% and symptomatic responses of approximately 75% (111). A three-arm randomized clinical trial comparing bland embolization, chemoembolization, and drug-eluting beads is currently enrolling patients.

Radioembolization is a newer liver-directed treatment that delivers ^{90}Y beads embedded either in a glass microsphere (TheraSphere) or resin microsphere (SIR-Spheres) intra-arterially. Response rates appear comparable to bland embolization or chemoembolization (114,115). Although short-term toxicity rates tend to be lower, long-term liver dysfunction is increasingly recognized as a complication of radioembolization (116).

Liver transplantation is performed rarely in highly select patients with disease confined to the liver. Studies show that recurrence rates are lowest in patients with low tumor burden and grade (117,118). In one nonrandomized study that compared patients who met strict transplant criteria and subsequently underwent liver transplant versus those who were screened but chose to forego transplantation, survival outcomes were substantially improved in the transplant group (119).

CONCLUSIONS

The treatment landscape for patients with advanced NETs has improved significantly in the past decade. Multiple phase 3 randomized clinical trials have met their primary end point leading to the approval of new treatments for tumor and symptom control. The challenge of the next decade will be to learn how to appropriately sequence these treatments, selecting the optimal therapy for the appropriate patient at the right time.

REFERENCES

1. Dasari A, Shen C, Halperin D, et al. Trends in the incidence, prevalence, and survival outcomes in patients with neuroendocrine tumors in the United States. *JAMA Oncol.* 2017;3:1335–1342. doi:10.1001/jamaoncol.2017.0589
2. Williams ED, Sandler M. The classification of carcinoid tum ours. *Lancet.* 1963;1:238–239. doi:10.1016/S0140-6736(63)90951-6
3. Klimstra DS, Modlin IR, Coppola D, et al. The pathologic classification of neuroendocrine tumors: a review of nomenclature, grading, and staging systems. *Pancreas.* 2010;39:707–712. doi:10.1097/MPA.0b013e3181ec124e
4. Velayoudom-Cephise FL, Duvillard P, Foucan L, et al. Are G3 ENETS neuroendocrine neoplasms heterogeneous? *Endocr Relat Cancer.* 2013;20:649–657. doi:10.1530/ERC-13-0027
5. Yang Z, Tang LH, Klimstra DS. Effect of tumor heterogeneity on the assessment of Ki67 labeling index in well-differentiated neuroendocrine tumors metastatic to the liver: implications for prognostic stratification. *Am J Surg Pathol.* 2011;35:853–860. doi:10.1097/PAS.0b013e31821a0696
6. Moertel CG. Karnofsky memorial lecture. An odyssey in the land of small tumors. *J Clin Oncol.* 1987;5:1502–1522. doi:10.1200/JCO.1987.5.10.1502
7. Eckhauser FE, Argenta LC, Strodel WE, et al. Mesenteric angiopathy, intestinal gangrene, and midgut carcinoids. *Surgery.* 1981;90:720–728.
8. Thorson A, Biorck G, Bjorkman G, et al. Malignant carcinoid of the small intestine with metastases to the liver, valvular disease of the right side of the heart (pulmonary stenosis and tricuspid regurgitation without septal defects), peripheral vasomotor symptoms, bronchoconstriction, and an unusual type of cyanosis; a clinical and pathologic syndrome. *Am Heart J.* 1954;47:795–817. doi:10.1016/0002-8703(54)90152-0
9. Cunningham JL, Janson ET, Agarwal S, et al. Tachykinins in endocrine tumors and the carcinoid syndrome. *Eur J Endocrinol.* 2008;159:275–282. doi:10.1530/EJE-08-0196
10. Smith AG, Greaves MW. Blood prostaglandin activity associated with noradrenaline-provoked flush in the carcinoid syndrome. *Br J Dermatol.* 1974;90:547–551. doi:10.1111/j.1365-2133.1974.tb06451.x
11. Matuchansky C, Launay JM. Serotonin, catecholamines, and spontaneous midgut carcinoid flush: plasma studies from flushing and nonflushing sites. *Gastroenterology.* 1995;108:743–751. doi:10.1016/0016-5085(95)90447-6
12. Pellikka PA, Tajik AJ, Khandheria BK, et al. Carcinoid heart disease. Clinical and echocardiographic spectrum in 74 patients. *Circulation.* 1993;87:1188–1196. doi:10.1161/01.CIR.87.4.1188
13. Strosberg JR, Weber JM, Feldman M, et al. Prognostic validity of the American Joint Committee on Cancer staging classification for midgut neuroendocrine tumors. *J Clin Oncol.* 2013;31:420–425. doi:10.1200/JCO.2012.44.5924
14. Modlin IM, Gilligan CJ, Lawton GP, et al. Gastric carcinoids. The Yale Experience. *Arch Surg.* 1995;130:250–255; discussion 255–256. doi:10.1001/archsurg.1995.01430030020003

15. Thomas RM, Baybick JH, Elsayed AM, et al. Gastric carcinoids. An immunohistochemical and clinicopathologic study of 104 patients. *Cancer*. 1994;73:2053–2058. doi:10.1002/1097-0142(19940415)73:8<2053::AID-CNCR2820730807>3.0.CO;2-0

16. Moses RE, Frank BB, Leavitt M, et al. The syndrome of type A chronic atrophic gastritis, pernicious anemia, and multiple gastric carcinoids. *J Clin Gastroenterol*. 1986;8:61–65. doi:10.1097/00004836-198602000-00013

17. Ahlman H, Kolby L, Lundell L, et al. Clinical management of gastric carcinoid tumors. *Digestion*. 1994;55 Suppl 3:77–85. doi:10.1159/000201206

18. Kulke MH, Shah MH, Benson AB 3rd, et al. Neuroendocrine tumors, version 1.2015. *J Natl Compr Canc Netw*. 2015;13:78–108. doi:10.6004/jnccn.2015.0011

19. Delle Fave G, Capurso G, Milione M, et al. Endocrine tumours of the stomach. *Best Pract Res Clin Gastroenterol*. 2005;19:659–673. doi:10.1016/j.bpg.2005.05.002

20. Saund MS, Al Natour RH, Sharma AM, et al. Tumor size and depth predict rate of lymph node metastasis and utilization of lymph node sampling in surgically managed gastric carcinoids. *Ann Surg Oncol*. 2011;18:2826–2832. doi:10.1245/s10434-011-1652-0

21. Moertel CG, Weiland LH, Nagorney DM, et al. Carcinoid tumor of the appendix: treatment and prognosis. *N Engl J Med*. 1987;317:1699–1701. doi:10.1056/NEJM198712313172704

22. Shaw PA. Carcinoid tumours of the appendix are different. *J Pathol*. 1990;162:189–190. doi:10.1002/path.1711620303

23. Grozinsky-Glasberg S, Alexandraki KI, Barak D, et al. Current size criteria for the management of neuroendocrine tumors of the appendix: are they valid? Clinical experience and review of the literature. *Neuroendocrinology*. 2013;98:31–37. doi:10.1159/000343801

24. Pape UF, Perren A, Niederle B, et al. ENETS Consensus Guidelines for the management of patients with neuroendocrine neoplasms from the jejuno-ileum and the appendix including goblet cell carcinomas. *Neuroendocrinology*. 2012;95:135–156. doi:10.1159/000335629

25. Jetmore AB, Ray JE, Gathright JB Jr, et al. Rectal carcinoids: the most frequent carcinoid tumor. *Dis Colon Rectum*. 1992;35:717–725. doi:10.1007/BF02050318

26. Naunheim KS, Zeitels J, Kaplan EL, et al. Rectal carcinoid tumors--treatment and prognosis. *Surgery*. 1983;94:670–676.

27. Fahy BN, Tang LH, Klimstra D, et al. Carcinoid of the Rectum Risk Stratification (CaRRs): a strategy for preoperative outcome assessment. *Ann Surg Oncol*. 2007;14:1735–1743. doi:10.1245/s10434-006-9311-6

28. Federspiel BH, Burke AP, Sobin LH, et al. Rectal and colonic carcinoids. A clinicopathologic study of 84 cases. *Cancer*. 1990;65:135–140. doi:10.1002/1097-0142(19900101)65:1<135::AID-CNCR2820650127>3.0.CO;2-A

29. Anthony LB, Strosberg JR, Klimstra DS, et al. The NANETS consensus guidelines for the diagnosis and management of gastrointestinal neuroendocrine tumors (nets): well-differentiated nets of the distal colon and rectum. *Pancreas*. 2010;39:767–774. doi:10.1097/MPA.0b013e3181ec1261

30. Strosberg JR, Cheema A, Weber J, et al. Prognostic validity of a novel American Joint Committee on Cancer Staging Classification for pancreatic neuroendocrine tumors. *J Clin Oncol*. 2011;29:3044–3049. doi:10.1200/JCO.2011.35.1817

31. Halfdanarson TR, Rubin J, Farnell MB, et al. Pancreatic endocrine neoplasms: epidemiology and prognosis of pancreatic endocrine tumors. *Endocr Relat Cancer*. 2008;15:409–427. doi:10.1677/ERC-07-0221

32. Service FJ, McMahon MM, O'Brien PC, et al. Functioning insulinoma--incidence, recurrence, and long-term survival of patients: a 60-year study. *Mayo Clin Proc*. 1991;66:711–719. doi:10.1016/S0025-6196(12)62083-7

33. Whipple AO. Islet cell tumors of the pancreas. *Can Med Assoc J*. 1952;66:334–342.

34. Jensen RT. Gastrinomas: advances in diagnosis and management. *Neuroendocrinology*. 2004;80 Suppl 1:23–27. doi:10.1159/000080736

35. Gibril F, Jensen RT. Advances in evaluation and management of gastrinoma in patients with Zollinger-Ellison syndrome. *Curr Gastroenterol Rep*. 2005;7:114–121. doi:10.1007/s11894-005-0049-2

36. Wolfe MM, Jensen RT. Zollinger-Ellison syndrome. Current concepts in diagnosis and management. *N Engl J Med*. 1987;317:1200–1209. doi:10.1056/NEJM198711053171907

37. Zollinger RM, Ellison EH. Primary peptic ulcerations of the jejunum associated with islet cell tumors of the pancreas. *Ann Surg*. 1955;142:709–723; discussion, 724–728. doi:10.1097/00000658-195510000-00015

38. Zollinger RM, Ellison EC, Fabri PJ, et al. Primary peptic ulcerations of the jejunum associated with islet cell tumors. Twenty-five-year appraisal. *Ann Surg*. 1980;192:422–430. doi:10.1097/00000658-198009000-00018

39. Metz DC, Strader DB, Orbuch M, et al. Use of omeprazole in Zollinger-Ellison syndrome: a prospective nine-year study of efficacy and safety. *Aliment Pharmacol Ther*. 1993;7:597–610. doi:10.1111/j.1365-2036.1993.tb00140.x

40. Verner JV, Morrison AB. Islet cell tumor and a syndrome of refractory watery diarrhea and hypokalemia. *Am J Med*. 1958;25:374–380. doi:10.1016/0002-9343(58)90075-5

41. Bloom SR, Polak JM, Pearse AG. Vasoactive intestinal peptide and watery-diarrhoea syndrome. *Lancet*. 1973;2:14–16. doi:10.1016/S0140-6736(73)91947-8

42. Grier JF. WDHA (watery diarrhea, hypokalemia, achlorhydria) syndrome: clinical features, diagnosis, and treatment. *South Med J*. 1995;88:22–24. doi:10.1097/00007611-199501000-00002

43. McGavran MH, Unger RH, Recant L, et al. A glucagon-secreting alpha-cell carcinoma of the pancreas. *N Engl J Med*. 1966;274:1408–1413. doi:10.1056/NEJM196606232742503

44. Wermers RA, Fatourechi V, Wynne AG, et al. The glucagonoma syndrome. Clinical and pathologic features in 21 patients. *Medicine (Baltimore)*. 1996;75:53–63. doi:10.1097/00005792-199603000-00002

45. Wermer P. Genetic aspects of adenomatosis of endocrine glands. *Am J Med*. 1954;16:363–371. doi:10.1016/0002-9343(54)90353-8

46. Agarwal SK, Lee Burns A, Sukhodolets KE, et al. Molecular pathology of the MEN1 gene. *Ann N Y Acad Sci*. 2004;1014:189–198. doi:10.1196/annals.1294.020

47. Thompson NW. Current concepts in the surgical management of multiple endocrine neoplasia type 1 pancreatic-duodenal disease. Results in the treatment of 40 patients with Zollinger-Ellison syndrome, hypoglycaemia or both. *J Intern Med*. 1998;243:495–500. doi:10.1046/j.1365-2796.1998.00307.x

48. Norton JA, Fraker DL, Alexander HR, et al. Surgery to cure the Zollinger-Ellison syndrome. *N Engl J Med*. 1999;341:635–644. doi:10.1056/NEJM199908263410902

49. Richards FM, Maher ER, Latif F, et al. Detailed genetic mapping of the von Hippel-Lindau disease tumour suppressor gene. *J Med Genet*. 1993;30:104–107. doi:10.1136/jmg.30.2.104

50. Hammel PR, Vilgrain V, Terris B, et al. Pancreatic involvement in von Hippel-Lindau disease. The Groupe Francophone d'Etude de la Maladie de von Hippel-Lindau. *Gastroenterology*. 2000;119:1087–1095. doi:10.1053/gast.2000.18143

51. Gortz B, Roth J, Krahenmann A, et al. Mutations and allelic deletions of the MEN1 gene are associated with a subset of sporadic endocrine pancreatic and neuroendocrine tumors and not restricted to foregut neoplasms. *Am J Pathol*. 1999;154:429–436. doi:10.1016/S0002-9440(10)65289-3

52. Jiao Y, Shi C, Edil BH, et al. DAXX/ATRX, MEN1, and mTOR pathway genes are frequently altered in pancreatic neuroendocrine tumors. *Science*. 2011;331:1199–1203. doi:10.1126/science.1200609

53. Banck MS, Kanwar R, Kulkarni AA, et al. The genomic landscape of small intestine neuroendocrine tumors. *J Clin Invest*. 2013;123:2502–2508. doi:10.1172/JCI67963

54. Karpathakis A, Dibra H, Thirlwell C. Neuroendocrine tumours: cracking the epigenetic code. *Endocr Relat Cancer*. 2013;20:R65–R82. doi:10.1530/ERC-12-0338

55. Strosberg J, Nasir A, Coppola D, et al. Correlation between grade and prognosis in metastatic gastroenteropancreatic neuroendocrine tumors. *Hum Pathol*. 2009;40:1262–1268. doi:10.1016/j.humpath.2009.01.010

56. O'Toole D, Grossman A, Gross D, et al. ENETS Consensus Guidelines for the Standards of Care in Neuroendocrine Tumors: biochemical markers. *Neuroendocrinology*. 2009;90:194–202. doi:10.1159/000225948

57. Bajetta E, Ferrari L, Martinetti A, et al. Chromogranin A, neuron specific enolase, carcinoembryonic antigen, and hydroxyindole acetic acid evaluation in patients with neuroendocrine tumors. *Cancer*. 1999;86:858–865. doi:10.1002/(SICI)1097-0142(19990901)86:5<858::AID-CNCR23>3.0.CO;2-8

58. Yao JC, Pavel M, Phan AT, et al. Chromogranin A and neuron-specific enolase as prognostic markers in patients with advanced pNET treated with everolimus. *J Clin Endocrinol Metab*. 2011;96:3741–3749. doi:10.1210/jc.2011-0666

59. Paulson EK, McDermott VG, Keogan MT, et al. Carcinoid metastases to the liver: role of triple-phase helical CT. *Radiology*. 1998;206:143–150. doi:10.1148/radiology.206.1.9423664

60. Legmann P, Vignaux O, Dousset B, et al. Pancreatic tumors: comparison of dual-phase helical CT and endoscopic sonography. *AJR Am J Roentgenol*. 1998;170:1315–1322. doi:10.2214/ajr.170.5.9574609

61. Dromain C, de Baere T, Baudin E, et al. MR imaging of hepatic metastases caused by neuroendocrine tumors: comparing four techniques. *AJR Am J Roentgenol*. 2003;180:121–128. doi:10.2214/ajr.180.1.1800121

62. Morse B, Jeong D, Thomas K, et al. Magnetic resonance imaging of neuroendocrine tumor hepatic metastases: does hepatobiliary phase imaging improve lesion conspicuity and interobserver agreement of lesion measurements? *Pancreas*. 2017;46:1219–1224. doi:10.1097/MPA.0000000000000920

63. Sadowski SM, Neychev V, Millo C, et al. Prospective study of 68Ga-DOTATATE positron emission tomography/computed tomography for detecting gastro-entero-pancreatic neuroendocrine tumors and unknown primary sites. *J Clin Oncol.* 2016;34:588–596. doi:10.1200/JCO.2015.64.0987

64. Kratochwil C, Stefanova M, Mavriopoulou E, et al. SUV of [68Ga]DOTATOC-PET/CT Predicts Response Probability of PRRT in Neuroendocrine Tumors. *Mol Imaging Biol.* 2015;17:313–318. doi:10.1007/s11307-014-0795-3

65. Sadot E, Reidy-Lagunes DL, Tang LH, et al. Observation versus resection for small asymptomatic pancreatic neuroendocrine tumors: a matched case-control study. *Ann Surg Oncol.* 2016;23:1361–1370. doi:10.1245/s10434-015-4986-1

66. Onozato Y, Kakizaki S, Iizuka H, et al. Endoscopic treatment of rectal carcinoid tumors. *Dis Colon Rectum.* 2010;53:169–176. doi:10.1007/DCR.0b013e3181b9db7b

67. Murray SE, Sippel RS, Lloyd R, et al. Surveillance of small rectal carcinoid tumors in the absence of metastatic disease. *Ann Surg Oncol.* 2017;19:3486–3490. doi:10.1245/s10434-012-2442-z

68. Schindl M, Niederle B, Hafner M, et al. Stage-dependent therapy of rectal carcinoid tumors. *World J Surg.* 1998;22:628–633; discussion 634. doi:10.1007/s002689900445

69. Caplin M, Sundin A, Nillson O, et al. ENETS Consensus Guidelines for the management of patients with digestive neuroendocrine neoplasms: colorectal neuroendocrine neoplasms. *Neuroendocrinology.* 2012;95:88–97. doi:10.1159/000335594

70. Maurer R, Reubi JC. Somatostatin receptors. *JAMA.* 1985;253:2741. doi:10.1001/jama.1985.03350420155035

71. Kvols LK, Moertel CG, O'Connell MJ, et al. Treatment of the malignant carcinoid syndrome. Evaluation of a long-acting somatostatin analogue. *N Engl J Med.* 1986;315:663–666. doi:10.1056/NEJM198609113151102

72. Maton PN. Use of octreotide acetate for control of symptoms in patients with islet cell tumors. *World J Surg.* 1993;17:504–510. doi:10.1007/BF01655110

73. Rubin J, Ajani J, Schirmer W, et al. Octreotide acetate long-acting formulation versus open-label subcutaneous octreotide acetate in malignant carcinoid syndrome. *J Clin Oncol.* 1999;17:600–606. doi:10.1200/JCO.1999.17.2.600

74. Strosberg J, Weber J, Feldman M, et al. Above-label doses of octreotide-LAR in patients with metastatic small intestinal carcinoid tumors. *Gastrointest Cancer Res.* 2013;6:81–85.

75. Rinke A, Muller HH, Schade-Brittinger C, et al. Placebo-controlled, double-blind, prospective, randomized study on the effect of octreotide LAR in the control of tumor growth in patients with metastatic neuroendocrine midgut tumors: a report from the PROMID Study Group. *J Clin Oncol.* 2009;27:4656–4663. doi:10.1200/JCO.2009.22.8510

76. Caplin ME, Pavel M, Ćwikła JB, et al. Lanreotide in metastatic enterpancreatic neuroendocrine tumors. *N Engl J Med.* 2014;371(3):224–233. doi:10.1056/nejmoa1316158

77. Qian ZR, Ter-Minassian M, Chan JA, et al. Prognostic significance of MTOR pathway component expression in neuroendocrine tumors. *J Clin Oncol.* 2013;31:3418–3425. doi:10.1200/JCO.2012.46.6946

78. Pavel ME, Hainsworth JD, Baudin E, et al. Everolimus plus octreotide long-acting repeatable for the treatment of advanced neuroendocrine tumours associated with carcinoid syndrome (RADIANT-2): a randomised, placebo-controlled, phase 3 study. *Lancet.* 2011;378:2005–2012. doi:10.1016/S0140-6736(11)61742-X

79. Pavel ME, Baudin E, Oberg KE, et al. Efficacy of everolimus plus octreotide LAR in patients with advanced neuroendocrine tumor and carcinoid syndrome: final overall survival from the randomized, placebo-controlled phase 3 RADIANT-2 study. *Ann Oncol.* 2017;28:1569–1575. doi:10.1093/annonc/mdx193

80. Yao JC, Shah MH, Ito T, et al. Everolimus for advanced pancreatic neuroendocrine tumors. *N Engl J Med.* 2011;364:514–523. doi:10.1056/NEJMoa1009290

81. Yao JC, Pavel M, Lombard-Bohas C, et al. Everolimus for the treatment of advanced pancreatic neuroendocrine tumors: overall survival and circulating biomarkers from the randomized, phase III RADIANT-3 study. *J Clin Oncol.* 2016;34:3906–3913. doi:10.1200/JCO.2016.68.0702

82. Yao JC, Fazio N, Singh S, et al. Everolimus for the treatment of advanced, non-functional neuroendocrine tumours of the lung or gastrointestinal tract (RADIANT-4): a randomised, placebo-controlled, phase 3 study. *Lancet.* 2016;387:968–977. doi:10.1016/S0140-6736(15)00817-X

83. Yao JC, Phan A, Hoff PM, et al. Targeting vascular endothelial growth factor in advanced carcinoid tumor: a random assignment phase II study of depot octreotide with bevacizumab and pegylated interferon alpha-2b. *J Clin Oncol.* 2008;26:1316–1323. doi:10.1200/JCO.2007.13.6374

84. Kulke MH, Lenz HJ, Meropol NJ, et al. Activity of sunitinib in patients with advanced neuroendocrine tumors. *J Clin Oncol.* 2008;26:3403–3410. doi:10.1200/JCO.2007.15.9020

85. Raymond E, Dahan L, Raoul JL, et al. Sunitinib malate for the treatment of pancreatic neuroendocrine tumors. *N Engl J Med.* 2011;364:501–513. doi:10.1056/NEJMoa1003825

86. Moertel CG, Kvols LK, O'Connell MJ, et al. Treatment of neuroendocrine carcinomas with combined etoposide and cisplatin. Evidence of major therapeutic activity in the anaplastic variants of these neoplasms. *Cancer*. 1991;68:227–232. doi:10.1002/1097-0142(19910715)68:2<227::AID-CNCR2820680202>3.0.CO;2-I

87. Mitry E, Baudin E, Ducreux M, et al. Treatment of poorly differentiated neuroendocrine tumours with etoposide and cisplatin. *Br J Cancer*. 1999;81:1351–1355. doi:10.1038/sj.bjc.6690325

88. Sorbye H, Welin S, Langer SW, et al. Predictive and prognostic factors for treatment and survival in 305 patients with advanced gastrointestinal neuroendocrine carcinoma (WHO G3): the NORDIC NEC study. *Ann Oncol*. 2013;24:152–160. doi:10.1093/annonc/mds276

89. Hentic O, Hammel P, Couvelard A, et al. FOLFIRI regimen: an effective second-line chemotherapy after failure of etoposide-platinum combination in patients with neuroendocrine carcinomas grade 3. *Endocr Relat Cancer*. 2012;19:751–757. doi:10.1530/ERC-12-0002

90. Zhu J, Strosberg JR, Dropkin E, et al. Treatment of high-grade metastatic pancreatic neuroendocrine carcinoma with FOLFIRINOX. *J Gastrointest Cancer*. 2015;46:166–169. doi:10.1007/s12029-015-9689-0

91. Kouvaraki MA, Ajani JA, Hoff P, et al. Fluorouracil, doxorubicin, and streptozocin in the treatment of patients with locally advanced and metastatic pancreatic endocrine carcinomas. *J Clin Oncol*. 2004;22:4762–4271. doi:10.1200/JCO.2004.04.024

92. Chan JA, Stuart K, Earle CC, et al. Prospective study of bevacizumab plus temozolomide in patients with advanced neuroendocrine tumors. *J Clin Oncol*. 2012;30:2963–2968. doi:10.1200/JCO.2011.40.3147

93. Kulke MH, Stuart K, Enzinger PC, et al. Phase II study of temozolomide and thalidomide in patients with metastatic neuroendocrine tumors. *J Clin Oncol*. 2006;24:401–406. doi:10.1200/JCO.2005.03.6046

94. Strosberg JR, Fine RL, Choi J, et al. First-line chemotherapy with capecitabine and temozolomide in patients with metastatic pancreatic endocrine carcinomas. *Cancer*. 2011;117:268–275. doi:10.1002/cncr.25425

95. Fine RL, Gulati AP, Krantz BA, et al. Capecitabine and temozolomide (CAPTEM) for metastatic, well-differentiated neuroendocrine cancers: The Pancreas Center at Columbia University experience. *Cancer Chemother Pharmacol*. 2013;71:663–670. doi:10.1007/s00280-012-2055-z

96. Cives M, Ghayouri M, Morse B, et al. Analysis of potential response predictors to capecitabine/temozolomide in metastatic pancreatic neuroendocrine tumors. *Endocr Relat Cancer*. 2016;23:759–767. doi:10.1530/ERC-16-0147

97. Sun W, Lipsitz S, Catalano P, et al. Phase II/III study of doxorubicin with fluorouracil compared with streptozocin with fluorouracil or dacarbazine in the treatment of advanced carcinoid tumors: Eastern Cooperative Oncology Group Study E1281. *J Clin Oncol*. 2005;23:4897–4904. doi:10.1200/JCO.2005.03.616

98. Ekeblad S, Sundin A, Janson ET, et al. Temozolomide as monotherapy is effective in treatment of advanced malignant neuroendocrine tumors. *Clin Cancer Res*. 2007;13:2986–2991. doi:10.1158/1078-0432.CCR-06-2053

99. Cros J, Hentic O, Rebours V, et al. MGMT expression predicts response to temozolomide in pancreatic neuroendocrine tumors. *Endocr Relat Cancer*. 2016;23:625–633. doi:10.1530/ERC-16-0117

100. Campana D, Walter T, Pusceddu S, et al. Correlation between MGMT promoter methylation and response to temozolomide-based therapy in neuroendocrine neoplasms: an observational retrospective multicenter study. *Endocrine*. 2017;60(3):490–498. doi:10.1007/s12020-017-1474-3

101. van der Zwan WA, Bodei L, Mueller-Brand J, et al. GEPNETs update: radionuclide therapy in neuroendocrine tumors. *Eur J Endocrinol*. 2015;172:R1–R8. doi:10.1530/EJE-14-0488

102. Imhof A, Brunner P, Marincek N, et al. Response, survival, and long-term toxicity after therapy with the radiolabeled somatostatin analogue [90Y-DOTA]-TOC in metastasized neuroendocrine cancers. *J Clin Oncol*. 2011;29:2416–2423. doi:10.1200/JCO.2010.33.7873

103. Brabander T, van der Zwan WA, Teunissen JJM, et al. Long-Term Efficacy, Survival, and Safety of [(177)Lu-DOTA(0),Tyr(3)]octreotate in Patients with Gastroenteropancreatic and Bronchial Neuroendocrine Tumors. *Clin Cancer Res*. 2017;23:4617–4624. doi:10.1158/1078-0432.CCR-16-2743

104. Bodei L, Kidd M, Paganelli G, et al. Long-term tolerability of PRRT in 807 patients with neuroendocrine tumours: the value and limitations of clinical factors. *Eur J Nucl Med Mol Imaging*. 2015;42:5–19. doi:10.1007/s00259-014-2893-5

105. Strosberg J, El-Haddad G, Wolin E, et al. Phase 3 Trial of 177Lu-Dotatate for Midgut Neuroendocrine Tumors. *N Engl J Med*. 2017;376:125–135. doi:10.1056/NEJMoa1607427

106. van Essen M, Krenning EP, Kam BL, et al. Salvage therapy with (177)Lu-octreotate in patients with bronchial and gastroenteropancreatic neuroendocrine tumors. *J Nucl Med*. 2010;51:383–390. doi:10.2967/jnumed.109.068957

107. Kulke MH, Horsch D, Caplin ME, et al. Telotristat Ethyl, a Tryptophan Hydroxylase Inhibitor for the Treatment of Carcinoid Syndrome. *J Clin Oncol.* 2017;35:14–23. doi:10.1200/JCO.2016.69.2780

108. Que FG, Nagorney DM, Batts KP, et al. Hepatic resection for metastatic neuroendocrine carcinomas. *Am J Surg.* 1995;169:36–42; discussion 42–43. doi:10.1016/S0002-9610(99)80107-X

109. Sarmiento JM, Heywood G, Rubin J, et al. Surgical treatment of neuroendocrine metastases to the liver: a plea for resection to increase survival. *J Am Coll Surg.* 2003;197:29–37. doi:10.1016/S1072-7515(03)00230-8

110. Hellman P, Ladjevardi S, Skogseid B, et al. Radiofrequency tissue ablation using cooled tip for liver metastases of endocrine tumors. *World J Surg.* 2002;26:1052–1056. doi:10.1007/s00268-002-6663-3

111. Kvols LK, Turaga KK, Strosberg J, et al. Role of interventional radiology in the treatment of patients with neuroendocrine metastases in the liver. *J Natl Compr Canc Netw.* 2009;7:765–772. doi:10.6004/jnccn.2009.0053

112. Therasse E, Breittmayer F, Roche A, et al. Transcatheter chemoembolization of progressive carcinoid liver metastasis. *Radiology.* 1993;189:541–547. doi:10.1148/radiology.189.2.7692465

113. Ruszniewski P, Rougier P, Roche A, et al. Hepatic arterial chemoembolization in patients with liver metastases of endocrine tumors. A prospective phase II study in 24 patients. *Cancer.* 1993;71:2624–2630. doi:10.1002/1097-0142(19930415)71:8<2624::AID-CNCR2820710830>3.0.CO;2-B

114. Kennedy AS, Dezarn WA, McNeillie P, et al. Radioembolization for unresectable neuroendocrine hepatic metastases using resin 90Y-microspheres: early results in 148 patients. *Am J Clin Oncol.* 2008;31:271–279. doi:10.1097/COC.0b013e31815e4557

115. Rhee TK, Lewandowski RJ, Liu DM, et al. 90Y Radioembolization for metastatic neuroendocrine liver tumors: preliminary results from a multi-institutional experience. *Ann Surg.* 2008;247:1029–1035. doi:10.1097/SLA.0b013e3181728a45

116. Sangro B, Gil-Alzugaray B, Rodriguez J, et al. Liver disease induced by radioembolization of liver tumors: description and possible risk factors. *Cancer.* 2008;112:1538–1546. doi:10.1002/cncr.23339

117. Lehnert T. Liver transplantation for metastatic neuroendocrine carcinoma: an analysis of 103 patients. *Transplantation.* 1998;66:1307–1312. doi:10.1097/00007890-199811270-00007

118. Le Treut YP, Gregoire E, Belghiti J, et al. Predictors of long-term survival after liver transplantation for metastatic endocrine tumors: an 85-case French multicentric report. *Am J Transplant.* 2008;8:1205–1213. doi:10.1111/j.1600-6143.2008.02233.x

119. Mazzaferro V, Sposito C, Coppa J, et al. The long-term benefit of liver transplantation for hepatic metastases from neuroendocrine tumors. *Am J Transplant.* 2016;16:2892–2902. doi:10.1111/ajt.13831

Early-Stage Anal Cancer

Clayton A. Smith, Nitesh Rana, and Lisa A. Kachnic

INTRODUCTION

Anal carcinoma is a rare malignancy of the gastrointestinal tract. The majority of cases are squamous cell carcinomas (SCCs) that develop in association with human papillomavirus (HPV) infection. A multidisciplinary team of colorectal surgeons, medical oncologists, and radiation oncologists are the key to diagnosis, management, and surveillance of patients with anal cancer. While SCC is the most common variant and is treated typically with concurrent chemotherapy and radiation therapy (chemo-RT), rarer histologies including adenocarcinoma and melanoma may also present a management dilemma. This chapter focuses primarily on the diagnosis and treatment of anal SCC with brief overviews of the management of less common histologies.

ANATOMY

The anal region consists of the perianal skin (also known as the anal margin) and the anal canal. Anatomically, the anal margin is defined as the 5 cm of perianal skin extending radially from the squamous mucocutaneous junction, also known as the anal verge. The anal canal, which measures approximately 4 cm in length, is the mucosal area between the anal verge inferiorly and the anorectal ring superiorly. The anorectal ring, also known as anorectal flexure, is a palpable muscular bundle at the junction of the rectum and anal canal, and is composed of the puborectalis sling, external sphincter, and the internal sphincter.

Histologically, the anal margin is characterized by keratinized squamous epithelium (epidermis). The anal canal, on the other hand, is characterized predominantly by nonkeratinized squamous epithelium (mucosa). The anal verge is the area of transition between the epidermis of the anal margin and the mucosa of the anal canal. The proximal part of the anal canal is lined by columnar epithelium, while the distal portion of the canal is lined by nonkeratinized stratified squamous epithelium. The area of transition between the columnar and squamous epithelium within the anal canal is the dentate line, also known as the pectinate line. This is an important anatomical landmark as the lymphatic drainage differs above and below the line. Tumors arising superior to the dentate line have lymphatic drainage to mesorectal and internal iliac nodal basins, whereas tumors arising inferior to the dentate line have lymphatic drainage to superficial inguinal and external iliac nodal basins.

EPIDEMIOLOGY

Anal cancers are a relatively rare malignancy with an estimated incidence of 8,580 new cases and 1,160 deaths in 2018 (1). Anal cancer represents 0.5% of all new cancer cases in the United States and is the 27th most common type of cancer (2). The median age at diagnosis is 61 with an estimated 48% of new diagnoses localized to primary site, 32% with regional spread to lymph nodes, and 13% with distant metastases. The incidence of anal cancer has been steadily increasing on an average rate of 2.2% each year over the past decade, likely due to the rise in HPV infection (2).

PATHOGENESIS AND ANAL CANCER BIOLOGY

There are several risk factors for the development of anal SCC including HPV infection, immunosuppression (including HIV infection and organ transplantation), and cigarette smoking. HPV

A Clinical Vignette is included at the end of the chapter.

infection has the strongest association with anal cancer, particularly from high-risk HPV types such as HPV 16 and HPV 18. Although a number of HPV subtypes can potentially be found in the anogenital tract, HPV 16 is the most frequently encountered and predictive subtype for anal SCC (3). The HPV-mediated changes that occur in anal squamous epithelium are similar to those that lead to the progression to cervical cancer. HPV viral proteins E6 and E7 bind to host proteins, which results in suppression of cell cycle arrest and of apoptosis. Through accumulation of DNA errors over time, the involved epithelium transitions from benign condylomata to high-grade squamous intraepithelial lesions to invasive SCC. Chronic immunosuppression is associated with increased incidence of squamous dysplasia and anal cancer, which is attributed to decreased ability to clear HPV infection. HIV-positive individuals have an increased incidence of anal SCC. An analysis of 13 North American cohorts comprising >34,000 HIV-positive and >114,000 HIV-negative individuals with follow-up from 1996 to 2007 in the highly active antiretroviral therapy (HAART) era revealed that HIV-positive men who have sex with men have an estimated 80 times greater chance of developing anal cancer than HIV-negative men (4). Other HIV-positive groups were also at an increased risk relative to the general population. Despite this increased incidence, HIV-positive patients with anal cancer do not appear to have significantly worse cancer-specific survival relative to HIV-negative patients (5). In addition, renal transplant patients also have an estimated 10-fold increase in the risk of developing anal cancer relative to the general population (6). Finally, cigarette smoking has also been noted to increase the risk of developing anal SCC, though the mechanism is unclear (3). The question has been investigated more thoroughly in cervical cancer, which also shares the same associated risk factors of HPV infection and cigarette smoking (7). It has been proposed that smoking acts as a cocarcinogen and is associated with increased HPV viral load in HPV-positive women who smoke (8,9).

EVALUATION AND STAGING

The most common presenting symptoms of anal cancer are rectal bleeding, pain, and sensation of mass. Rectal bleeding is often assumed to be caused by hemorrhoids and may lead to a delay in diagnosis. Other symptoms include pruritus, narrowing of stool caliber, tenesmus, abnormal anal discharge, and inguinal lymphadenopathy.

During physical examination, detailed attention should be directed toward examination of the abdomen, inguinal region, anus, and rectum. On visual inspection of the anus, the primary tumor may be visible if it is at or distal to the anal verge. The perianal skin should also be carefully inspected for involvement. If there is tissue involved by anal intraepithelial neoplasia (AIN), the extent of involvement should be noted to ensure coverage during treatment. It is important to make a distinction between a primary lesion of the perianal skin versus the anal canal, as treatment approaches may vary based on location. On digital rectal examination (DRE), the anal tone should be assessed; the extent and location of the primary should also be noted. An inguinal examination should be performed to assess for inguinal lymphadenopathy. Anoscopy should also be performed to fully visualize the primary lesion, to accurately determine the size for T staging, and to determine relationship of the mass to the dentate line. All females should have a gynecologic exam to evaluate for vulvar or vaginal involvement and undergo screening for cervical cancer. If HIV status is unknown, HIV testing should be performed.

Diagnosis is made by biopsy to determine histology, which directly guides management. Additionally, any suspicious inguinal lymphadenopathy should undergo a fine-needle aspiration to confirm malignant involvement. Histologically, the vast majority of anal cancers are SCCs (10,11). Other potential histologies include adenocarcinoma, melanoma, neuroendocrine tumor, Kaposi sarcoma, lymphoma, basal cell carcinoma, SCC in situ, or extramammary Paget disease. Given the association with HPV infection, surrogate marker p16 testing via immunohistochemistry should be performed on all anal SCC specimens.

After diagnosis of anal SCC is established, diagnostic imaging to assess the extent of disease should be obtained. This includes a CT scan of the chest, abdomen, and pelvis with intravenous (IV) and oral contrast. A PET scan from skull base to midthigh should also be obtained. It is important to note that PET/CT does not replace diagnostic CT imaging. MRI of the pelvis with contrast may also be considered to provide additional information on tumor extent, sphincter involvement, and adjacent organ involvement, since these features may be difficult to determine on CT or PET.

Staging of anal SCC is in accordance with the eighth edition of the American Joint Committee on Cancer (AJCC) to include separate tumor (T), nodal (N), and metastatic (M) assessments based on clinical findings from exam and diagnostic imaging (12). T stage is based on size (T1: ≤2 cm, T2: 2 to ≤5 cm, T3: >5 cm) and degree of invasion (T4: invading adjacent organs including vagina, urethra, and bladder) and has not changed from the seventh edition. N stage has been modified in the eighth edition to node-negative (N0) or node-positive (N1), with N1 disease subclassified by location (N1a: inguinal, mesorectal, or internal iliac nodes, N1b: external iliac nodes, N1c: external iliac nodes and N1a nodes). Prognostic grouping has also been revised to reflect the changes in the N stage categories.

MANAGEMENT

Prior to the 1970s, the mainstay of treatment for anal SCC involved abdominoperineal resection (APR) with a permanent colostomy, resulting in 5-year overall survival (OS) rates of 50% (13,14). Due to poor outcomes with radical surgery alone, Nigro and colleagues first reported in 1974 on surgical outcomes of three patients treated with neoadjuvant radiation with concurrent 5-fluorouracil (5-FU) and mitomycin C (MMC) who were found to have a pathologic complete response at the time of surgery (15). This report sparked interest in utilizing definitive chemo-RT alone in the treatment of anal cancer in order to preserve sphincter function and avoid permanent colostomy. Although definitive chemo-RT has never been prospectively compared with APR alone, subsequent series demonstrated significant complete response rates with chemoradiation such that it was soon adopted as the primary treatment of anal SCC (16,17). Although the majority of anal cancers are of squamous histology, less common histologies including adenocarcinoma and melanoma exhibit a different natural history response to therapies. Figure 49.1 provides a broad outline of the management algorithm by histology for locoregional anal carcinomas.

Small (<2 cm) SCC of the perianal region is approached as a skin cancer, with wide local excision (WLE) being the preferred management. Five-year survival after WLE is reported up to 88% (18). The recommended cancer-free margins are 1 cm (19). Cancer involving only the perianal skin without extension into the canal primarily drains to the inguinal nodal basins. With T1 lesions, WLE alone of the primary site is sufficient for disease control since the risk of

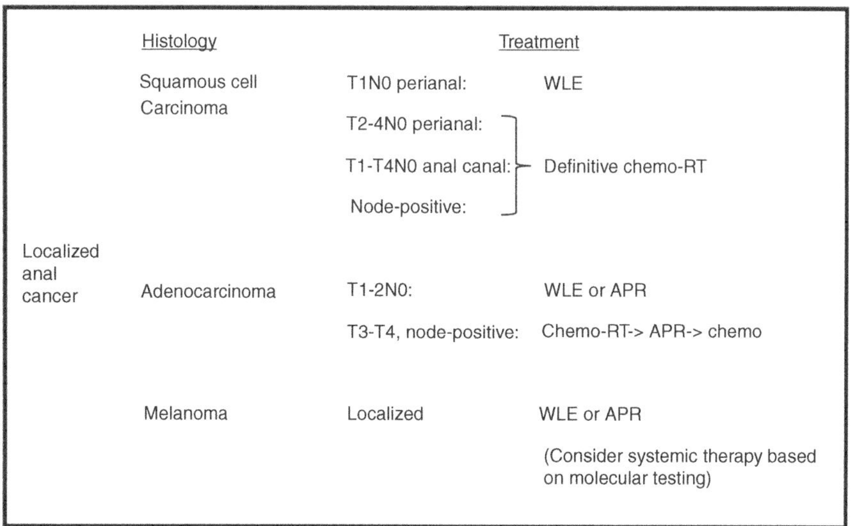

FIGURE 49.1   Treatment algorithm for localized anal cancer by histologic diagnosis.

APR, abdominoperineal resection; chemo-RT, concurrent chemotherapy and radiation therapy; WLE, wide local excision.

lymphatic metastases is very low. In patients with T2–T4 disease or T1 lesions requiring APR for complete resection, concurrent chemo-RT is the preferred approach for sphincter preservation and to treat at-risk lymphatic basins to reduce regional recurrence.

For patients with nonmetastatic anal canal SCC or T2-T4 perianal SCC, the recommended treatment is definitive chemo-RT. Chemotherapy consists of continuous infusion (CI) 5-FU (1,000 mg/m^2/day IV on days 1–4 and 29–32) and bolus MMC (10 mg/m^2 IV on days 1 and 29). Radiation is delivered using intensity-modulated radiation therapy (IMRT) with a dose painting technique. In this cT2 cN1 anal canal SCC, the doses used would be 54 Gy to the primary tumor, 50.4 Gy to involved <3 cm nodes, and 45 Gy to elective nodal basins. The intent of treatment is both cure and sphincter preservation.

Combined Modality Therapy Is Superior to Radiation Therapy Alone

Two randomized trials have assessed the benefit of chemo-RT over radiation alone. The United Kingdom Coordinating Committee on Cancer Research (UKCCCR) Anal Cancer Trial I (ACT I) randomized 585 patients to either 45 Gy in 20 to 25 fractions delivered with anteroposterior–posteroanterior (AP–PA) fields alone or to the same radiation therapy (RT) with concurrent administration of MMC 12 mg/m^2 bolus on day 1 and CI 5-FU 1,000 mg/m^2/day IV on days 1 to 4 or CI 5-FU 750 mg/m^2/day on days 1 to 5. An additional cycle of 5-FU was given during the final week of radiation therapy. Following completion of initial therapy, clinical assessment of response was made 6 weeks later. Patients with <50% response were referred for resection while patients with >50% response received either external beam boost of 15 Gy in six fractions or brachytherapy boost of 25 Gy over 2 to 3 days. There was no difference in the number of patients with >50% response rate between arms (92% for both arms) (20). The chemo-RT arm did have greater acute hematologic, skin, gastrointestinal, and genitourinary toxicity (48%) compared to radiation alone (39%; *p* = .03). With long-term follow-up of 13 years, concurrent chemo-RT demonstrated superior 5-year locoregional failure (32% vs. 57%; *p* < .001), 5-year cancer-specific survival (70% vs. 58%; *p* = .004), and 5-year colostomy-free survival (47% vs. 37%; *p* = .004) (21). There was no difference in OS between arms (58% vs. 53%; *p* = .12) or in late morbidity.

In a smaller trial of 110 patients with locally advanced (T3–T4 or node-positive) disease, the European Organisation for Research and Treatment of Cancer (EORTC) 22861 trial also compared chemo-RT to radiation alone. Outcomes were similar to ACT I with improvements in locoregional control and colostomy-free survival but no difference in OS with the addition of chemotherapy (22). Collectively, these trials support the current recommendation of combined modality chemo-RT in patients who can tolerate treatment.

Selection and Sequencing of Chemotherapy

Due to significant hematologic toxicity associated with MMC, the U.S. Intergroup (Radiation Therapy Oncology Group [RTOG] 8704/Eastern Cooperative Oncology Group [ECOG] 1289) trial evaluated whether MMC could be safely omitted from the chemo-RT regimen. Initial chemotherapy was administered as CI 5-FU 1,000 mg/m^2/day on days 1 to 4 and 29 to 32 in both the 5-FU + MMC arm and 5-FU only arm. The dose of MMC was 10 mg/m^2 bolus on days 1 and 29. Radiation treatment was given to 45–50.4 Gy in 25 to 28 fractions with shrinking field technique after 30.6 Gy. Similar to the ACT I trial, assessment was made 4 to 6 weeks after completion of initial radiation to determine if residual disease was present. If there was palpable inguinal adenopathy or if disease remained on biopsy, an additional 9 Gy radiation boost was delivered along with 5-FU and cisplatin 100 mg/m^2. Four-year outcomes demonstrated the superiority of MMC combined with 5-FU with reduced colostomy rates (9% vs. 22%; *p* =.002), increased colostomy-free survival (71% vs. 59%; *p* = .014), and increased disease-free survival (73% vs. 51%; *p* = .0003) (23). There was no difference in OS. As expected, grade 4 acute toxicity was worse with the addition of MMC (23% vs. 7%). Based on these results, concurrent single-agent chemotherapy is not recommended except in patients who may not tolerate multiagent and/or reduced dose chemotherapy.

Two trials have investigated the substitution of cisplatin for MMC, albeit with differing designs that make direct comparisons difficult. RTOG 9811 compared standard chemo-RT with 5-FU and MMC (the experimental arm from RTOG 8704) to induction chemotherapy with CI 5-FU 1,000 mg/m^2/day on days 1 to 4, 29 to 32, 57 to 60, and 85 to 88 with bolus cisplatin 75 mg/m^2 on days 1, 29, 57, and 85 (24). Radiation was given concurrently with the control 5-FU/MMC and with the third cycle (day 57) on the experimental 5-FU/cisplatin arm. In a departure from prior trials, a delay between initial radiation and boost was no longer built into the protocol. Radiation was given as 45 Gy in 25 fractions with AP–PA fields with a reduction in the superior field border after 30.6 Gy. After 45 Gy, a boost of 10 to 14 Gy in 2 Gy/fraction was given to patients with T2 residual disease, T3–T4 disease, or involved inguinal nodes. Although initial outcomes appeared to be similar between treatment groups, with long-term follow-up, the cisplatin arm had poorer outcomes (25). Compared to induction and concurrent 5-FU/cisplatin, 5-FU/MMC resulted in improved 5-year disease-free survival (68% vs. 58%; p = .006), colostomy-free survival (72% vs. 65%; p = .05), and OS (78% vs. 71%; p = .026). Although acute grade 3–4 hematologic toxicity was worse with concurrent MMC (61% vs. 42%; p < .001), overall late grade 3–4 toxicity did not differ between groups (13% MMC vs. 11% cisplatin; p = .35). Due to differences in both chemotherapy and use of induction between the arms, the outcomes may be interpreted in several ways. One interpretation is that cisplatin has decreased efficacy in comparison to MMC as a radiosensitizer for treating anal SCC. An alternative explanation is that induction chemotherapy delays definitive treatment and adversely affects outcomes. Based on these results, chemo-RT with concurrent 5-FU/ MMC without induction chemotherapy remains the standard of care in the United States for patients who are candidates for MMC.

The UKCCCR ACT II trial also assessed the use of concurrent 5-FU/MMC versus 5-FU/ cisplatin in addition to whether maintenance chemotherapy could improve outcomes (26). In a 2 × 2 factorial design, patients were randomized to (a) 5-FU/cisplatin with radiation and no maintenance, (b) 5-FU/cisplatin with radiation followed by maintenance 5-FU/cisplatin, (c) 5-FU/MMC with radiation and no maintenance, or (d) 5-FU/MMC with radiation followed by maintenance 5-FU/cisplatin. Chemotherapy was given as CI 5-FU 1,000 mg/m²/day on days 1 to 4 and 29 to 32 with either bolus cisplatin 60 mg/m² on days 1 and 29 or MMC 12 mg/ m² on day 1. Maintenance chemotherapy was delivered as two cycles of CI 5-FU on days 71 to 74 and 92 to 95 and cisplatin on days 71 and 92. Radiation therapy was given as 50.4 Gy in 28 fractions by AP–PA fields with reduction after 30.6 Gy. No planned boost was delivered in this trial. In comparing the 5-FU/MMC arms with 5-FU/cisplatin, there was no difference in 5-year colostomy-free survival (68% vs. 67%) or OS (79% vs. 77%). There was also no benefit to maintenance chemotherapy for progression-free survival (74% vs. 73% no maintenance). Although overall acute grade 3–4 toxicity was similar between MMC and cisplatin arms (71% vs. 72%), there were increased hematologic events with the use of MMC (26% vs. 16%; p < .001). Given the lack of benefit with concurrent cisplatin or maintenance chemotherapy, chemo-RT with concurrent 5-FU/MMC remains the standard of care for locoregional anal SCC; nevertheless, the ACT II trial results demonstrate the efficacy of a cisplatin-based regimen for patients who may not tolerate MMC due to concerns for hematologic toxicity.

Radiation Therapy Delivery and Planning
The aforementioned randomized trials administered radiation therapy with traditional AP–PA or three-dimensional (3D) conformal techniques that resulted in significant dose to bladder, bowel, bone marrow, and skin. IMRT is now the standard of care for anal cancer based on the results of RTOG 0529. IMRT employs advanced technology to fluctuate beam intensities and target radiation dose to tumor and nodal basins at risk while sparing dose to adjacent normal organs (Figure 49.2). RTOG 0529 was a phase II trial assessing acute toxicity in patients treated with standard concurrent 5-FU/MMC and radiation delivered by IMRT, with differential dosing up to 54 Gy for patients based on the tumor stage (27). Toxicity outcomes were compared to patients treated on the 5-FU/MMC arm from RTOG 9811. Patients treated with IMRT experienced significantly lower grade 2 or higher hematologic (73% vs. 85%; p = .032), grade 3 or higher gastrointestinal (21% vs. 36%; p = .0082), and grade 3 or higher dermatologic (23% vs. 49%; p < .0001) acute toxicity. Patients treated with IMRT also underwent a shorter duration of radiation therapy in comparison with patients treated with 3D-conformal treatment on RTOG 9811 (median 42.5 days vs. 49 days; p < .0001).

Radiation therapy planning is based on CT imaging of the patient in the treatment position, which is typically prone with radiopaque markers placed around gross disease extending outside of the anal verge. Targets include gross target volume (GTV), clinical target volume (CTV), and planning target volume (PTV). The GTV is contoured based on information provided by physical exam, endoscopy reports, and imaging such as PET/CT or MRI. This includes both the primary tumor as well as involved inguinal or pelvic lymphadenopathy. The CTV of the primary site consists of 1.5 to 2 cm isotropic expansion around the GTV and includes the entire

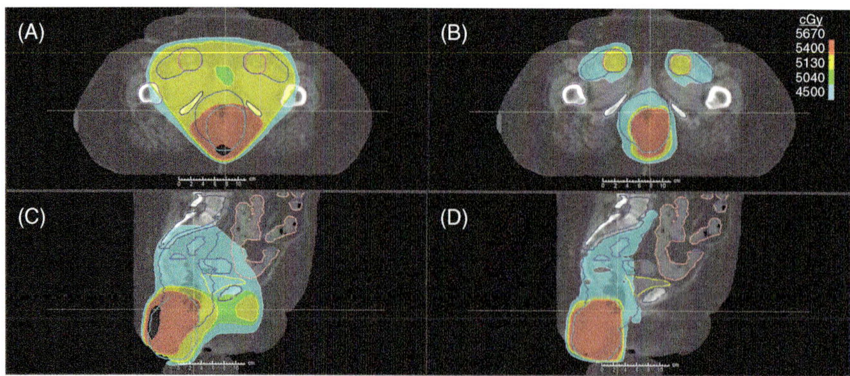

FIGURE 49.2   Comparative radiation treatment plans with dose distributions for a female patient with stage IIIA (T2 N1a M0) anal canal squamous cell carcinoma simulated supine due to body habitus. Representative axial (A and B) and sagittal (C and D) CT images are displayed. Traditional 3D-conformal planning (A and C) delivers significant dose to bowel and bone marrow relative to modern IMRT planning (B and D).

3D, three-dimensional; IMRT, intensity-modulated radiation therapy.

anal canal. The elective CTV includes bilateral inguinal, internal and external iliac, mesorectum, and presacral lymph node regions. Multiple atlases are available for assistance with contouring the primary and elective targets (28,29). The PTV accounts for daily setup error and is typically 0.5 to 0.7 cm when daily image guidance is used. In addition to target volumes, organs at risk (OARs) should be contoured, which include the small bowel, femoral heads, bladder, external genitalia, pelvic bone marrow, and large bowel.

Differential dosing to targets is delivered with a dose painting technique. For T1–T2 N0 nonbulky patients, the primary tumor PTV is treated to 50.4 Gy in 28 fractions while elective nodal basins are treated to 42 Gy at the same time. For T3–T4 tumors, the primary tumor PTV is treated to 54 Gy in 30 fractions, while involved nodes receive either 50.4 Gy or 54 Gy based on size less than or greater than 3 cm, respectively. Elective nodal regions are treated to 45 Gy in 30 fractions in the setting of T3–T4 or node-positive disease. For plan optimization of target coverage and sparing of OARs, we follow the guidelines of RTOG 0529 protocol.

Treatment of HIV-positive patients may present a management dilemma due to hematologic toxicity. For HIV-positive patients who are on HAART with CD4 counts >200, we offer standard radiation and chemotherapy with 5-FU/MMC. In HIV-positive patients who are not on HAART and have CD4 counts <200, we recommend initiation of HAART prior to beginning definitive chemo-RT as CD4 counts will likely decrease during treatment. They should also be placed on appropriate antibiotic prophylaxis for impaired immunity. As part of radiation treatment planning, the pelvic bone marrow is prioritized to limit the risk of myelosuppression. Additionally, cisplatin may be considered in place of MMC to further reduce this risk. During treatment, granulocyte colony-stimulating factors may be required in the setting of neutropenia; it is recommended that chemotherapy and radiation be held during administration as concomitant use may potentiate myelosuppression and adversely affect treatment outcomes (30).

Anal adenocarcinoma represents approximately 5% to 10% of anal carcinomas (10,31). Anal adenocarcinoma carries a significantly worse prognosis relative to anal SCC (HR: 0.66, 95% CI: 0.59–0.75, p < .01) or rectal adenocarcinoma (HR: 0.68, 95% CI: 0.61–0.77, p < .01) with median OS of 33, 118, and 68 months, respectively (32). Given the low incidence, there are no randomized data to directly guide treatment; however, many cases are thought to arise from the adjacent rectum with distal extension to the anal canal, making determination of the site of origin difficult. Since there is extensive literature to guide treatment of rectal adenocarcinoma, a similar approach is followed for anal adenocarcinoma. Transanal excision alone may be considered for small, well-differentiated T1 lesions if negative margins can be achieved. For larger lesions, APR is the recommended definitive treatment since the ability to undergo APR is the strongest predictor of survival (32,33). For locally advanced disease (cT3–T4 or node-positive), we offer neoadjuvant long-course radiation to 50.4–54 Gy in 28 to 30 fractions with concurrent CI 5-FU or capecitabine based on improved local control, decreased toxicity, and potential for downstaging of neoadjuvant therapy for locally advanced rectal cancer (34,35). While rectal cancer has historically been treated with 3D-conformal radiotherapy, for anal adenocarcinoma, we deliver treatment with IMRT as described earlier to cover the more extensive at-risk nodal basins that drain from the anal canal while limiting dose to OARs.

Anal mucosal melanoma accounts for approximately 1% to 2% of anal malignancies. Incidence increases with age, with mean age at diagnosis of 69 years (10,36). It is more common in Caucasians and females. Common presenting symptoms are not specific to the histology and include anal pain or discomfort, pruritus, bleeding, anal mass, or inguinal mass. Anal melanoma is not included in the AJCC staging system, but retrospective series have generally divided patients into localized, regional (lymphatic spread), or metastatic disease. At presentation, approximately 40% have localized disease, 35% have regional, and 25% have distant metastases (36).

First-line therapy for localized or regional disease is surgical resection. Primary resection may be with WLE or APR. The type of resection has been retrospectively analyzed in several series without clear survival benefit for APR over local excision (36–38). Positive resection margin is a negative prognostic factor for recurrence (39). Therefore WLE with negative margins is preferred over APR to limit morbidity.

Adjuvant radiation therapy has not been tested prospectively. In one of the largest retrospective series of 54 patients, Kelly and colleagues (2011) observed a 5-year local failure rate of 18% and sphincter preservation in 96% of patients treated with WLE and hypofractionated radiation therapy (40). Most patients received a dose of 30 to 36 Gy in 5 to 6 fractions delivered twice weekly. Patients treated with more extended fields covering the inguinal nodes did not demonstrate improved outcomes in comparison with primary site RT only. Despite improved local control with this approach, 5-year OS remained low at 30% due to distant failure. Without evidence of a survival benefit, adjuvant radiation therapy should be discussed with patients considered at a high risk for local recurrence, but it is not recommended as standard for all patients.

Adjuvant systemic therapy is undefined for anorectal mucosal melanoma. Unlike cutaneous melanoma, approximately 6% of patients harbor BRAF mutations while up to 36% may have c-kit mutations (41,42). The literature on efficacy is limited to case reports and case series, so no specific recommendation for systemic therapy can be made at this time.

TOXICITY AND SYMPTOM MANAGEMENT

Patients undergoing definitive chemo-RT should be counseled on the potential acute side effects including dermatitis and desquamation, cytopenias and sepsis, diarrhea, nausea, vomiting, tenesmus, fecal leakage or urgency, urinary frequency, and dysuria. Late side effects should also be discussed, including vaginal stenosis, dyspareunia and dryness in women, erectile dysfunction in men, infertility and sterility, hematuria, hematochezia, fistulas, anorectal dysfunction, and decreased bone density that may result in sacral or femoral head fractures.

During treatment, acute dermatitis and desquamation may result in significant treatment breaks, which are detrimental to outcomes. IMRT treatment planning is key to limiting the risk of this toxicity, particularly in the elective inguinal folds. As skin toxicity advances, progressive treatments with barrier creams, sitz baths, topical lidocaine mixtures, silver sulfadiazine, and Domeboro soaks are employed for symptomatic relief. Acute gastrointestinal toxicity presenting as diarrhea is generally managed with loperamide or prescription atropine/diphenoxylate. Proctofoam may be prescribed for severe tenesmus. Dietary modifications including low fat and low residue diets may also reduce the risk and severity of bowel and anorectal symptoms. Urinary frequency may be managed with antispasmodics, while dysuria typically responds to phenazopyridine. As mentioned earlier, cytopenias prompting use of growth stimulating factors will necessitate a treatment break from chemotherapy and radiation. We typically resume radiation at the conclusion of growth factor administration.

Late side effects can be more difficult to manage and may offer chronic morbidity. Rectal bleeding may occur as a result of telangiectasias. This should be evaluated with endoscopic exam and may be managed with sulfasalazine or in severe cases, argon laser coagulation. Treatment may also worsen anorectal function and fecal continence, which may be addressed conservatively with dietary modification, bulking agents, and pelvic floor exercises, or in severe cases prompt attempted surgical sphincter repair or palliative colostomy.

We offer female patients receiving pelvic radiotherapy a vaginal dilator at the end of treatment to prevent vaginal stenosis. Topical estrogen may also be useful in treating both vaginal stenosis and dryness. In men who develop new or worsening erectile dysfunction, we offer oral phosphodiesterase inhibitors. Given the increased risk of insufficiency fractures following pelvic radiation, postmenopausal females in particular should be counseled on vitamin D and calcium supplementation.

SURVEILLANCE

The National Comprehensive Cancer Network has established guidelines for follow-up and surveillance of anal SCC (43). Visual and digital rectal exam are recommended 8 to 12 weeks following definitive treatment. For patients who have a complete clinical response, DRE and inguinal nodal palpation are recommended every 3 to 6 months for 5 years, anoscopy every 6 to 12 months for 3 years, and CT chest, abdomen, and pelvis with contrast annually for 3 years for T3–T4 or node-positive disease. Though not part of the guidelines, we typically obtain PET/CT 3 months following treatment as complete metabolic response is predictive of improved cancer-specific survival (44). For patients with stable or partial response on initial assessment, the recommendation is to continue with clinical assessments for up to 26 weeks. This is based on post hoc analysis of the ACT II trial, which called for assessments at 11, 18, and 26 weeks posttreatment (45). It was observed that 64% of patients had complete response at the 11-week assessment, but with further follow-up 85% eventually demonstrated a complete response by 26-week assessment. Development of complete clinical response by final assessment was a predictor of survival. Biopsies are not recommended prior to 6 months except in patients for whom there is concern of progressive disease, as this may increase the risk of developing radiation necrosis.

Patients who develop progressive local disease following initial definitive chemo-RT should be considered for surgical resection if disease remains limited. Complete restaging scans with PET/CT and MRI should be used to determine the extent of disease and suitability for resection (APR vs. pelvic exenteration). Following surgical salvage, reported 5-year OS ranges ~50% to 60% (46–48). For patients who are not surgical candidates or for whom an R0 resection may be difficult to obtain, accelerated hyperfractionated reirradiation to 39 Gy in 1.5 Gy fractions given twice daily has been reported for both anal and rectal cancer patients with acceptable toxicity risk (49,50).

CONCLUSION

Diagnosis and treatment of anal carcinomas requires multidisciplinary input from colorectal surgeons, medical oncologists, and radiation oncologists. Histology and stage of the tumor directs management, with the majority of anal SCC responding to sphincter-preservation therapy with definitive chemo-RT. Anal adenocarcinoma is less responsive to chemo-RT, so patients should undergo definitive surgical resection +/– neoadjuvant chemo-RT similar to a distal rectal cancer. Anal melanoma is very rare and carries a high risk for distant metastases, so WLE with negative margins is the preferred surgical approach with consideration of adjuvant systemic therapy based on molecular testing. Management of acute toxicity during definitive chemo-RT is important to reduce treatment breaks. Surveillance following standard guidelines is imperative since early locoregional recurrences may undergo surgical salvage.

Clinical Vignette 49.1

Case 1: Anal Margin Squamous Cell Carcinoma. *A 47-year-old female with a history of HPV infection and vulvar/perianal squamous dysplasia presents with pain and pruritus involving a 1.5 cm ulcerated lesion with red borders approximately 2 cm distal to the anal verge along the anal margin. Punch biopsy reveals invasive well-differentiated squamous cell carcinoma.*

Case 2: Anal Canal Squamous Cell Carcinoma. *A 51-year-old female underwent screening colonoscopy and was found to have a 3.5 cm hemicircumferential lesion in the anal canal at 0 cm to 3.5 cm from the verge just distal to the dentate line. Biopsy revealed moderately differentiated squamous cell carcinoma. Inguinal nodal exam was significant for a right-sided 2 cm firm node. PET/CT was obtained and revealed uptake in the primary anal canal lesion as well as bilateral inguinal nodes, the largest measuring 2.0 cm. Fine-needle aspiration of the right inguinal node was positive for malignant cells.*

Case 3: Anal Cancer and HIV. *A 42-year-old male with a history of HIV infection and prior excision of perianal condyloma presents with a 6 cm ulcerated, fungating mass extending from the anal verge. He has palpable bilateral inguinal adenopathy. His CD4 count is 74. Upon further questioning, he has not been taking his prescribed antiretroviral medications.*

Case 4: Anal Adenocarcinoma. *A 61-year-old male was referred to a gastroenterologist after presenting with a 6-month history of anorectal pain, bleeding, and decreased stool caliber. Colonoscopy was notable for a 3 cm raised friable mass in the anal canal. Biopsy revealed moderately differentiated adenocarcinoma.*

Case 5: Anal Melanoma. *A 67-year-old Caucasian female presents to a colorectal surgeon for progressive discomfort and pruritus of a presumed hemorrhoid refractory to medical management. On exam, she has an ulcerated, hyperemic lesion involving the anal verge. Biopsy reveals mucosal melanoma with the presence of melanocytes.*

REFERENCES

1. Siegel RL, Miller KD, Jemal A. Cancer statistics, 2018. *CA Cancer J Clin*. 2018;68(1):7–30. doi:10.3322/caac.21442
2. National Cancer Institute. Anal Cancer - Cancer Stat Facts. 2018; https://seer.cancer.gov/statfacts/html/anus.html
3. Daling JR, Madeleine MM, Johnson LG, et al. Human papillomavirus, smoking, and sexual practices in the etiology of anal cancer. *Cancer*. 2004;101(2):270–280. doi:10.1002/cncr.20365
4. Silverberg MJ, Lau B, Justice AC, et al. Risk of anal cancer in HIV-infected and HIV-uninfected individuals in North America. *Clin Infect Dis*. 2012;54(7):1026–1034. doi:10.1093/cid/cir1012
5. Coghill AE, Shiels MS, Suneja G, et al. Elevated cancer-specific mortality among HIV-infected patients in the United States. *J Clin Oncol*. 2015;33(21):2376–2383. doi:10.1200/JCO.2014.59.5967
6. Patel HS, Silver ARJ, Northover JMA. Anal cancer in renal transplant patients. *Int J Colorectal Dis*. 2006;22(1):1–5. doi:10.1007/s00384-005-0023-3
7. International Collaboration of Epidemiological Studies of Cervical Cancer, Appleby P, Beral V, et al. Carcinoma of the cervix and tobacco smoking: collaborative reanalysis of individual data on 13,541 women with carcinoma of the cervix and 23,017 women without carcinoma of the cervix from 23 epidemiological studies. *Int J Cancer*. 2006;118(6):1481–1495. doi:10.1002/ijc.21493
8. Xi LF, Koutsky LA, Castle PE, et al. Relationship between cigarette smoking and human papilloma virus types 16 and 18 DNA load. *Cancer Epidemiol Biomarkers Prev*. 2009;18(12):3490–3496. doi:10.1158/1055-9965.EPI-09-0763
9. Haverkos HW, Haverkos GP, O'Mara M. Co-carcinogenesis: human papillomaviruses, coal tar derivatives, and squamous cell cervical cancer. *Front Microbiol*. 2017;8:2253. doi:10.3389/fmicb.2017.02253
10. Shiels MS, Kreimer AR, Coghill AE, et al. Anal cancer incidence in the United States, 1977-2011: distinct patterns by histology and behavior. *Cancer Epidemiol Biomarkers Prev*. 2015;24(10):1548–1556. doi:10.1158/1055-9965.EPI-15-0044
11. Shiels MS, Pfeiffer RM, Chaturvedi AK, et al. Impact of the HIV epidemic on the incidence rates of anal cancer in the United States. *J Natl Cancer Inst*. 2012;104(20):1591–1598. doi:10.1093/jnci/djs371
12. Amin MB, Edge SB, American Joint Committee on Cancer. *AJCC Cancer Staging Manual*. 2018; https://www.springer.com/us/book/9783319406176
13. Pintor MP, Northover JM, Nicholls RJ. Squamous cell carcinoma of the anus at one hospital from 1948 to 1984. *Br J Surg*. 1989;76(8):806–810. http://www.ncbi.nlm.nih.gov/pubmed/2765832

14. Brown DK, Oglesby AB, Scott DH, et al. Squamous cell carcinoma of the anus: a twenty-five year retrospective. *Am Surg*. 1988;54(6):337–342. http://www.ncbi.nlm.nih.gov/pubmed/2454044

15. Nigro ND, Vaitkevicius VK, Considine B. Combined therapy for cancer of the anal canal: a preliminary report. *Dis Colon Rectum*. 1974;17(3):354–356. http://www.ncbi.nlm.nih.gov/pubmed/4830803

16. Nigro ND, Seydel HG, Considine B, et al. Combined preoperative radiation and chemotherapy for squamous cell carcinoma of the anal canal. *Cancer*. 1983;51(10):1826–1829. http://www.ncbi.nlm.nih.gov/pubmed/6831348

17. Leichman L, Nigro N, Vaitkevicius VK, et al. Cancer of the anal canal. Model for preoperative adjuvant combined modality therapy. *Am J Med*. 1985;78(2):211–215. http://www.ncbi.nlm.nih.gov/pubmed/3918441

18. Greenall MJ, Quan SH, Stearns MW, et al. Epidermoid cancer of the anal margin. Pathologic features, treatment, and clinical results. *Am J Surg*. 1985;149(1):95–101. http://www.ncbi.nlm.nih.gov/pubmed/3966647

19. Steele SR, Varma MG, Melton GB, et al. Practice parameters for anal squamous neoplasms. *Dis Colon Rectum*. 2012;55(7):735–749. doi:10.1097/DCR.0b013e318255815e

20. Northover JMA, Arnott SJ, Cunningham D, et al. Epidermoid anal cancer: results from the UKCCCR randomised trial of radiotherapy alone versus radiotherapy, 5-fluorouracil, and mitomycin. *Lancet*. 1996;348(9034):1049–1054. doi:10.1016/S0140-6736(96)03409-5

21. Northover J, Glynne-Jones R, Sebag-Montefiore D, et al. Chemoradiation for the treatment of epidermoid anal cancer: 13-year follow-up of the first randomised UKCCCR Anal Cancer Trial (ACT I). *Br J Cancer*. 2010;102(7):1123–1128. doi:10.1038/sj.bjc.6605605

22. Bartelink H, Roelofsen F, Eschwege F, et al. Concomitant radiotherapy and chemotherapy is superior to radiotherapy alone in the treatment of locally advanced anal cancer: results of a phase III randomized trial of the European Organization for Research and Treatment of Cancer Radiotherapy and Gastrointestinal Cooperative Groups. *J Clin Oncol*. 1997;15(5):2040–2049.

23. Flam M, John M, Pajak TF, et al. Role of mitomycin in combination with fluorouracil and radiotherapy, and of salvage chemoradiation in the definitive nonsurgical treatment of epidermoid carcinoma of the anal canal: results of a phase III randomized intergroup study. *J Clin Oncol*. 1996;14(9):2527–2539. doi:10.1200/JCO.1996.14.9.2527

24. Ajani JA. Fluorouracil, mitomycin, and radiotherapy vs fluorouracil, cisplatin, and radiotherapy for carcinoma of the anal canal. *JAMA*. 2008;299(16):1914. doi:10.1001/jama.299.16.1914

25. Gunderson LL, Winter KA, Ajani JA, et al. Long-term update of US GI intergroup RTOG 98-11 Phase III trial for anal carcinoma: survival, relapse, and colostomy failure with concurrent chemoradiation involving fluorouracil/mitomycin versus fluorouracil/cisplatin. *J Clin Oncol*. 2012;30(35):4344–4351. doi:10.1200/JCO.2012.43.8085

26. James RD, Glynne-Jones R, Meadows HM, et al. Mitomycin or cisplatin chemoradiation with or without maintenance chemotherapy for treatment of squamous-cell carcinoma of the anus (ACT II): a randomised, phase 3, open-label, 2×2 factorial trial. *Lancet Oncol*. 2013;14(6):516–524. doi:10.1016/S1470-2045(13)70086-X

27. Kachnic LA, Winter K, Myerson RJ, et al. RTOG 0529: a phase 2 evaluation of dose-painted intensity modulated radiation therapy in combination with 5-fluorouracil and mitomycin-C for the reduction of acute morbidity in carcinoma of the anal canal. *Int J Radiat Oncol Biol Phys*. 2013;86(1):27–33. doi:10.1016/j.ijrobp.2012.09.023

28. Myerson RJ, Garofalo MC, El Naqa I, et al. Elective clinical target volumes for conformal therapy in anorectal cancer: a Radiation Therapy Oncology Group consensus panel contouring atlas. *Int J Radiat Oncol*. 2009;74(3):824–830. doi:10.1016/j.ijrobp.2008.08.070

29. Ng M, Leong T, Chander S, et al. Australasian Gastrointestinal Trials Group (AGITG) contouring atlas and planning guidelines for intensity-modulated radiotherapy in anal cancer. *Int J Radiat Oncol*. 2012;83(5):1455–1462. doi:10.1016/j.ijrobp.2011.12.058

30. Bunn PA, Crowley J, Kelly K, et al. Chemoradiotherapy with or without granulocyte-macrophage colony-stimulating factor in the treatment of limited-stage small-cell lung cancer: a prospective phase III randomized study of the Southwest Oncology Group. *J Clin Oncol*. 1995;13(7):1632–1641. doi:10.1200/JCO.1995.13.7.1632

31. Nelson RA, Levine AM, Bernstein L, et al. Changing patterns of anal canal carcinoma in the United States. *J Clin Oncol*. 2013;31(12):1569–1575. doi:10.1200/JCO.2012.45.2524

32. Franklin RA, Giri S, Valasareddy P, et al. Comparative survival of patients with anal adenocarcinoma, squamous cell carcinoma of the anus, and rectal adenocarcinoma. *Clin Colorectal Cancer*. 2016;15(1):47–53. doi:10.1016/j.clcc.2015.07.007

33. Kounalakis N, Artinyan A, Smith D, et al. Abdominal perineal resection improves survival for nonmetastatic adenocarcinoma of the anal canal. *Ann Surg Oncol*. 2009;16(5):1310–1315. doi:10.1245/s10434-009-0392-x

34. Sauer R, Becker H, Hohenberger W, et al. Preoperative versus postoperative chemoradiotherapy for rectal cancer. *N Engl J Med*. 2004;351(17):1731–1740. doi:10.1056/NEJMoa040694

35. Sauer R, Liersch T, Merkel S, et al. Preoperative versus postoperative chemoradiotherapy for locally advanced rectal cancer: results of the German CAO/ARO/AIO-94 randomized phase III trial after a median follow-up of 11 years. *J Clin Oncol*. 2012;30(16):1926–1933. doi:10.1200/JCO.2011.40.1836

36. Chen H, Cai Y, Liu Y, et al. Incidence, Surgical Treatment, and Prognosis of Anorectal Melanoma From 1973 to 2011: A Population-Based SEER Analysis. *Medicine (Baltimore)*. 2016;95(7):e2770. doi:10.1097/MD.0000000000002770

37. Kiran RP, Rottoli M, Pokala N, et al. Long-term outcomes after local excision and radical surgery for anal melanoma: data from a population database. *Dis Colon Rectum*. 2010;53(4):402–408. doi:10.1007/DCR.0b013e3181b71228

38. Matsuda A, Miyashita M, Matsumoto S, et al. Abdominoperineal resection provides better local control but equivalent overall survival to local excision of anorectal malignant melanoma: a systematic review. *Ann Surg*. 2015;261(4):670–677. doi:10.1097/SLA.0000000000000862

39. Nilsson PJ, Ragnarsson-Olding BK. Importance of clear resection margins in anorectal malignant melanoma. *Br J Surg*. 2010;97(1):98–103. doi:10.1002/bjs.6784

40. Kelly P, Zagars GK, Cormier JN, et al. Sphincter-sparing local excision and hypofractionated radiation therapy for anorectal melanoma: a 20-year experience. *Cancer*. 2011;117(20):4747–4755. doi:10.1002/cncr.26088

41. Heppt MV, Roesch A, Weide B, et al. Prognostic factors and treatment outcomes in 444 patients with mucosal melanoma. *Eur J Cancer*. 2017;81:36-44. doi:10.1016/j.ejca.2017.05.014

42. Santi R, Simi L, Fucci R, et al. KIT genetic alterations in anorectal melanomas. *J Clin Pathol*. 2015;68(2):130–134. doi:10.1136/jclinpath-2014-202572

43. Deborah Freedman-Cass N, Gregory KM, Al Benson OB, et al. NCCN Guidelines Version 1.2018 Anal Carcinoma. 2018; https://www.nccn.org/professionals/physician_gls/pdf/anal.pdf

44. Schwarz JK, Siegel BA, Dehdashti F, et al. Tumor response and survival predicted by post-therapy FDG-PET/CT in anal cancer. *Int J Radiat Oncol*. 2008;71(1):180–186. doi:10.1016/j.ijrobp.2007.09.005

45. Glynne-Jones R, Sebag-Montefiore D, Meadows HM, et al. Best time to assess complete clinical response after chemoradiotherapy in squamous cell carcinoma of the anus (ACT II): a post-hoc analysis of randomised controlled phase 3 trial. *Lancet Oncol*. 2017;18(3):347–356. doi:10.1016/S1470-2045(17)30071-2

46. Mariani P, Ghanneme A, De la Rochefordière A, et al. Abdominoperineal resection for anal cancer. *Dis Colon Rectum*. 2008;51(10):1495–1501. doi:10.1007/s10350-008-9361-x

47. Lefèvre JH, Corte H, Tiret E, et al. Abdominoperineal resection for squamous cell anal carcinoma: survival and risk factors for recurrence. *Ann Surg Oncol*. 2012;19(13):4186–4192. doi:10.1245/s10434-012-2485-1

48. Guerra GR, Kong JC, Bernardi M-P, et al. Salvage surgery for locoregional failure in anal squamous cell carcinoma. *Dis Colon Rectum*. 2018;61(2):179–186. doi:10.1097/DCR.0000000000001010

49. Osborne EM, Eng C, Skibber JM, et al. Hyperfractionated accelerated reirradiation for patients with recurrent anal cancer previously treated with definitive chemoradiation. *Am J Clin Oncol*. 2018;41(7):632–637. doi:10.1097/COC.0000000000000338

50. Tao R, Tsai CJ, Jensen G, et al. Hyperfractionated accelerated reirradiation for rectal cancer: an analysis of outcomes and toxicity. *Radiother Oncol*. 2017;122(1):146–151. doi:10.1016/J.RADONC.2016.12.015

Metastatic Anal Cancer

Saivaishnavi Kamatham, Faisal Shahjehan, and Pashtoon M. Kasi

INTRODUCTION

Anal cancer comprises about 2.7% of all gastrointestinal cancers in the United States (1). Its incidence, however, has been increasing over the past few decades. According to American Cancer Society, the expected number of new anal cancer cases and deaths in 2018 are estimated to be 8,580 and 1,160, respectively (1). According to Surveillance, Epidemiology, and End Results (SEER 18 2008–2014), 13% of patients have metastatic anal cancer at diagnosis with a 5-year survival rate of 29.8% (2). While definitive chemoradiation offers curative intent therapy for most including those that can be salvaged with surgery for residual disease, a proportion of these individuals later develop metastatic disease. Treatment in these situations revolves around systemic therapy and is usually palliative in intent. Here we review the current standards of care and recent developments in the management of metastatic anal cancer.

As noted earlier, the predominant histology and the discussion here for anal cancer is for squamous cell carcinomas (3). They are associated with human papillomavirus (HPV) in 65% to 89% of cases, with the viral type HPV-16 being the most frequently detected, followed by HPV-18 (4). Given the risk factors including the number of lifetime sexual partners, sexual behavior, homosexuality, smoking, race, and age, it is important to test for coexisting HIV infection.

Anal cancers often have a delayed diagnosis or misdiagnosis because of the symptoms with which they present, including bleeding from the anus, mass at anal opening, and change in bowel habits, being mistaken for other diagnoses (e.g., hemorrhoids). The most common sites of metastasis from anal cancer include lungs, liver, and bones. Patients who develop distant metastasis are staged M1 according to the tumor, node, and metastasis (TNM) staging system, irrespective of the tumor size. Metastatic anal cancers fall under overall stage IV of American Joint Committee on Cancer (AJCC) staging (version 7). An important distinction of advanced versus metastatic disease when it comes to anal cancer with respect to nodal spread is the fact that unilateral and/or bilateral metastases to inguinal and/or internal iliac lymph nodes are considered N2 or N3 disease and not M1.

TREATMENT OF METASTATIC ANAL CANCER

Treatment for metastatic anal cancer revolves around systemic therapy and includes the following two classes of drugs:

- Chemotherapy
- Immunotherapy

Radiation is often employed up front or later in the disease course to primary and/or metastatic sites of disease if they are symptomatic. Otherwise systemic chemotherapy or immunotherapy is the mainstay of management of patients with metastatic anal cancer. Here we outline the commonly used and recommended regimens including recent updates.

Chemotherapy

Chemotherapy has been the main first-line treatment modality for metastatic anal cancer. The current National Comprehensive Cancer Network (NCCN) guidelines version 2.2018 includes various chemotherapy combination regimens as the mainstay for frontline and/or later treatment for patients with metastatic anal cancer. Simplistically, these drugs fall into three main classes (Table 50.1):

TABLE 50.1 Systemic Therapy for Metastatic Anal Cancer

First-Line Therapy	Platinum Drugs	Taxanes	Fluoropyrimidines	Immunotherapy
Carboplatin/Paclitaxel (preferred)*	Carboplatin	Paclitaxel		
5-FU/Cisplatin	Cisplatin		5-Fluorouracil	
mFOLFOX6	Oxaliplatin		5-Fluorouracil	
Modified DCF regimen[†] vs. DCF regimen	Cisplatin	Docetaxel	5-Fluorouracil	
Taxanes as monotherapy		Paclitaxel		
Second-line therapy				
Immunotherapy: immune checkpoint inhibitors (anti-PD1 drugs)				Nivolumab or pembrolizumab
Chemotherapy options	Chemotherapy options second line or later depend on what drugs and/or combinations were used earlier *(Clinical trials are always preferable regardless of the line of therapy)*			

*A recent trial using carboplatin and paclitaxel reported at the European Society for Medical Oncology (ESMO) 2018 meeting employed carboplatin at an AUC of 5 and paclitaxel weekly. This is based on extrapolation on the dose-dense regimens employed for ovarian cancer. However, both iterations (weekly or every 3-week regimens) are acceptable. The latter is often helpful for patients who have to travel a distance to go to their cancer center for treatment.

[†]Modified DCF is preferred over the historical DCF regimen due to better tolerability (see section on triplet regimens of chemotherapy in this chapter for dosing and details).

5-FU, 5-fluorouracil; DCF, docetaxel, cisplatin, and 5-FU.

1. Fluoropyrimidines (5-fluorouracil [5-FU], capecitabine)]
2. Platinum drugs (cisplatin, carboplatin, oxaliplatin)
3. Taxanes (paclitaxel, docetaxel)

The significance of chemotherapy and multidisciplinary management in metastatic anal cancer has been well-documented by Eng et al. Of the 77 patients included in the study, 42 received 5-FU + cisplatin; 24 patients received carboplatin and paclitaxel; 11 received an alternative regimen. All the patients had a median progression-free survival (PFS) of 7 months and a median overall survival (OS) of 22 months. Multidisciplinary treatment for 33 patients resulted in a median PFS of 16 months and a median OS of 53 months (5).

FLUOROPYRIMIDINE AND PLATINUM DRUG REGIMENS

Doublet Regimens

Treatment with **5-FU and cisplatin** as a combination therapy has been a well-documented treatment for metastatic anal cancer as evident from several studies (6–8). Common adverse drug reactions (ADRs) with this regimen include nausea, vomiting, anorexia, mucositis, and myelosuppression. Specific to the platinum part of chemotherapy are peripheral neuropathy, kidney injury (acute and cumulative from), hearing loss, and tinnitus due to damage to the cochlear hair cells. Different dosing recommendations and iterations exist for every 3- versus every 4-week regimen (9). Some institutions have biweekly regimens as well.

Similar to colorectal cancer, oxaliplatin is often utilized by institutions as the platinum chemotherapy backbone, every 2 weeks for better tolerability. Typically this is in the form of **mFOLFOX6** (10). Feasibility of capecitabine as an oral drug alternative to the intravenous (IV) 5-FU chemotherapy has been shown in different studies (both in combination with oxaliplatin and cisplatin). It has not been widely adopted due to relatively increased toxicity. However, since its increasing use in colorectal cancer recently, it is an option to consider in patients deemed candidates for such an approach.

Treatment with fluoropyrimidine/platinum based therapy as the first line was considered pretty much the standard of care till recently. At the European Society for Medical Oncology (ESMO) 2018 meeting, Eng and colleagues reported the results of a randomized trial comparing 5-FU/cisplatin based therapy with carboplatin/paclitaxel (Table 50.1) (11). The latter showed better tolerability as well as efficacy and represents the new standard for first-line therapy; see details in the Taxanes section—"InterAACT" Study: An international multicenter open label randomized phase II advanced anal cancer trial comparing cisplatin (CDDP) plus 5-fluorouracil (5-FU) versus carboplatin (CBDCA) plus weekly paclitaxel (PTX) in patients with inoperable locally recurrent (ILR) or metastatic disease (11).

Triplet Regimens

Triplet chemotherapies, for example, the DCF regimen (docetaxel, cisplatin, and 5-FU), have not been employed due to greater toxicity (Table 50.1). However, the French group in July 2018 reported in *Lancet Oncology* the results of a modified DCF regimen with different dosing and a biweekly rather than every 3-week approach that had manageable toxicity profile [details noted in the Taxanes section (12)]. What was really exciting was the number of individuals who had complete as well as partial responses that were deep as well as durable. In a person with good performance status and/or where response may be a goal, the modified DCF represents yet another treatment option.

TAXANES

Monotherapy

According to a case series by Abbas et al., seven patients with metastatic or recurrent anal cancer who had progressive disease after 5-FU and cisplatin therapy were treated with **paclitaxel monotherapy** weekly. Four of the seven patients had a radiographic objective response and one had stabilization of the disease. A 12- to 14-month improvement in OS was noted (13). Common adverse events with paclitaxel therapy include low blood counts, hair loss, arthralgias, myalgias, and peripheral neuropathy. This may be a consideration who may not tolerate doublet or triplet regimens. It also depends on what the patients received earlier (Table 50.1).

Doublet Regimens

Kim et al. conducted a study in which 12 patients with metastatic squamous cell anal cancer received **carboplatin plus paclitaxel** as first-line treatment. They documented a response rate of 53% and a median OS of 12.19 months (14). Current NCCN guidelines version 2.2018 recommend administering carboplatin AUC 5 IV and paclitaxel 175 mg/m^2 IV on day 1 and repeating the regimen every 21 days (9).

InterAACT, an open-label, multicenter, randomized phase II **International Rare Cancers Initiative (IRCI) trial**, was conducted to compare the efficacy of carboplatin plus weekly paclitaxel versus 5-FU plus cisplatin. The study included inoperable locally recurrent or metastatic anal cancer (n = 91) from four countries including the United Kingdom, Norway, United States, and Australia. The results showed that the response rates in the carboplatin/paclitaxel arm and 5-FU/cisplatin arm were 59% and 57.1%, respectively (11). It was also found that patients who received carboplatin plus paclitaxel had favorably longer median OS (20 months) compared to those who received 5-FU plus cisplatin (12.3 months). Furthermore, the carboplatin plus paclitaxel regimen had a better toxicity profile. Grade ≥3 toxicity was reported in 71% patients on carboplatin/paclitaxel and 76% patients on 5-FU plus cisplatin. Also, serious adverse events (SAEs) were noted in only 36% of patients on carboplatin/paclitaxel compared to 62% of patients on 5-FU/cisplatin (11). It was presented at the ESMO Congress 2018 asserting that the carboplatin plus paclitaxel combination is more effective and better tolerated than the 5-FU and cisplatin regimen, recommending **carboplatin plus paclitaxel as first-line therapy for advanced/metastatic anal cancer**. This represents a recent new change in the standard of care moving forward. As noted earlier, every 3-week paclitaxel dosing may also be employed for practical considerations.

Triplet Regimens

Triplet chemotherapies in general are not utilized frequently and have not been adopted due to toxicity concerns.

Previously, a phase II trial conducted by Hainsworth et al. evaluated the efficacy of combination therapy with paclitaxel, carboplatin, and long-term 5-FU infusion. While it did demonstrate a significant overall response rate of 90%, grade 3 and/or 4 adverse events were seen often including leukopenia, mucositis, and portacath-related events (15).

More recently as noted earlier (Table 50.1), Kim et al. reported the results of a phase 2, multicenter clinical trial, NCT02402842, to demonstrate the effects of DCF chemotherapy for patients with metastatic or unresectable locally recurrent anal cancer. Of the 66 patients, 36 received the standard DCF regimen and 30 received dose modified DCF regimen (12). While again grade 3 and/or 4 events were seen (neutropenia, diarrhea, asthenia, anemia, lymphopenia, vomiting, and mucositis), they were seen less frequently and manageable with the modified DCF regimen (docetaxel 40 mg/m^2 and cisplatin 40 mg/m^2 on day 1 and fluorouracil 2,400 mg/m^2 per day over 46 hours biweekly). What was really impressive was the number of patients who had complete or partial responses (44% complete responses; 86% overall responses) (12). While doublet chemotherapy regimens are the standard of care, the modified version of the triplet DCF chemotherapy (every 2-week dosing) represents yet another option to consider in the patients who have good performance status and/or where response is a key variable.

Other Historical Regimens

The efficacy of the TIP regimen (Taxol, ifosfamide, and platinum) in recurrent, metastatic anal cancer was studied by Golub et al. They administered TIP chemotherapy to three patients who developed recurrent disease with chemoradiotherapy with 5-FU and cisplatin and analyzed the treatment outcomes, which showed complete remission per CT/PET after three to four cycles according to Response Evaluation Criteria in Solid Tumors (RECIST). Toxicities included alopecia, anemia, thrombocytopenia, and peripheral neuropathy (16).

Jhawer et al. conducted a study on 20 patients with advanced anal cancer who were not responsive to radiotherapy or surgery. They were administered mitomycin C, Adriamycin, and cisplatin (MAP) followed by bleomycin–CCNU and demonstrated a partial response rate of 60% and a median survival of 15 months. Moderate toxicities of vomiting, respiratory distress, leg cramps, and hematological adverse events were noted (17).

These regimens, however, are no longer employed since there are more tolerable regimens with similar if not better efficacy.

IMMUNOTHERAPY (IMMUNE CHECKPOINT INHIBITORS—ANTI-PD1 DRUGS)

Immunotherapy as treatment for patients with metastatic anal cancer is in the refractory setting with immune checkpoint inhibitors. These are the antiprogrammed cell death-1 (anti-PD1) antibodies: nivolumab and pembrolizumab. With immunotherapy showing excellent and promising results in other solid tumor types, the initial enthusiasm for immunotherapy given the viral basis and/or association with immunosuppression was very high. While activity was seen as noted in the following and it has been recommended for use in the refractory setting (Table 50.1), it was not as effective and/or durable as initially thought of.

Nivolumab

The first phase II trial, NCI9673, to validate the effectiveness of immunotherapy for metastatic anal cancer patients was done by Morris et al. through the National Cancer Institute Experimental Therapeutics Clinical Trials Network (ETCTN) at 10 centers in the United States. It was a single-arm trial to determine the efficacy of nivolumab, an anti-PD1 monoclonal antibody in patients with progressive, metastatic/advanced, histologically confirmed squamous cell anal cancer. Nivolumab at a dose of 3 mg/kg was administered intravenously every 2 weeks. Thirty-seven patients received a median of six doses of nivolumab and were followed up for median 10.1 months. They reported that single-drug therapy with nivolumab in metastatic anal cancer patients resulted in an objective response rate (partial or complete radiographic response as per RECIST 1.1) of 24% and a disease control rate of 72%. The median PFS was 4.1 months, 6-month PFS of 38%, median OS of 11.5 months, and 1-year OS of 48%. The most common ADRs with nivolumab were anemia (70%), fatigue (68%), and rash (30%) as summarized in Table 50.2 (18). The guidelines and the current recommended dosing is the fixed dose of 240 mg every 2 weeks or 3 mg/kg every 2 weeks (9).

Pembrolizumab

Similarly, Otta et al. conducted the KEYNOTE-028 study, which was a multicenter, multicohort, phase Ib trial to demonstrate the safety and efficacy of pembrolizumab, humanized anti-PD1 antibody in patients with programmed death ligand-1 (PD-L1) positive (greater than or equal to 1%—22C3 prototype assay) advanced solid tumors (Table 50.2). The anal cancer cohort comprised patients with programmed death ligand-1 (PDL-1) positive advanced anal cancer from Europe and the United States. They were administered 10 mg/kg of pembrolizumab intravenously every 2 weeks. They received treatment for a median duration of 92 days (1–449 days) and were followed for a median duration of 10.6 months (0.3–15 months). Immune-related adverse events (e.g., hypothyroidism) were seen at similar frequencies as reported previously in other tumor types and were manageable. The antitumor activity was explained by the overall response rate of 17% and stable disease in 42% of patients with a median duration of 3.6 months. Median and 1-year OS were similar to the other study (9.3 months and 47.6%, respectively) (19). The current recommend dosing of pembrolizumab is a fixed dose of 200 mg every 3 weeks or 2 mg/kg every 3 weeks instead of the study dosing (9).

ONGOING AND FUTURE TRIALS

While anti-PD1 based immune checkpoint inhibitors did not show as much activity as initially anticipated, current and future trials are exploring immunotherapy combinations (e.g., anti-PD + anti-CTLA4), chemo + immunotherapy combinations, and/or immune adjuncts (e.g., vaccine-based approaches). Given the recent advances and continued interest of immunotherapy for patients with metastatic anal cancer, **treatment of these patients ideally should be on a**

TABLE 50.2 Summary of Studies Utilizing Antiprogrammed Cell Death (Anti-PD1) Immune Checkpoint Inhibitors

Study	Immunotherapy (Anti-PD1)	Outcomes	Comments/AEs
Morris et al. (NCI9673) (18) N = 37	Nivolumab	• Objective response rate (partial or complete radiographic response as per RECIST 1.1): 24% • Disease control rate: 72% • Median PFS time: 4.1 months • 6-month PFS: 38% • Median OS: 11.5 months • 1-year OS: 48%	No serious AEs reported. Grade 3 anemia was seen in 2 patients; rash (n = 1), hypothyroidism (n = 1), and fatigue (n = 1) were the other side effects seen
Otta et al. (KEYNOTE-028 study) (19) N = initial 43; 32 (74%) had PD-L1 positive tumors 24 patients with anal squamous cell cancer histology	Pembrolizumab; criteria: PD-L1 positive tumors ≥1%	• Overall response rate: 17% • Stable disease in 42% of patients • Disease control rate 58% • 6- and 12-month PFS rates of 31.6% and 19.7%, respectively • Median OS of 9.3 months • 6- and 12-month OS rates of 64.5% and 47.6%, respectively	Grade 3 AEs similar and manageable

AE, adverse event; OS, overall survival; PFS, progression-free survival; RECIST, Response Evaluation Criteria in Solid Tumors.

clinical trial. Given anal cancers are relatively rare, accrual to these trials is even more important. Some examples include:

- **NCT02314169**—ongoing, multi-institutional, phase 2 study of **nivolumab** or nivolumab
  in combination with **ipilimumab** in refractory metastatic squamous cell carcinoma of the
  anal canal. Nivolumab is administered once every 4 weeks and ipilimumab once every
  8 weeks. Outcomes of the trial are PFS as the primary outcome and OS alongside incidence of SAEs as secondary outcomes (20).
- **NCT02919969**—multicenter, phase II clinical trial to study the safety and efficacy of **pembrolizumab** in patients with refractory metastatic anal cancer with 200 mg of pembrolizumab administered as 30-minute IV infusion every 3 weeks. Overall response rate is the
  primary outcome, and PD-L1 positive response rate, OS, PFS, and incidence of SAEs are
  secondary outcomes (21).
- **NCT03519295**—**SCARCE study** is a randomized 2:1 phase II study to assess long-term
  PFS of chemotherapy + immunotherapy (**docetaxel, cisplatin, and 5-FU** in combination
  with **atezolizumab**) in patients with metastatic or unresectable locally advanced squamous cell anal carcinoma (22).

OTHER THERAPIES/TRIALS

- **Anti–epidermal growth factor receptor (anti-EGFR) drugs**

In a study by Rogers et al., anti-EGFR drugs like cetuximab or panitumumab when combined
with chemotherapy in 17 patients with metastatic anal cancer resulted in a response in 35%
of the patients and stable disease in 24%. They also reported 7.3 months of PFS and 24.7
months of OS in these patients (23).

- **T-cell receptor (TCR) gene therapy/tumor-infiltrating lymphocyte (TIL) therapy**

Draper et al. studied TIL cultures from a metastatic anal cancer patient with HLA*02:01, who
had a prolonged disease-free interval after her second resection of distant metastases to the
portal lymph node. They found that the resected tumor harbored HPV-16 E6 T-cells and the
frequency was about 400 times greater in the tumor than in the peripheral blood. Furthermore,
the genetically engineered T-cells to express TCR from that tumor revealed specific recognition
of a panel of HPV-16+ tumors from cervical and head and neck cancers signifying that E6 TCR
possessed reactivity against the patient's tumor (24). This was followed by a phase I/II clinical
trial (NCT02280811) by Hinrichs et al. to determine the safety and efficacy of anti-HPV E6 T-cells
in shrinkage of HPV-16+ tumors, which included cervical, anal, oropharyngeal, and vaginal ori-
gins. E6 TCR T-cells up to doses of 2×10^{11} cells were administered. Two of the four patients
with anal cancer had partial tumor responses, which lasted for 6 and 3 months post treatment.
In the patient with a 6-month response, one tumor showed complete regression and two tumors
showed partial regression and were resected upon progression, with no evidence of disease
22 months after therapy. Effectiveness of TCR therapy was 45% to 51% in the responders and
revealed high levels of E6 TCR T-cell memory (30%–46% of circulating T-cells 1 month after
treatment) (25).

- **ADXS11-001 Listeria-based immunotherapy**

ADXS11-001 immunotherapy is a live attenuated, bioengineered Listeria monocytogenes that
produces tumor antigen specific T-cells against the E7 peptide of HPV-16. Eng et al. conducted
the first trial (NCT02399813) to assess the efficacy and safety of ADXS11-001 in metastatic anal
cancer. Patients with histologically confirmed squamous cell anal cancer who had advanced
disease with previous therapies were administered 1×10^9 colony forming units of ADXS as
monotherapy intravenously every 3 weeks for up to 2 years. Preliminary stage 1 results revealed
favorable outcomes with a disease control rate and a 6-month PFS rate of 28% and 22%
respectively. Adverse events were infusion related and were managed with supportive care (26).

Radiation
Radiation is often employed up front or later in the disease course to primary and/or metastatic
sites of disease if they are symptomatic (27). Outside of a clinical trial and/or for treating symptomatic disease, therapy for patients with metastatic anal cancer is usually with chemotherapy

and/or immunotherapy. For the ones who are truly oligometastatic, it is reasonable to consider radiation therapy to help consolidate response and local control, in addition to systemic chemotherapy.

TREATING PATIENTS WITH CONCURRENT HIV AND ANAL CANCER

The incidence of anal cancer among HIV infected patients has been increasing despite treatment with antiretroviral therapy (28). Also, several studies have documented that patients with HIV experience more severe adverse events and profound toxicities from chemotherapy and radiation therapy (29,30). Recommendations in general for treatment of cancers in patients with HIV do not necessarily recommend any dose modifications. The adverse events reported in some of these trials are similar. However, in practice, patients who are sick often do not necessarily qualify for some of these trials and side effects with chemotherapies are generally higher. Given the palliative intent of therapy in the metastatic setting, it is advisable to monitor closely and consider dose reductions where appropriate. The doses of chemotherapy and/or radiation in the metastatic setting may therefore be modified depending on the level of immune compromise (pretreatment CD4 counts), performance status, and presence of opportunistic infections in patients with HIV (31). Close ongoing follow-up with infectious disease for ongoing treatment of HIV is important. Drug–drug interactions are also important to consider with highly active antiretroviral therapy (HAART).

PROGNOSIS

The observed 5-year survival for patients with metastatic squamous cell anal cancer is 15% in accordance with data by the American Cancer Society. The prognosis has improved over the years because of the advancement in treatment strategies. However, in each individual, outcomes depend on several factors in addition to histology, severity/disease burden, and comorbid conditions including HIV, performance status, and overall general health of the individual. Other health-related disparities also play a role. It has been shown that socioeconomic status of patients does play a role in the prognosis of anal cancer patients. It might be related to lack of access to facility, delayed diagnosis, and poor education. A recent study conducted on squamous cell type anal cancer patients (n = 9,550) reported that patients belonging to lower median household income areas were associated with poor OS and cancer-specific survival compared to those belonging to high median household income areas (32). However, there were only 6.1% stage IV anal cancer patients in the aforementioned study and the majority were stage II and III anal cancer. Similarly, African Americans have worse survival compared to Caucasians (33). Coupled with advances in immunotherapy and novel clinical trials, these health-related disparities are important to consider as well.

REFERENCES

1. Siegel RL, Miller KD, Jemal A. Cancer statistics, 2018. *CA Cancer J Clin*. 2018;68(1):7–30. doi:10.3322/caac.21442
2. National Institutes of Health National Cancer Institute - Surveillance, Epidemiology, and End Results Program, Cancer Stat Facts: Anal Cancer. https://seer.cancer.gov/statfacts/html/anus.html
3. Flejou JF. An update on anal neoplasia. *Histopathology*. 2015;66(1):147–160. doi:10.1111/his.12574
4. Frisch M, Fenger C, van den Brule AJ, et al. Variants of squamous cell carcinoma of the anal canal and perianal skin and their relation to human papillomaviruses. *Cancer Res*. 1999;59(3):753–757.
5. Eng C, Chang GJ, You YN, et al. The role of systemic chemotherapy and multidisciplinary management in improving the overall survival of patients with metastatic squamous cell carcinoma of the anal canal. *Oncotarget*. 2014;5(22):11133–11142. doi:10.18632/oncotarget.2563
6. Tanum G. Treatment of relapsing anal carcinoma. *Acta Oncol*. 1993;32(1):33–35. doi:10.3109/02841869309083882
7. Faivre C, Rougier P, Ducreux M, et al. [5-fluorouracile and cisplatinum combination chemotherapy for metastatic squamous-cell anal cancer]. *Bull Cancer*. 1999;86(10):861–865.

8. Ajani JA, Carrasco CH, Jackson DE, et al. Combination of cisplatin plus fluoropyrimidine chemotherapy effective against liver metastases from carcinoma of the anal canal. *Am J Med*. 1989;87(2):221–224. doi:10.1016/S0002-9343(89)80702-8

9. National Comprehensive Cancer Network. *NCCN Guidelines Version 2.2018 Anal Carcinoma*. 2018.

10. Matsunaga M, Miwa K, Oka Y, et al. Successful treatment of metastatic anal canal adenocarcinoma with mFOLFOX6 + Bevacizumab. *Case Rep Oncol*. 2016;9(1):249–254. doi:10.1159/000446107

11. ESMO, European Society For Medical Oncology. Carboplatin Plus Paclitaxel Represents a New Standard of Care for Patients with Squamous Cell Carcinoma of the Anal Canal. 2018; https://www.esmo.org/Oncology-News/InterAACT-inoperable-locally-recurrent-metastatic-anal-cancer-Rao

12. Kim S, François E, André T, et al. Docetaxel, cisplatin, and fluorouracil chemotherapy for metastatic or unresectable locally recurrent anal squamous cell carcinoma (Epitopes-HPV02): a multicentre, single-arm, phase 2 study. *Lancet Oncol*. 2018;19(8):1094–1106. doi:10.1016/S1470-2045(18)30321-8

13. Abbas A, Nehme E, Fakih M. Single-agent paclitaxel in advanced anal cancer after failure of cisplatin and 5-fluorouracil chemotherapy. *Anticancer Res*. 2011;31(12):4637–4640.

14. Kim R, Byer J, Fulp WJ, et al. Carboplatin and paclitaxel treatment is effective in advanced anal cancer. *Oncology*. 2014;87(2):125–132. doi:10.1159/000361051

15. Hainsworth JD, Burris HA, Meluch AA, et al. Paclitaxel, carboplatin, and long-term continuous infusion of 5-fluorouracil in the treatment of advanced squamous and other selected carcinomas: results of a phase II trial. *Cancer*. 2001;92(3):642–649. doi:10.1002/1097-0142(20010801)92:3<642::AID-CNCR1365>3.0.CO;2-Z

16. Golub DV, Civelek AC, Sharma VR. A regimen of taxol, Ifosfamide, and platinum for recurrent advanced squamous cell cancer of the anal canal. *Chemother Res Pract*. 2011;2011:163736. doi:10.1155/2011/163736

17. Jhawer M, Mani S, Lefkopoulou M, et al. Phase II study of mitomycin-C, adriamycin, cisplatin (MAP) and Bleomycin-CCNU in patients with advanced cancer of the anal canal: an eastern cooperative oncology group study E7282. *Invest New Drugs*. 2006;24(5):447–454. doi:10.1007/s10637-006-7667-x

18. Morris VK, Salem ME, Nimeiri H, et al. Nivolumab for previously treated unresectable metastatic anal cancer (NCI9673): a multicentre, single-arm, phase 2 study. *Lancet Oncol*. 2017;18(4):446–453. doi:10.1016/S1470-2045(17)30104-3

19. Ott PA, Piha-Paul SA, Munster P, et al. Safety and antitumor activity of the anti-PD-1 antibody pembrolizumab in patients with recurrent carcinoma of the anal canal. *Ann Oncol*. 2017;28(5):1036–1041. doi:10.1093/annonc/mdx029

20. National Institutes of Health U.S. National Library of Medicine. Nivolumab With or Without Ipilimumab in Treating Patients With Refractory Metastatic Anal Canal Cancer. ClinicalTrials.gov Identifier: NCT02314169. https://clinicaltrials.gov/ct2/show/NCT02314169

21. National Institutes of Health U.S. National Library of Medicine. Pembrolizumab in Refractory Metastatic Anal Cancer. ClinicalTrials.gov Identifier: NCT02919969. https://clinicaltrials.gov/ct2/show/NCT02919969

22. National Institutes of Health U.S. National Library of Medicine. A Study of mDCF in Combination or Not With Atezolizumab in Advanced Squamous Cell Anal Carcinoma (SCARCE). ClinicalTrials.gov Identifier: NCT03519295. https://clinicaltrials.gov/ct2/show/NCT03519295

23. Rogers JE, Ohinata A, Silva NN, et al. Epidermal growth factor receptor inhibition in metastatic anal cancer. *Anticancer Drugs*. 2016;27(8):804–808. doi:10.1097/CAD.0000000000000383

24. Draper LM, Kwong MLM, Gros A, et al. Targeting of HPV-16+ Epithelial Cancer Cells by TCR Gene Engineered T Cells Directed against E6. *Clin Cancer Res*. 2015;21(19):4431–4439. doi:10.1158/1078-0432.CCR-14-3341

25. Hinrichs CS, Doran SL, Stevanovic S, et al. A phase I/II clinical trial of E6 T-cell receptor gene therapy for human papillomavirus (HPV)-associated epithelial cancers. *J Clin Oncol*. 2017;35(15_suppl):3009–3009. doi:10.1200/jco.2017.35.15_suppl.3009

26. Eng C, Fakih M, Amin M, et al. 537PP2 study of ADXS11-001 Immunotherapy in patients with persistent/recurrent, surgically unresectable locoregional, or metastatic squamous cell anal cancer. *Ann Oncol*. 2017. 28(suppl_5):mdx393.063–mdx393.063. doi:10.1093/annonc/mdx393.063

27. Heinze C, Omari J, Othmer M, et al. Image-guided interstitial brachytherapy in the management of metastasized anal squamous cell carcinoma. *Anticancer Res*. 2018;38(9):5401–5407. doi:10.21873/anticanres.12870

28. Piketty C, Selinger-Leneman H, Grabar S, et al. Marked increase in the incidence of invasive anal cancer among HIV-infected patients despite treatment with combination antiretroviral therapy. *Aids*. 2008;22(10).1203–1211. doi:10.1097/QAD.0b013e3283023f78

29. Chadha M, Rosenblatt EA, Malamud S, et al. Squamous-cell carcinoma of the anus in HIV-positive patients. *Dis Colon Rectum*. 1994;37(9):861–865. doi:10.1007/BF02052589
30. Holland JM, Swift PS. Tolerance of patients with human immunodeficiency virus and anal carcinoma to treatment with combined chemotherapy and radiation therapy. *Radiology*. 1994;193(1):251–254. doi:10.1148/radiology.193.1.8090901
31. Hoffman R, Welton ML, Klencke B, et al. The significance of pretreatment CD4 count on the outcome and treatment tolerance of HIV-positive patients with anal cancer. *Int J Radiat Oncol Biol Phys*. 1999;44(1):127–131. doi:10.1016/S0360-3016(98)00528-8
32. Lin D, Gold HT, Schreiber D, et al. Impact of socioeconomic status on survival for patients with anal cancer. *Cancer*. 2018;124(8):1791–1797. doi:10.1002/cncr.31186
33. Bojko MM, Kucejko RJ, Poggio JL. Racial disparities and the effect of county level income on the incidence and survival of young men with anal cancer. *Health Equity*. 2018;2(1):193–198. doi:10.1089/heq.2018.0018

Gastrointestinal Stromal Tumors

Kantha Ratnam Kolla and Mahesh Seetharam

INTRODUCTION

Gastrointestinal stromal tumors (GISTs) are the most common mesenchymal tumors of the gastrointestinal tract and arise from interstitial cells of Cajal. GISTs most commonly occur due to activating mutations in KIT or platelet-derived growth factor receptor alpha (PDGFRα). Mutations in BRAF gene and succinate dehydrogenase gene occur infrequently. For small GISTs, surgical resection is the preferred treatment and is frequently curative. For advanced and metastatic GISTs, systemic therapy with tyrosine kinase inhibitors (TKIs) is the recommended approach with frontline imatinib followed by sunitinib and regorafenib as subsequent therapies. Newer molecular targeted therapies evaluated in studies include second-generation KIT/PDGFR inhibitors, drugs targeting mitogen activating protein (MAP) kinase, BRAF, insulin growth factor-1 receptor, switch pocket kinase, PI3K, mammalian target of rapamycin (mTOR), heat shock protein 90, immune checkpoint, and vascular endothelial growth factor receptors (VEGFRs) to name a few. In this chapter, we review pathobiology, diagnostics, significance of mutation testing, approved and investigational therapies in GIST.

EPIDEMIOLOGY

Mesenchymal tumors constitute approximately 1% of primary gastrointestinal tumors. GISTs constitute the most common nonepithelial neoplasms, which account for an annual incidence of 14 to 20 cases per million.

GISTs are the most common mesenchymal tumors of the gastrointestinal tract. GISTs commonly occur in the stomach and proximal small intestine, but may also be found in any part of the alimentary tract, omentum, mesentery, and peritoneum (1–3). Lipomas, liposarcomas, leiomyosarcomas, desmoid tumors, schwannomas, and peripheral nerve sheath tumors are also seen but are less common than GISTs.

GISTs develop most often due to mutations in *KIT* or in *PDGFRA* genes, while mutations in *BRAF* gene and succinate dehydrogenase are less common.

As per the Surveillance, Epidemiology, and End Results (SEER) analysis of histologically confirmed GISTs, 6,142 cases were diagnosed annually between 2001 and 2011, with an incidence of 0.68 per 100,000 (3). Results of autopsy data showed small GISTs (<1 mm–1 cm) in 22.5% to 35% of cases. Only a few microscopic tumors eventually become significant and acquire malignant potential, which might be the reason for the relatively low incidence of clinically significant GISTs. Transformation or progression of micro-GISTs (GISTlets) is linked to progressive acquisition of genomic abnormalities as depicted in Figure 51.1.

GISTs commonly occur in the older population (median age 60–65 years), with similar incidence rates in men and women. GISTs arise from interstitial cells of Cajal, which are spindle-shaped pacemaker cells of the gut. The most common imaging modalities used to monitor GIST are CT, MRI, and PET. Mutations in *KIT* gene or in *RTK PDGFRA* gene are found in 85% of GISTs, and are termed type I GISTs (4). Ten to fifteen percent of GISTs that lack mutations in *KIT* and *PDGFRA* show poor response to imatinib therapy and are referred to as wild-type GIST. Gain of function V600E mutation in the *BRAF* gene has been reported in 7% of GISTs, which lack *KIT/PDGFRA* mutations. Neurofibromatosis-1 (NF1) related GISTs account for 1.5% of total GISTs. Deficiency or mutations in the succinate dehydrogenase (SDH) complex account for 40% of wild-type GISTs, and are referred to as type II GISTs (Figure 51.2) (5,6).

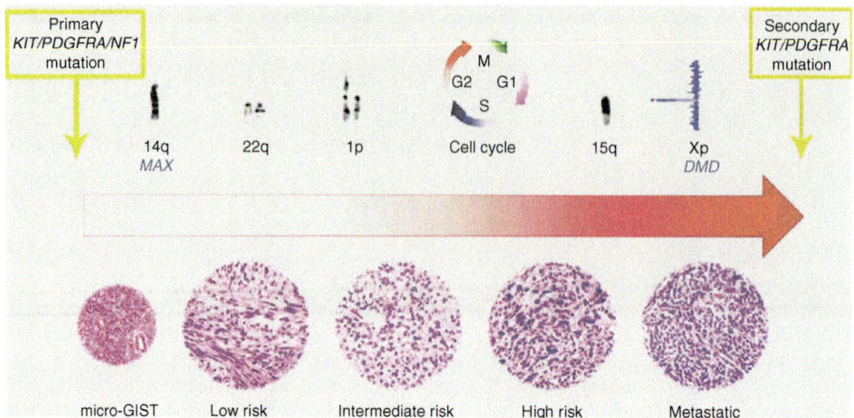

FIGURE 51.1   Genomic progression of GIST.

GIST, gastrointestinal stromal tumor.

Source: Reproduced with permission from Schaefer IM, Mariño-Enríquez A, Fletcher JA. What is new in gastrointestinal stromal tumor? *Adv Anat Pathol.* 2017;24(5):259–267. doi:10.1097/pap.0000000000000158 Licensed under the terms and conditions of the Creative Commons Attribution license (http://creativecommons.org/licenses/by/3.0/).

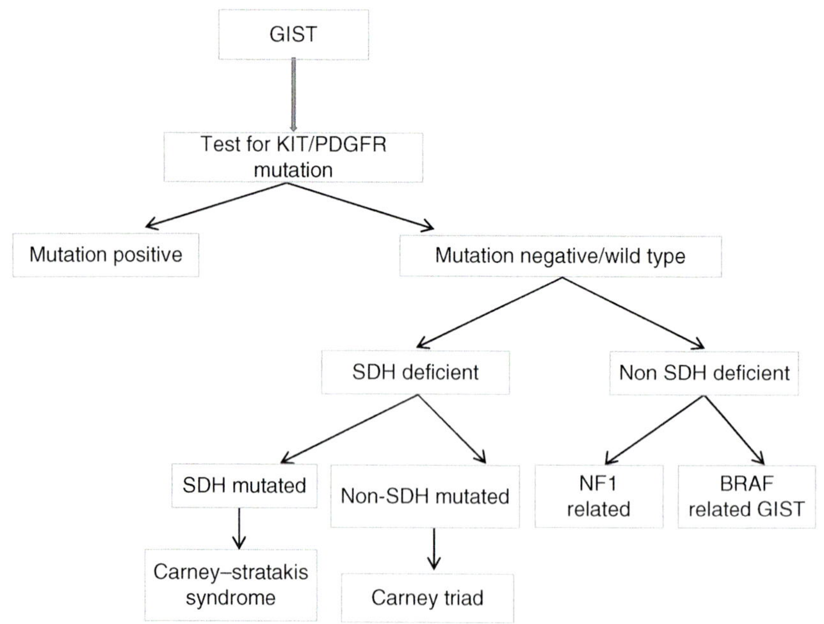

FIGURE 51.2   Classification of GIST.

GIST, gastrointestinal stromal tumor.

Source: From Shi E, Chmielecki J, Tang CM, et al. FGFR1 and NTRK3 actionable alterations in "Wild-Type" gastrointestinal stromal tumors. *J Transl Med.* 2016;14(1):339.

Imatinib was initially approved for chronic myelogenous leukemia in 2001. It was approved by the U.S. Food and Drug Administration (FDA) for GIST in 2002 (7). For imatinib refractory or intolerant GISTs, sunitinib was approved in 2006, and in 2013 regorafenib, an oral multikinase inhibitor, was approved for advanced GIST. Sunitinib and regorafenib are approved for second-line and beyond treatment of GIST (8).

RISK STRATIFICATION OF GIST

The decision to administer adjuvant therapy is based on a patient's risk of recurrence based on prognostic factors. Although traditional American Joint Committee on Cancer (AJCC) based tumor, node, and metastasis (TNM) classification is used for staging, because of the difference in outcomes based on other factors, a few different risk stratification criteria have been developed. The most commonly used are National Institutes of Health (NIH) consensus criteria, Armed Forces Institute of Pathology (AFIP), and modified NIH criteria. These criteria help select appropriate patients for treatment and avoid overtreatment of patients with early-stage or low-risk disease who are potentially cured with surgery alone.

Table 51.1 summarizes the risk of recurrence of localized GIST based on tumor size, location, and mitotic rate.

MOLECULAR CHARACTERIZATION OF GIST

GISTs mostly result due to activation mutations in the receptor tyrosine kinase gene *KIT* or *PDGFRα*. The location of tyrosine kinase gene mutations plays a role in biological behavior and determines risk category, clinical outcome, and drug response.

In KIT/PDGFRA wild-type GISTs, mutations in rat sarcoma oncogene (*RAS*) signaling pathogenesis, such as KRAS and BRAF have been reported. Patients with *NF1* mutations have a higher risk of developing GISTs. Through induction of aberrant DNA methylation, altered expression, or mutation of members, SDH heterotetramer results in GIST development. GISTs with no alterations in *KIT*, *PDGFRA*, *RAS* signaling genes, or *SDH* family genes are considered as true wild-type GISTs.

Discovery of DOG1, also known as TMEM16A or ANO1, serves as a novel diagnostic marker of GISTs, and is typically positive in about 95% of GISTs. Thus, positive DOG1 and KIT are generally considered to be diagnostic of GISTs, which also stain for interstitial cells of cajal (ICCs). Upregulation of protein kinase-C theta (PKCθ) has also been noted in GISTs, compared to other soft-tissue tumors.

TABLE 51.1 Risk Stratification of GISTs

Tumor Parameters		Risk of Progressive Disease (%)			
Mitotic rate	**Size**	**Gastric**	**Duodenum**	**Jejunum/ Ileum**	**Rectum**
≤5 per 5 mm²	≤2 cm	None (0%)	None (0%)	None (0%)	None (0%)
	2.1–5 cm	Very low (1.9%)	Low (8.3%)	Low (4.3%)	Low (8.5%)
	5.1–10 cm	Low (3.6%)	Inadequate data	Moderate (24%)	Inadequate data
	>10 cm	Moderate (10%)	High (34%)	High (52%)	High (57%)
>5 per 5 mm²	≤ 2 cm	None	Inadequate data	High	High (54%)
	2.1–5 cm	Moderate (16%)	High (50%)	High (73%)	High (52%)
	5.1–10 cm	High (55%)	Inadequate data	High (85%)	Inadequate data
	>10 cm	High (86%)	High (86%)	High (90%)	High (71%)

GIST, gastrointestinal stromal tumor.

Wild-type GISTs are characterized by overexpression of CALCRL/COL 22A1, tyrosine kinase NTRK 2, the cyclin dependent kinase CDK 6, and ERG, a member of the ETS- transcription factor family (9).

Mutations in *TP53*, *MEN1*, or *MAX* are seen in a subset of wild-type GISTs (10). KIT belongs to the type III receptor tyrosine kinase K family and encodes a 145 KDa receptor tyrosine kinase c-kit. Through autoinhibition of the kinase domain, KIT is maintained in an inactive form. Stem cell factor (SCF) acts as a KIT ligand. The SCF-KIT signal results in activation of downstream pathways, including (a) MAP kinase cascade: leading to upregulation of transcriptional factors such as MYC, ELK, CREB, and FOS, and (b) PE3K/AKT pathway: causing downregulation of cell cycle inhibitors and promotion of antiapoptotic effects.

KIT mutations in GISTs can be seen in exons 9, 11, 13, 14, 17, and 18 (Figure 51.3). Seventy percent of mutations are in exon 11, while 5% to 10% are in exon 9. Mutation in exon 11 leads to disruption of autoinhibition, which subsequently leads to activation of KIT (11).

KIT exon 13 and *17* mutations are seen in 1% to 2% of GISTs. Mutations in *exon 8* are rare, and are characterized by extragastric and distant metastatic tumors (12).

PDGFR Mutation in GIST

PDGFRA mutations are seen in 10% to 15% of GISTs. *PDGFRA* mutation results in activation of signal transduction molecules including MAPK, AKT, STAT 1, and STAT (13). *D842V* mutation on *exon 18* is seen in 60% to 65% of *PDGFRA* mutations (14). *PDGFR exon 14* mutation is seen in about 1% of all GISTs.

Familial GIST

Familial GIST results from germline mutation of *KIT* or *PDGFRA*. This can present with multiple GISTs, hyperpigmentation, mast cell tumors, and ICC hyperplasia associated dysphagia. Familial GISTs commonly occur in middle age, and the tumors exhibit histological features similar to sporadic GISTs.

SDH Deficient GIST

SDH deficiency is the most frequent molecular alteration in wild-type KIT/PDGFRA GISTs. SDH deficiency can result in paraganglioma, GIST, renal cell carcinoma, and pituitary adenoma (15). SDH deficient GISTs can be part of the Carney triad or Carney–Stratakis syndrome. The Carney triad constitutes gastric stromal sarcoma, paraganglioma, and pulmonary chondroma. Carney–Stratakis syndrome includes gastric GISTs and paragangliomas.

RAS Gene Mutations in GIST

In a subset of GISTs, mutations occur in the *RAS* family of genes and *BRAF*. In a study by Miranda et al. (16), *KRAS* mutations were detected at codon 12 and/or 13 (G12D, G13D, and G12A/G13D). Deletions at exon 11 of KIT (Δ570-576 and Δ579) were detected in tumors carrying the *G12D* and *G12A/G13D* mutations, while *PDGFRA* mutation at *exon 18* (*D842V*) was found in tumors with *G13D* mutation. *BRAFV600E* mutations were identified in GISTs with wild-type KIT/ PDGFRA (17).

Other Gene Mutations in GIST

EGFR mutations are seen in less than 1% of GISTs. It is more common in females, the stomach region, and generally has a low recurrence rate.

Some of the other mutations seen in wild-type GISTs include genes *ARIDIB*, *ATR*, *FGFRI*, *LTK*, *SUFU*, *PARK 2*, and *ZNF217* (18). Mutations in *PP2R1A* were found in 18% of GISTs (19).

Tumor Suppressor Genes in GIST

Neurofibromin negatively regulates RAS signaling. A high risk of developing GISTs is found in patients with *NF1* mutations. NF1 associated GISTs mostly occur in younger age and are characterized by small multiple tumors with an indolent clinical course and frequently affect the small intestine and duodenum. Dystrophin (DMD) acts as a tumor suppressor by inhibiting invasion, migration, anchorage independence, and invadopodia formation. Intragenic deletion of dystrophin is commonly seen in metastatic GISTs (2).

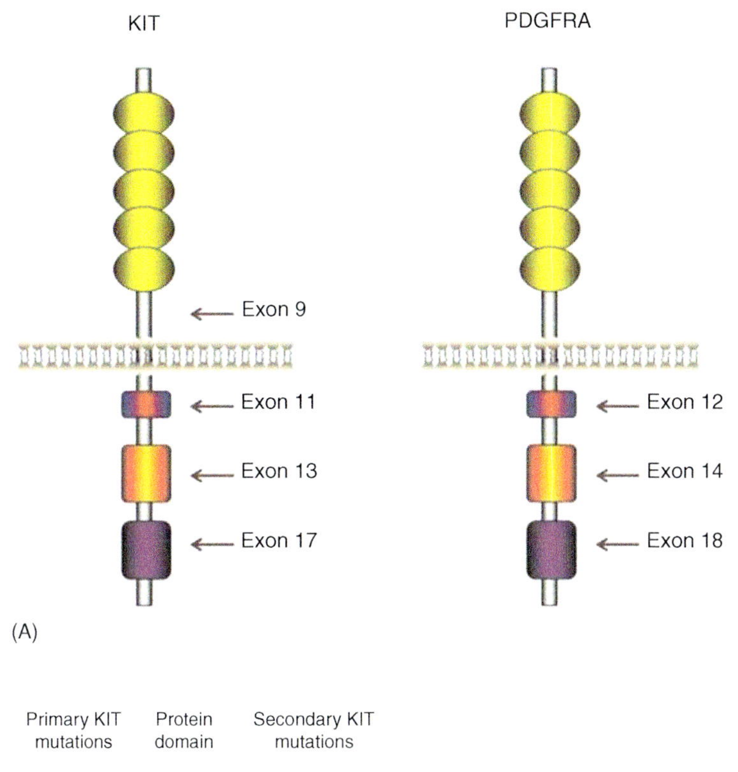

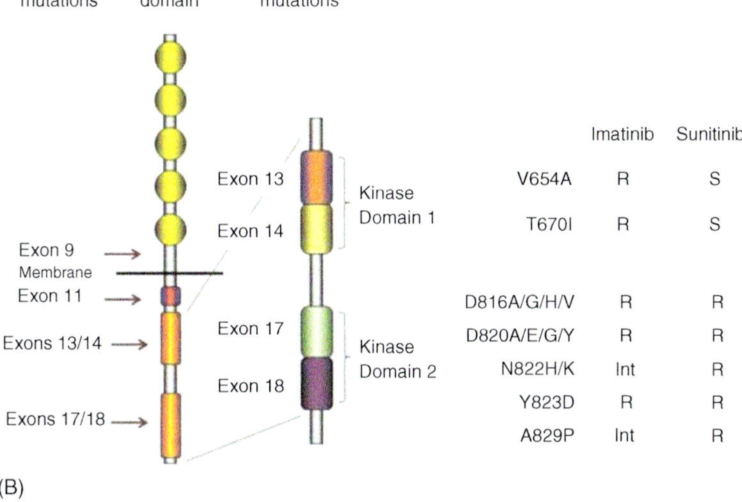

FIGURE 51.3 KIT mutations in GIST.

GIST, gastrointestinal stromal tumor; Int, intermediate; R, resistant; S, sensitive.

Source: Reproduced with permission from Li K, Cheng H, Li Z, et al. Genetic progression in gastrointestinal stromal tumors: mechanisms and molecular interventions. *Oncotarget.* 2017;8(36):60589–60604. doi:10.18632/oncotarget.16014 Licensed under the terms and conditions of the Creative Commons Attribution license (http://creativecommons.org/licenses/by/3.0/).

DIAGNOSIS OF GIST

Gastrointestinal bleeding, anemia, early satiety, abdominal satiety, abdominal distension, and discomfort are the common symptoms in GIST. Based on morphological and immunohistochemical findings, pathological diagnosis of GIST is done. Before initiating TKIs, mutational testing to detect abnormalities in *KIT* or *PDGFRA* genes is recommended for appropriate treatment selection.

Commonly used imaging techniques to diagnose GIST are CT, MRI, and PET. CT is the preferred initial imaging study to screen and stage GIST, except for patients who cannot receive intravenous contrast agents. PET/CT scans are helpful to evaluate metabolic activity of tumor, and decrease in uptake can help with early detection of treatment activity. Although CT scans are commonly used for evaluation of response, sometimes it may not be entirely reliable due to the possibility of pseudo-progression with tyrosine kinase inhibitors.

Other diagnostic modalities to detect and confirm GIST are upper endoscopy, endoscopic ultrasound (EUS), and EUS-guided fine-needle aspiration (EUS-FNA) biopsy (20).

STAGING OF GIST TUMORS

GISTs are staged based on the conventional TNM classification as outlined in Tables 51.2 and 51.3 with slight differences based on origin.

TREATMENT OF GIST

Localized GIST
The main treatment approach for localized GISTs is surgical resection (21).

Neoadjuvant Therapy in the Management of Locally Advanced GIST
Patients with localized disease, who are unable to undergo upfront complete surgical resection or borderline resectable, could be considered for neoadjuvant TKI therapy in an attempt to downstage the tumor. The goal with preoperative treatment is to reduce tumor size to allow complete resection. It is important to understand the genotype of the tumor before starting treatment to allow selection of the most effective therapy. If *KIT exon 9* mutation is identified, a higher dose of imatinib (800 mg per day) should be considered. If the tumor harbors a *PDGFR D842V* mutation or is of wild-type genotype, the current approved TKIs are ineffective, and so proceeding with surgery is likely the best approach. Neoadjuvant imatinib is also beneficial in patients with primary localized rectal GIST to minimize the extent of surgery. Although there are potential benefits with neoadjuvant therapy, this approach may not allow accurate recurrence risk assessment due to the inability to estimate the mitotic rate post therapy.

Based on the Radiation Therapy Oncology Group (RTOG) 0132/ACRIN6665 prospective trial with 52 patients, the benefit with preoperative imatinib was seen in patients treated for at least 16 weeks to attain partial response (PR), and radiographic response was seen after 3 to 9

TABLE 51.2 Staging of Gastric and Omental GIST (i)

Stage		N	M	Mitotic Rate
IA	T1 or T2	N0	M0	Low
IB	T3	N0	M0	Low
II	T1	N0	M0	High
	T2	N0	M0	High
	T4	N0	M0	Low
IIIA	T3	N0	M0	High
IIIB	T4	N0	M0	High
IV	Any T	N1	M0	Any rate
	Any T	Any N	M1	Any rate

GIST, gastrointestinal stromal tumor.

TABLE 51.3 GIST Staging (ii)

Small Intestinal, Esophageal, Colorectal, Mesenteric, and Peritoneal Staging				
Stage I	T1 or T2	N0	M0	Low
Stage II	T3	N0	M0	Low
Stage IIIA	T1	N0	M0	High
	T4	N0	M0	Low
Stage IIIB	T2	N0	M0	High
	T3	N0	M0	High
	T4	N0	M0	High
Stage IV	Any T	N1	M0	Any rate
	Any T	Any N	M1	Any rate

GIST, gastrointestinal stromal tumor.

months of treatment (22). In this trial, at 5 years of median follow-up, the progression-free survival (PFS) was 57% and disease-specific survival was 77%. It is important to understand the genotype of the tumor to exclude imatinib insensitive tumors, which include KIT wild-type, SDH and neurofibromatosis related GIST, *PDGFR D842V* mutated tumors as they are not expected to respond to imatinib. In patients who receive neoadjuvant imatinib, the recommendation is to continue adjuvant imatinib for a total of 3 years including pre- and postoperative therapy.

Adjuvant Therapy in Management of Resected GISTs
The benefit of adjuvant therapy in higher risk GIST was confirmed in phase III clinical trials.

a. *Imatinib vs. placebo*
   A randomized, double-blind phase III trial was conducted in patients who had undergone complete resection of localized GIST to evaluate the efficacy of imatinib (400 mg/day for 1 year). Results showed that the recurrence-free survival (RFS) was 98% and 83%, respectively, among imatinib and placebo groups respectively (hazard ratio [HR]: 0.35, 95% confidence interval [CI]; $p < .0001$). RFS was noted across all three tumor size categories in the imatinib group (tumor size $\geq$3 to <6 cm: HR: 0.23, $p = .011$; tumor size $\geq$6 to 10 cm, HR: 0.5, $p = .041$; for $\geq$ 10 cm: HR: 0.29, $p < .001$ for $\geq$ 10 cm) (23).

b. *Imatinib 1 year vs. 3 years*
   A randomized phase 3 study was conducted to evaluate the efficacy of imatinib for adjuvant therapy in patients with a high risk of GIST recurrence after surgery. Patients were assigned to receive 400 mg/day imatinib started within 12 weeks of surgery for either 12 months or 36 months. Results found that 5-year RFS was 65.6% versus 47.9% and overall survival (OS) was 92% versus 81.7% among patients who received imatinib for 36 months and 12 months, respectively ($p < .001$, 95% CI) (24).

MANAGEMENT OF METASTATIC GIST

The three FDA approved drugs for metastatic GIST are imatinib, sunitinib, and regorafenib. The drugs are approved based on the molecular mechanism of activity to inhibit c-kit and PDGFRA. In addition, sunitinib has activity against VEGFR 1, 2, and 3, and regorafenib has activity against RET and FGFR 1 and 3. Outlined in Table 51.4 are the relevant clinical trials and results that led to the approval of these drugs. The data in Table 51.5 outline data with nilotinib, which showed PFS improvement in the intention-to-treat population and OS in patients who had one line of imatinib and sunitinib, but was not significant for the overall cohort of patients.

a. *Imatinib*
   A phase III study was conducted on patients with metastatic/refractory GIST to evaluate the efficacy of imatinib. Results found that median OS was 49 months and median PFS was 20 months. Fluid retention, nausea, fatigue, and skin rash were the common adverse events noted.

b. *Sunitinib*
   In patients with imatinib resistant GIST, the phase I/II trial with sunitinib showed median OS of 26.9 months and 12.3 months in those with *KIT exon 9* and *KIT 11* mutation, respectively. The median PFS was 19 months and 5 months in patients with KIT exon 9 mutation and KIT 11 mutation, respectively. Common adverse events noted were fatigue, diarrhea, nausea, and anorexia (25).

c. *Regorafenib*
   The phase III GRID study was conducted in patients with imatinib and sunitinib resistant GIST to evaluate the efficacy of regorafenib. The disease control rate was 58% in the regorafenib group versus 20% in the placebo group. The most commonly noted adverse effects were hypertension, hand–foot skin reaction, and maculopapular rash (26).

d. *Nilotinib*
   Nilotinib is a selective TKI that has inhibitory potency against KIT, PDGFR, and BCR-ABL. The phase III open-label trial compared patients treated with nilotinib or placebo in patients after progression with imatinib and sunitinib. Results from post hoc subset analysis showed a significant difference in median OS of >4 months in the nilotinib group (405 vs. 280 days; p = .02) in intention-to-treat analysis patients based on central radiology review (CRR); no significant difference in PFS was noted.

TABLE 51.4 Clinical Trials of Interest

Drug	Phase of Study	Patient Group	Results
Nivolumab	Phase II	Patients with advanced/metastatic GIST resistant to imatinib	Nivolumab only gp: 3/7—SD, CBR—42.8%, PFS—8 weeks
			Nivolumab + imatinib: PR— 20%, 1/5—SD, CBR—40%, PFS—8.43 weeks
Masitinib	Phase II	Patients with imatinib resistant GIST	CR—3.3%, PR—50%, SD—43.3%, PFS was 59.7% and 55.4% at 2 and 3 years, respectively; OS 1 and 3 years was 89.9%
Dovitinib	Phase II (DOVIGIST trial)	Patients with imatinib and sunitinib resistant GIST	DCR at 24 weeks—13%, PR—3%, PFS—3.6 months (95% CI), median OS—9.7 months (95% CI)
BIIB021 (Hsp90 inhibitor)	Phase II trial	23 patients with imatinib and sunitinib resistant GIST	PR—5 patients, overall response rate—22%, duration of response: 25–138 days
Imatinib + onalespib (AT13387, non-ansamycin Hsp 90 inhibitor)	Phase II	TKI resistant GIST patients	DCR at 4 months—19%, median PFS—112 days
Olaratumab (anti-PDGF alpha monoclonal antibody)	Phase II	Patients with metastatic GIST with *PDGFRA* mutations	SD—50%, 12-week clinical benefit (CR, PR, SD)—50%
Linsitinib (OSI-906, IGF 1R inhibitor)	Phase II	KIT/PDGFRA wild-type GIST	PR and stable FDG metabolic response—35%, CBR (CR, PR, SD) at 9 months—45%; PFS—52%, OS at 9 months—80%

(continued)

TABLE 51.4 Clinical Trials of Interest (*continued*)

Drug	Phase of Study	Patient Group	Results
Sorafenib	Phase II	Patients with imatinib or imatinib/sunitinib resistant GIST	PR—13%; SD—55%, DCR (SD + PR)—68%; PFS—5.2 months (95% CI), median OS—11.6 months (95% CI)
Dasatinib	Phase II	Patients with TKI-naïve GIST	FDG-PET response rate (CR + PR) at 4 weeks—67%; median PFS—11.1 months
Vatalanib	Phase II	Patients with imatinib or sunitinib resistant GIST	Clinical benefit—45%; partial remissions—4.4%; SD—35.6 %; median time to progression—3.2 months (95% CI)
Ponatinib	Phase II	Patients with advanced GIST with *KIT exon 11* mutation	CBR at >/=16 weeks—55%; objective response rate—8%

CBR, clinical benefit rate; CI, confidence interval; CR, complete response; DCR, disease control rate; FDG, fluorodeoxyglucose; GIST, gastrointestinal stromal tumor; OS, overall survival; PFS, progression-free survival; PR, partial response; SD, stable disease; TKI, tyrosine kinase inhibitor.

Drug	Phase 1 Clinical Trial	Patient Group	Results
BLU-285	Phase I trial	Patients with unresectable GIST	17 PDGFR-alpha D842V patients: 7 had PR; 10 had SD
			Of 11 *KIT* mutation patients: 2 had PR; 5 had SD
DCC-2618	Phase I trial	Patients with GIST	Partial metabolic response—78%
Retaspimycin (IPI-504)	Phase I trial	Patients with metastatic and/or unresectable GIST	SD—70%, metabolic PR—38%
Cabozantinib (MET inhibitor)	Phase I trial	Four patients who were pretreated with imatinib and sunitinib	SD for 6–20 months
Imatinib + panobinostat (histone deacetylase inhibitor)	Phase I trial	Patients with imatinib and sunitinib resistant GIST	Metabolic PR—1/11; metabolic SD—7/11

GIST, gastrointestinal stromal tumor; PDGFR, platelet-derived growth factor receptor; PR, partial response; SD, stable disease.

Management of Intermediate-Risk GIST

The benefit of adjuvant TKIs in improving outcomes has been proven in randomized clinical trials. Imatinib for 36 months for adjuvant therapy of high-risk GIST is the standard of care endorsed by U.S. and European regulatory agencies and also the National Comprehensive Cancer Network (NCCN). Also well understood is the lack of need for adjuvant treatment in low-risk GIST due to low likelihood of recurrence.

TABLE 51.5 Pivotal Trials and Results for Approved Tyrosine Kinase Inhibitors

Drug	Clinical Trial	Patient Population	Median OS	Median PFS	Other Results	Adverse Events
Imatinib	Phase III	Patients with metastatic/ refractory GIST	49 months	20 months		Fluid retention, nausea, fatigue, skin rash
Sunitinib	Phase I/II trial	Patients with imatinib resistant GIST	*KIT exon 9 muta-tion: 26.9* months	*KIT exon 9* mutation/ *PDGFRA* mutation: 19 months		
			KIT exon 11 muta-tion: 12.3 months	*KIT exon 11* mutation: 5 months		Fatigue, diarrhea, nausea, anorexia
Regorafenib	Phase III study (GRID)	Imatinib and sunitinib resistant GIST	17.4 months in both arms (crossover design)	Regorafenib: 4.8 months Placebo: 0.9 months ($p <$ .0001)	Disease control rate: 58% in regorafenib group vs. 20% in placebo group	Hypertension, hand–foot skin reaction, maculopapular rash

GIST, gastrointestinal stromal tumor; OS, overall survival; PFS, progression-free survival.

The European Organisation for Research and Treatment of Cancer (EORTC) 62024 trial assigned 908 patients with high and intermediate risk (based on NIH 2002 classification) to adjuvant imatinib for two years of observation. The results showed no benefit of adjuvant imatinib in intermediate risk GIST, and their outcomes were similar to those with low-risk GIST (27). The results were similar when patients were restratified based on the modified NIH risk stratification.

Another study included 44 intermediate-risk patients who received imatinib and were followed prospectively. The results showed recurrence-free benefit at 1 year, 1 to 3 years, and >3 years with treatment, but the difference was not statistically significant (28).

Interestingly, in a study by Quek et al. with 105 patients harboring KIT abnormalities, 60 patients had KIT exon 11 deletion, and 25 out of the 60 patients were classified as intermediate-risk GIST based on traditional risk stratification criteria. Multivariate analysis confirmed KIT exon 11 deletion as an independent adverse prognostic feature for relapse-free survival (29).

KIT exon 11 deletions affecting codons 557–558 are seen in 23% to 28% of all GIST cases. The published literature suggests this genomic abnormality may be associated with an aggressive biology with increased tendency for metastasis and poor prognosis. Even in tumors that are categorized as intermediate risk by modified NIH criteria and arising from the stomach, the presence of KIT exon 11 deletions has less favorable outcomes (30).

In essence, the understanding of management of intermediate-risk GIST is evolving. Even though the traditional risk stratification based treatment approach is generally helpful in deciding the treatment for this patient population, incorporation of genomic information based on the aforementioned studies may help us identify a subset of intermediate-risk patients who are at higher risk for recurrence and may benefit from adjuvant therapy. At this time until we have new information, the treatment decision for intermediate-risk GIST on the use of adjuvant therapy is based on clinical and patient characteristics with help from genomic information.

RELEVANT CLINICAL TRIALS

Phase II Clinical Trials

a. *Nivolumab*

A phase II study was conducted on patients with advanced/metastatic GIST resistant to imatinib to evaluate the efficacy of nivolumab. Patients with advanced/metastatic GIST resistant to imatinib were randomly assigned to receive nivolumab and nivolumab plus imatinib, respectively. Results found that disease stability, clinical benefit rate (CBR), and PFS were noted in 3/7, 42.8 %, and 8 weeks in the nivolumab group versus 1/5, 40%, and 8.43 weeks in the nivolumab plus imatinib group. Fatigue and diarrhea are the commonly noted adverse events (31).

b. *Masitinib*

A phase 2 study was conducted on imatinib-naïve patients with advanced GIST to evaluate the effect of masitinib. Results were complete response (CR; 3.3%), PR (50%), and stable disease (SD) in 43.3% patients. At 2 months, the response rate was 20% according to Response Evaluation Criteria in Solid Tumors (RECIST) and 86% according to FDG-PET response criteria. PFS was 59.7% and 55.4% at 2 and 3 years, respectively; OS at 2 and 3 years was stable at 89.9% (71.8; 96.6). Rash (10%) and neutropenia (7%) were the most commonly noted grade 3–4 toxicities. Thus, masitinib appears as an effective first-line option for advanced GIST (32).

c. *Dovitinib*

A prospective phase II study was conducted on patients with metastatic and/or unresectable GISTs (having a history of failure to imatinib and sunitinib) to evaluate the efficacy of dovitinib. Results showed that the disease control rate at 24 weeks was noted in 13% patients and PR was noted in 3% patients. PFS was 3.6 months (95% CI: 3.5–3.7 months); median OS was 9.7 months (95% CI: 6–13.4 months). Asthenia (20%), neutropenia (13%), and thrombocytopenia (10%) were the commonly noted side effects.

d. *HSP90 inhibitor (BIIB021)*

HSP90 inhibition through proteasomal degradation of activated KIT exerts efficacy against GISTs. A phase II study was conducted on 23 patients with GIST refractory to imatinib and sunitinib, to evaluate the efficacy of HSP90 inhibitor, BIIB021. Results showed that PR was observed in five patients, for an overall response rate of 22%. The duration of response was 25 to 138 days. Mild–moderate adverse events were noted. Thus, results found that BIIB021 led to objective response in refractory GIST and the study met its primary end point, thus warranting further evaluation of BIIB021 in GIST patients.

e. *Onalespib (AT 13387)*

GIST treated with TKI imatinib may develop additional mutations in the receptor tyrosine kinase *KIT* or *PDGFRA* and become resistant to imatinib. To maintain stability and activity, mutated *KIT* requires the molecular chaperone heat shock protein 90 (Hsp 90). Onalespib (AT 13387) acts as a potent non-ansamycin Hsp 90 inhibitor. Wagner et al. conducted a dose escalation phase II study to evaluate the safety and efficacy of a combination of onalespib and imatinib in TKI resistant GIST patients. Results showed that disease control at 4 months was achieved in 19% patients and median PFS was 112 days (95% CI: 43–165). Diarrhea (58%), nausea (50%), injection site events (46%), and vomiting (39%) were the commonly reported side effects.

f. *Olaratumab, IMC-3G3 (anti-PDGF alpha monoclonal antibody)*

A phase II study was conducted on previously treated patients with metastatic GIST to evaluate the impact of a human anti-PDGF alpha monoclonal antibody (olaratumab, IMC-3G3). Patients with or without *PDGFRA* alpha mutations were grouped into cohorts 1 and 2, respectively, and received olaratumab. SD was noted in 50% of cohort 1 patients and 14.3% of cohort 2 patients. Progressive disease (PD) was noted in 50% of cohort 1 patients and 85.7% of cohort 2 patients. The 12-week clinical benefit (which includes CR, PR, and SD; 90% CI) was 50% in cohort 1 patients and 14.3% in cohort 2 patients. Median OS was 24.9 weeks in cohort 2 patients and was not reached in cohort 1 patients. Olaratumab related adverse events such as fatigue, nausea, and peripheral edema were noticed in all cohort 1 patients and 64.3% of cohort 2 patients. Thus, these results show that patients with PDGF alpha mutant GIST expressed longer disease control, with acceptable adverse event profiles.

g. *Linsitinib (OSI-906), IGF1R inhibitor*
A phase II study was conducted on pediatric and adult patients with KIT/PDGFRA wild-type GIST to evaluate the efficacy of IGF 1R inhibitor linsitinib (OSI-906). Results found that qualitative partial and stable FDG metabolic responses were seen in 35% patients; CBR (CR, PR, and SD) at 9 months was 45%; PFS was 52%; OS at 9 months was noted in 80% patients. Tolerable adverse events were noted (33).

h. *Dasatinib*
Dasatinib is a second-generation TKI, which exerts inhibitory activity against Bcr-abl, Src family kinases, and KIT. In a phase II study, patients with TKI-naïve GIST received dasatinib. Results showed that FDG-PET response rate (CR + PR) at 4 weeks was 67% (13 CR, 16 PR, 7 SD, and 3 PD). Median PFS was 11.1 months. Thus, dasatinib demonstrated promising results in TKI-naïve patients with FDG-PET positive GIST.

i. *Vatalanib:* Vatalanib exerts inhibitory activity against KIT, PDGFRs, and VEGFRs. A phase II study was conducted on patients with advanced GIST to evaluate the efficacy of vatalanib. Forty-five patients had imatinib resistant metastatic GIST and nineteen of them also had prior resistance to sunitinib. Results found that 40% (95% CI) patients had clinical benefit; 4.4% patients had partial remissions; 35.6% patients had stabilized disease. Median time to progression was 5.8 months (95% CI) in the patient group that did not receive prior sunitinib and 3.2 months (95% CI) in the patient group that had prior resistance to imatinib and sunitinib ($p = .992$).

j. *Ponatinib:* Ponatinib, an oral TKI, exhibits inhibitory activity against mutant isoforms of *KIT* (including secondary *exon 17* resistance mutants) and *PDGFRA*. A phase II study was conducted on patients with advanced GIST to evaluate the efficacy of ponatinib. Patients with or without primary mutations in KIT exon 11 were assigned to group A and group B, respectively. Results found that CBRs at ≥16 weeks were 55% (in group A; 1/11 had PR and 10/11 had SD) and 22% (in group B). Objective response rates were 8% (group A) and 0% (group B). Rash, fatigue, myalgia, dry skin, headache, and abdominal pain were the most commonly noted adverse events (34).

Relevant Phase I Clinical Studies
a. *BLU-285*
A phase I study was conducted on patients with unresectable GIST to evaluate the efficacy of BLU-285, a dual inhibitor of KIT receptor and PDGFRAα. Of 17 patients with PDGFR-alpha D842V mutations, seven had PR and 10 had disease stability. Nausea, fatigue, and peripheral neuropathy were the commonly noted adverse events (35).

b. *DCC-2618*
Patients with GIST were enrolled for phase I trial to evaluate the efficacy of DCC-2618, a pan-KIT and PDGFRα inhibitor. Results found a partial metabolic response of 78%. Anemia, increased lipase, and hypertension were the commonly noted adverse events (36).

c. *Retaspimycin (IPI-504)*
A phase I study was conducted on patients with metastatic and/or unresectable GIST to determine the efficacy of retaspimycin hydrochloride (IPI-504), a potent Hsp90 inhibitor. Results showed that SD was noted in 70% patients and metabolic PR in 38% patients. Fatigue (59%), headache (44%), and nausea (43%) were the commonly noted side effects.

d. *Cabozantinib*
A phase I trial was conducted on four patients with GIST who were pretreated with imatinib and sunitinib to evaluate the efficacy of cabozantinib, a MET inhibitor. Results found SD for 6 to 20 months. The commonly found adverse events were palmar–plantar erythrodysesthesia, hypertension, diarrhea, and stomatitis.

e. *Histone deacetylase inhibitors*
In in vitro and in vivo studies, it was found that histone deacetylase inhibition (HDACI) resulted in proteasomal degradation and transcriptional downregulation of KIT. A phase I trial was conducted on patients with metastatic GIST refractory to imatinib and sunitinib. Patients

received a combination of imatinib and panobinostat, a third-generation pan-HDAC inhibitor. Results found that 1/11 patients had metabolic PR, 7/11 patients had metabolic disease stabilization, and 3/11 demonstrated metabolically progressive disease. Thrombocytopenia, fatigue, creatinine elevation, and nausea were the common adverse events.

f. *MEK inhibitor (Binimetinib)*
In a phase Ib/II trial, patients with imatinib resistant advanced GIST received a combination of imatinib and MEK inhibitor binimetinib (MEK162). Results found that 5/15 patients (33%) had PR; 9/15 had SD at an 8-week period. Asymptomatic CPK elevation, peripheral edema, and rash were the common adverse events.

g. *Crenolanib*
Crenolanib is a potent inhibitor of PDGFRα, with in vitro inhibitory activity against PDGFRA D842V. A phase I/II study was conducted on patients having advanced GIST with PDGFRA D842V mutations to assess the efficacy of crenolanib. Results found that the CBR was 31% (5/16 patients, of whom two had PR and three had SD). Anemia and reversible liver function test (LFT) elevations were the common adverse events noted.

h. *Everolimus (mTOR inhibitor)*
A phase I–II study was conducted on patients with imatinib resistant GIST to assess the efficacy of a combination regimen of everolimus, an mTOR inhibitor, and imatinib. Results show that the progression-free rate was 37% at 4 months with a median PFS of 3.5 months. One patient had PR. Diarrhea, nausea, fatigue, and anemia were the commonly noted adverse events.

i. *Immune checkpoint inhibitor (ipilimumab)*
In a phase Ib study, patients with GIST and other sarcomas received dasatinib and CTLA-4 inhibitor (immune checkpoint inhibitor), ipilimumab. Results found that 7/20 patients had PR as per the Choi criteria.

IMMUNOTHERAPY IN GIST

The frequently found tumor-infiltrating immune cells in GIST are tumor-associated macrophages (TAMs), CD3+ T lymphocytes, tumor-infiltrating neutrophils (TINs), dendritic cells (DCs), natural killer (NK) cells, natural killer T (NKT) cells, gamma delta T-cells and B cells, and Tregs.

In a study conducted by Balachandran et al. on GIST bearing mice, it was found that a combination of imatinib and immune checkpoint inhibitor CTLA-4 blockade resulted in a significant reduction in tumor size, compared to either treatment alone.

Using DNA microarray studies, the heterogeneous expression of PDL1 across GISTs was found by Bertucci et al. (37).

Patients with a history of soft tissue sarcoma (STS) or GIST received cyclophosphamide and PD-1 targeting agent pembrolizumab in a phase II study. Results showed that 6-month nonprogression rates were noted in 11.1% of patients with GIST. Fatigue, diarrhea, and anemia were the most commonly reported side effects (38).

Chimeric antigen receptor (CAR) T-cells are genetically modified tumor-specific T lymphocytes that act against specific tumor antigens. A study was conducted on a mouse model employing GIST xenografts. A significant reduction in the tumor growth rate resulted due to treatment with anti-KIT CAR T-cells. Thus, these results suggest the significant role of CAR T-cells in the immunotherapeutic management of GIST patients.

Results from preclinical studies found that 10% to 27% of GISTs express cancer testis antigens (CTAs). It was also found that expression of CTAs is closely related to a higher recurrence risk, increased mitotic activity, and a significantly shorter RFS. These findings suggest CTAs as potential targets for immunotherapy.

GLOBAL EVIDENCE AND IMPLEMENTATION SUMMIT GUIDELINES

Recommendations for Localized GIST
a. The standard treatment for localized GISTs is complete surgical resection.
b. Spontaneous or intraoperative capsule rupture is considered a poor prognostic factor.
c. Three years of adjuvant treatment with imatinib is recommended for high-risk patients with resected primary tumors.

Recommendations for Unresectable or Metastatic Disease

a. The recommended first-line treatment option for advanced/metastatic GIST is imatinib 400 mg/day.
b. In *exon 9* mutants, the recommended dose is 800 mg/day.
c. For patients with failure on imatinib therapy, sunitinib 50 mg orally once a day for 4 weeks on followed by 2 weeks off is the recommended strategy.
d. The recommended standard therapy for patients with intolerance or progression on imatinib or sunitinib is regorafenib 160 mg a day.
e. Other treatment options for patients with progression or intolerance on imatinib are sorafenib, pazopanib, and ponatinib.

ADDITIONAL READING/BIBLIOGRAPHY

Debiec-Rychter M, Sciot R, Le Cesne A, et al. KIT mutations and dose selection for imatinib in patients with advanced gastrointestinal stromal tumours. *Eur J Cancer.* 2006;42(8):1093–1103. doi:10.1016/j.ejca.2006.01.030

Gramza AW, Corless CL, Heinrich MC, et al. Resistance to tyrosine kinase inhibitors in gastrointestinal stromal tumors. *Clin Cancer Res.* 2009;15(24):7510–7518. doi:10.1158/1078-0432.CCR-09-0190

Reichardt P, Blay JY, Gelderblom H, et al. Phase III study of nilotinib versus best supportive care with or without a TKI in patients with gastrointestinal stromal tumors resistant to or intolerant of imatinib and sunitinib. *Ann Oncol.* 2012;23(7):1680–1687. doi:10.1093/annonc/mdr598

Wagner AJ, Agulnik M, Heinrich MC, et al. Dose-escalation study of a second-generation non-ansamycin HSP90 inhibitor, onalespib (AT13387), in combination with imatinib in patients with metastatic gastrointestinal stromal tumour. *Eur J Cancer.* 2016;61:94–101. doi:10.1016/j.ejca.2016.03.076

Wagner AJ, Kindler H, Gelderblom H, et al. A phase II study of a human anti-PDGFR alpha monoclonal antibody (olaratumab, IMC-3G3) in previously treated patients with metastatic gastrointestinal stromal tumors. *Ann Oncol.* 2017;28(3):541–546. doi:10.1093/annonc/mdw659

West RB, Corless CL, Chen X, et al. The novel marker, DOG1, is expressed ubiquitously in gastrointestinal stromal tumors irrespective of KIT or PDGFRA mutation status. *Am J Pathol.* 2004;165(1):107–113. doi:10.1016/S0002-9440(10)63279-8

REFERENCES

1. Rubin BP, Fletcher JA, Fletcher CDM. Molecular insights into the histogenesis and pathogenesis of gastrointestinal stromal tumors. *Int J Surg Pathol.* 2000;8(1):5–10. doi:10.1177/106689690000800105
2. Miettinen M, Lasota J. Gastrointestinal stromal tumors--definition, clinical, histological, immunohistochemical, and molecular genetic features and differential diagnosis. *Virchows Arch.* 2001;438(1):1–12. doi:10.1007/s004280000338
3. Ma GL, Murphy JD, Martinez ME, et al. Epidemiology of gastrointestinal stromal tumors in the era of histology codes: results of a population-based study. *Cancer Epidemiol Biomarkers Prev.* 2015;24(1):298–302. doi:10.1158/1055-9965.EPI-14-1002
4. Heinrich MC, Corless CL, Demetri GD, et al. Kinase mutations and imatinib response in patients with metastatic gastrointestinal stromal tumor. *J Clin Oncol.* 2003;21(23):4342–4349. doi:10.1200/JCO.2003.04.190
5. Belinsky MG, Rink L, von Mehren M, et al. Succinate dehydrogenase deficiency in pediatric and adult gastrointestinal stromal tumors. *Front Oncol.* 2013;3:117. doi:10.3389/fonc.2013.00117
6. Killian JK, Miettinen M, Walker RL, et al. Recurrent epimutation of SDHC in gastrointestinal stromal tumors. *Sci Transl Med.* 2014;6(268):268ra177. doi:10.1126/scitranslmed.3009961
7. Dagher R, Cohen M, Williams G, et al. Approval summary: imatinib mesylate in the treatment of metastatic and/or unresectable malignant gastrointestinal stromal tumors. *Clin Cancer Res.* 2002;8(10):3034–3038.
8. Goodman VL, Rock EP, Dagher R, et al. Approval summary: sunitinib for the treatment of imatinib refractory or intolerant gastrointestinal stromal tumors and advanced renal cell carcinoma. *Clin Cancer Res.* 2007;13(5):1367–1373. doi:10.1158/1078-0432.CCR-06-2328
9. Nannini M, Astolfi A, Urbini M, et al. Integrated genomic study of quadruple-WT GIST (KIT/PDGFRA/SDH/RAS pathway wild-type GIST). *BMC Cancer.* 2014;14:685. doi:10.1186/1471-2407-14-685
10. Pantaleo MA, Urbini M, Indio V, et al. Genome-wide analysis identifies MEN1 and MAX mutations and a neuroendocrine-like molecular heterogeneity in quadruple WT GIST. *Mol Cancer Res.* 2017;15(5):553–562. doi:10.1158/1541-7786.MCR-16-0376

11. Gajiwala KS, Wu JC, Christensen J, et al. KIT kinase mutants show unique mechanisms of drug resistance to imatinib and sunitinib in gastrointestinal stromal tumor patients. *Proc Natl Acad Sci U S A.* 2009;106(5):1542–1547. doi:10.1073/pnas.0812413106

12. Ito T, Yamamura M, Hirai T, et al. Gastrointestinal stromal tumors with exon 8 c-kit gene mutation might occur at extragastric sites and have metastasis-prone nature. *Int J Clin Exp Pathol.* 2014;7(11):8024–8031.

13. Heinrich MC, Corless CL, Duensing A, et al. PDGFRA activating mutations in gastrointestinal stromal tumors. *Science.* 2003;299(5607):708–710. doi:10.1126/science.1079666

14. Wozniak A, Rutkowski P, Schoffski P, et al. Tumor genotype is an independent prognostic factor in primary gastrointestinal stromal tumors of gastric origin: a European multicenter analysis based on ConticaGIST. *Clin Cancer Res.* 2014;20(23):6105–6116. doi:10.1158/1078-0432.CCR-14-1677

15. Gill AJ, Lipton L, Taylor J, et al. Germline SDHC mutation presenting as recurrent SDH deficient GIST and renal carcinoma. *Pathology.* 2013;45(7):689–691. doi:10.1097/PAT.0000000000000018

16. Miranda C, Nucifora M, Molinari F, et al. KRAS and BRAF mutations predict primary resistance to imatinib in gastrointestinal stromal tumors. *Clin Cancer Res.* 2012;18(6):1769–1776. doi:10.1158/1078-0432.CCR-11-2230

17. Rossi S, Gasparotto D, Miceli R, et al. KIT, PDGFRA, and BRAF mutational spectrum impacts on the natural history of imatinib-naive localized GIST: a population-based study. *Am J Surg Pathol.* 2015;39(7):922–930. doi:10.1097/PAS.0000000000000418

18. Shi E, Chmielecki J, Tang CM, et al. FGFR1 and NTRK3 actionable alterations in "Wild-Type" gastrointestinal stromal tumors. *J Transl Med.* 2016;14(1):339.

19. Toda-Ishii M, Akaike K, Suehara Y, et al. Clinicopathological effects of protein phosphatase 2, regulatory subunit A, alpha mutations in gastrointestinal stromal tumors. *Mod Pathol.* 2016;29(11):1424–1432. doi:10.1038/modpathol.2016.138

20. Nishida T, Blay J-Y, Hirota S, et al. The standard diagnosis, treatment, and follow-up of gastrointestinal stromal tumors based on guidelines. *Gastric Cancer.* 2016;19(1):3–14. doi:10.1007/s10120-015-0526-8

21. Demetri GD, von Mehren M, Blanke CD, et al. Efficacy and safety of imatinib mesylate in advanced gastrointestinal stromal tumors. *N Engl J Med.* 2002;347(7):472–480. doi:10.1056/NEJMoa020461

22. Abbeele V, Gatsonis C, de Vries DJ, et al. ACRIN 6665/RTOG 0132 phase II trial of neoadjuvant imatinib mesylate for operable malignant gastrointestinal stromal tumor: monitoring with 18F-FDG PET and correlation with genotype and GLUT4 expression. *J Nucl Med.* 2012;53(4):567–574. doi:10.2967/jnumed.111.094425

23. Dematteo RP, Ballman KV, Antonescu CR, et al. Adjuvant imatinib mesylate after resection of localised, primary gastrointestinal stromal tumour: a randomised, double-blind, placebo-controlled trial. *Lancet.* 2009;373(9669):1097–1104. doi:10.1016/S0140-6736(09)60500-6

24. Joensuu H, Eriksson M, Hatrmann J, et al. Twelve versus 36 months of adjuvant imatinib (IM) as treatment of operable GIST with a high risk of recurrence: final results of a randomized trial (SSGXVIII/AIO). *J Clin Oncol.* 2011;29(18_suppl):LBA1–LBA1. doi:10.1200/jco.2011.29.18_suppl.lba1

25. Heinrich MC, Maki RG, Corless CL, et al. Primary and secondary kinase genotypes correlate with the biological and clinical activity of sunitinib in imatinib-resistant gastrointestinal stromal tumor. *J Clin Oncol.* 2008;26(33):5352–5359. doi:10.1200/JCO.2007.15.7461

26. Komatsu Y, Doi T, Sawaki A, et al. Regorafenib for advanced gastrointestinal stromal tumors following imatinib and sunitinib treatment: a subgroup analysis evaluating Japanese patients in the phase III GRID trial. *Int J Clin Oncol.* 2015;20(5):905–912. doi:10.1007/s10147-015-0790-y

27. DeMatteo RP, Ballman KV, Antonescu CR, et al. Long-term results of adjuvant imatinib mesylate in localized, high-risk, primary gastrointestinal stromal tumor: ACOSOG Z9000 (Alliance) intergroup phase 2 trial. *Ann Surg.* 2013;258(3):422–429. doi:10.1097/SLA.0b013e3182a15eb7

28. Casali PG, Le Cesne A, Velasco AP, et al. Time to definitive failure to the first tyrosine kinase inhibitor in localized GI stromal tumors treated with imatinib as an adjuvant: a European Organisation for Research and Treatment of Cancer Soft Tissue and Bone Sarcoma Group Intergroup Randomized Trial in Collaboration With the Australasian Gastro-Intestinal Trials Group, UNICANCER, French Sarcoma Group, Italian Sarcoma Group, and Spanish Group for Research on Sarcomas. *J Clin Oncol.* 2015;33(36):4276. doi:10.1200/JCO.2015.62.4304

29. Lin JX, Chen Q-F, Zheng C-H, et al. Is 3-years duration of adjuvant imatinib mesylate treatment sufficient for patients with high-risk gastrointestinal stromal tumor? a study based on long-term follow-up. *J Cancer Res Clin Oncol.* 2017;143(4):727–734. doi:10.1007/s00432-016-2334-x

30. Quek R, Farid M, Kanjanapan Y, et al. Prognostic significance of KIT exon 11 deletion mutation in intermediate-risk gastrointestinal stromal tumor. *Asia Pac J Clin Oncol.* 2014;13(3):115–124. doi:10.1111/ajco.12603

31. Singh AS, Chmielowski B, Hecht JR, et al. A randomized phase 2 study of nivolumab monotherapy versus nivolumab combined with ipilimumab in patients with metastatic or unresectable gastrointestinal stromal tumor (GIST). *J Clin Oncol.* 2018;36(4_suppl):55–55. doi:10.1200/jco.2018.36.4_suppl.55

32. Lv A, Li Z, Tian X, et al. SKP2 high expression, KIT exon 11 deletions, and gastrointestinal bleeding as predictors of poor prognosis in primary gastrointestinal stromal tumors. *PLoS One.* 2013;8(5):e62951. doi:10.1371/journal.pone.0062951

33. Mehren MV, George S, Heinrich MC, et al. Results of SARC 022, a phase II multicenter study of linsitinib in pediatric and adult wild-type (WT) gastrointestinal stromal tumors (GIST). *J Clin Oncol.* 2014;32(15_suppl):10507–10507. doi:10.1200/jco.2014.32.15_suppl.10507

34. Heinrich MC, von Mehren M, Demetri GD, et al. A phase 2 study of ponatinib in patients (pts) with advanced gastrointestinal stromal tumors (GIST) after failure of tyrosine kinase inhibitor (TKI) therapy: Initial report. *J Clin Oncol.* 2014;32(15_suppl):10506–10506. doi:10.1200/jco.2014.32.15_suppl.10506

35. Heinrich MC, Jones RL, von Mehren M, et al. Clinical activity of BLU-285 in advanced gastrointestinal stromal tumor (GIST). *J Clin Oncol.* 2017;35(15_suppl):11011–11011. doi:10.1200/jco.2017.35.15_suppl.11011

36. Janku F, Abdul Razak AR, Gordon MS, et al. Pharmacokinetic-driven phase I study of DCC-2618 a pan-KIT and PDGFR inhibitor in patients (pts) with gastrointestinal stromal tumor (GIST) and other solid tumors. *J Clin Oncol.* 2017;35(15_suppl):2515–2515. doi:10.1200/jco.2017.35.15_suppl.2515

37. Bertucci F, Finetti P, Mamessier E, et al. PDL1 expression is an independent prognostic factor in localized GIST. *Oncoimmunology.* 2015;4(5):e1002729. doi:10.1080/2162402X.2014.1002729

38. Toulmonde M, Penel N, Adam J, et al. Use of PD-1 targeting, macrophage infiltration, and IDO pathway activation in sarcomas: a phase 2 clinical trial. *JAMA Oncol.* 2018;4(1):93–97. doi:10.1001/jamaoncol.2017.1617

VI

Special Clinical Considerations for Gastrointestinal Cancer Patients

52

Nutritional Needs for Gastrointestinal Cancer Patients

Tiffany Barrett

NUTRITION

Patients with gastrointestinal cancer are at risk for malnutrition. This is due to both metabolic changes from the disease and side effects of cancer therapies. Inflammation, insulin resistance, increased protein catabolism, and anorexia are associated with cancer-related malnutrition. The metabolic changes in carbohydrates, lipids, and proteins are related to the tumor and inflammatory cytokines. Malnutrition leads to decreased wound healing, impaired immune response, reduced muscle strength, fatigue, impaired psychosocial function, reduced quality of life, and reduced response and tolerance to prescribed oncology treatment (1). Malnutrition during cancer is a result of increased nutrient requirements, inadequate intake, decreased gastrointestinal absorption, and impaired digestion of nutrients. Malnutrition has been demonstrated at 39% in hospital cancer patients. In addition, 55% had reduced oral food intake due to anorexia, loss of taste, nausea, pain, constipation, diarrhea, and abdominal pain (2). Nutrition risk is high in patients with gastrointestinal cancers, reducing their ability to tolerate treatment. Early symptoms can often be unclear leading to delayed diagnosis and nutrition decline. In a study of geriatric gastrointestinal cancer patients, 37.9% were malnourished and 34.6% at malnutrition risk at diagnosis. After chemotherapy, 46.4% were malnourished (3). Due to metabolic changes, cancer patients have elevated resting energy expenditure (REE). Cao et al. found elevated energy needs of cancer patients: 46.7% were hypermetabolic, 43.5% were normal metabolic, and 9.8% were hypometabolic (4). To maintain weight and prevent worsening malnutrition, nutrition intake needs to meet energy requirements (Table 52.1). Commonly used equations to estimate nutrient needs include: Harris–Benedict, Mifflin–St Jeor, Ireton-Jones, Penn State (critically ill), and kcal/kg (5,6).

Nutrition screening identifies patients who may have a malnutrition diagnosis and benefit from an assessment by a registered dietitian. Validated tools in oncology patients include the Malnutrition Screening Tool (MST), the Malnutrition Universal Screening Tool (MUST), Patient-Generated Subjective Global Assessment (PG-SGA), and Subjective Global Assessment.

In 2009, the American Society for Parenteral and Enteral Nutrition (ASPEN) and the Academy of Nutrition and Dietetics developed a workgroup to standardize an approach to the diagnosis of malnutrition. The identification of two or more of the six characteristics is recommended for diagnosis of either severe or nonsevere malnutrition: weight loss, insufficient energy intake, loss of muscle mass, loss of body fat, fluid accumulation, and diminished functional status as measured by hand grip strength. When calculating BMI height and weight should be measured and not estimated (7).

NUTRIENT ABSORPTION

The gastrointestinal tract is essential to digest food to provide macronutrients and micronutrients. Normal gut function can be affected at diagnosis but surgical treatment, radiation, and chemotherapy can further impact digestion and absorption (Table 52.2) (8).

TABLE 52.1 Energy and Protein Needs in Gastrointestinal Cancer

Nutrient	Nutrition Assessment
Energy	30–35 kcal/kg cancer repletion 35 kcal/kg hypermetabolic
Protein (with normal renal function)	1–1.5 grams/kg bodyweight
Fluid needs	1 mL fluid per 1 kcal of estimated energy needs Based on bodyweight, 20–40 mL/kg/day

Source: From Hamilton KK. Oncology nutrition for clinical practice: nutritional needs of the adult oncology patient. Oncology Nutrition Dietetic Practice Group of the Academy of Nutrition and Dietetics; 2013;33–40.

COLORECTAL CANCER

Treatment for colorectal cancer typically involves surgery, chemotherapy, radiation, or immunotherapy. Side effects leading to changes in appetite and weight loss include diarrhea, nausea, vomiting, mucositis, taste changes, and fatigue. Miyamoto et al. evaluated the association of skeletal muscle mass loss during chemotherapy. Progression-free survival and overall free survival were better in patients without skeletal muscle loss (9). Decreased skeletal muscle mass (sarcopenia) was found in 71% of colorectal patients and grade 3 to 4 chemotherapy toxicities (10). Loss of lean body mass affects treatment tolerance. Postoperative complications can be associated with reduced muscle mass and a diagnosis of malnutrition (11). During surgery, an opening of the small or large intestine called a stoma is performed. Absorption of fluid and nutrients depends on the ostomy location (ileostomy or colostomy) and amount of colon removed. During the first 6 to 8 weeks after surgery, patients need to avoid high-fiber foods. It is advised to introduce new foods one at a time to assess tolerance and changes in stool. Monitor increase in gas production or bloating as lactose and/or fat intolerance should be determined. Patients should be encouraged to drink an additional 1 L more than their output daily (12).

Pancreatic Cancer

Malnutrition is common due to the wide variety of symptoms. At diagnosis of pancreatic cancer, 80% present with weight loss (13). Nemer et al. found weight loss at diagnosis present in 71.5% of patients. Weight loss also correlated with a longer duration of symptoms (14). A nutrition assessment is important to determine current symptoms that are impacting nutrition status and assist with diagnosis with exocrine and endocrine pancreatic insufficiency. The prevalence of exocrine pancreatic insufficiency is estimated greater than 50% with locally advanced or metastatic pancreatic cancer (15). Pancreatic enzyme replacement was recommended to patients with weight and without weight loss, 39.8% and 31.4%, respectively (14). Surgery, chemotherapy, and radiation increase pancreatic insufficiency prevalence. Symptoms

TABLE 52.2 GI Tract Absorption

GI Tract Location	Nutrients
Stomach	Water, copper, iodide, fluoride, molybdenum
Duodenum	Biotin, calcium, copper, folate, iron, magnesium, niacin, phosphorus, selenium, thiamin, vitamins A, D, E, K
Ileum	Folate, magnesium, vitamins C, D, K, B_{12}, bile salts
Jejunum	Amino acids, biotin, calcium, chromium, folate, iron, lipids, magnesium, manganese, molybdenum, monosaccharides, niacin, pantothenate, phosphorus, riboflavin, thiamin, vitamins B6, C, D, E, K
Large intestine	Biotin, chloride, potassium, short-chain fatty acids, sodium, water, vitamin K

GI, gastrointestinal.

Source: From Gropper S, Smith JL. *Advanced nutrition and metabolism.* Boston, MA: Wadsworth Cengage Learning; 2012.

of exocrine pancreatic insufficiency include steatorrhea, malnutrition, and weight loss. A small study demonstrated pancreatic enzyme replacement therapy during 16 weeks of chemotherapy improved nutrition status (16). Another recent small study found pancreatic patients with increased energy expenditure and decreased intestinal absorption. The measured REE was 33% higher when compared to predicted calculations (17). Tests to diagnose pancreatic exocrine insufficiency include fecal elastase, 13C mixed triglyceride breath test, fecal fat excretion, and fecal chymotrypsin level (18). However, pancreatic insufficiency is more often diagnosed based on symptoms: bloating, fatty stools, excessive gas, foul smelling stools or gas, floating stools, indigestion, and unexplained weight loss (19). Patients can be underdiagnosed and undertreated leading to worsening malnutrition. Pancreatic enzyme replacement therapy is the primary treatment and individually dosed. Dosage is started low and titrated up based on symptoms, stool output, and fat content of meals. Enzyme is taken at the start of a meal and continued throughout the meal. Appropriate dosing plays a critical role in improving bowel function and quality of life (18). Micronutrient deficiency studies are limited in this population long term. Daily intake of micronutrients should be evaluated with a protocol in place for repletion (20).

Hepatocellular Carcinoma

Patients diagnosed with hepatocellular cancer are at an increased risk for malnutrition. Decline in nutrition is caused by decreased nutrient intake but also impaired liver function. The liver is involved with metabolism of nutrients, and these patients often suffer from hepatitis and liver cirrhosis. Malnutrition is associated with mortality and reduced quality of life, and tumor progression and tumor-directed therapies may further worsen liver function (21,22). Patients suffer from anorexia, weight loss, lean muscle wasting, anemia, fluid overload, and impaired albumin synthesis (23). The REE is increased in this population, and patients should follow a high energy, high protein diet. Guidelines suggest daily energy intakes of 35 to 40 kcal/kg and optimal protein intakes of 1.2 to 1.5 g/kg of ideal bodyweight (24). The source of protein and timing of consuming protein during the day need to be addressed when assessing these patients. It has been observed that branched-chain amino acids (BCAAs) improve liver function and have the potential to improve overall survival (25). BCAAs have been found to be effective in reducing ascites and elevating albumin levels (26,27). Additional nutrition studies in this population are warranted.

GASTRIC CANCER

Common symptoms of gastric cancer are early satiety, heartburn, abdominal pain, nausea, and vomiting. There is a high prevalence of malnutrition prior to surgery but nutrition support preoperatively for 10 days was associated with reduced surgical site infections. In this study, patients were provided ≥25 kcal/kg ideal bodyweight per day (28). After partial or total gastrectomy, a diet of small frequent meals and reducing intake of simple carbohydrates are recommended. When oral intake is insufficient, enteral tube feeding is provided to meet nutrient needs. Nutrition deficiencies are common after gastric surgery: anemia, vitamin B_{12}, vitamin A, vitamin D, and vitamin E. Following a total gastrectomy, anemia develops in 50% of patients. Vitamin and mineral deficiencies need to be monitored and replenished based on tested blood levels. It is recommended to have a protocol in place to prevent such deficiencies, which can have long-term consequences (29,30).

Esophageal Cancer

Weight loss before the start of treatment has been shown to occur in up to 74% of patients and during treatment in 40% to 57% (31). A retrospective study of esophageal patients treated with chemotherapy or radiation found a decline in weight loss of 3.5% (32). Dysphagia and weight loss associated with diagnosis will continue to worsen during neoadjuvant therapy (chemotherapy alone or concurrent with radiation). In patients hospitalized with dysphagia, placement of feeding tubes is the most common intervention (33). Prior to the initiation of neoadjuvant therapy, nutrition therapy restores normal swallowing, maintains weight, and may prevent feeding tube placement. Patients were provided an individualized plan as determined by a specialized upper gastrointestinal cancer nutritionist. Of the 130 patients treated, 78 reported dysphagia at baseline. Weight did not significantly change after one cycle of chemotherapy. Intense nutrition support prior to and during treatment assisted with resuming oral intake (34).

Rare Gastrointestinal Cancers

As with other gastrointestinal cancers, side effects are often increased when therapies are combined. Common symptoms include anorexia, nausea, vomiting, pain, taste aversions, and changes in bowels resulting in unintentional weight loss. Neuroendocrine tumors are rare, but their symptoms of diarrhea, steatorrhea, weight loss, and vitamin deficiencies result in malnutrition. A thorough assessment by a specialist dietitian working with a multidisciplinary team is recommended.

Perioperative Nutrition

Enhanced Recovery After Surgery (ERAS) guidelines are protocols to achieve early recovery after surgery. Nutrition protocols include limiting pre-operative fasting, oral carbohydrate load, and early initiation of oral or enteral nutrition postoperatively. The strongest evidence exists for colon and rectal surgeries (35). ERAS patients provided an oral nutrition supplement had reduced length of stay and complications. Protein intakes were higher in the ERAS group but lower in the subjects with extreme nausea (36). Education by a dietitian is an important tool to increase energy and protein intake.

Immunonutrition including omega-3 fatty acids, glutamine, and arginine has gained interest following gastrointestinal surgery. The benefits of immune enhancing enteral nutrition have been reviewed in a meta-analysis of upper gastrointestinal surgery. When immunonutrition was administered postoperatively, wound infection and length of stay were reduced (37). Cheng et al. performed a review of seven studies with gastric cancer diagnosis. Reduced postoperative complications, enhanced immune function, and inflammatory response were found in the immunonutrition elemental subjects (38). Immunonutrients also have the potential to reduce infections in the preoperative setting when combined postoperatively (39,40). A combination of ERAS and immunonutrients was also shown to have reduced infections and complications

TABLE 52.3 Medical Nutrition Therapy for Gastrointestinal Cancer

Complication/Issue	Nutrition Intervention
Dumping syndrome	Small frequent meals Increase soluble fiber Limit liquids with meals High protein, complex carbohydrates Pancreatic enzymes
Reflux	Avoid high fat meals Small volume at meals Moist, soft foods Add high calorie, protein foods
Anorexia	Protein source at every small meal Sip on small amount of fluids during meals Smoothies, protein shakes
Nausea/Vomiting	Bland, soft easy-to-digest foods Small meals on a schedule Consume foods and liquids at room temperature Avoid strong food odor Sip on liquids during meals Talk to medical team about medications
Mucositis	Soft and tender cooked foods Moisten foods with broth, sauces, oil, yogurt Foods at room temperature Good mouth care with baking soda mixture, avoid alcohol-based mouthwash Use a straw, suck on ice chips Avoid citrus, spicy foods
Enteral or parenteral nutrition	If oral food intake is inadequate orally, enteral preferred

Source: From National Cancer Institute at the National Institutes of Health, March 16th 2018.

following colorectal surgery (41). Further studies in the gastric population and other gastrointestinal surgeries are needed.

SUMMARY

Gastrointestinal cancer patients should be followed by a multidisciplinary team including nutrition therapy, followed closely by a nutrition expert. Individual dietary counseling by a dietitian improved both energy and protein intake in patients with gastric and esophageal cancer. Subjects in the intervention group lost less weight during the treatment period (42). Assessment by a registered dietitian includes patient history, laboratory values, prior and current weight changes, diet history, and symptoms. Provide intervention to meet nutrient needs with changes in food intake and adding supplements of alternate forms of nutrition (Table 52.3) (43).

REFERENCES

1. Barker LA, Gout BS, Crowe TC. Hospital malnutrition: prevalence, identification and impact on patients and the healthcare system. *Int J Environ Res Public Health*. 2011;8(2):514–527. doi:10.3390/ijerph8020514
2. Hebuterne X, Lemarie E, Michallet M, et al. Prevalence of malnutrition and current use of nutrition support in patients with cancer. *J Parenter Enteral Nutr*. 2014;38(2):196–204. doi:10.1177/0148607113502674
3. Bicakli DH, Ozveren A, Uslu R, et al. The effect of chemotherapy on nutritional status and weakness in geriatric gastrointestinal system cancer patients. *Nutrition*. 2018;47:39–42. doi:10.1016/j.nut.2017.09.013
4. Cao D, Wu G, Zhang B, et al. Resting energy expenditure and body composition in patients with newly detected cancer. *Clin Nutr*. 2010;29(1):72–77. doi:10.1016/j.clnu.2009.07.001
5. Academy of Nutrition and Dietetics, Evidence Anaylsis Library; 2014. www.andeal.org
6. Hamilton KK. Oncology Nutrition for Clinical Practice: Nutritional Needs of the Adult Oncology Patient. Oncology Nutrition Dietetic Practice Group of the Academy of Nutrition and Dietetics; 2013:33–40.
7. White JV, Guenter P, Jensen G, et al. Consensus statement: Academy of Nutrition and Dietetics and American Society for Parenteral and Enteral Nutrition: characteristics recommended for the identification and documentation of adult malnutrition (undernutrition). *J Parenter Enteral Nutr*. 2012;36(3):275–283. doi:10.1177/0148607112440285
8. Gropper S, Smith JL. *Advanced nutrition and metabolism*. Boston, MA: Wadsworth Cengage Learning; 2012.
9. Miyamoto Y, Baba Y, Sakamoto Y, et al. Negative impact of skeletal muscle mass after systemic chemotherapy in patients with unresectable colorectal cancer. *Plos One*. 2015;10(6):e0129742. doi:10.1371/journal.pone.0129742
10. Barret M, Antoun S, Dalban C, et al. Sarcopenia is linked to treatment toxicity in patients with metastatic colorectal cancer. *Nutr Cancer*. 2014;66(4):583–589. doi:10.1080/01635581.2014.894103
11. Maurico SF, Xiao J, Prado CM, et al. Different nutritional assessment tools as predictors of postoperative complications in patients undergoing colorectal cancer resection'. *Clin Nutr*. 2018;37(5):1505–1511. doi:10.1016/j.clnu.2017.08.026
12. United Ostomy Associations of America; n.d. https://www.ostomy.org
13. Olson S, Xu Y, Herzog K, et al. Weight loss, diabetes, fatigue, and depression preceding pancreatic cancer. *Pancreas*. 2016;45(7):986–991.doi:10.1097/MPA.00000000000000590
14. Nemer L, Krishna SG, Shah ZK, et al. Predictors of pancreatic cancer-associated weight loss and nutritional interventions. *Pancreas*. 2017;46(9):1152–1157. doi:10.1097/MPA.0000000000000898
15. Laquente B, Calsina-Berna A, Carmona-Bayonas A, et al. Supportive care in pancreatic ductal adenocarcinoma. *Clin Tranl Oncol*. 2017;19(11):1293–1302. doi:10.1007/s12094-017-1682-6
16. Saito T, Hirano K, Isayama H, et al. The role of pancreatic enzyme replacement therapy in unresectable pancreatic cancer. *Pancreas*. 2017;46(3):341–346. doi:10.1097/MPA.0000000000000767
17. Nierop JW-v, Lochtenberg-Potjess C, Wierdsma N, et al. Assessment of nutritional status, digestion and absorption, and quality of life in patients with locally advanced pancreatic cancer. *Gastroenterol Res Pract*. 2017;2017:1–7. doi:10.1155/2017/6193765
18. Sabater L, Ausania F, Bakker O. Evidence based guidelines for the management of exocrine pancreatic insufficiency after pancreatic surgery. *Ann Surg*. 2016;264(6):949–958. doi:10.1097/SLA.0000000000001732

19. Lindkvist B, Phillips M, Dominguez-Munoz J. Clinical, anthropometric and laboratory nutritional markers of pancreatic exocrine insufficiency: prevelance and diagnostic use. *Pancreatology*. 2015;15(6):589–597. doi:10.1016/j.pan.2015.07.001

20. Petzel MQ, Hoffman L. Nutrition implications for long-term survivors of pancreatic cancer surgery. *Nutr Clin Pract*. 2017;32(5):588–598. doi:10.1177/0884533617722929

21. Hsu W, Tsai A, Chan S-C, et al. Mini-nutritional assessment predicts functional status and quality of life of patients with hepatocellular carcinoma in Taiwan. *Nutr Cancer*. 2012;64(4):543–549. doi:10.1080/01635581.2012.675620

22. Montano-Loza AJ, Duarte-Rojo A, Meza-Junco J, et al. Inclusion of Sarcopenia within MELD (MELD-sarcopenia) and the prediction of mortality in patients with cirrhosis. *Clin Transl Gastroenterol*. 2015;6:102. doi:10.1038/ctg.2015.31

23. Plauth M, Cabré E, Riggio O, et al. ESPEN guidelines on enteral nutrition: liver disease. *Clin Nutr*. 2006;25(2):285–294. doi:10.1016/j.clnu.2006.01.018

24. Amodio P, Bemeur C, Butterworth R, et al. The nutritional management of hepatic encephalopathy in patients with cirrhosis: International society for hepatic encephalopathy and nitrogen metabolism consensus. *Hepatalogy*. 2013;58(1):325–336. doi:10.1002/hep.26370

25. Nojiri S, Fujiwara K, Shinkai N, et al. Effects of branched-chain amino acid supplementation after radiofrequency ablation for hepatocellular carcinoma: a randomized trial. *Nutrition*. 2017;33:20–27. doi:10.1016/j.nut.2016.07.013

26. Kikuchi Y, Hiroshima Y, Matsuo K, et al. A randomized clinical trial of preoperative administration of branched-chain amino acids to prevent postoperative ascites in patients with liver resection for hepatocellular carcinoma. *Ann Surg Onc*. 2016;23:3727–3735. doi:10.1245/s10434-016-5348-3

27. Schütte K, Tippelt B, Schulz C, et al. Malnutrition is a prognostic factor in patients with hepatocellular carcinoma (HCC). *Clin Nutr*. 2015;34:1122–1127. doi:10.1016/j.clnu.2014.11.007

28. Fukuda Y, Yamamoto K, Hirao M, et al. Prevelance of malnutrition among gastric cancer patients undergoing gastrectomy and optimal preoperative nutrition al support for preventing surgical site infections. *Ann Surg Oncol*. 2015;22:S778–S785. doi:10.1245/s10434-015-4820-9

29. Rino Y, Oshima T, Yoshikawa T. Changes in fat soluble vitamin levels after gastrectomy for gastric cancer. *Surg Today*. 2017;47:145–150. doi:10.1007/s00595-016-1341-5

30. Hu Y, Kim H-I, Hyung WJ, et al. Vitamin B12 deficiency after Gastrectomy for gastric cancer. *Ann Surg*. 2013;258(6):970–975. doi:10.1097/SLA.0000000000000214

31. Rietveld SC, Nierop JW-v, Ottens-Oussoren K, et al. The prediction of deterioration of nutritional status during chemoradiation therapy in patients with esophageal cancer. *Nutr Cancer*. 2018;70:229–235. doi:10.1080/01635581.2018.1412481

32. Mak M, Bell K, Ng W, et al. Nutritional status, management and clinical outcomes in patients with esophageal and gastro-oesophageal cancers: a descriptive study. *Nutr Diet*. 2017;74:229–235. doi:10.1111/1747-0080.12306

33. Modi RM, Mikhail S, Ciombor K, et al. Outcomes of nutritional interventions to treat dysphagia in esophageal cancer: a population based study. *Dis Esophagus*. 2017;30(11):1–8. doi:10.1093/dote/dox101

34. Cools-Lartigue J, Jones D, Spicer J, et al. Management of dysphagia in esophageal adenocarcinoma patients undergoing neoadjuvant chemotherapy: can invasive tube feeding be avoided? *Ann Surg Oncol*. 2015;22:1858–1865. doi:10.1245/s10434-014-4270-9

35. Sandrucci S, Beets G, Braga M, et al. Perioperative nutrition and enhanced recovery after surgery in gastrointestinal cancer patients. A position paper by the ESSO task force in collaboration with the ERAS society (ERAS coalition). *Eur J Clin Oncol*. 2018;44:509–514. doi:10.1016/j.ejso.2017.12.010

36. Yeung S, Hilkewich L, Gillis C, et al. Protein intakes are associated with reduced length stay: a comparison of Enhanced Recovery After Surgery (ERAS) and conventional care after elective colorectal surgery. *Am J Clin Nutr*. 2017;106(1):44–51. doi:10.3945/ajcn.116.148619

37. Wong CS, Aly EH. The effects of enteral immunonutrition in upper gastrointestinal surgery: a systematic review and meta-analysis. *Int J Surg*. 2016;29:137–150. doi:10.1016/j.ijsu.2016.03.043

38. Cheng Y, Zhang J, Zhang L, et al. Enteral immunonutrition versus enteral nutrition for gastric cancer patients undergoing a total gastrectomy: a systematic review and meta-analysis. *BMC Gastroenterol*. 2018;18(1):11. doi:10.1186/s12876-018-0741-y

39. Osland E, Hossain M, Khan S, et al. Effect of timing of pharmaconutrition (immunonutrition) administration on outcomes of elective surgery for gastrointestinal malignancies: a systematic review and meta-analysis. *J Parenter Enter Nutr*. 2014;38:53–69. doi:10.1177/0148607112474825

40. Song GM, Tian X, Zhang L, et al. Immunonutrition support for patients undergoing surgery for gastrointestinal malignancy: preoperative, postoperative, or perioperative? A Bayesian network meta-analysis of randomized controlled trials. *Medicine*. 2015;94:1225. doi:10.1097/MD.0000000000001225

41. Moya P, Soriano-Irigaray L, Ramirez JM, et al. Perioperative Standard oral nutrition supplements versus immunonutrition in patients undergoing colorectal resection in an Enhanced Recovery (ERAS) protocol: a multicenter randomized clinical trial (SONVI Study). *Medicine*. 2016;95:3704. doi:10.1097/MD.0000000000003704
42. Poulsen GM, Pedersen LL, Osterlind K, et al. Randomized trial of the effects of individual nutritional counseling in cancer patients. *Clin Nutr*. 2014;33:749–753. doi:10.1016/j.clnu.2013.10.019
43. National Cancer Institute at the National Institutes of Health, March 16th 2018

Palliative Care for Gastrointestinal Cancer Patients

Kimberly Angelia Curseen

PALLIATIVE CARE

Palliative care is defined by the Center for Advancement of Palliative Care as follows:

> Specialized medical care for people with serious illness. This type of care is focused on providing relief from the symptoms and stress of a serious illness. The goal is to improve quality of life for both the patient and the family. Palliative care is provided by a specially trained team of doctors, nurses, and other specialists who work together with a patient's other doctors to provide an extra layer of support. It is appropriate at any age and at any stage in a serious illness, and it can be provided along with curative treatment (1).

Palliative care is whole person care that manages patients as multidimensional beings addressing physical, psychological, and spiritual distress to improve patient quality of life, improve clinical outcomes, and assist patients in reaching their clinical goals. There is a growing body of literature that recognizes the importance of incorporating palliative care in the management of patients with cancer (2). The ideal model is the early integration of palliative care into the oncology clinical model. Early integration of palliative care allows for anticipatory symptom management, prevention of suffering, as well as improved communication concerning patient goals of care, treatment preferences, and prognosis (3). The American Society of Clinical Oncology (ASCO) has supported the integration of early palliative care in patients with advanced cancer and high symptom burden. In 2016, ASCO partnering with the American Academy of Hospice and Palliative Medicine published guidance on what qualifies as the *high-quality palliative care* that should be delivered in oncology practices. The recommendations were developed by consensus with a group of interprofessional clinical experts using a modified Delphi methodology. The group identified nine domains that should be addressed in patient care when delivering palliative care for patients with cancer. They are listed as follows:

1. Symptom assessment and management
2. Psychosocial assessment and management
3. Spiritual and cultural assessment and management
4. Communication and shared decision making
5. Advanced care planning
6. Coordination and continuity of care
7. Appropriate palliative care and hospice referrals
8. Caregiver support
9. End-of-life (EOL) care (4)

The goal is for oncology practices to address these domains with patients and provide primary palliative care. Oncology should also have access to dedicated palliative care teams for consultation to address these domains for patients with advanced cancer and high symptom burden. During a palliative care consultation, patients are evaluated by an interprofessional team that focuses on aggressive physical, spiritual, and emotional symptom management. Palliative care consultation teams are available to both inpatients and outpatients. The team is usually composed of a clinical provider with expertise in symptom management and communication; social work; nursing; and a spiritual health clinician. Palliative care services are not a substitute for the patient's primary management team, but they are collaborative support for the patient, the family, and the treatment team (2,4).

There is a growing body of research in multiple cancers and other chronic conditions showing the benefit of early palliative care intervention. In January 2017, ASCO published clinical practice guidelines that recommended particularly, patients with advanced cancer and high symptom burden be specifically referred to dedicated interdisciplinary palliative care consultation teams. It also stressed the importance of oncology and palliative care team collaboration in providing patients with the best patient-centered care. The recommendations also included that patients with advanced cancer receive palliative care consultation within 8 weeks of diagnosis (2,5). This recommendation came from one of the sentinel studies in palliative care in which patients with non–small cell lung cancer were randomized to an early outpatient palliative care intervention versus standard clinical oncology care. The early intervention group showed improved quality of life and depression scores. In addition, patients in the early intervention group had less aggressive interventions of EOL. Also the palliative care, early intervention group showed a 2.7-month survival versus the standard oncology practice group (6). In the ENABLE III trial, the goal was to identify the optimal time to enroll patients in early palliative care versus delayed palliative care. The study did not find significant differences in quality-of-life scores. However, the early intervention group did show a 15% survival benefit after 1 year. The patient mix consisted of advance stage solid tumor or hematologic malignancy with a prognosis of 6 to 24 months (7). In a study evaluating the effects of early integration of palliative care in lung and gastrointestinal cancers, the randomized clinical controlled trial showed that patients with gastrointestinal cancers had improvements in mood as well as quality of life with early palliative care interventions within the first 12 weeks of the intervention. However, unlike lung cancer, this benefit did not appear to sustain within 3 months prior to death. If their conditions were terminal, they were more likely to communicate their concerns and wishes around EOL to their oncology team (5).

In the Cochran review, it was found that early palliative interventions showed benefit in symptom management and improved quality of life for patients with advanced cancer, although the effect size found was small at the time of the analysis (8). There is a study that shows that patients who receive education on palliative care early in their diagnosis are more willing to attend and want outpatient palliative care appointments. Some programs have developed palliative care triggers using distress scales to ensure that patients are screened properly and routed to palliative care services as the standard of care. For cancer institutions and clinical practices that lack access to on-site palliative care teams, there is ongoing research to evaluate the efficacy of virtual support, which can include telemedicine and telephone evaluations (2). Also, there is an increasing trend toward the development of in-home palliative care programs that fill in the gaps for patients who have limited access to transportation and palliative care services. These palliative care services also serve as a bridge to hospice care as well as support for patients who are undergoing aggressive interventions but have significant debility. Early integration of palliative care in newly diagnosed gastrointestinal and lung cancer also improves psychological symptoms and experience for caregivers (9). Although it is ideal to have independent palliative care teams, whether embedded or freestanding, there are not enough palliative specialists to meet the demand currently and likely in the future. It is important for all clinical specialists to have skills in primary palliative care, which includes training in rudimentary symptom management, communication, and advance care planning. Studies have shown that hematology/oncology fellows are open to this training and see clinical competency in this area as important to practicing patient care (10,11). Palliative care consultation should not be limited, however, to patients receiving only palliative therapy. Patients with curative intent can receive benefit from the support palliative care provides as well as aggressive symptom management to help them and their family cope during and after treatments.

HOSPICE

Palliative care is different from hospice care. *All hospice care is palliative care, but not all palliative care is hospice.* Hospice is the medical service that manages the palliative care needs of patients who are at the EOL and who have a life expectancy of less than 6 months. Patients and family usually elect hospice services when the decision has been made to forego curative therapy and aggressive life prolonging interventions. The goals shift to focusing primarily on the management of symptoms of their illness. Hospice service traditionally provides care, using Medicare benefit as the example, as given in Table 53.1.

TABLE 53.1 Medicare Hospice Benefit

1. Routine nursing care and assessment and emergent evaluations accessible 24 hours a day
2. Social work and spiritual health clinician support
3. Certified nursing assistants to assist with personal care needs
4. Durable medical equipment and medications related to the hospice diagnosis
5. 13 months of bereavement for family and caregivers, which may be important in family grieving and recovery

Hospices are delivered through independent agencies, which function similarly according to Medicare rules, but there are nuanced differences in agencies that may dictate what services outside of the basic requirements they provide. Hospice uses interprofessional teams to deliver EOL care. Hospice care can reduce the cost in the last year of life for patients. For Medicare beneficiaries, costs for patients newly enrolled in hospice and nonhospice programs were not significantly different. However, after hospice began, it was noted that the total cost of the last year of life significantly decreased in the hospice group by approximately $8,700 dollars. Hospice can also lower the patients'/caregivers' out-of-pocket cost reducing the financial burden on families (12).

It is important when referring to a hospice agency to have the referral include the goals of care and special requirements that may be unique to the patient's comfort. For example, routinely hospices have not provided intravenous (IV) fluid or total parental nutrition. However, for some patients these measures may be important to help them reach a well-defined goal. It is agreed that these interventions will not significantly prolong their lives and will eventually have to be discontinued, secondary to medical reasons. However, with clear explanations of how the proposed interventions will benefit patients in the short term, some hospices may be open to what is considered to be more traditional aggressive therapy.

There is research supporting the use of interprofessional team members, including RN case managers and social workers to assist patients and families with decision making and transition to hospice care. There is a higher rate of transition to hospice versus just being counseled by the physician alone. Also, outpatient palliative care consults can be helpful with explaining the details of hospice services to the patients within the proper context (13).

COMMUNICATION

Palliative care consultants are trained in communication techniques to help counsel patients concerning their prognosis, goals of care, and existential distress they may be experiencing through the course of their illness. Dedicated palliative care teams focus on building relationships with patients and families, assisting with exploring the understanding of prognosis as well as clarification of goals, care coordination with other providers, and assessment of coping, in addition to primary symptom management. Effective communication has several benefits not only for patients but also for the healthcare system. A study showed that palliative care consultation that focused on advance care planning and patient and family coping with illness and treatment decisions resulted in improved quality of life for patients, improved depression scores, and hospitalizations, as well as a decreased rate of chemotherapy initiation within 2 weeks prior to death. Discussions about advance care planning also correlated with increased use of hospice in these patients (14). In the age of immunotherapy, palliative care consultants are being trained to address prognosis, symptom management, and disease trajectory for patients who are using these agents.

Palliative care uses several structured communication techniques that improve communication between patient/family and clinical providers. The use of structured communication techniques can improve patient satisfaction, understanding of prognosis, quality of life, and can have a positive impact on clinical outcomes. The use of structured communication techniques is not limited to palliative care providers; other specialists can use it to improve patient communication.

There are several validated techniques for patient communication. One of the standard tools is the SPIKES protocol. The SPIKES protocol stands for: (a) **Setting**: identify a comfortable setting for patient and family; (b) **Perception**: identify what a patient/family understands; (c) **Invitation**: identify how much a patient wants to know; (d) **Knowledge**: share information the patient wishes and needs to know about any medical decision; (e) **Empathy**: identify emotions and respond to empathically to the patient's feelings; (f) **Summary**: provide a summary of the information discussed and identify the need for a follow-up meeting (15). A study shows that using the SPIKES protocol to have difficult family discussions and to relay difficult news has the effect of strengthening the doctor–patient relationship and maintaining the quality of the relationship. Structured communication techniques are skills that can be taught to trainees and other clinical providers to improve their communication outcomes with their patients (16). OncoTalk is communication training specifically for oncologists to develop and improve communication skills (17). As part of their education, palliative care clinicians and interprofessional team members receive training in cultural competency and cultural humility. Cultural humility is self-reflection and emotional/intellectual curiosity concerning others and their cultural identity and experience. This concept goes beyond cultural competency and may be a more effective tool in communication with patients and families at the EOL. Cultural humility is an essential tool that is required to communicate with diverse patient populations. Treatment plans and advance care plans have increased success when they fit into the construct of a patient's culture and personal value system (18). For patients who are open to knowing, discussion of patient prognosis has been shown in several studies to improve patient understanding of illness (19). A multicenter observational study of greater than 500 patients with solid tumors found that prognostic discussions lead to patients having a more realistic understanding of their life expectancy without adversely affecting the doctor–patient relationship. These discussions in this study did not increase depression or anxiety in patients routinely (20). Discussion of prognosis should be routinely integrated into clinical care. This information is not intended to be forced on patients who have expressed a desire to not discuss it, but patients should be offered the opportunity to have frank discussions concerning prognosis. The literature also showed that patients want prognosis to be given in a nonbiased way. They do not want information to be delivered in an overly optimistic or pessimistic manner, but they do want the information delivered with empathy. They also want the information given without the use of medical jargon and be given the opportunity to ask questions and have subsequent discussions (21).

ADVANCE CARE PLANNING

Advance care planning is a very important component of providing adequate palliative care. Advance care planning should be tailored to the patient's communication style, willingness to discuss a plan, prognosis, disease, and clinical needs. Advance care planning not only includes assisting the patients with developing a living will, which usually consists of treatment preferences in the case of advanced/terminal and irreversible illness and identification of healthcare proxies but also facilitating conversations between patients and their surrogate decision makers. Advance care planning uses the model of shared decision making between patients and their healthcare providers, and the process is designed to be patient centered (22). Advance care planning should start early for patients who have terminal illness. The ideal is to have these conversations develop over time to allow patients a chance to consider their choices carefully. Also, advance care planning is dynamic and not static. As a patient's clinical situation changes, his or her treatment preferences may change. Advance care planning should be readdressed routinely as patients progress through their illness. Depending on the geographical location of the patients, there can be variations in standard advance care planning forms. It is important to collaborate with social work and/or palliative care to assist patients with planning. A study showed that there was a greater rate of advanced directive completion if facilitated by a nonphysician member of the team (23). For patients who have a prognosis of less than a year, many states will have a variation of *physician orders for life-sustaining treatment* (POLST) forms. These forms are designed to serve as medical orders that can be carried out during a serious illness when patients are unable to speak for themselves. These orders are meant to be portable between institutions and to be honored by medical staff. Another purpose, however, is to facilitate conversations concerning treatment preferences of patients with terminal illness between patients, their healthcare providers, and/or surrogate decision makers. POLST must be established in states by legislation and, in 2018, 49 states have endorsed or developed POLST programs. Standard POLST forms address: (a) determination of code status and mechanical ventilation preferences; (b) treatment preferences concerning medical treatment and hospitalization; (c) treatment preferences concerning artificial nutrition and hydration; and (d) other elements that may include preferences concerning antibiotics and other life-sustaining treatments (24).

These forms are designed to be reviewed annually to assess that they are still representative of a patient's treatment preferences and that the forms are still appropriate based on the patient's clinical progress. The POLST form promotes clarification of treatment preferences at the EOL and facilitates what can be difficult discussions concerning code status (25). It has been studied widely that patients and families have misconceptions concerning resuscitation rates and outcomes and overestimate chance of survival and functional recovery (26–28). A study evaluating in-hospital cardiac resuscitation rates showed that patients with advanced cancer had lower multivariable-adjusted rates of return of spontaneous circulation 52.3% versus 56.6% in noncancer patients but survival to discharge for these groups was 7.4% versus 13.4% in the noncancer group. POLST discussions can allow for an opportunity to explain not only resuscitation statistics, but also discuss outcomes in the context of patient goals (29).

There can be concerns among clinical practitioners that addressing advance care planning and goals of care may cause patients to lose hope. However, several studies have shown advanced care planning and goals of care discussions do not routinely cause patients to lose hope. A study evaluating an online advance care planning tool for patients with cancer resulted in greater satisfaction with the advanced care planning process, and improved self-determination. This study also showed that there was no increase in hopelessness or anxiety (30). In a systematic review of advanced care planning, it showed that it improves compliance with patient's EOL wishes, increases hospice use, and decreases aggressive medical interventions and hospitalizations at the EOL (14,31).

A significant part of advanced care planning is an assessment of a patient's understanding of his or her prognosis and clinic condition. In a study of patients with gastrointestinal malignancies admitted to the hospital with malignant bowel obstructions, most patients understood that they had advanced cancer, but only 39% of patients in the study acknowledge or understood their poor prognosis and that they may no longer be chemotherapy candidates (32). Palliative care consultation can assist patients and families with advance care planning within the framework of the patient's prognosis and diagnosis. Using the interdisciplinary team allows information to be framed in a variety of models, which may help patient and family understanding, subsequently leading to improved advanced care planning. Identification of patient preferences can save the cost of medical interventions that are not congruent with patient goals or would add to a patient's quality of life. One primary drive of cost is unnecessary hospitalizations (12,32,33).

EOL CARE

EOL care is defined as the intensive medical care that a patient receives prior to death. This care focuses on aggressive symptom management and emotional/spiritual support of patients and families. During the active dying process, patients may develop high symptom burden, which includes dyspnea, depression, terminal delirium, pain, and nausea. Also, there can be significant emotional and spiritual distress. The role of palliative care at the EOL is using the expertise of trained interprofessional team members (physician, spiritual health clinician, and counselor) to mitigate the suffering from some uncontrolled symptoms. Partnering with palliative care and ideally with a hospice can improve a patient's EOL care outcomes as well as outcomes for the patient's caregiver and family (3). The discussion concerning artificial nutrition and hydration can be particularly difficult in gastrointestinal malignancies. A study evaluating the attitudes and preferences of patients and caregivers with advanced cancer towards artificial nutrition and hydration showed that patients were more comfortable with the decision to forego artificial nutrition and hydration at the EOL than their caregivers (34). There is a lack of evidence to support that artificial nutrition and hydration improves clinical or quality-of-life outcomes for patients at the EOL. There is concern that during the last days of life artificial nutrition and hydration could contribute to harm by causing volume overload resulting in edema and respiratory distress. In a review of cancer patients receiving artificial nutrition and hydration, the EOL of the five studies reviewed two found patients had less chronic nausea and less signs of dehydration. Two found increased ascites and intestinal drainage. Four studies showed no improvement in delirium, thirst, chronic nausea, and increase fluid overload (35).

However, caregivers and families who are concerned that their family member may experience feelings of starvation and thirst can have feelings of moral distress when deciding to forego artificial nutrition and or hydration. This can be true even in cases where they would choose to forego the option for themselves. Patients and families can also have outside pressure from distant family members, friends, and religious relationships that makes the decisions concerning discontinuing artificial nutrition and hydration complicated and difficult. Patient, caregiver, and family education is important in this case. Artificial nutrition is not recommended because of its invasive nature, while artificial hydration may be considered on a case-by-case basis (11,35). The concept of the *time limit trial* is important in EOL care because it can allow traditionally aggressive interventions to proceed with clear parameters that will allow its discontinuation if certain criteria are not met. For example, a patient has advanced metastatic pancreatic cancer and a bowel obstruction, and the patient/family is requesting total parenteral nutrition (TPN) and comfort measures. In this instance, a hospice may discuss what the patient's expectations are concerning TPN and help the patient and family develop realistic expectations of the intervention. They will counsel the patient and family concerning that TPN is not likely to significantly prolong survival and can have significant side effects. The hospice may agree to time a limited trial for 2 months to determine if the patient will have any benefit to support the patient's and the family's goal. They do this with the understanding that if adverse side effects develop, TPN will be discontinued during the trial. The time limited trial approach allows for flexibility in the management of EOL and honors the shared decision-making process. Time limited trials can strengthen the trust in the doctor–patient relationship (36–38).

Palliative care consultation for management of pain and shortness of breath at the EOL can help the family and treating staff become more comfortable with the use of opioids for symptom management at the EOL. Use of opioids for symptom management in the actively dying patient has not been shown to hasten death. When used appropriately in the care of an expert team, opioids can improve the quality of life for patients and families. Families who witness difficult deaths or suffering in their love ones at the EOL may be susceptible to posttraumatic stress disorder symptoms and complicated bereavement (39,40).

SYMPTOM MANAGEMENT PEARLS

This section focuses on symptoms that may not be covered in other chapters.

Pain

Pain in gastrointestinal malignancies can be multifactorial. The cancer pain patients experience is usually a combination of visceral, somatic, and neuropathic pain, which may require a multimodal approach using several interventions to manage the pain properly. Palliative care consultation and cancer pain management consultation are beneficial in controlling these symptoms. About 30% to 50% of cancer patients will experience moderate to severe pain. Approximately, 55% will experience moderate to severe pain during cancer therapy and 66% of advance care cancer patients have moderate to severe pain at baseline (41,42). Oral opioids/opiates are the mainstay of treatment for malignant pain. However, it is important to use these medications judiciously. It is appropriate to follow the World Health Organization (WHO) analgesic ladder when managing cancer pain; see Table 53.2 (43).

TABLE 53.2 World Health Organization Analgesic Ladder

Step 1: for mild pain, start with nonsteroidal anti-inflammatories and acetaminophen +/− adjuvants
Step 2: for mild to moderate pain, add a weak opioid, which is defined as codeine, tramadol, and hydrocodone +/− adjuvants
Step 3: for moderate to severe pain, add a strong opioid, i.e., morphine or fentanyl +/− adjuvants (1)

Source: Table adapted from World Health Organization.

The WHO analgesic ladder does include at each step adjuvant therapy and nonopioid therapy. This is particularly important for pain caused by gastrointestinal malignancies; such a pain syndrome can arise from a variety of factors including local disease, treatment effect, metastasis, and organ dysfunction.

For patients with liver failure or renal dysfunction, nonsteroidal anti-inflammatories may not be a safe option. The choice of opioid therapy is dictated not only by the severity of pain; but by organ function, side-effect profile, and potential medication interactions (44). The conventional thinking has been that because most pains caused by gastrointestinal malignancies will have a neuropathic component, starting adjuvant neuropathic agents is a consideration to incorporate early into treatment plans. Examples of these agents are tricyclic antidepressants, gabapentin, pregabalin, and serotonin–norepinephrine reuptake inhibitors (SNRIs). However, a recent systematic review and meta-analysis of opioid use with antidepressants or antiepileptic drugs for cancer pain did not show improvement in pain control versus monotherapy, and additional adverse events were found more frequent in the combination arms. The four studies evaluated gabapentin and pregabalin in combination with opioid therapy. There was a significant amount of heterogeneity in patients in the study, so more research on these combinations is warranted. Deciding to start a neuropathic adjuvant is a clinical decision based on patient symptoms, risk factors, and presentation (45). Consider ordering naloxone to prevent accidental overdose for patients on these combinations.

Inflammation is a contributing factor for pain in gastrointestinal/pancreatic/hepatic malignancies. If there are no other contraindications, the addition of nonsteroidal anti-inflammatories or steroids closely monitored for short courses can be an effective adjuvant and can serve for some patients as the primary treatment based on the etiology of their pain and goals of care.

Nonpharmacological therapy should be considered early in the treatment of malignant pain. Patients with pancreatic cancer or metastatic colon cancer should consider a celiac plexus block or hypogastric nerve block, respectively. These interventions can reduce acute pain. It was not sure that these interventions will improve quality of life or reduce opioid therapy, but in a recent study it showed patients with good performance status and low opioid use prior to celiac plexus block/neurolysis had better pain outcomes. The median survival was significantly lower for patients with poor analgesia after celiac plexus neurolysis. Painful cancerous masses that are amenable to radiation and/or cryotherapy should be referred for evaluation (46,47).

For patients with pain and shortness of breath from ascites, paracentesis and placement of peritoneal drains (for patients at EOL) can be effective for pain management. For patients who develop malignant gastroparesis and/or bowel obstructions, high-dose opioid therapy may become counterproductive, secondary to the side effect of gastrointestinal dysmotility. Use of steroids, prokinetic agents, and antispasmodics may be appropriate. Also, response to cancer therapy may also improve pain (48).

There is a growing body of research literature to determine the place of cannabinoids in cancer pain management. The current medical literature does not consist of strong studies, which is supported by multiple reviews and meta-analysis. Most of the research confirms that there is a likely benefit in neuropathic pain, but more research is required (45,49–52). A literature review analyzed studies from 1975 and 2017 and identified five clinical studies that evaluated the effect of THC or CBD on controlling cancer pain. Five studies that evaluated THC oil capsules, THC:CBD oromucosal spray (nabiximols), or THC oromucosal sprays found some evidence of cancer pain reduction associated with these therapies (53). Effective doses ranging from 2.7 to 43.2 mg/day THC and 0 to 40 mg/day CBD were administered. Higher doses of THC correlated with significant improvement in pain. One study found that significant pain control was achieved at doses as low as 2.7 to 10.8 mg THC in combination with 2.5 to 10.0 mg CBD, but there was conflicting evidence on whether increasing doses continue to provide improved pain relief. Side effects include drowsiness, hypotension, confusion, and paradoxical nausea and vomiting if used in excess. There is some evidence that suggests that medical cannabis reduces chronic and neuropathic pain in advanced cancer patients. However, the results of many studies lacked statistical power, due to a limited number of study subjects. There is a clear need for randomized, double-blind, placebo-controlled clinical trials with large sample sizes (53).

The Centers for Disease Control and Prevention (CDC) recommends that patients who are prescribed opioids with a history of substance abuse, overdose history, on greater than 50 mg oral morphine equivalent daily, and concurrent benzodiazepine use should be prescribed naloxone for treatment of unintentional overdose (54). Patients on opioid therapy should be on a bowel regimen consisting of a stimulant laxative and stool softener. The standard of care is senna and polyethylene glycol one to two times daily. Docusate has been shown in several studies to be ineffective (55). For constipation that is refractory to standard therapy, methylnaltrexone, which is subcutaneous, or naloxegol, which is oral, may be appropriate options. Constipation can contribute to nausea, abdominal pain, fatigue, anorexia, and irritability (55–57).

ANOREXIA/CACHEXIA

One of the most distressing symptoms of cancer is cachexia, secondary to it being a visible sign of illness and patient decline. It adversely affects a patient's quality of life. This symptom is also associated with poor survival and lower chemotherapy response rates. Cancer cachexia is a syndrome affects most all cancer patients (58). The etiology of this symptom is complex and requires individualized multimodal management including a formal nutritional assessment. Patients with cachexia syndrome have accelerated muscle and tissue mass breakdown because of a variety of factors; thus increasing appetite alone is not sufficient treatment. Evaluating for other causes of weight loss and anorexia is important, for example, nausea, constipation, dysgeusia, depression, and medication effect. Treatment response to cancer may improve this symptom. Incorporating exercise consisting of resistance and aerobic muscle training may be beneficial in cachexia and should be incorporated into cachexia treatment programs (59).

Choosing pharmacological therapy should be based on patient goals, current treatment plan, side-effect profile, and efficacy of the medication. Megestrol in a dose of 400mg to 800mg improves appetite and weight, secondary to increasing fat stores, but does improve lean muscle pain and does not incur a survival benefit. Megestrol may also improve a patient's sense of well-being. However, megestrol may increase thrombosis in patients on chemotherapy. Megestrol also can increase edema and cause suppression of the hypothalamic pituitary axis and androgen deficiency in men. The benefit of megestrol is also transient (60). Steroids improve appetite and can improve a sense of well-being, but its side-effect profile prevents long-term use. However, it can be a good option for patients at the EOL with a prognosis in weeks to months. Like megestrol, the benefits of steroids are transient in increasing appetite. Mirtazapine and cyproheptadine have relatively safer side-effect profiles. These medications increase appetite, though their antihistamine and serotonin antagonist effect on histamine and serotonin receptors in the brain. Cyproheptadine 8 mg can counteract increased serotonin and may be a better choice in carcinoid syndrome (56,61). It improves appetite, but has not been shown to improve weight. Mirtazapine at a dose of 15 to 30 mg has been associated with an increase in weight and appetite, but has not been proven in a randomized, placebo-controlled trial (62).

Quality research on the use of cannabinoids in cancer anorexia is growing, but more evidence is needed to fully understand its place in the treatment of cancer anorexia and cachexia. Cannabinoid nabilone was recently studied, which showed that after 8 weeks of treatment, it improved caloric intake in patients with non–small cell lung cancer as well as quality of life. Its long-term effect on weight gain and life expectancy is not clear (63). Dronabinol has not been shown to be effective consistently in the literature for treatment of cancer anorexia but does improve associated cancer-related dysgeusia and nausea, which may improve appetite (61,64). Other pharmacological options such as thalidomide, which has been shown to increase lean muscle mass and slow weight loss but has a difficult side-effect profile, have been studied as an option. Eicosapentaenoic acid showed promise but has not proven to be efficacious in phase III clinical trials. Melatonin showed improvement and cachexia in patients with advanced non–small cell lung cancer (58,61). A research medication (ACT-1 trial) espindolol (nonselective beta-blocker with central 5-HT1A and partial β2 receptor agonist effects) 10mg twice a day showed improved weight loss, fat free mass, and maintenance of fat mass in advanced colorectal cancer and non–small cell lung cancer related cachexia (65). Traditional Japanese medicine rikkunshito has been shown to improve anorexia, gastrointestinal dysmotility, muscle wasting, and anxiety. Other medications such as ACE inhibitors, nonsteroidal anti-inflammatory medication, and beta-blockers may have some limited benefits as well, but are not appropriate for all patients as the primary treatment (58).

Depression and Anxiety

The rate of depression in cancer patients ranges between 15% and 30%, at a rate of 3 to 5 times that of the general population. Depression and anxiety have adverse effects on patients' quality of life and can affect treatment outcomes. There are several studies reporting the role of depression as a precursor to pancreatic cancer (66,67). The standard of care is to start a selective serotonin reuptake inhibitor (SSRI) with the expectation of effect in 3 to 4 weeks. Some patients benefit from the addition of an atypical antipsychotic as adjuvant therapy. Addition of olanzapine to an SSRI may be a good choice for patients with concomitant nausea, anxiety, and anorexia. Patients with concomitant neuropathic and myofascial pain may benefit from an SNRI. If the patient is at the EOL with a prognosis in weeks, a psychostimulant may be a better option, secondary to its rapid onset of action (68). More recent treatments of depression have been identified, but they are not yet mainstream. There is a growing body of literature supporting the use of ketamine/esketamine and psilocybin for use in treatment resistant depression (69). They may have good utility for patients with advance illness secondary to the rapidity onset. A recent clinical trial showed that in conjunction with psychotherapy, psilocybin produced rapid and lasting anxiolytic and antidepressant effects in patients with cancer-related psychological distress (70). These agents are limited by availability, potential side-effect profile, and lack of familiarity with use among providers. For refractory depression, electroconvulsive therapy may be a good option for some patients.

Low-dose benzodiazepines can be effective for acute anxiety, but an SSRI for maintenance is the appropriate treatment long term. Buspirone, cyproheptadine, trazodone, and gabapentin can be used as alternatives for the management of anxiety especially for patients with contraindications to benzodiazepines. These are often off-label uses with limited evidence in the literature (68,70–72). Patients can have improved outcomes with psychological therapy, particularly cognitive behavioral therapy, to help control anxiety. Patients may benefit from integrative modalities such as acupuncture, yoga, mindfulness, and exercise. Patients with advanced cancer benefit from the emotional and spiritual support given by palliative care teams (68,73). Patients should be routinely screened at each visit for anxiety and depression. A study evaluated that patients diagnosed with depression prior to or postcancer were less likely to receive aggressive EOL care than patients without depression (74). Cancer patients are at increased risk for suicidal ideation when compared to the general population. Mental health screening and access are important in this population (75).

Fatigue

Patients often identify fatigue as a symptom that adversely affects their quality of life. It is the most common cancer-related symptom and one of the most difficult to manage. Treatment plans should be tailored to individual patient needs. Cancer-related fatigue (CRF) not only affects patients in active treatment, but patients posttreatment and survivors. A stepwise approach to management can be helpful. In a study evaluating a CRF clinic, patients showed clinical benefit within 2 weeks (76). The clinic focused on evaluating for physical etiologies contributing to fatigue, such as anemia, depression, sleep disturbance, underlying cardiopulmonary screening, and medication effects. Interventions focused on the treatment of underlying medical conditions contributing to fatigue. Energy conservation and exercise plans were developed for appropriate patients. Exercise has been shown to improve CRF in appropriate candidates (77).

If nonpharmacological management is not effective, then the addition of psychostimulants may be an appropriate option. Studies evaluating the effects of stimulants methylphenidate, dexmethylphenidate, and modafinil are mixed, but they are fairly well-tolerated. Used in low doses, patients can tolerate them well. Side effects to monitor are tachycardia, anxiety, irritability, constipation, and sleep disturbance, which are the most common. Steroids can be beneficial in the short term and are used often as the medication of choice for fatigue at the EOL. The side-effect profile makes them not appropriate for long-term use. Herbal treatments have shown benefit in CRF as well. American ginseng at a dose of 2,000 mg daily showed improvement in symptoms after 8 weeks, primarily in patients undergoing active treatment; less effect was seen in patients posttreatment. However, it does have a risk of drug interactions; ginseng is an inhibitor of CYP3A4 and should be avoided in patients on imatinib. It should also be avoided in patients on warfarin, thrombolytic agents, and hormonal agents (78). Guarana at 100 mg daily has shown improvement in fatigue in a small study of cancer patients after about 21 days, but further research concerning efficacy and long-term safety is required (79). All herbal supplements should be evaluated by nutrition and/or oncology pharmacologists. Integrative oncology therapies such as acupuncture, yoga, and mindfulness may be helpful tools to integrate into a patient's treatment plan (80–82).

Nausea and Vomiting

Nausea and vomiting are common symptoms in patients with cancer, and the etiology is often multifactorial. Because these symptoms are ubiquitous and many cancer therapies cause nausea, patients often receive well-established treatment protocols pre- and postchemotherapy to manage for anticipatory and chemotherapy-induced nausea and vomiting. However, even with this innovation, about 40% of patients may experience breakthrough nausea and vomiting; which may not always be directly secondary to treatment. There is a lack of strong evidence to manage nausea and vomiting based on mechanism. Understanding of the etiology can help guide treatment, especially when it is secondary to a reversible condition such as uncontrolled constipation, medication side effect, gastric reflux disease, gastrointestinal dysmotility or obstruction, and anticipatory nausea caused by psychological distress. In these cases, tailoring the treatment plan to the mechanism may be the most appropriate way to start (83). Olanzapine 5 to 10 mg/day has been shown to be more beneficial in the management of chemotherapy-induced nausea and vomiting (CINV) and for the prevention of nausea and vomiting as compared with other standard agents. CINV treatment plans should consider its routine inclusion (84,85). Cannabinoids for CINV and nausea studies have shown mixed results despite public perception of efficacy and animal model evidence (86).

Palliative management goals for malignant bowel obstruction in patients with advanced disease are to control pain, nausea/vomiting; decrease secretions; and clarify the goals of care. In patients who are going to forego interventions and are not candidates for surgery or stenting, medical management is the key to quality of life. Patients may initially require a nasogastric tube, especially if they are having significant vomiting and abdominal pain from distention (87). The medical management should include initially:

1. IV fluid hydration electrolyte replacement with bowel rest
2. IV steroids, that is, 6 to 16 mg of dexamethasone daily to decrease bowel wall edema
3. Analgesia: the mainstay has been opioids; haloperidol for nausea
4. Somatostatin analogs can be beneficial in reducing the release of gastrointestinal hormones resulting in decreased gut secretion and may be added early in treatment if the patient is not a surgical candidate
5. Advance care planning and goals of care discussion because a patient with malignant bowel obstruction has a high rate of in-hospital mortality regardless of the intervention (88,89)

If a patient's obstruction is not resolving with conservative management or he or she is not a candidate for surgical intervention or a stent, then a palliative plan of care has to be developed. The palliative care consultation will need to include discussions concerning (a) prognosis and disease trajectory; (b) long-term management of symptoms including duration of IV hydration, parental nutrition, and candidacy for venting gastrostomy tube, which relieves symptoms by decompressing the stomach and small bowel; and (c) hospice care and disposition, secondary to the patient's anticipated high clinical needs posthospitalization. Hospices are capable of managing these symptoms in the home or inpatient setting (87). One widely used treatment for constipation in partial bowel obstruction is oral petroleum jelly, "Vaseline balls." The theory is that patients freeze small balls of petroleum jelly covered in confection sugar and swallow 2 to 3 of them to lubricate the stool to produce a bowel movement. Although used routinely in hospice care, the reports of efficacy are still anecdotal (90).

Integration of palliative care into oncology care has become the standard of care for patients with advanced cancer early in their diagnosis. Palliative care clearly has benefits for patient quality of life, caregiver experience, and may have some survival benefits under certain clinical conditions. Oncology providers and treatment teams should be trained to provide primary palliative care to their patients, but should routinely refer to integrated or dedicated palliative care teams for patients with high symptom burden and advanced cancer (Table 53.3).

TABLE 53.3 Palliative Management and Prognosis of Common Gastrointestinal Malignancies

Cancer	Common Symptoms of Advanced Disease	Palliative Management Pearls	Median Survival: Advanced Disease With Treatment
Pancreatic	Pain from local disease Malignant gastroparesis Peritoneal carcinomatosis Obstructive jaundice/biliary obstruction: pruritus, cholangitis Gastric outlet obstruction Anorexia/cachexia, fatigue, depression	Pain: celiac plexus block, systemic opioid with neuropathic agent, anti-inflammatories, palliative radiation Malignant gastroparesis: metoclopramide, erythromycin Peritoneal carcinomatosis: steroid/NSAIDs, opioids Bowel obstruction: stent, venting percutaneous gastrostomy tube, goal oriented artificial nutrition and hydration time limited trials (e.g., the FARGO trial) Obstructive jaundice: biliary stent placement; pruritus: bile acid binders, paroxetine, steroids; in monitored inpatient palliative care setting naloxone treatment Peritoneal carcinomatosis: steroid/NSAIDs, opioids	6 months
Gastric	Malignant gastroparesis Peritoneal carcinomatosis Refractory bleeding Dysphagia for cancer (at GE junction) Gastric outlet obstruction Abdominal pain Nausea/vomiting Early satiety Hiccups	Malignant gastroparesis: metoclopramide, erythromycin Peritoneal carcinomatosis: steroid/NSAIDs, opioids Bowel obstruction: stent, venting percutaneous gastrostomy tube, goal oriented artificial nutrition and hydration time limited trials Refractory bleeding: radiation therapy/laser therapy Dysphagia for cancer (at GE junction): radiation, esophageal stent Gastric outlet obstruction: gastrojejunostomy/stent, venting gastrostomy tube Abdominal pain: opioids Nausea/vomiting: olanzapine, haloperidol, ondansetron; if obstructed, avoid metoclopramide Hiccups: chlorpromazine, baclofen, metoclopramide, gabapentin	8–10 months
Neuroendocrine tumor	Carcinoid syndrome: flushing, diarrhea Abdominal cramping; wheezing, fatigue Heart failure: cardiac infiltration	Carcinoid syndrome: octreotide Liver capsular pain: steroids, NSAIDS, transarterial chemoembolization Diarrhea: lomotil, tincture of opioid, codeine Abdominal cramping: hyoscyamine, dicyclomine	>5 years

(continued)

TABLE 53.3 Palliative Management and Prognosis of Common Gastrointestinal Malignancies (*continued*)

Cancer	Common Symptoms of Advanced Disease	Palliative Management Pearls	Median Survival: Advanced Disease With Treatment
Hepatocellular	Abdominal pain Ascites Anorexia Fatigue, peripheral edema Liver dysfunction Obstructive jaundice: pruritus, cholangitis Nausea	Abdominal pain/capsular pain: steroids/NSAIDs Systemic opioids (adjust for liver dysfunction) Refractory ascites at end of life: recurrent paracentesis +/– albumin, peritoneal drainage catheter placement, spironolactone (off-label dose) starting at 100 mg q day titrate up to 3–5 days (maximum 400 mg daily) Liver failure: avoid long-acting opioids (including fentanyl transdermal patches) in favor of short-acting preparations, monitor for neurotoxicity Nausea: olanzapine, haloperidol, ondansetron, metoclopramide Obstructive jaundice: biliary stent placement; pruritus: bile acid binders, paroxetine, steroids; monitored inpatient palliative care setting/consultation IV naloxone or oral naltrexone	6–8 months
Esophageal	Dysphagia Radiation esophagitis/mucositis Candida esophagitis Pain Weight loss Fatigue Dehydration	Dysphagia: radiation/stent, percutaneous gastrostomy tube Esophagitis: Magic Mouthwash, topical anesthetics, systemic opioids, topical opioids (viscous morphine) Mucositis: palifermin Hydration schedule: goal oriented artificial nutrition and hydration time limited trials	8–10 months

(*continued*)

TABLE 53.3 Palliative Management and Prognosis of Common Gastrointestinal Malignancies (*continued*)

Cancer	Common Symptoms of Advanced Disease	Palliative Management Pearls	Median Survival: Advanced Disease With Treatment
Colorectal	Abdominal pain: metastatic and local disease Bowel obstruction Malignant gastroparesis Peritoneal carcinomatosis Treatment induced diarrhea Treatment induced mucositis	Abdominal pain: systemic opioid therapy with neuropathic agent, anti-inflammatories Evaluation by intervention pain management to consider hypogastric nerve block or intrathecal pain pump, referral for cryotherapy Bowel obstruction: palliative surgical intervention, bowel stents, palliative radiation Malignant gastroparesis: (caution: rule out obstruction) metoclopramide, erythromycin Peritoneal carcinomatosis: Steroid/NSAIDs, opioids Bowel obstruction: stent, goal oriented artificial nutrition and hydration time limited trials Diarrhea (grade 3–4): hospitalization with intravenous hydration, octreotide IV 25–50 ug/hr vs. SC 100–150 ug TID, evaluate for need for antibiotics, hold cytotoxic chemotherapy Mucositis: Magic Mouthwash, topical anesthetics, systemic opioids, topical opioids (viscous morphine) Mucositis: palifermin	2+ years

GE, gastroesophageal; IV, intravenous; NSAID, nonsteroidal anti-inflammatory drug; SC, subcutaneous.
Source: From Wong GY, Schroeder DR, Carns PE, et al. Effect of neurolytic celiac plexus block on pain relief, quality of life, and survival in patients with unresectable pancreatic cancer: a randomized controlled trial. JAMA. 2004;291(9):1092–1099. doi:10.1001/jama.291.9.1092; Goldberg J, Goldman D, McCaskey S, et al. Illness understanding, prognostic awareness and end of life care after drainage percutaneous endoscopic gastrostomy for malignant bowel obstruction in metastatic gastrointestinal cancer (FR481C). J Pain Symptom Manage. 2018;55(2):633. doi:10.1016/j.jpainsymman.2017.12.154; Hardy J, Haberecht J. Palliative care: core skills and clinical competencies. - by LL Emanuel and SL Librach. Intern Med J. 2008;38(12):933. doi:10.1111/j.1445-5994.2008.01839.x; Mercadante S, Chen W. Palliative care of bowel obstruction in cancer patients. 2017.

REFERENCES

1. Connor SR. *Hospice and Palliative Care: The Essential Guide*. New York: Taylor & Francis; 2017.
2. Ferrell BR, Temel JS, Temin S, et al. Integration of palliative care into standard oncology care: American Society of Clinical Oncology clinical practice guideline update. *J Clin Oncol*. 2016;35(1):96–112. doi:10.1200/JCO.2016.70.1474
3. Dalal S, Bruera E. End-of-Life care matters: palliative cancer care results in better care and lower costs. *Oncologist*. 2017;22(4):361–368. doi:10.1634/theoncologist.2016-0277
4. Bickel KE, McNiff K, Buss MK, et al. Defining high-quality palliative care in oncology practice: an American Society of Clinical Oncology/American Academy of Hospice and Palliative Medicine guidance statement. *J Oncol Pract*. 2016;12(9):e828–e838. doi:10.1200/JOP.2016.010686
5. Temel JS, Greer JA, El-Jawahri A, et al. Effects of early integrated palliative care in patients with lung and GI cancer: a randomized clinical trial. *J Clin Oncol*. 2017;35(8):834–841. doi:10.1200/JCO.2016.70.5046
6. Temel JS, Greer JA, Muzikansky A, et al. Early palliative care for patients with metastatic non–small-cell lung cancer. *N Engl J Med*. 2010;363(8):733–742. doi:10.1056/NEJMoa1000678
7. Bakitas MA, Tosteson TD, Li Z, et al. Early versus delayed initiation of concurrent palliative oncology care: patient outcomes in the ENABLE III randomized controlled trial. *J Clin Oncol*. 2015;33(13):1438. doi:10.1200/JCO.2014.58.6362
8. Haun MW, Estel S, Rücker G, et al. Early palliative care for adults with advanced cancer. *The Cochrane Library*. 2017. doi:10.1002/14651858.CD011129.pub2
9. El-Jawahri A, Greer JA, Pirl WF, et al. Effects of early integrated palliative care on caregivers of patients with lung and gastrointestinal cancer: a randomized clinical trial. *Oncologist*. 2017;22(12):1528–1534. doi:10.1634/theoncologist.2017-0227
10. Buss MK, Lessen DS, Sullivan AM, et al. Hematology/oncology fellows' training in palliative care. *Cancer*. 2011;117(18):4304–4311. doi:10.1002/cncr.25952
11. Hui D, Dev R, Bruera E. The last days of life: symptom burden and impact on nutrition and hydration in cancer patients. *Curr Opin Support Palliat Care*. 2015;9(4):346. doi:10.1097/SPC.0000000000000171
12. Obermeyer Z, Makar M, Abujaber S, et al. Association between the Medicare hospice benefit and health care utilization and costs for patients with poor-prognosis cancer. *JAMA*. 2014;312(18):1888–1896. doi:10.1001/jama.2014.14950
13. Gidwani R, Joyce N, Kinosian B, et al. Gap between recommendations and practice of palliative care and hospice in cancer patients. *J Palliat Med*. 2016;19(9):957–963. doi:10.1089/jpm.2015.0514
14. Houben CH, Spruit MA, Groenen MT, et al. Efficacy of advance care planning: a systematic review and meta-analysis. *J Am Med Dir Assoc*. 2014;15(7):477–489. doi:10.1016/j.jamda.2014.01.008
15. Kaplan MR. SPIKES: a framework for breaking bad news to patients with cancer. *Clin J Oncol Nurs*. 2010;14(4):514–516. doi:10.1188/10.cjon.514-516
16. de Sousa FH, Valenti VE, Hamaji MP, et al. The use of spikes protocol in cancer: an integrative review. *Int Arch Med*. 2017;10. doi:10.3823/2324
17. Baer L, Weinstein E. Improving oncology nurses' communication skills for difficult conversations. *Clin J Oncol Nurs*. 2013;17(3):E45–E51. doi:10.1188/13.cjon.e45-e51
18. Foronda C, Baptiste D-L, Reinholdt MM, et al. Cultural humility: a concept analysis. *J Transcult Nurs*. 2016;27(3):210–217. doi:10.1177/1043659615592677
19. Epstein AS, Prigerson HG, O'Reilly EM, et al. Discussions of life expectancy and changes in illness understanding in patients with advanced cancer. *J Clin Oncol*. 2016;34(20):2398–2403. doi:10.1200/JCO.2015.63.6696
20. Enzinger AC, Zhang B, Schrag D, et al. Outcomes of prognostic disclosure: associations with prognostic understanding, distress, and relationship with physician among patients with advanced cancer. *J Clin Oncol*. 2015;33(32):3809. doi:10.1200/JCO.2015.61.9239
21. Bernacki RE, Block SD. Communication about serious illness care goals: a review and synthesis of best practices. *JAMA Intern Med*. 2014;174(12):1994–2003. doi:10.1001/jamainternmed.2014.5271
22. Sudore RL, Lum HD, You JJ, et al. Defining advance care planning for adults: a consensus definition from a multidisciplinary Delphi panel. *J Pain Symptom Manage*. 2017;53(5):821–832.e1. doi:10.1016/j.jpainsymman.2016.12.331
23. Clark MA, Ott M, Rogers ML, et al. Advance care planning as a shared endeavor: completion of ACP documents in a multidisciplinary cancer program. *Psycho-Oncology*. 2017;26(1):67–73. doi:10.1002/pon.4010
24. Zive DM, Fromme EK, Schmidt TA, et al. Timing of POLST form completion by cause of death. *J Pain Symptom Manage*. 2015;50(5):650–658. doi:10.1016/j.jpainsymman.2015.06.004

25. Lammers AJ, Zive DM, Tolle SW, et al. The oncology specialist's role in POLST form completion. *Am J Hosp Palliat Med*. 2018;35:297–303. doi:10.1177/1049909117702873
26. Sundar S, Hoong TTC, Alharganee A. A confirmatory survey regarding public misconception about cardiopulmonary resuscitation (CPR) in advanced cancer patients. *J Clin Oncol*. 2016;34(15_suppl):e21507. doi:10.1200/jco.2016.34.15_suppl.e21507
27. Ouellette L, Puro A, Weatherhead J, et al. Public knowledge and perceptions about cardiopulmonary resuscitation (CPR): results of a multicenter survey. *Am J Emerg Med*. 2018;36:1900–1901. doi:10.1016/j.ajem.2018.01.103
28. Osinski A, Vreugdenhil G, de Koning J, et al. Do-not-resuscitate orders in cancer patients: a review of literature. *Support Care Cancer*. 2017;25(2):677–685. doi:10.1007/s00520-016-3459-9
29. Bruckel JT, Wong SL, Chan PS, et al. Patterns of resuscitation care and survival after in-hospital cardiac arrest in patients with advanced cancer. *J Oncol Pract*. 2017;13(10):e821–e830. doi:10.1200/JOP.2016.020404
30. Green MJ, Schubart JR, Whitehead MM, et al. Advance care planning does not adversely affect hope or anxiety among patients with advanced cancer. *J Pain Symptom Manage*. 2015;49(6):1088–1096. doi:10.1016/j.jpainsymman.2014.11.293
31. Brinkman-Stoppelenburg A, Rietjens JA, van der Heide A. The effects of advance care planning on end-of-life care: a systematic review. *Palliat Med*. 2014;28(8):1000–1025. doi:10.1177/0269216314526272
32. Gonzalez-Saenz de Tejada M, Bilbao A, Baré M, et al. Association between social support, functional status, and change in health-related quality of life and changes in anxiety and depression in colorectal cancer patients. *Psycho-Oncology*. 2017;26(9):1263–1269. doi:10.1002/pon.4303
33. Narang AK, Nicholas LH. Out-of-pocket spending and financial burden among Medicare beneficiaries with cancer. *JAMA Oncol*. 2017;3(6):757–765. doi:10.1001/jamaoncol.2016.4865
34. Bükki J, Unterpaul T, Nübling G, et al. Decision making at the end of life—cancer patients' and their caregivers' views on artificial nutrition and hydration. *Support Care Cancer*. 2014;22(12):3287–3299. doi:10.1007/s00520-014-2337-6
35. Raijmakers NJH, van Zuylen L, Costantini M, et al. Artificial nutrition and hydration in the last week of life in cancer patients. A systematic literature review of practices and effects. *Ann Oncol*. 2011;22(7):1478–1486. doi:10.1093/annonc/mdq620
36. Hudoba C, Hwang DY. Goals of care and difficult conversations. In: Sheth KN and White JL, eds. Neurocritical Care for the Advanced Practice Clinician. New York: Springer International Publishing AG; 2017: 343–361.
37. Quill TE, Holloway R. Time-limited trials near the end of life. *JAMA*. 2011;306(13):1483–1484. doi:10.1001/jama.2011.1413
38. Hickson M, Smith S, Whelan K. Advanced nutrition and dietetics in nutrition support. In: Schwartz DB, ed. *Nutrition Support in Palliative Care*. Hoboken: John Wiley & Sons; 2018: 389–397. doi:10.1002/9781118993880.ch5.18
39. Shinjo T, Morita T, Hirai K, et al. Why people accept opioids: role of general attitudes toward drugs, experience as a bereaved family, information from medical professionals, and personal beliefs regarding a good death. *J Pain Symptom Manage*. 2015;49(1):45–54. doi:10.1016/j.jpainsymman.2014.04.015
40. Alexander S. *A Project to Improve Nurses' Knowledge of, and Attitudes Towards, Pain Management at End of Life*. Amherst: University of Massachusetts; 2016.
41. van den Beuken-van MH, Hochstenbach LM, Joosten EA, et al. Update on prevalence of pain in patients with cancer: systematic review and meta-analysis. *J Pain Symptom Manage*. 2016;51(6):1070–1090.e9. doi:10.1016/j.jpainsymman.2015.12.340
42. Wiffen PJ, Wee B, Derry S, et al. Opioids for cancer pain—an overview of Cochrane reviews. *Cochrane Database Syst Rev*. 2017 Jul 6;7:CD012592. doi: 10.1002/14651858.CD012592.pub2.
43. World Health Organization. *WHO pain relief ladder for cancer pain relief*. 2017.
44. Fredheim O, Brelin S, Hjermstad M, et al. Prescriptions of analgesics during complete disease trajectories in patients who are diagnosed with and die from cancer within the five-year period 2005–2009. *Eur J Pain*. 2017;21(3):530–540. doi:10.1002/ejp.956
45. Kane CM, Mulvey MR, Wright S, et al. Opioids combined with antidepressants or antiepileptic drugs for cancer pain: systematic review and meta-analysis. *Palliat Med*. 2018;32:276–286. doi:10.1177/0269216317711826
46. Nedeljkovic SS, Ali SIQ. Celiac plexus block. In: Yong R., Nguyen M., Nelson E., Urman R, eds. *Pain Medicine*. New York: Springer Publishing; 2017: 289–291.
47. Wong GY, Schroeder DR, Carns PE, et al. Effect of neurolytic celiac plexus block on pain relief, quality of life, and survival in patients with unresectable pancreatic cancer: a randomized controlled trial. *JAMA*. 2004;291(9):1092–1099. doi:10.1001/jama.291.9.1092

48. Portenoy RK, Copenhaver DJ, Fishman S, et al. Cancer pain management: interventional therapies. Retrieved from com/contents/cancer-pain-management-interventional-therapies; 2017: 8.
49. Brown MR, Farquhar-Smith WP. Cannabinoids and cancer pain: a new hope or a false dawn? *Eur J Intern Med*. 2018;49:30–36. doi:10.1016/j.ejim.2018.01.020
50. Häuser W, Fitzcharles M-A, Radbruch L, et al. Cannabinoids in pain management and palliative medicine: an overview of systematic reviews and prospective observational studies. *Dtsch Ärztebl Int*. 2017;114(38):627. doi:10.3238/arztebl.2017.0627
51. Tateo S. State of the evidence: cannabinoids and cancer pain—a systematic review. *J Am Assoc Nurse Pract*. 2017;29(2):94–103. doi:10.1002/2327-6924.12422
52. Pergolizzi JJ, Lequang J, Taylor JR, et al. The role of cannabinoids in pain control: the good, the bad, and the ugly. *Minerva Anestesiol*. 2018;84(8):955–969. doi:10.23736/S0375-9393.18.12287-5
53. Blake A, Wan BA, Malek L, et al. A selective review of medical cannabis in cancer pain management. *Ann Palliat Med*. 2017;6(S2):S215–S222. doi:10.21037/apm.2017.08.05
54. Dowell D, Haegerich T, Chou R. CDC guideline for prescribing opioids for chronic pain—United States, 2016. *MMWR Recomm Rep*. 2016;65(1);1–49. doi:10.15585/mmwr.rr6501e1
55. Muldrew DH, Hasson F, Carduff E, et al. Assessment and management of constipation for patients receiving palliative care in specialist palliative care settings: a systematic review of the literature. *Palliat Med*. 2018;32:930–938. doi:10.1177/0269216317752515
56. Abramowitz L, Béziaud N, Labreze L, et al. Prevalence and impact of constipation and bowel dysfunction induced by strong opioids: a cross-sectional survey of 520 patients with cancer pain: DYONISOS study. *J Med Econ*. 2013;16(12):1423–1433. doi:10.3111/13696998.2013.85 1082
57. Dong ST, Costa DS, Butow PN, et al. Symptom clusters in advanced cancer patients: an empirical comparison of statistical methods and the impact on quality of life. *J Pain Symptom Manage*. 2016;51(1):88–98. doi:10.1016/j.jpainsymman.2015.07.013
58. Aoyagi T, Terracina KP, Raza A, et al. Cancer cachexia, mechanism and treatment. *W J Gastrointest Oncol*. 2015;7(4):17. doi:10.4251/wjgo.v7.i4.17
59. Argilés JM, Busquets S, López-Soriano FJ, et al. Are there any benefits of exercise training in cancer cachexia? *J Cachexia Sarcopenia Muscle*. 2012;3(2):73–76. doi:10.1007/s13539-012-0067-5
60. Ruiz-García V, López-Briz E, Carbonell-Sanchis R, et al. Megestrol acetate for cachexia–anorexia syndrome. A systematic review. *J Cachexia Sarcopenia Muscle*. 2018;9(3):444–452. doi:10.1002/jcsm.12292
61. Ronga I, Gallucci F, Riccardi F, et al. Anorexia–cachexia syndrome in pancreatic cancer: recent advances and new pharmacological approach. *Adv Med Sci*. 2014;59(1):1–6. doi:10.1016/j.advms.2013.11.001
62. Riechelmann RP, Burman D, Tannock IF, et al. Phase II trial of mirtazapine for cancer-related cachexia and anorexia. *Am J Hosp Palliat Med*. 2010;27(2):106–110. doi:10.1177/1049909109345685
63. Turcott JG, Núñez MdRG, Flores-Estrada D, et al. The effect of nabilone on appetite, nutritional status, and quality of life in lung cancer patients: a randomized, double-blind clinical trial. *Support Care Cancer*. 2018;26(9):3029–3038. doi:10.1007/s00520-018-4154-9
64. Davis MP. Cannabinoids for symptom management and cancer therapy: the evidence. *J Natl Compr Canc Netw*. 2016;14(7):915–922. doi:10.6004/jnccn.2016.0094
65. Stewart Coats AJ, Ho GF, Prabhash K, et al. Espindolol for the treatment and prevention of cachexia in patients with stage III/IV non-small cell lung cancer or colorectal cancer: a randomized, double-blind, placebo-controlled, international multicentre phase II study (the ACT-ONE trial). *J Cachexia Sarcopenia Muscle*. 2016;7(3):355–365. doi:10.1002/jcsm.12126
66. Kenner BJ. Early detection of pancreatic cancer. *Pancreas*. 2018;47(4):363–367. doi:10.1097/MPA.0000000000001024
67. Parker G, Brotchie H. Pancreatic cancer and depression: a narrative review. *J Nerv Ment Dis*. 2017;205(6):487–490. doi:10.1097/NMD.0000000000000593
68. Irwin S, Hirst J, Block S, et al. *Overview of anxiety in palliative care*. 2017.
69. Daly EJ, Singh JB, Fedgchin M, et al. Efficacy and safety of intranasal esketamine adjunctive to oral antidepressant therapy in treatment-resistant depression: a randomized clinical trial. *JAMA Psychiatry*. 2018;75(2):139–148. doi:10.1001/jamapsychiatry.2017.3739
70. Ross S, Bossis A, Guss J, et al. Rapid and sustained symptom reduction following psilocybin treatment for anxiety and depression in patients with life-threatening cancer: a randomized controlled trial. *J Psychopharmacol*. 2016;30(12):1165–1180. doi:10.1177/0269881116675512
71. Berlin RK, Butler PM, Perloff MD. Gabapentin therapy in psychiatric disorders: a systematic review. *Prim Care Companion for CNS Disord*. 2015;17(5). doi:10.4088/PCC.15r01821
72. Bossini L, Coluccia A, Casolaro I, et al. Off-label trazodone prescription: evidence, benefits and risks. *Curr Pharm Des*. 2015;21(23):3343–3351. doi:10.2174/1381612821666150619092236

73. Butow P, Price MA, Shaw JM, et al. Clinical pathway for the screening, assessment and management of anxiety and depression in adult cancer patients: Australian guidelines. *Psycho-Oncology*. 2015;24(9):987–1001. doi:10.1002/pon.3920

74. Doan KC, Levy BR, Gross CP, et al. *Associations of pre-and post-cancer depression with end-of-life cancer care intensity*. J Clin Oncol. 2016;34(15_suppl):10031-10031. doi:10.1200/JCO.2016.34.15_suppl.10031

75. Alves M, Tavares A. Suicide risk in cancer patients–are we prepared? *Eur Psychiatry*. 2017;41:S667. doi:10.1016/j.eurpsy.2017.01.1137

76. Escalante CP, Manzullo E, Valdres R. A cancer-related fatigue clinic: opportunities and challenges. *J Natl Compr Canc Netw*. 2003;1(3):333–343. doi:10.6004/jnccn.2003.0030

77. Hilfiker R, Meichtry A, Eicher M, et al. Exercise and other non-pharmaceutical interventions for cancer-related fatigue in patients during or after cancer treatment: a systematic review incorporating an indirect-comparisons meta-analysis. *Br J Sports Med*. 2018;52:651–658. doi:10.1136/bjsports-2016-096422

78. Chang Y, Smith J, Portman DG, et al. *The combination therapy with methylphenidate and American ginseng in cancer-related fatigue*. J Clinical Oncol. 2016;34(26_suppl):215. doi:10.1200/jco.2016.34.26_suppl.215

79. de Oliveira Campos MP, Riechelmann R, Martins LC, et al. Guarana (Paullinia cupana) improves fatigue in breast cancer patients undergoing systemic chemotherapy. *J Altern Complement Med*. 2011;17(6):505–512. doi:10.1089/acm.2010.0571

80. Bower JE. Cancer-related fatigue—mechanisms, risk factors, and treatments. *Nat Rev Clin Oncol*. 2014;11(10):597. doi:10.1038/nrclinonc.2014.127

81. Wang XS, Woodruff JF. Cancer-related and treatment-related fatigue. *Gynecol Oncol*. 2015;136(3):446–452. doi:10.1016/j.ygyno.2014.10.013

82. Yennurajalingam S, Bruera E. Review of clinical trials of pharmacologic interventions for cancer-related fatigue: focus on psychostimulants and steroids. *Cancer J*. 2014;20(5):319–324. doi:10.1097/PPO.0000000000000069

83. Del Fabbro E, Bruera E, Savarese D. *Palliative care: assessment and management of nausea and vomiting*. UpToDate, Waltham, MA; 2017.

84. Chiu L, Chow R, Popovic M, et al. Efficacy of olanzapine for the prophylaxis and rescue of chemotherapy-induced nausea and vomiting (CINV): a systematic review and meta-analysis. *Support Care Cancer*. 2016;24(5):2381–2392. doi:10.1007/s00520-016-3075-8

85. Navari RM, Qin R, Ruddy KJ, et al. Olanzapine for the prevention of chemotherapy-induced nausea and vomiting. *N Engl J Med*. 2016;375(2):134–142. doi:10.1056/NEJMoa1515725

86. Madras BK. Update of Cannabis and Its Medical Use. Report to the WHO Expert Committee on Drug Dependence. http://www.who int/medicines/access/controlled-substances/6_2_cannabis_update pdf; 2015.

87. Goldberg J, Goldman D, McCaskey S, et al. Illness understanding, prognostic awareness and end of life care after drainage percutaneous endoscopic gastrostomy for malignant bowel obstruction in metastatic gastrointestinal cancer (FR481C). *J Pain Symptom Manage*. 2018;55(2):633. doi:10.1016/j.jpainsymman.2017.12.154

88. Hardy J, Haberecht J. Palliative care: core skills and clinical competencies. - by LL Emanuel and SL Librach. *Intern Med J*. 2008;38(12):933. doi:10.1111/j.1445-5994.2008.01839.x

89. Mercadante S, Chen W. *Palliative care of bowel obstruction in cancer patients*. 2017.

90. Tavares CN, Kimbrel JM, Protus BM, et al. Petroleum jelly (vaseline balls) for the treatment of constipation: a survey of hospice and palliative care practitioners. *Am J Hosp Palliat Med*. 2014;31(8):797–803. doi:10.1177/1049909113502578

54

Care for Elderly Gastrointestinal Cancer Patients

Grant R. Williams and Hanna K. Sanoff

INTRODUCTION

The incidence of all gastrointestinal (GI) cancers increases steadily with age. For example, in the United States, the incidence rate of colorectal cancer in those under 65 years is 18 per 100,000 persons compared with 185.7 per 100,000 in those 65 years and older, which mirrors the incidence rates of most malignancies in the United States (Figure 54.1) (1). The median age at diagnosis of most GI cancers is over 65, with notable exceptions of anal cancer with a median age of 62 and liver cancers with a median age of 64 (1). Thus, more than half of GI cancers are diagnosed in people over 65, making care of older adults a central part of the job of the GI oncologist. The importance of geriatric oncology is not likely to decrease in coming years. As of 2017, people over 65 years comprised 15% of the U.S. population, a proportion which will steadily grow to 25% by 2060, equating to a doubling of the number of elderly Americans (2). Even among cancers with a declining incidence rate such as colorectal cancer, this decline will be counterbalanced by the marked aging of our population. We are likely to see a considerable increase in the absolute number of cases of all GI cancers in the decades to come.

The care of an older patient is not inherently different than the care of a younger patient: Decisions about treatment should focus on the anticipated benefit in light of the patient's tumor characteristics, performance status, and comorbidities. However, clinically relevant comorbid disease is substantially more common among older individuals, and age-related decline in organ function may alter drug pharmacokinetics and thereby adversely affect tolerability of chemotherapy (3,4); both of these physiologic changes should be taken into account during treatment decision making. In addition, while on average older patients are just as likely as younger patients to want to try treatment for cancer, they are less willing to take treatments that result in severe adverse effects than are younger patients (5). This preference for giving greater weight to quality of life over life prolongation makes incorporating the patient's voice into treatment decision making absolutely critical.

In this chapter, we highlight best practices in assessing and evaluating older adults with GI malignancies to better inform treatment decision making and individualize cancer therapies.

ASSESSING THE OLDER PATIENT WITH CANCER

Chronologic age alone and performance status assessments are insufficient in appraising the significant variability in overall health status of older adults. Two-thirds of older adults with "normal" performance status may have geriatric assessment (GA) identified impairments that can influence treatment outcomes (6). As individuals of the same chronologic age may vary widely in their ability to tolerate cancer treatments, more comprehensive evaluations are needed to appropriately personalize therapies in older adults with any cancer.

GA is a multidimensional diagnostic process to assess the medical, functional, and psychosocial abilities of an older person (7). GA evaluates a broad array of health domains that include physical function, functional status, comorbidity, nutrition, cognition, social support, and psychological health (see Table 54.1) in order to develop a coordinated and integrated plan for treatment. Traditionally, GAs were performed by geriatricians and as part of a multidisciplinary evaluation that could take several hours, but this is frequently not realistic nor feasible due to lack of resources, challenging logistics, and the overwhelming number of older adults with cancer in most centers. Therefore, shortened versions of the GA that are predominately patient-reported have been developed for ease of use in busy oncology clinics (8). These

---

A Clinical Vignette is included at the end of the chapter.

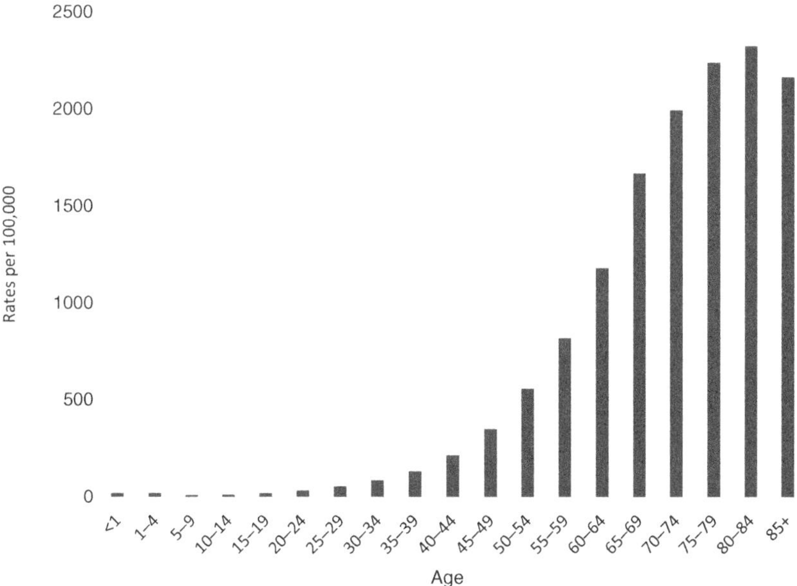

FIGURE 54.1 Cancer incidence rates by age.

Source: From Surveillance, Epidemiology, and End Results (SEER) Cancer Statistics Review. National Cancer Institute; 1975–2015. http://seer.cancer.gov/faststats/index.php

abbreviated tools have been shown to be feasible in different clinical settings and often take on average 20 to 30 minutes to complete and only about 5 minutes of healthcare provider time (8–10). The most commonly employed GAs are composed of an assortment of well-validated individual instruments to assess the health domains of the GA. See Table 54.1 for a list of commonly utilized measures for each GA domain. Deciding on which specific measures to employ can be tailored to provider preference/familiarity and local resources. The exact tools incorporated into a GA may vary between centers and different studies, but all GAs should address the following key domains: functional status, physical performance, comorbidity/polypharmacy, cognition, nutrition, social support, and psychological status (11).

There are several benefits to incorporating a GA in the management of older adults with cancer. First, GA can reveal areas of vulnerability that often go unrecognized by traditional oncologic evaluations. For example, the presence of impairments in instrumental activities of daily living (IADLs) and/or falls are frequently overlooked by routine oncologic evaluations, yet are important indicators of health and have been associated with increased chemotherapy toxicities and mortality (12,13). In one study of older patients with cancer and normal performance status, over two-thirds of patients had a GA-identified impairment, and a quarter of older patients had three or more impairments (6). A GA has also been shown to be superior to oncologists' clinical judgment in identifying frail older adults who are at risk for increased adverse outcomes (14). Second, these identified impairments and areas of vulnerability can aid in the prediction of several key outcomes such as risk of surgical complications, prognosis, and tolerability of systemic chemotherapy (15). Using falls and IADL impairments as examples, both are independently predictive of severe chemotherapy toxicity (12). In a recent study of predominately older patients with GI malignancies, patients with a high GA-based chemotherapy toxicity risk score treated with standard therapy (full dose combinational chemotherapy) had remarkably high rates of severe chemotherapy toxicities and hospitalizations (88% and 50%, respectively) (16). An improved understanding of the likelihood of severe chemotherapy toxicities, surgical complications, and overall survival can aid in the treatment decision-making process when weighing the potential risk/benefits of cancer treatments (17). Last, many of the impairments identified by a GA are amenable to interventions, such as physical and occupational therapy, nutritional guidance, geriatrician consultation, and improved management of comorbid conditions (see Table 54.1). These GA-based interventions have been shown to

TABLE 54.1 Domains Assessed in a Typical Geriatric Assessment and Potential Interventions for Impairments

Domain	What Is Measured?	Commonly Used Measures	Interventions for Impairments
Functional status	ADLs and IADLs	OARS, Katz ADL scale, Lawton IADL scale	Referral to physical or occupational therapy
Physical function	Ability to ambulate, walk stairs, and history of falls	MOS Physical Function	Referral to physical or occupational therapy, geriatrician, home safety assessment
Comorbidity	Number of any coexisting conditions in addition to cancer, hearing/vision, number/type of medications including potential interactions	Charlson Comorbidity Index, OARS Physical Health Subscale, CIRS-G	Referral to geriatrician and/or pharmacist
Nutritional status	History of weight loss, BMI	BMI, weight loss, PG-SGA, MNA	Referral to nutritionist
Psychological state	Assessment of anxiety and depression	MHI, GDS, PHQ-9, HADS	Referral to psychologist and/or social worker
Social support	Availability of social support	MOS Social Support Survey	Referral to social worker
Cognition	Measure of cognitive function	Mini-Cog, MMSE, or MoCA, BOMC test	Referral to geriatrician, neurologist

ADL, activity of daily living; BMI, body mass index; BOMC, Blessed Orientation-Memory-Concentration; CIRS-G, Cumulative Illness Rating Scale for Geriatrics; GDS, Geriatric Depression Scale; HADS, Hospital Anxiety and Depression Scale; IADL, instrumental activity of daily living; MHI, Mental Health Index; MMSE, Mini-Mental State Exam; MNA, Mini Nutritional Assessment; MoCA, Montreal Cognitive Assessment; MOS, Medical Outcomes Survey; OARS, Older Americans Resources and Services; PG-SGA, Patient-Generated Subjective Global Assessment; PHQ-9, Patient Health Questionnaire-9.

improve health-related quality of life and even potentially survival in noncancer populations, and the impact of these interventions on the long-term outcomes of older adults with cancer is an area of ongoing focus (18,19).

Other assessments and biomarkers, such as body composition metrics and inflammatory/senescence markers, can be potentially useful in assessing older adults with cancer to improve prognostication and assess tolerability of potential cancer treatments (20,21). Most notably, low muscle mass, commonly known as sarcopenia within oncology, is highly associated with severe chemotherapy toxicities, surgical complications, and increased mortality (22–24). This is a particularly attractive measure for use in older patients with GI malignancies as body composition metrics can be easily obtained from the CT imaging used as part of routine staging and disease monitoring for nearly all GI malignancies (25). Skeletal muscle measures can also potentially aid in identifying frail older adults and those with physical function limitations (26,27). Moreover, body composition variables may better inform chemotherapy dosing strategies in older and overweight patients as body surface area based dosing may result in higher drug levels, particularly in sarcopenia obese patients (28–30). However, these biomarkers and measures are not yet a part of routine oncologic care and remain primarily tools for future research (21).

INCORPORATING ASSESSMENTS INTO ONCOLOGIC PRACTICE

Performing a GA is recommended in all patients 75 years or older or in younger patients with specific age-related concerns (11). Although many of these assessments have been designed specifically for use in busy oncology clinics, performing a GA in all older patients can be resource- and time-consuming. In order to better target those older patients who may benefit most from a full GA, screening tools have been developed (31). Using screening tools such as the Geriatric 8 (G8) or the Vulnerable Elders Survey 13 (VES-13) takes only a few minutes to complete (32,33). Any older patient with a positive screening evaluation warrants further evaluation with a full GA. In settings where performing a full GA is not feasible, screening tools can themselves provide useful and prognostic information (34). In a study of older adults with late-stage colorectal cancer, the VES-13 was predictive of mortality (35). In addition, targeted questions that fit on a single page and can be completed within a few short minutes in the waiting room can provide considerable information regarding chemotherapy toxicity and survival prognostication. Incorporating the five questions found to be independently predictive of chemotherapy toxicity can allow for easy calculation of the chemotherapy toxicity risk score (12). In addition, three items from within the full GA were recently found to significantly improve estimation of overall survival in older adults with cancer (13). Using these more abbreviated tools can complement routine oncologic practice and help personalize the care of older adults with cancer. Table 54.2 highlights some selected online resources for geriatric oncology that include online access to the commonly employed Cancer and Aging Research Group (CARG) geriatric assessment and CARG toxicity calculator.

OLDER ADULT SPECIFIC GI TRIALS

Older adults have been consistently underrepresented on therapeutic clinical trials in cancer (36). Few elderly specific trials have been conducted, and even fewer that incorporate a refined assessment of physiologic aging or end points of particular importance to decision making in the older cancer patient such as health-related quality of life and functional independence. As such, we do not have robust data on the optimal treatment approach for older patients with GI cancers.

In colorectal cancer, the FOCUS2 trial is notable in that it was designed to specifically evaluate not just the efficacy, but also the tolerability of chemotherapy as measured by a comprehensive health assessment, global quality of life, and standard toxicity measures. FOCUS2

TABLE 54.2 Useful Online Resources for Managing Older Adults With Cancer

Site	Web Address	Highlighted Resources
SIOG	www.siog.org	• Links to published guidelines on management of older adults with cancer • Screening tools and geriatric assessment measures
CARG	www.mycarg.org	• Access to geriatric assessments (in a variety of different languages) and an online chemotherapy toxicity calculator
Moffitt Cancer Center SAOP Tools	https://moffitt.org/for-healthcare-providers/clinical-programs-and-services/senior-adult-oncology-program/senior-adult-oncology-program-tools/	• CRASH chemotherapy toxicity score • Online access to the CIRS-G
ASCO Geriatric Oncology website	www.asco.org/practice-guidelines/cancer-care-initiatives/geriatric-oncology	• Geriatric oncology resources and updates with links on a variety of different aging related topics including cancer-specific information

ASCO, American Society of Clinical Oncology; CARG, Cancer and Aging Research Group; CIRS-G, Cumulative Illness Rating Scale for Geriatrics; CRASH, Chemotherapy Risk Assessment Scale for High-Age Patients; SAOP, Senior Adult Oncology Program; SIOG, International Society of Geriatric Oncology.

specifically enrolled only patients considered "unfit" for standard combination chemotherapy (37). In this trial, patients were randomized via two-by-two design to receive 5-fluorouracil and leucovorin on a modified de Gramont schedule, FOLFOX, capecitabine, or capecitabine and oxaliplatin. All drugs were initiated at 80% of the standard dose, and escalated as tolerated after 6 weeks of therapy. This approach resulted in a small improvement in progression-free survival (median 5.8 vs. 4.5 months) for the addition of oxaliplatin without any clinically significant decline in overall health. Capecitabine's efficacy was no different than 5-fluorouracil but was associated with a greater number of severe adverse effects.

More studies specifically tailored to the needs of older cancer patients, such as FOCUS2, are greatly needed in GI cancers as our other means of assessing treatment in older adults are unable to provide adequate information for treatment decision making. Subgroup analyses of older patients treated in large randomized clinical trials provide valuable information on how well the fittest of elderly patients tolerate treatment and the efficacy in that subgroup, yet the results are not often generalizable to the entire population of older patients with GI cancers. Observational comparative effectiveness studies also offer an estimate of the safety and effectiveness of drugs in a more representative population; however, the nonrandomized nature of such studies and lack of patient specific information on physiologic age make it difficult to interpret the treatment effect estimates provided. Both of these approaches can provide general guidance to patients and their physicians, but offer much less precise information than trials such as FOCUS2.

CLINICAL APPROACH TO THE OLDER ADULT PATIENT WITH A GI MALIGNANCY

Older adults considered for systemic chemotherapy should undergo a screening evaluation with either the VES-13 or G8 upon first consultation with their medical oncologist (see Figure 54.2). For patients identified as fit and screen negative, no further evaluation is required and they can proceed with routine oncologic care. For patients who test positive on a screening tool, a full GA should be pursued. Any modifiable impairments identified on GA should be treated as appropriate (see Table 54.1). In the context of considering chemotherapy treatment,

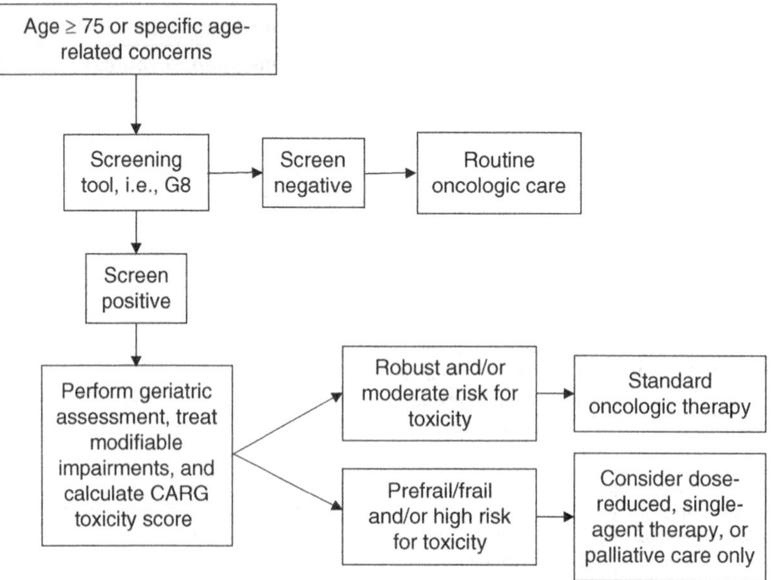

FIGURE 54.2 Suggested treatment algorithm for approaching chemotherapy decision making in older adults with GI malignancies.

CARG, Cancer and Aging Research Group; GI, gastrointestinal.

we suggest scoring the CARG toxicity score based on GA and routine laboratory variables (available online at the CARG website) (12). When using the CARG toxicity score in the clinic to assist in decision making, we suggest imputing as standard dose and polychemotherapy as part of initial chemotherapy toxicity evaluation using the CARG tool (16). Of note, all older adults with GI malignancies being considered for combinational chemotherapy are at least at moderate risk of severe chemotherapy toxicity. For patients identified as robust and/or with a moderate risk for chemotherapy (≤9), proceed with standard guideline treatment recommendations. For patients identified as prefrail/frail or at high risk of chemotherapy toxicity (≥10), consider dose-reduced therapy, single-agent therapy, or palliative treatment alone. Although this algorithm represents an oversimplification of the complex decision making surrounding chemotherapy in older adults, this framework can be helpful as an initial approach. Furthermore, patient preferences and treatment goals should be elicited during initial consultation and used to inform all treatment decisions.

CONCLUSION

Although the treatment of older adults with GI malignancies is frequently complicated by comorbid conditions and functional impairments, many tools are available to assist in providing personalized and comprehensive care. As chronologic age and physiologic age are distinct entities, a GA may assist cancer providers in assessing the overall fitness of older adults and/or those with geriatric syndromes such as functional and cognitive impairments for cancer treatments and facilitate their treatment decision making with their caregivers. Performing a GA provides more than only prognostic information and can be used to guide intervention strategies for patients with identified impairments. Screening tools can be easily performed in busy clinics and are useful in identifying which patients warrant a full GA. More studies are needed to provide specific guidance surrounding certain treatment decisions in older adults with GI malignancies, but existing clinical trials, such as FOCUS2, provide a framework for clinical trial design and chemotherapy dosing in older frail patients.

Clinical Vignette 54.1

To demonstrate the nuances of treating older adults with gastrointestinal malignancies, we present two cases of stage IV colon cancer. Mr. Smith and Mr. Johnson are 76-year-old men who presented to the emergency room with abdominal pain, and CT imaging revealed bilobar hepatic lesions and several pulmonary nodules as well as a right-sided colonic mass. Both patients underwent CT-guided liver biopsies that confirmed moderately differentiated adenocarcinoma with immunohistochemistry staining consistent with metastatic colon cancer (CK 20 and CDX2 positive). The tumors were found to be KRAS and BRAF wild-type and microsatellite stable (MSS). Both patients are referred for consultation with their medical oncologist to discuss possible systemic chemotherapy.

Upon consultation with their medical oncologist to discuss systemic therapy, Mr. Smith undergoes a G8 screening tool and scores a 16 out of 17 (notable only for more than three daily medications), indicating a negative screen for vulnerability (total score ≤14 = vulnerable). He remains active with no functional status limitations and minimal comorbid conditions. He prefers aggressive treatment of his cancer and is recommended to undergo systemic therapy with 5-fluorouracil and oxaliplatin (FOLFOX) with bevacizumab. On the other hand, Mr. Johnson undergoes the same screening assessment but scores a 9 out of 17 (below the ≤14 cutoff), and therefore has a full geriatric assessment performed that reveals significant weight loss, history of falls, limitations in ability to walk 1 block, and impairments in IADL. His CARG chemotherapy toxicity score is calculated at a 94% risk of developing a grade 3 to 5 toxicity. Mr. Smith is referred for physical and occupational therapy (for his IADL and mobility limitations) and to see a nutritionist (for weight loss). After discussion of the risks/benefits of systemic therapy and the patient's preferences/goals for treatment, he is started on single-agent infusional 5-fluorouracil. As he appeared to tolerate the treatment without significant side effects, at his toxicity check 2 weeks later, oxaliplatin was added with a 20% dose reduction.

REFERENCES

1. Surveillance Epidemiology and End Results (SEER) Cancer Statistics Review. National Cancer Institute; 1975–2015. http://seer.cancer.gov/faststats/index.php
2. Vespa J, Armstrong D, Medina L. Demographic turning points for the United States: population projections for 2020 to 2060. *United States Census Bureau.* 2018:25–1144.
3. Sawhney R, Sehl M, Naeim A. Physiologic aspects of aging: impact on cancer management and decision making, part I. *Cancer J.* 2005;11(6):449–460. doi:10.1097/00130404-200511000-00004
4. Sehl M, Sawhney R, Naeim A. Physiologic aspects of aging: impact on cancer management and decision making, part II. *Cancer J.* 2005;11(6):461–473. doi:10.1097/00130404-200511000-00005
5. Yellen SB, Cella DF, Leslie WT. Age and clinical decision making in oncology patients. *J Natl Cancer Inst.* 1994;86(23):1766–1770. doi:10.1093/jnci/86.23.1766
6. Jolly TA, Deal AM, Nyrop KA, et al. Geriatric assessment-identified deficits in older cancer patients with normal performance status. *Oncologist.* 2015;20(4):379–385. doi:10.1634/theoncologist.2014-0247
7. Wildiers H, Heeren P, Puts M, et al. International society of geriatric oncology consensus on geriatric assessment in older patients with cancer. *J Clin Oncol.* 2014;32(24):2595–2603. doi:10.1200/jco.2013.54.8347
8. Hurria A, Gupta S, Zauderer M, et al. Developing a cancer-specific geriatric assessment: a feasibility study. *Cancer.* 2005;104(9):1998–2005. doi:10.1002/cncr.21422
9. Williams GR, Deal AM, Jolly TA, et al. Feasibility of geriatric assessment in community oncology clinics. *J Geriatr Oncol.* 2014;5(3):245–251. doi:10.1016/j.jgo.2014.03.001
10. Hurria A, Cirrincione CT, Muss HB, et al. Implementing a geriatric assessment in cooperative group clinical cancer trials: CALGB 360401. *J Clin Oncol.* 2011;29(10):1290–1296. doi:10.1200/JCO.2010.30.6985
11. Mohile SG, Velarde C, Hurria A, et al. Geriatric assessment-guided care processes for older adults: a delphi consensus of geriatric oncology experts. *J Natl Compr Cancer Netw.* 2015;13(9):1120–1130. doi:10.6004/jnccn.2015.0137
12. Hurria A, Togawa K, Mohile SG, et al. Predicting chemotherapy toxicity in older adults with cancer: a prospective multicenter study. *J Clin Oncol.* 2011;29(25):3457–3465. doi:10.1200/JCO.2011.34.7625
13. Nishijima TF, Deal AM, Lund JL, et al. The incremental value of a geriatric assessment-derived three-item scale on estimating overall survival in older adults with cancer. *J Geriatr Oncol.* 2018;9(4):329–336. doi:10.1016/j.jgo.2018.01.007
14. Kirkhus L, Saltyte Benth J, Rostoft S, et al. Geriatric assessment is superior to oncologists' clinical judgement in identifying frailty. *Br J Cancer.* 2017;117(4):470–477. doi:10.1038/bjc.2017.202
15. Puts MT, Santos B, Hardt J, et al. An update on a systematic review of the use of geriatric assessment for older adults in oncology. *Ann Oncol.* 2014;25(2):307–315. doi:10.1093/annonc/mdt386
16. Nishijima TF, Deal AM, Williams GR, et al. Chemotherapy toxicity risk score for treatment decisions in older adults with advanced solid tumors. *Oncologist.* 2018;23(5):573–579. doi:10.1634/theoncologist.2017-0559
17. Mohile SG, Magnuson A, Pandya C, et al. Community oncologists' decision-making for treatment of older patients with cancer. *J Natl Compr Cancer Netw.* 2018;16(3):301–309. doi:10.6004/jnccn.2017.7047
18. Magnuson A, Allore H, Cohen HJ, et al. Geriatric assessment with management in cancer care: current evidence and potential mechanisms for future research. *J Geriatr Oncol.* 2016;7(4):242–248. doi:10.1016/j.jgo.2016.02.007
19. Rubenstein LZ, Stuck AE, Siu AL, et al. Impacts of geriatric evaluation and management programs on defined outcomes: overview of the evidence. *J Am Geriatr Soc.* 1991;39(9 Pt 2):8S–16S; discussion 17S–18S. doi:10.1111/j.1532-5415.1991.tb05927.x
20. Hubbard JM, Cohen HJ, Muss HB. Incorporating biomarkers into cancer and aging research. *J Clin Oncol.* 2014;32(24):2611–2616. doi:10.1200/JCO.2014.55.4261
21. Williams GR, Muss HB, Shachar SS. Research methods: translational research in geriatric oncology. In: Extermann M, ed. *Geriatric Oncology.* Cham, Switzerland: Springer International Publishing; 2017:1–20.
22. Rier HN, Jager A, Sleijfer S, et al. The prevalence and prognostic value of low muscle mass in cancer patients: a review of the literature. *Oncologist.* 2016;21(11):1396–1409. doi:10.1634/theoncologist.2016-0066
23. Shachar SS, Williams GR, Muss HB, et al. Prognostic value of sarcopenia in adults with solid tumours: a meta-analysis and systematic review. *Eur J Cancer.* 2016;57:58–67. doi:10.1016/j.ejca.2015.12.030

24. Kazemi-Bajestani SM, Mazurak VC, Baracos V. Computed tomography-defined muscle and fat wasting are associated with cancer clinical outcomes. *Sem Cell Dev Biol.* 2016;54:2–10. doi:10.1016/j.semcdb.2015.09.001

25. Mourtzakis M, Prado CMM, Lieffers JR, et al. A practical and precise approach to quantification of body composition in cancer patients using computed tomography images acquired during routine care. *Appl Physiol Nutr Me.* 2008;33(5):997–1006. doi:10.1139/H08-075

26. Williams GR, Deal AM, Muss HB, et al. Frailty and skeletal muscle in older adults with cancer. *J Geriatr Oncol.* 2018;9(1):68–73. doi:10.1016/j.jgo.2017.08.002

27. Williams GR, Deal AM, Muss HB, et al. Skeletal muscle measures and physical function in older adults with cancer: sarcopenia or myopenia? *Oncotarget.* 2017;8(20):33658–33665. doi:10.18632/oncotarget.16866

28. Mir O, Coriat R, Blanchet B, et al. Sarcopenia predicts early dose-limiting toxicities and pharma-cokinetics of sorafenib in patients with hepatocellular carcinoma. *Plos One.* 2012;7(5):e37563. doi:10.1371/journal.pone.0037563

29. Prado CM, Maia YL, Ormsbee M, et al. Assessment of nutritional status in cancer–the relationship between body composition and pharmacokinetics. *Anti-cancer Agents Med Chem.* 2013;13(8):1197–1203. doi:10.2174/18715206113139990322

30. Williams GR, Deal AM, Shachar SS, et al. The impact of skeletal muscle on the pharmacokinetics and toxicity of 5-fluorouracil in colorectal cancer. *Cancer Chemother Pharmacol.* 2018;81(2):413–417. doi:10.1007/s00280-017-3487-2

31. Decoster L, Van Puyvelde K, Mohile S, et al. Screening tools for multidimensional health problems warranting a geriatric assessment in older cancer patients: an update on SIOG recommendationsdagger. *Ann Oncol.* 2015;26(2):288–300. doi:10.1093/annonc/mdu210

32. Mohile SG, Bylow K, Dale W, et al. A pilot study of the vulnerable elders survey-13 compared with the comprehensive geriatric assessment for identifying disability in older patients with prostate cancer who receive androgen ablation. *Cancer.* 2007;109(4):802–810. doi:10.1002/cncr.22495

33. Soubeyran P, Bellera C, Goyard J, et al. Validation of the G8 screening tool in geriatric oncology: the ONCODAGE project. *J Clin Oncol.* 2011;29(15S):550S. doi:10.1200/jco.2011.29.15_suppl.9001

34. Loh KP, Soto-Perez-de-Celis E, Hsu T, et al. What every oncologist should know about geriatric assessment for older patients with cancer: Young International Society of Geriatric Oncology Position Paper. *J Oncol Pract.* 2018;14(2):85–94. doi:10.1200/jop.2017.026435

35. Ramsdale E, Polite B, Hemmerich J, et al. The Vulnerable Elders Survey-13 predicts mortality in older adults with later-stage colorectal cancer receiving chemotherapy: a prospective pilot study. *J Am Geriatr Soc.* 2013;61(11):2043–2044. doi:10.1111/jgs.12536

36. Talarico L, Chen G, Pazdur R. Enrollment of elderly patients in clinical trials for cancer drug registration: a 7-Year experience by the US Food and Drug Administration. *J Clin Oncol.* 2004;22(22):4626–4631. doi:10.1200/JCO.2004.02.175

37. Seymour MT, Thompson LC, Wasan HS, et al. Chemotherapy options in elderly and frail patients with metastatic colorectal cancer (MRC FOCUS2): an open-label, randomised factorial trial. *Lancet.* 2011;377(9779):1749–1759. doi:10.1016/S0140-6736(11)60399-1

Survivorship Care for Gastrointestinal Cancer Patients

Nataliya V. Uboha, Mary Mulkerin, Stephanie L. Fricke, and Noelle K. LoConte

BACKGROUND ON SURVIVORSHIP

The American Cancer Society defines a cancer survivor as, "any person with a history of cancer, from the time of diagnosis through the remainder of life" (1). As we continue to make progress against the wide variety of gastrointestinal cancers, including better treatments and hopefully more cures, there will be more cancer survivors. In 2019, there are expected to be over 1,500,000 colorectal cancer survivors alone, and these numbers are increasing over time (1). Optimal survivorship care for cancer survivors is a critical skill for oncologists who care for patients with gastrointestinal malignancies.

The Institute of Medicine (IOM) report *From Cancer Patient to Cancer Survivor: Lost in Transition* detailed deficits in posttreatment cancer care delivery (2). To address these deficits, the IOM recommended that a survivorship care plan (SCP), consisting of a treatment summary and a plan for long-term follow-up care, be given to each cancer survivor treated with curative intent. Since this report, there has been increased focus and research directed at the development of SCPs and their effect on patient satisfaction and outcomes, though there has been a relative paucity of research in nonbreast cancer survivors, including gastrointestinal cancer patients. Wide variations in SCP content, format, delivery, and metrics for outcome evaluation exist. For example, Palmer et al. created a metric scorecard to assess concordance with IOM recommendations for SCPs in breast cancer patients. The scorecard consists of 92 total items, 60 for the treatment summary and 32 for the follow-up plan (3).

The American Cancer Society has created guidelines for SCP for colorectal cancer survivors (4). Key elements include surveillance for colorectal cancer recurrence, screening for new primary cancers, assessment and management of physical and psychosocial effects of cancer treatments, and general health promotion such as tobacco cessation. The SCP is much less studied in other gastrointestinal malignancies, and this is a critical area for future research. Nonetheless, the content of a sample SCP for colorectal cancer provides an ideal framework for reviewing the relevant issues for gastrointestinal cancer survivors. In this chapter, we review the survivorship issues by modality—surgery, radiation and finally, chemotherapy.

POSTSURGICAL ISSUES

Surgical treatment of gastrointestinal cancers is frequently the only curative therapy and is often offered to patients with localized or even oligometastatic disease. However, there are many long-term consequences of these surgeries of which the medical oncologist should be aware.

Gastroesophageal Surgery

Esophagectomy and gastrectomy are part of the treatment for locoregional gastroesophageal malignancies. These operations are associated with significant impairment of health-related quality of life (HRQOL) in survivors, both during the short-term postsurgical recovery period and during longer term follow-up. Two years after esophagectomy, survivors may still have significant fatigue, decreased appetite, and respiratory issues (5). Swallowing dysfunction, reflux, and coughing have been reported to be major long-term complications of esophagectomy, with swallowing problems having the largest impact on HRQOL (6). Patients who undergo esophagectomy or gastrectomy are at risk for long-term nutritional disorders resulting from inadequate intake, absorption, or digestion. Survivors may develop osteoporosis, anemia, and select vitamin deficiencies (7). Gastrectomy patients should receive prophylactic vitamin B_{12} injections to prevent megaloblastic anemia resulting from decreased intrinsic factor, which is normally produced by gastric mucosa (8). Iron-deficiency anemia is seen in up to 50% of patients and should be treated with ferrous sulfate, which was shown to be superior to ferrous glycinate chelate (9). Gastrectomy patients are also at risk for dumping syndrome, which is associated with palpitations, abdominal cramping, diarrhea, and dizziness 0.5 to 3 hours after a meal. These symptoms are usually treated with dietary changes (frequent smaller meals, higher fiber intake, low carbohydrate diet). Octreotide has been used in more severe cases of dumping syndrome and resulted in quality of life (QOL) improvement (10).

Pancreatic Surgery

Pancreatic resection is used for both adenocarcinoma and neuroendocrine tumors, as well as much rarer types of pancreas cancers. Short-term postoperative complications are seen in about 50% of patients, including infections and pancreatic leaks. Long-term sequelae of the operation stem from the physiological effects of pancreas removal, such as impaired glucose tolerance or diabetes, pancreatic insufficiency, and delayed gastric emptying. Late sequelae of the resection (over 3 years) may also include ulcer disease, biliary stricture, postsplenectomy syndrome, and metachronous malignancies (11). Despite long-term persistence of physiological symptoms, recurrence-free survivors report favorable quality of life after pancreatic surgery (12).

Colorectal Surgery

Almost all colorectal cancer survivors undergo bowel surgery as part of their treatment, and nearly half experience long-term issues with bowel symptoms as a result. Bowel dysfunction may be an ongoing issue for many years after the cancer diagnosis and is the main determinant of QOL in this patient population (13). Close to half of all colorectal cancer survivors have problems with chronic diarrhea after the completion of their treatment (14,15). Antidiarrhea medications (such as loperamide or diphenoxylate/atropine) and fiber are typically the first-line treatments for persistent diarrhea. Patients with cancer in their middle or upper third of the rectum who undergo low-anterior resection (LAR) are at risk for developing LAR syndrome, especially if they received neoadjuvant radiation therapy (RT). LAR syndrome is defined by a combination of increased stool frequency, clustering, urgency, incomplete evacuation, and incontinence in some cases (15). Although these symptoms decrease over time in the majority of patients, a significant fraction of patients suffer from long-term symptoms and disability (16). Currently, there are no standard treatment options for LAR syndrome. Encouraging results were seen with sacral or tibial nerve stimulation or transanal irrigation and biofeedback, but prospective randomized data are needed to confirm these benefits (17–21). Both patients with primary anastomosis and patients with permanent ostomies are at risk for late surgical complications. For patients with ostomies, these include hernia formation, urinary retention, skin conditions, infection, and fistula formation, all of which are associated with lower HRQOL (22). Patients with permanent ostomy face a range of other issues that physicians must be aware. Ostomy and appliance care is one of the greatest challenges, requiring significant lifestyle changes (23). The many other HRQOL issues reported include problems with physical activity, intimacy and sexuality, travel, and psychological well-being (24). Ostomy-specific concerns persist for more than 5 years in colorectal cancer survivors, which highlights the need for long-term support programs for this patient population.

Liver Surgery

Hepatectomy is being used for treatment of hepatocellular carcinoma, cholangiocarcinoma, as well as colorectal cancer metastases to the liver. There are immediate risks after resection of the liver, including bleeding, liver failure, infection, coagulopathy, hyperglycemia, and portal hypertension (25). The perioperative mortality rates at large-volume medical centers are generally in the 3% or less range (25). All of these complications are more likely if the patient has a prior history of cirrhosis or diabetes (26). Importantly, however, the liver does regrow after the surgery, which lessens the risk of these complications over time. Patients with pre-existing renal failure also appear to be at higher risk of postoperative morbidity and mortality. It is important to counsel patients who have had a liver resection to limit their alcohol intake as well as monitoring their acetaminophen usage (27).

POST-RT ISSUES

RT is an integral treatment modality in the management of gastrointestinal cancers to prolong disease-free survival and reduce local recurrence rates. Long-term effects of RT are dependent on the area involved in the radiation field and the dose and volume of radiation delivered (28). Long-term side effects of RT may occur as soon as 3 to 6 months after completing treatment, but may also occur many years after completion of RT (29), requiring the oncology team to remain vigilant for the development of these side effects.

Pelvic Radiation

Chronic radiation proctitis (CRP) occurs in 5% to 10% of patients who receive pelvic RT (30). The most common presenting symptom of CRP is bleeding from the rectum (either with or independent of bowel movements) (29). Other symptoms include diarrhea, mucus discharge, fecal urgency, and tenesmus (29). The following symptoms related to strictures may also occur: constipation, rectal pain, urgency, fecal incontinence, and decreased stool caliber (29). Endoscopy is necessary to evaluate the extent of radiation disease (31). Management of CRP is largely based on experiential data rather than evidence-based practice as there are few randomized controlled trials, and no consistent guidelines for the treatment of CRP exist (30). Mild forms of CRP with minimal bleeding may be treated with loperamide, fiber, stool bulking agents, and corticosteroids (32). Several treatments are used to manage rectal bleeding. Topical anti-inflammatory enemas and suppositories are used as first-line therapy but their effectiveness has yielded mixed results (31). Endoscopic therapy with cryoablation and argon plasma coagulation is used to control bleeding but must be done with caution due to the potential risk for fistulas or ulcerations (29). CRP is often self-limiting and responds well to medical management (29). Surgical treatments are reserved for patients who develop nonhealing fistulas, sepsis, perforation, or refractory bleeding (31).

Radiation cystitis varies in severity but often negatively impacts HRQOL. Symptoms include frequency, dysuria, urgency, nocturia, suprapubic pain, bladder infection, fatigue, and microscopic and/or macroscopic hematuria (33). Urinalysis with culture and cytology should be done to rule out infection and malignancy (33). There are no guidelines or standard-of-care therapy for radiation cystitis. Treatment is based on current knowledge (33). Mild cystitis may be treated with anticholinergic drugs (33). Moderate cystitis is treated with clot evacuation, hyperbaric oxygen therapy, or bladder instillations (33). Surgical intervention is reserved for severe or refractory cystitis (33).

Pelvic RT has been associated with sexual dysfunction in both males and females (34). Vaginal stenosis (VS) is a common long-term effect from pelvic RT. Manifestations of VS include dyspareunia and postcoital bleeding (35). Symptoms are often exacerbated by decreased lubrication and thinning of vaginal tissues associated with menopause (35). Little scientific evidence exists regarding the prevention and management of VS (35). A Cochrane review concluded that there is no evidence that regular vaginal dilation prevents VS or improves quality of life (36). Despite lack of evidence, vaginal dilators remain highly used in clinical practice (35). A Delphi consensus panel recommended that dilator use should start 4 weeks post-RT, performed two to three times per week for 1 to 3 minutes, and continue for 9 to 12 months after the completion of pelvic RT (37). Further studies are needed to evaluate efficacy and use of topical treatments and hormone replacement therapy (35). Males who received pelvic RT for anorectal cancer reported increased rates of erectile dysfunction (38,39). Phosphodiesterase type 5 inhibitors were shown to be beneficial in treating erectile dysfunction in prostate cancer patients (34). For those patients who do not respond to phosphodiesterase type 5 inhibitors, a referral to a urologist is clinically indicated.

Radiation to the Central Chest

RT for esophageal cancer can lead to the development of strictures or stenosis resulting in dysphagia, odynophagia, and compromised nutritional status. Endoscopic dilation provides improvement of the stricture, but there is up to a 33% recurrence rate requiring repeat dilation (40). For those patients who become refractory to dilation, esophageal stent placement is considered (41).

While advancements in cancer treatments have resulted in improved overall survival, there is increasing concern about the long-term carcinogenic potential of RT. The risk of developing a new malignancy is 14% higher among cancer survivors compared to the general population (42). However, less than 10% of these secondary malignancies are likely related to RT (43). In addition to anticancer treatments (particularly radiation and specific chemotherapy agents), many factors are suspected in the development of secondary malignancies including age, gender, environmental exposures, genetic predisposition, and lifestyle (44,45). Survivors should continue to receive age- and gender-appropriate cancer screenings, and lifestyle modifications should be encouraged (46). Individuals at increased risk due to genetic factors should undergo more intensive screening regimens (4).

Cardiopulmonary Toxicity

Increased survivorship has also raised concerns about radiation-induced cardiopulmonary toxicity. A review by Beukema et al. estimated the incidence of symptomatic cardiac toxicity after RT for esophageal cancer to be as high as 10.8% with the most frequent complications including pericardial effusions, cardiac ischemia, and heart failure (47). Radiation-induced lung injury occurs frequently as well and limits dose escalations for treatment of thoracic malignancies (48). Radiation pneumonitis, often presenting as mild–severe dyspnea, can occur within 1 to 3 months of treatment and can evolve into progressive pulmonary fibrosis (48). There is a lack of high-quality evidence regarding the utility of screening cancer survivors for late cardiopulmonary effects (49). However, the emergence of the field of cardio-oncology serves as an important tool in the promotion of cardiovascular health among survivors.

POSTCHEMOTHERAPY ISSUES

Neuropathy

Chemotherapy-induced peripheral neuropathy can lead to permanent disability in more than 50% of cancer survivors (50). In the treatment of early-stage gastrointestinal malignancies, oxaliplatin-induced peripheral neuropathy (OIPN) is of greatest concern. Acute oxaliplatin-related neurotoxicity results in reversible cold sensitivity. Prolonged use can lead to paresthesias, dysesthesias, and numbness in the hands and feet that can be progressive and irreversible in nature. These symptoms may continue to worsen even after oxaliplatin is discontinued ("coasting" phenomenon), stressing the importance of close clinical evaluations while patients are on active treatment. OIPN is dose dependent, with severe symptoms typically seen when the cumulative dose exceeds 750 mg/m^2 (51). Although neuropathy diminishes in most patients after treatment completion and time away from oxaliplatin, a significant percentage of patients report persistent symptoms for years posttreatment (52,53). As far out as 7 years from treatment completion, OIPN impacts physical and emotional health and HRQOL in survivors (54). At present, there are no proven neuroprotective treatments to prevent OIPN. Duloxetine can be used to treat neuropathy symptoms and has been shown to significantly reduce pain compared to placebo in patients with chemotherapy-induced neuropathy in a multi-institutional, double-blind crossover trial (55). Physical and occupational therapy may be useful for patients with neuropathy-related gait instability and balance issues. Other platinum agents as well as taxanes can also cause neuropathy.

Infertility

Many chemotherapy agents are gonadotoxic, which can lead to premature menopause and impaired fertility. The possibility of infertility and fertility preservation options should be promptly discussed with all patients of reproductive age anticipating treatment (56). Established fertility preservation methods include sperm, oocyte, and embryo cryopreservation (57). Ovarian transposition may be considered for pelvic RT (57). Ovarian tissue cryopreservation and ovarian suppression remain experimental as data on efficacy are limited (56–58). Manifestations of premature menopause include vasomotor symptoms (hot flashes, night sweats), which can be managed with hormone replacement therapy (HRT), medications (selective serotonin reuptake inhibitor [SSRI]/serotonin–norepinephrine reuptake inhibitor [SNRI], gabapentin, clonidine), and avoidance of triggers (58). Symptoms of atrophic vaginitis (vaginal dryness, dyspareunia) can be improved with topical estrogens, moisturizers/lubricants, and dilators for stenosis. Insomnia and mood changes can be addressed with sleep hygiene and appropriate counseling (58).

LIFE AFTER CANCER

The 2005 release of the IOM seminal publication *From Cancer Patient to Cancer Survivor: Lost in Transition* exposed the posttreatment phase as a neglected area of cancer care and identified several gaps in care delivery (59). Historically, survivorship has been characterized by fragmentation of care, lack of emphasis on prevention of recurrence and secondary cancers, poor attention to long-term and late effects of cancer treatment, and insufficient communication and care coordination between providers (59). Based on this report, the IOM recommends that all patients treated with curative intent should receive a cancer treatment summary and follow-up care plan (SCP) with the purpose of guiding and coordinating care, managing treatment effects, and the adoption of healthy lifestyle behaviors by patients (59).

Poor physical and mental HRQOL were reported by 1 in 4 and 1 in 10 of cancer survivors, respectively (59). Most cancer survivors report moderate-intensity fear of cancer recurrence that does not diminish over time (60,61). Cancer-related posttraumatic stress disorder (CR-PTSD) has been documented in survivors (62,63). Risk factors for CR-PTSD include diagnosis at a younger age, advanced disease at diagnosis, and recent completion of treatment (62). Further research is needed to predict vulnerability and design intervention strategies. Awareness of CR-PTSD is necessary, and a referral to cancer health psychology or other mental health providers should be made if warranted.

The adoption of healthy behaviors, such as physical activity, smoking cessation, and optimizing nutrition and maintaining a healthy body weight, is recommended for cancer survivors. Physical activity after a colorectal cancer diagnosis reduces the risk of colorectal cancer–specific and all-cause mortality (64). Patients with colorectal cancer have a high rate (more than 40% of patients) of comorbid conditions such as diabetes, chronic obstructive pulmonary disease, and congestive heart failure (65). The benefits of diet and physical activity have been well-documented in lowering the risk of cardiovascular disease and diabetes. Therefore, improving diet and exercise among colorectal cancer survivors may have overall health benefits for these patients. Physical activity has been shown to shorten the recovery time from treatment-related side effects and improve HRQOL (66–68). Exercise has led to improved fatigue, anxiety, depression, self-esteem, and happiness in cancer survivors (67,69). The American Cancer Society and American Institute for Cancer Research have published guidelines for physical activity for all cancer survivors (70).

While the IOM and the Commission on Cancer (CoC) endorse the implementation of SCPs, improved patient outcomes have not been linked to the SCP document in randomized control trials (71,72). Several descriptive studies have demonstrated high levels of patient satisfaction with SCPs (73–75). Further, randomized controlled clinical trials assessing patient outcomes targeted by SCPs are needed. Since most SCP research has involved breast and gynecological cancers, future studies conducted in other cancer groups are warranted. The literature review suggests that in addition to the SCP document content, research opportunities should also focus on the delivery process of the SCP. Strategies such as motivational interviewing and counseling sessions may improve patient-reported outcomes (76).

CONCLUSION

In conclusion, there are many unique and pervasive issues for medical oncologists to be aware of as they care for gastrointestinal cancer patients. Each cancer treatment modality has its own long-term potential side effects. These include neuropathy, digestive issues like chronic diarrhea, radiation fibrosis, heart disease, sexual dysfunction, and infertility. The SCP is one strategy an oncology team can implement to raise awareness of these issues with patients, while also improving the patients' satisfaction with their care.

REFERENCES

1. American Cancer Society. Cancer Treatment and Survivorship Facts and Figures 2016-2017. https://cancercontrol.cancer.gov/ocs/statistics/statistics.html
2. Institute of Medicine and National Research Council. From Cancer Patient to Cancer Survivor: Lost in Transition. https://www.nap.edu/catalog/11468/from-cancer-patient-to-cancer-survivor-lost-in-transition
3. Palmer SC, Javobs LA, DeMichele A, et al. Metrics to evaluate treatment summaries and survivorship care plans: a scorecare. *Support Care Cancer.* 2014;22(6):1475–1483. doi:10.1007/s00520-013-2107-x
4. El-Shami K, Oeffinger KC, Erb NL, et al. American cancer society colorectal cancer survivorship care guidelines. *CA Cancer J Clin.* 2015;65(6):428–455. doi:10.3322/caac.21286

5. Scarpa M, Valente S, Alfieri R, et al. Systematic review of health-related quality of life after esophagectomy for esophageal cancer. *World J Gastroenterol*. 2011;17:4660–4674. doi:10.3748/wjg.v17.i42.4660

6. Donohoe CL, McGillycuddy E, Reynolds JV. Long-term health-related quality of life for disease-free esophageal cancer patients. *World J Surg*. 2011;35:1853–1860. doi:10.1007/s00268-011-1123-6

7. Davis JL, Ripley RT. Postgastrectomy syndromes and nutritional considerations following gastric surgery. *Surg Clin North Am*. 2017;97:277–293. doi:10.1016/j.suc.2016.11.005

8. Baker A, Wooten LA, Malloy M. Nutritional considerations after gastrectomy and esophagectomy for malignancy. *Curr Treat Options Oncol*. 2011;12:85–95. doi:10.1007/s11864-010-0134-0

9. Mimura EC, Bregano JW, Dichi JB, et al. Comparison of ferrous sulfate and ferrous glycinate chelate for the treatment of iron deficiency anemia in gastrectomized patients. *Nutrition*. 2008;24:663–668. doi:10.1016/j.nut.2008.03.017

10. Arts J, Caenepeel P, Bisschops R, et al. Efficacy of the long-acting repeatable formulation of the somatostatin analogue octreotide in postoperative dumping. *Clin Gastroenterol Hepatol*. 2009;7:432–437. doi:10.1016/j.cgh.2008.11.025

11. Chen KT, Devarajan K, Hoffman JP. Morbidity among long-term survivors after pancreatoduodenectomy for pancreatic adenocarcinoma. *Ann Surg Oncol*. 2015;22:1185–1189. doi:10.1245/s10434-014-3969-y

12. Cloyd JM, Tran Cao HS, Petzel MQ, et al. Impact of pancreatectomy on long-term patient-reported symptoms and quality of life in recurrence-free survivors of pancreatic and periampullary neoplasms. *J Surg Oncol*. 2017;115:144–150. doi:10.1002/jso.24499

13. Hart TL, Charles ST, Gunaratne M, et al. Symptom severity and quality of life among long-term colorectal cancer survivors compared with matched control subjects: a population-based study. *Dis Colon Rectum*. 2018;61:355–363. doi:10.1097/DCR.0000000000000972

14. Bregendahl S, Emmertsen KJ, Lous J, et al. Bowel dysfunction after low anterior resection with and without neoadjuvant therapy for rectal cancer: a population-based cross-sectional study. *Colorectal Dis*. 2013;15:1130–1139. doi:10.1111/codi.12244

15. Emmertsen KJ, Laurberg S, Rectal Cancer Function Study Group. Impact of bowel dysfunction on quality of life after sphincter-preserving resection for rectal cancer. *Br J Surg*. 2013;100:1377–1387. doi:10.1002/bjs.9223

16. Engel J, Kerr J, Schlesinger-Raab A, et al. Quality of life in rectal cancer patients: a four-year prospective study. *Ann Surg*. 2003;238:203–213. doi:10.1097/01.sla.0000080823.38569.b0

17. Kim KH, Yu CS, Yoon YS, et al. Effectiveness of biofeedback therapy in the treatment of anterior resection syndrome after rectal cancer surgery. *Dis Colon Rectum*. 2011;54:1107–1113. doi:10.1097/DCR.0b013e318221a934

18. Allgayer H, Dietrich CF, Rohde W, et al. Prospective comparison of short- and long-term effects of pelvic floor exercise/biofeedback training in patients with fecal incontinence after surgery plus irradiation versus surgery alone for colorectal cancer: clinical, functional and endoscopic/endosonographic findings. *Scand J Gastroenterol*. 2005;40:1168–1175. doi:10.1080/00365520510023477

19. Koch SM, Rietveld MP, Govaert B, et al. Retrograde colonic irrigation for faecal incontinence after low anterior resection. *Int J Colorectal Dis*. 2009;24:1019–1022. doi:10.1007/s00384-009-0719-x

20. Matzel KE, Stadelmaier U, Bittorf B, et al. Bilateral sacral spinal nerve stimulation for fecal incontinence after low anterior rectum resection. *Int J Colorectal Dis*. 2002;17:430–434. doi:10.1007/s00384-002-0412-9

21. Dulskas A, Smolskas E, Kildusiene I, et al. Treatment possibilities for low anterior resection syndrome: a review of the literature. *Int J Colorectal Dis*. 2018;33:251–260. doi:10.1007/s00384-017-2954-x

22. Liu L, Herrinton LJ, Hornbrook MC, et al. Early and late complications among long-term colorectal cancer survivors with ostomy or anastomosis. *Dis Colon Rectum*. 2010;53:200–212. doi:10.1007/DCR.0b013e3181bdc408

23. Sun V, Grant M, McMullen CK, et al. Surviving colorectal cancer: long-term, persistent ostomy-specific concerns and adaptations. *J Wound Ostomy Continence Nurs*. 2013;40:61–72. doi:10.1097/WON.0b013e3182750143

24. Krouse RS, Herrinton LJ, Grant M, et al. Health-related quality of life among long-term rectal cancer survivors with an ostomy: manifestations by sex. *J Clin Oncol*. 2009;27:4664–4670. doi:10.1200/JCO.2008.20.9502

25. Mullen JT, Ribero D, Reddy SK, et al. Hepatic insufficiency and mortality in 1,059 noncirrhotic patients undergoing major hepatectomy. *J Am Coll Surg*. 2007;204:854. doi:10.1016/j.jamcollsurg.2006.12.032

26. Shimada M, Matsumata T, Akazawa K, et al. Estimation of risk of major complications after hepatic resection. *Am J Surg*. 1994;167:399–403. doi:10.1016/0002-9610(94)90124-4

27. Hill-Kayser CE, Vachani C, Hampshire MK, et al. An internet tool for creation of cancer survivorship care plans for survivors and health care providers: design, implementation, use and user satisfaction. *J Med Internet Res*. 2009;11:e39. doi:10.2196/jmir.1223

28. Fiorino C, Valdagni R, Rancati G. Dose-volume effects for normal tissues in external radiotherapy: pelvis. *Radiother Oncol*. 2009;93:153–167. doi:10.1016/j.radonc.2009.08.004

29. Vanneste BGL, Van De Voorde L, de Ridder RJ, et al. Chronic radiation proctitis: tricks to prevent and treat. *Int J Colorectal Dis*. 2015;30:1293–1303. doi:10.1007/s00384-015-2289-4

30. Bansal N, Soni A, Kauer P, et al. Exploring the management of radiation proctitis in current clinical practice. *J Clin Diagn Res*. 2016;10:XEO1–XEO6. doi:10.7860/JCDR/2016/17524.7906

31. Ashburn JH, Kalady MF. Radiation-induced problems in colorectal surgery. *Clin Colon Rectal Surg*. 2016;29:85–91. doi:10.1055/s-0036-1580632

32. Andreyev HJ, Benton BE, Lalji A, et al. Algorithm-based management of patients with gastrointestinal symptoms in patients after pelvic radiation treatment (ORBIT): a randomized controlled trial. *Lancet*. 2013;382:2084–2092. doi:10.1016/S0140-6736(13)61648-7

33. Zwaans BM, Nicolai HG, Chancellor MB, et al. Challenges and opportunities in radiation-induced hemorrhagic cystitis. *Rev Urol*. 2016;18:57–65.

34. Incrocci L, Jensen PT: Pelvic radiotherapy and sexual function in men and women. *J Sex Med*. 2013;1:53–64. doi:10.1111/jsm.12010

35. Morris L, Do V, Chard J. Radiation-induced vaginal stenosis: current perspectives. *Int J Women's Health*. 2017;9:273–279. doi:10.2147/IJWH.S106796

36. Miles T, Johnson N. Vaginal dilator therapy for women receiving pelvic radiotherapy. *Cochrane Database Syst Rev*. 2014;9:CD0007291. doi:10.1002/14651858.cd007291.pub3

37. Bakker RM, ter Kuile MM, Vermeer WM, et al. Sexual rehabilitation after pelvic radiotherapy and vaginal dilator use: consensus using the Delphi method. *Int J Gynecol Cancer*. 2014;24:1499–1506. doi:10.1097/IGC.0000000000000253

38. Heriot AG, Tekkis PP, Fazio VW, et al. Adiuvant radiotherapy is associated with increased sexual dysfunction in male patients undergoing resection for rectal cancer. *Ann Surg*. 2005;242:502–511. doi:10.1097/01.sla.0000183608.24549.68

39. Bentzen AG, Balteskard L, Wanderwas EH, et al. Impaired health-related quality of life after chemoradiotherapy for anal cancer: late effects in a national cohort of 128 survivors. *Acta Oncologica*. 2013;52:736–744. doi:10.3109/0284186X.2013.770599

40. Agarwalla A, Small AJ, Mendelson AH, et al. Risk of recurrent or refractory strictures and outcome of endoscopic dilation for radiation-induced esophageal strictures. *Surg Endosc*. 2015;29:1903–1912. doi:10.1007/s00464-014-3883-1

41. Van Boeckel PG, Siersema PD. Refractory esophageal strictures: what to do when all else fails. *Curr Treat Options Gastroenterol*. 2015;13:47–58. doi:10.1007/s11938-014-0043-6

42. Fraumeni JF Jr, Curtis RE, Edwards BK, Tucker MA. Introduction. In: Curtis RE, Freedman DM, Ron E, et al. eds. New Malignancies Among Cancer Survivors: SEER Cancer Registries, 1973–2000. Bethesda, MD: National Cancer Institute; 2006.

43. Berrington de Gonzalez A, Curtis RE, Kry SF, et al. Proportion of second cancers attributable to radiotherapy treatment in adults: a cohort study in the US SEER cancer registries. *Lancet Oncol*. 2011;12(4):353–360. doi:10.1016/S1470-2045(11)70061-4

44. Kamran SC, Berrington de Gonzalez A, Ng A, et al. Therapeutic radiation and the potential risk of second malignancies. *Cancer*. 2016;122(12):1809–1821. doi:10.1002/cncr.29841

45. Bhatia S, Sklar C. Second cancers in survivors of childhood cancer. *Nat Rev Cancer*. 2002;2(2):124–132. doi:10.1038/nrc722

46. Schumacher JR, Witt WP, Palta M, et al. Cancer screening of long-term cancer survivors. *J Am Board Fam Med*. 2012;25(4):460–469. doi:10.3122/jabfm.2012.04.110118

47. Beukema JC, van Luijk P, Widder J, et al. Is cardiac toxicity a relevant issue in the radiation treatment of esophageal cancer? *Radiother Oncol*. 2015;114(1):85–90. doi:10.1016/j.radonc.2014.11.037

48. Graves PR, Siddiqui F, Anscher MS, et al. Radiation pulmonary toxicity: from mechanisms to management. *Semin Radiat Oncol*. 2010;20(3):201–207. doi:10.1016/j.semradonc.2010.01.010

49. Carver JR, Shapiro CL, Ng A, et al. American Society of Clinical Oncology clinical evidence review on the ongoing care of adult cancer survivors: cardiac and pulmonary late effects. *J Clin Oncol*. 2007;25(25):3991–4008. doi:10.1200/JCO.2007.10.9777

50. Park SB, Goldstein D, Krishnan AV, et al. Chemotherapy-induced peripheral neurotoxicity: a critical analysis. *CA Cancer J Clin*. 2013;63:419–37. doi:10.3322/caac.21204

51. de Gramont A, Figer A, Seymour M, et al. Leucovorin and fluorouracil with or without oxaliplatin as first-line treatment in advanced colorectal cancer. *J Clin Oncol*. 2000;18:2938–2947. doi:10.1200/JCO.2000.18.16.2938

52. Andre T, Boni C, Navarro M, et al. Improved overall survival with oxaliplatin, fluorouracil, and leucovorin as adjuvant treatment in stage II or III colon cancer in the MOSAIC trial. *J Clin Oncol*. 2009;27:3109–3116. doi:10.1200/JCO.2008.20.6771

53. Park SB, Lin CS, Krishnan AV, et al. Long-term neuropathy after oxaliplatin treatment: challenging the dictum of reversibility. *Oncologist*. 2011;16:708–716. doi:10.1634/theoncologist.2010-0248

54. Tofthagen C, Donovan KA, Morgan MA, et al. Oxaliplatin-induced peripheral neuropathy's effects on health-related quality of life of colorectal cancer survivors. *Support Care Cancer*. 2013;21:3307–3313. doi:10.1007/s00520-013-1905-5

55. Smith EM, Pang H, Cirrincione C, et al. Effect of duloxetine on pain, function, and quality of life among patients with chemotherapy-induced painful peripheral neuropathy: a randomized clinical trial. *JAMA*. 2013;309:1359–1367. doi:10.1001/jama.2013.2813

56. Loren AW, Mangu PB, Beck LN, et al. Fertility preservation for patients with cancer: American Society of Clinical Oncology clinical practice guideline update. *J Clin Oncol*. 2013;31(19):2500–2510. doi:10.1200/JCO.2013.49.2678

57. Marhhom E, Cohen I. Fertility preservation options for women with malignancies. *Obstet Gynecol Surv*. 2007;62(1):58–72. doi:10.1097/01.ogx.0000251029.93792.5d

58. Ruddy KJ, Partridge AH. Fertility (male and female) and menopause. *J Clin Oncol*. 2012;30(30):3705–3711. doi:10.1200/JCO.2012.42.1966

59. Weaver KE, Forsythe LP, Reeve BB, et al. Mental and physical health-related quality of life among U.S. cancer survivors: population estimates from the 2010 national health interview survey. *Cancer Epidemiol Biomarkers Prev*. 2012;21:2108–2117. doi:10.1158/1055-9965.EPI-12-0740

60. Kock L, Jansen L, Brenner H, et al. Fear of recurrence and disease progression in long-term (≥ 5 years) cancer survivors – a systematic review of quantitative studies. *Psychooncology*. 2013;22:1–11. doi:10.1002/pon.3022

61. Custers JAE, Gielissen MFM, Janssen SHV. Fear of cancer recurrence in colorectal cancer survivors. *Support Care Cancer*. 2016;24:555–562. doi:10.1007/s00520-015-2808-4

62. Abbey G, Thompson SB, Hickish T, et al. A meta-analysis of prevalence rates and moderating factors for cancer-related post-traumatic stress disorder. *Psychooncology*. 2015;24:371–381. doi:10.1002/pon.3654

63. Swartzman S, Booth JN, Munro A, et al. Posttraumatic stress disorder after cancer diagnosis in adults: a meta-analysis. *Depress Anxiety*. 2017;34:327–339. doi:10.1002/da.22542

64. Schmid D, Leitzmann MF. Association between physical activity and mortality among breast cancer and colorectal cancer survivors: a systematic review and meta-analysis. *Ann Oncol*. 2014;25:1293–1311. doi:10.1093/annonc/mdu012

65. Edwards BK, Noone AM, Mariotto AB, et al. Annual report to the nation on status of cancer 1975-2010, featuring prevalence of comorbidity and impact on survival among persons with lung, colorectal, breast, or prostate cancer. *Cancer*. 2014;120:1290–1314. doi:10.1002/cncr.28509

66. Blanchard CM, Stein KD, Baker F, et al. Association between current lifestyle behaviors and health-related quality of life in breast, colorectal, and prostate cancer survivors. *Psychology and Health*. 2004;19:1–13. doi:10.1080/08870440310001606507

67. Brown JC, Damjanov N, Courneya KS, et al. A randomized dose-response trial of aerobic exercise and health-related quality of life in colon cancer survivors. *Psychooncology*. 2018;27(4):1221–1228. doi:10.1002/pon.4655

68. Cabilan CJ, Hines S. The short-term impact of colorectal cancer treatment on physical activity, functional status and quality of life: a systematic review. *JBI Database System Rev Implement Rep*. 2017;15:517–566. doi:10.11124/JBISRIR-2016003282

69. Courneya KS, Mackey JR, Bell GJ, et al. Association between current lifestyle behaviors and health-related quality of life in breast, colorectal, and prostate cancer survivors. *Psychology & Health*. 2004;19:1–13. doi:10.1080/08870440310001606507

70. American Institute for Cancer Research. AICR's Guidelines for Cancer Survivors. http://www.aicr.org/patients-survivors/aicrs-guidelines-for-cancer.html

71. Grunfeld E, Julian JA, Pond G et al: Evaluating survivorship care plans: results of a randomized, clinical trial of patients with breast cancer. *J Clin Oncol*. 2011;29:4755–4762. doi:10.1200/JCO.2011.36.8373

72. Nicolaije KA, Ezendam NP, Vos MC, et al. Impact of an automatically generated cancer survivorship care plan on patient-reported outcomes in routine clinical practice: longitudinal outcomes of a pragmatic, cluster randomized trial. *J Clin Oncol*. 2015;33:3550–3559. doi:10.1200/JCO.2014.60.3399

73. Faul LA, Rivers B, Shibata D, et al. Survivorship care planning in colorectal cancer: feedback from survivors & providers. *J Psychosoc Oncol*. 2012;30:198–216. doi:10.1080/07347332.2011.651260

74. Blinder VS, Norris VW, Peacock NW, et al. Patient perspectives on breast cancer treatment and summary documents in community oncology care: a pilot program. *Cancer*. 2013;119:164–172. doi:10.1002/cncr.27856

75. Sprague BL, Dittus KL, Pace CM, et al. Patient satisfaction with breast and colorectal survivorship care plans. *Clin J Oncol Nurs*. 2013;17:266–272. doi:10.1188/13.CJON.17-03AP

76. Kvale EA, Huang CHS, Meneses KM, et al. Patient-centered support in the survivorship care transition: outcomes from the patient-owned survivorship care plan intervention. *Cancer*. 2016;122:3232–3242. doi:10.1002/cncr.30136

Index

ABC-02 trial, 375, 376
abdominal perineal resection, 49
abdominal ultrasound, pancreatic cancer, 159
abdominoperineal resection (APR), 409
ablation
    GEP-NETs, 400
    hepatocellular carcinoma, 242
    oligometastatic colorectal cancer, 71–76, 82–83
ACCENT-based web calculator, 26
acinar-to-ductal metaplasia (ADM), 149
adaptive immune response, biliary tract cancer,
    389
Adjuvant Chemoradiotherapy in Stomach Tumors
    (ARTIST) trial, 315–316, 326
Adjuvant Colon Cancer End Points (ACCENT)
    database, 20
adjuvant therapy
    biliary tract cancers
        clinical trials, 372–373
        historical perspective, 369–371
    resected pancreatic cancer
        biomarkers, 188–189
        chemotherapy, 184–188
        clinical trials, 186–187
        clinical vignette, 189–190
        radiation therapy, 185, 188
        supportive care, 188
        surveillance, 189
ADM. *See* acinar-to-ductal metaplasia
adoptive cell therapy, 212
adoptive immunotherapy, 299, 390
advanced hepatocellular cancer
    immunotherapy, 295–300
    multikinase inhibitors, 287–292
    targeted therapies, 287–292
ADXS11-001 listeria-based immunotherapy, 423
AFP. *See* alpha-fetoprotein
alcohol consumption
    hepatocellular carcinoma, 226
    pancreatic ductal adenocarcinoma, 143
Alliance A021101 trial, 198
alpha-fetoprotein (AFP)
    hepatocellular carcinoma, 236, 251
    nonalcoholic fatty liver disease, 226
alpha-smooth muscle actin (αSMA), 150, 151
ALPPS. *See* associating liver partition with portal
    vein ligation
American Joint Committee on Cancer (AJCC)
    criteria, 163–164
American Society for Parenteral and Enteral
    Nutrition (ASPEN), 444
American Society of Clinical Oncology (ASCO)
    clinical practice guidelines, 205
anal mucosal melanoma, 413
anaplastic lymphoma receptor tyrosine kinase
    (ALK), 11

anatomical-plane based pancreatic resection
    techniques, 172
angiogenesis, 287
anorexia/cachexia management, 458
anti-cytotoxic T-lymphocyte-associated protein 4
    (CTLA-4) antibody, 296, 298
anti-epidermal growth factor receptor (anti-EGFR),
    107, 423
anti-PD1. *See* antiprogrammed cell death
antiprogrammed cell death (anti-PD1)
    immune checkpoint inhibitors, 422
    protein 1 pathway antibodies, 296, 298
APC vaccine, 299
appendiceal NETs, 395
APR. *See* abdominoperineal resection
ARTIST trial. *See* Adjuvant Chemoradiotherapy in
    Stomach Tumors trial
ASCOT trial, 373
asialoglycoprotein receptor 1 (ASGR1), 299
ASPEN. *See* American Society for Parenteral and
    Enteral Nutrition
associating liver partition with portal vein ligation
    (ALPPS), 58, 241
ataxia telangiectasia mutation (ATM), 11
AVAGAST trial, 337

Barcelona Clinic Liver Cancer (BCLC) Staging
    System, 231, 236, 237, 250, 260, 262
BCAT trial, 371
BCLC Staging System. *See* Barcelona Clinic Liver
    Cancer Staging System
bevacizumab
    metastatic colorectal cancer, 107
    oligometastatic colorectal cancer, 63
BILCAP trial, 372
bile ducts and gallbladder cancer
    biliary strictures and molecular markers, 351
    comprehensive genomic profiling, 352
    epidemiology, 350
    immunohistochemistry and in situ hybridization,
        351
    risk factors, 350
    tumor markers, 350–351
biliary tract cancers (BTCs)
    DNA repair mutations, 388
    EGFR signaling pathways, 384–385
    FGFR signaling pathway, 386–387
    IDH1 and *IDH2* mutations, 387
    immunotherapy, 388–390
    molecular subtypes, 383
    surgical resection, 354–364
biomarkers
    pancreatic cancer, 158–159
    resected pancreatic cancer, 188–189
bispecific T-cell engagers (BiTEs), 211–212
bland embolization, colorectal cancer, 76–77

blinatumomab, 211
borderline resectable pancreatic cancer, 198–199, 202
BRAF gene mutation
  biliary tract cancers, 385
  gastrointestinal stromal tumors, 427
  metastatic colorectal cancer, 108
BRCA1/2 mutations
  metastatic pancreatic cancer, 206
  pancreatic cancer, 189
BTCs. *See* biliary tract cancers
B-type Raf kinase V600E (BRAF^{V600E}) mutations, 8, 108, 124–125

CA 19-9. *See* cancer antigen 19-9
cabiralizumab, 213
cabozantinib
  advanced hepatocellular cancer, 291
  gastrointestinal stromal tumors, 438
CAIRO3 trial, 118
calcium supplementation, colorectal cancer, 3
Cancer and Leukemia Group B (CALGB) trial, 313, 315
cancer antigen 19-9 (CA 19-9)
  metastatic pancreatic cancer, 204
  pancreatic cancer, 158
  resected pancreatic cancer, 189
Cancer of the Liver Italian Program (CLIP) Score, 231
cancer testis antigens (CTAs), 439
cancer vaccines, 212
cancer-associated fibroblasts (CAFs), 151
cancer-related fatigue (CRF), 459
cancer-related posttraumatic stress disorder (CR-PTSD), 480
cannabinoids, 458, 460
capecitabine, 20, 26, 117
capecitabine plus oxaliplatin (XELOX) regime, 21
carbohydrate antigen 19-9 (CA 19-9), 174–176, 350
carboplatin plus paclitaxel, 419
carcinoembryonic antigen (CEA)
  bile ducts and gallbladder cancer, 350
  early-stage colon cancer, 15
  metastatic pancreatic cancer, 204, 211
carcinoid heart disease (CHD), 394
Cardiovascular and Interventional Radiological Society of Europe (CIRSE) guidelines, 82
CARTs. *See* chimeric antigen receptor T-cells
caval replacement, 244
CCR2 blockade, 213
CDKN2 mutation, 213
CEA. *See* carcinoembryonic antigen
cell cycle inhibition, metastatic pancreatic cancer, 213
cetuximab, 7, 63–64
chemoembolization, oligometastatic colorectal cancer, 77
chemokine-associated signaling, 299
ChemoRadiotherapy for Oesophageal Cancer Followed by Surgery Study (CROSS), 313
chemotherapy
  anal cancer
    early-stage, 410–411
    metastatic, 418–421
  bile ducts and gallbladder, advanced cancers, 375–380

early-stage colon cancer, 17
elderly gastrointestinal cancer, 472
gastric and esophageal cancer
  clinical vignette, 339–340
  first-line chemotherapy regimens, 333–337
  second-line therapy, 337–338
gastroenteropancreatic neuroendocrine tumors, 399
metastatic colorectal cancer, 106–112
metastatic pancreatic cancer
  frontline treatment, 204–206
  initial assessment, 204
  second line treatment, 206–207
  third-line chemotherapy, 207
rectal cancer, 53–54
resected pancreatic cancer
  clinical trial participation, 184
  combination vs. single-agent chemotherapy, 184
  duration, 184–185
  post neoadjuvant treatment, 188
  with radiation therapy, 185–188
chemotherapy, adjuvant
  early-stage colon cancer
    circulating tumor DNA analysis, 26
    elderly patients, 25–26
    fluoropyrimidine-based regimens, 20
    intraperitoneal chemotherapy, 22
    liquid biopsy approaches, 26
    microsatellite instability and mutations, 22–23
    nodal involvement, 22
    not recommended regimens, 22
    optimal duration, 26–27
    oxaliplatin-based regimens, 20–21
    patient evaluation, 22
    portal vein infusion, 22
    risk assessment, 22
    risk stratification, 26
    stage II and III colon cancer, 23–25
    timing, 22
  oligometastatic colorectal cancer
    clinical vignette, 91–92
    ESMO and NCCN guidelines, 90
    hepatic arterial infusion plus systemic chemotherapy, 90
    irinotecan-based regimens, 89
    oxaliplatin-based regimens, 88–89
    single-agent fluoropyrimidines, 88
    targeted therapy, 89–90
chemotherapy-induced nausea and vomiting (CINV), 460
chemotherapy-induced peripheral neuropathy, 479
Child–Turcotte–Pugh (CTP) score, 240, 252–253
chimeric antigen receptor T-cells (CARTs), 212, 299, 439
cholangiocarcinoma (CC), 350
chromosomal instability (CIN), gastric cancer, 311, 312
chronic radiation proctitis (CRP), 478
chylothorax, 324
CINV. *See* chemotherapy-induced nausea and vomiting
circulating tumor DNA (ctDNA), 26
Clinical Outcomes of Surgical Therapy Study Group (COST) trial, 16
clinical target volume (CTV), 411
COIN trial, 116

colon cancer, early-stage
  CERAS protocol, 15–16, 18
  chemotherapy, 17, 22–27
  clinical vignette, 18
  initial workup, 15
  laparoscopic vs. robotic surgery, 17
  malignant polyp, 17
  medical history, 15
  open vs. minimally invasive surgery, 16–17
COlon cancer Laparoscopic or Open Resection
    (COLOR) trial, 16
colon enhanced recovery after surgery (CERAS)
    protocol, 15–16
colonoscopy, 2
colony stimulating factor-1 (CSF-1), 213
colorectal cancer (CRC). *See also* metastatic
    colorectal cancer; oligometastatic colorectal
    cancer
  in African Americans, 2
  behavioral and sedentary lifestyle, 3
  cancer survival, 5
  clinical vignette, 27–28
  colonoscopy screening, 2
  diagnosis and staging, 5
  family history, 2
  genetics, 2
  incidence rates, 2, 3
  molecular testing, 7–11
  mortality rates, 2, 3
  nutritional needs, 445
  risk factors, 2
  survivorship care, 477
  symptoms, 5
colorectal NETs, 395
comprehensive geriatric assessment (CGA), 25
computed tomography (CT) scan
  borderline resectable pancreatic cancer, 202
  early-stage colon cancer, 15
  gastric cancer, 309
  GEP-NETs, 396–397
  locally advanced pancreatic cancer, 202
  pancreatic adenocarcinoma, 159–162
  rectal cancer, early-stage, 45–46
conformal radiation therapy, 277–278
consensus molecular subtypes (CMSs), 135
conventional form transarterial chemoembolization
    (cTACE), 266
COUGAR-02 trial, 337
Couinaud classification, 240, 241
CRC. *See* colorectal cancer
crenolanib, gastrointestinal stromal tumors, 439
CR-PTSD. *See* cancer-related posttraumatic stress
    disorder
cryoablation
  colorectal cancer, 74–76
  hepatocellular carcinoma, LRT, 264–265
  NSCLC, 82, 83
cryoshock, 269
CRYSTAL trial, 107, 109
CTAs. *See* cancer testis antigens
CXCR4, 212–213
cyclin dependent kinase (CDK) inhibitors, 213
cytoreduction, 96–98, 100, 400
cytotoxic T-lymphocytes (CTLs), 233

dasatinib, 438
deceased donor liver transplantation (DDLT), 243

defective mismatch repair/microsatellite instability
    metastatic colorectal cancer (dMMR/MSI
    mCRC)
  cytotoxic lymphocyte infiltration, 132
  immune checkpoint therapy, 132
  immunotherapy (*see* immunotherapy, MSI/
    dMMR mCRC)
dendritic cell–based vaccines, biliary tract cancers,
    389–390
depression
  and anxiety management, 458–459
  resected pancreatic cancer, 188
diagnostic laparoscopy (DL), 97
diarrhea
  immune-related adverse events, 297
  midgut NETs, 394
  pancreatic NETs, 395–396
digital image analysis (DIA), 351
direct antiviral agents (DAA), 225
disease control rate (DCR), 133
distal extrahepatic cholangiocarcinoma, 361–362
distal subtotal gastrectomy, 327
dMMR/MSI mCRC. *See* defective mismatch
    repair/microsatellite instability metastatic
    colorectal cancer
DNA damage repair deficient tumors, 206, 214
DNA mismatch repair (MMR) proteins, 24
donation after circulatory death (DCD), 244
dovitinib, 437
drug-eluting beads-transarterial
    chemoembolization (DEB-TACE), 242, 266
dystrophin, 430

early-stage anal cancer
  clinical vignette, 414–415
  diagnosis, 408
  digital rectal examination, 408
  epidemiology, 407
  incidence, 407
  management, 409–414
  pathogenesis and biology, 407–408
  physical examination, 408
  radiation therapy, 411–413
  staging, 409
  surveillance, 414
  symptoms, 408
  visual inspection, 408
early-stage esophageal cancer
  neoadjuvant chemoradiation therapy, 313–318
  surgery, 321–325
early-stage gastric cancer
  neoadjuvant chemoradiation therapy, 313–318
  surgery, 325–329
early-stage hepatocellular cancer
  algorithm approach, 252
  clinical vignette, 245–246
  diagnostic evaluation and staging, 239–240
  liver transplantation, 243–244
  locoregional therapy, 242–243
  multidisciplinary approach, 244–245
  radiation therapy, 277–284
  resection, 240–241
  surgical resection, 251–256
  surveillance, 236–239
Eastern Cooperative Oncology Group (ECOG)
    score, 199, 230, 251
ECF. *See* epirubicin, cisplatin and fluorouracil

egalitarian approach, 244
EGFR. *See* epidermal growth factor receptor
EHCCA. *See* extrahepatic cholangiocarcinoma
eicosapentaenoic acid, 458
elderly gastrointestinal cancer
   assessments and biomarkers, 468–470
   clinical approach, 472–473
   clinical trials, 471–472
   clinical vignette, 473
   incidence, 468, 469
   screening tools, 471
endocrine insufficiency, 188
endoscopic mucosal resection (EMR), 321–322
endoscopic retrograde cholangiopancreatography
   (ERCP), 161, 163
endoscopic ultrasound (EUS)
   esophageal cancer, 309
   pancreatic cancer, 160, 162
   rectal cancer, early-stage, 46
Enhanced Recovery After Surgery (ERAS)
   guidelines, 447
epidermal growth factor receptor (EGFR), 7–8
epirubicin, cisplatin and fluorouracil (ECF), 333
Epstein–Barr virus (EBV), 311, 312
ERCP. *See* endoscopic retrograde
   cholangiopancreatography
esophageal cancer
   carcinogen exposure, 306
   cervical incision, 324
   chemotherapy and biological therapy, 333–340
   clinical staging, 321
   clinical vignette, 324–325
   clinical workup, 321
   diagnosis and staging, 309
   en bloc resection and nodal dissection, 323
   endoscopic mucosal resection, 321–322
   epidemiology, 306–307
   esophagectomy, 322
   immunotherapy, 343–346
   incidence, 306
   minimally invasive esophagectomy, 323
   molecular diagnostic guidelines, 311
   neoadjuvant chemoradiation therapy, 313–318,
      322
   nutritional needs, 446
   risk factors, 321
   risk reduction programs, 323
   squamous cell carcinoma (SCC), 321
   surgery, 321–325
   transhiatal approach, 322, 323
   transthoracic approach, 322
esophagectomy, 322
esophagogastric junction (EGJ) cancer staging,
   321
esophagogastroduodenoscopy (EGD), 321
ESPAC-3 trial, 371
European MOSAIC trial, 21
European Organisation for Research and Treatment
   of Cancer (EORTC) trial, 410, 435
EUS. *See* endoscopic ultrasound
everolimus, 398, 439
exocrine insufficiency, 188
Experimental Therapeutics Clinical Trials Network
   (ETCTN), 421
external body radiation therapy (EBRT), 243
extrahepatic cholangiocarcinoma (EHCCA), 350,
   362, 364

familial gastrointestinal stromal tumors, 430
familial pancreatic cancer, 145
farnesyl transferase inhibitor (FTI), 122–123
fatigue, 459
fibroblast growth factor receptor (FGFR)
   mutations, 10, 126
   signaling pathway, 386
5-fluorouracil/leucovorin (5-FU/LV), 20
FLAGS trial, 335
FLOT regimen, 335
fluorescence in situ hybridization (FISH), 351
fluoropyrimidine-based regimens, 20, 418–419
fluoropyrimidines, 20, 335
5-fluorouracil and cisplatin (FLP) regimen, 333
5-fluorouracil and oxaliplatin regimen (FLO), 333
fluorouracil, leucovorin, and oxaliplatin (FOLFOX4)
   regimen, 21, 27
5-fluorouracil, leucovorin, irinotecan, and
   oxaliplatin (FOLFIRINOX), 184
   borderline resectable pancreatic cancer, 198–199
   locally advanced pancreatic cancer, 200
   metastatic pancreatic cancer, 204–205
   resectable pancreatic cancer, 194, 195
focal adhesion kinase (FAK), 213
folate consumption, colorectal cancer, 3
FOLFIRINOX. *See* 5-fluorouracil, leucovorin,
   irinotecan, and oxaliplatin
FOLFOX chemotherapy. *See* folinic acid,
   fluorouracil, and oxaliplatin chemotherapy
folinic acid, fluorouracil, and irinotecan (FOLFIRI)
   chemotherapy, 63, 333
folinic acid, fluorouracil, and oxaliplatin (FOLFOX)
   chemotherapy
   metastatic colorectal cancer, 106
   oligometastatic colorectal cancer, 62
frameshift mutations, microsatellite instability high
   colorectal cancer, 9
French Prodige 7 trial, 101
future liver remnant (FLR), 57, 240–241, 253

gall-bladder cancer (GBC). *See also* bile ducts and
   gallbladder cancer
   adjuvant therapy, 369–373
   incidence rates, 350
gastrectomy, 326, 476–477
gastric cancer
   diagnosis and staging, 309
   epidemiology, 306–307
   Helicobacter pylori (H. pylori) infection, 306
   hereditary syndromes, 307
   incidence, 306
   molecular diagnostic guidelines, 311–312
   neoadjuvant chemoradiation therapy, 313–318
   nutritional and environmental factors, 306
   nutritional needs, 446
   surgery, 325–329
gastric NETs, 394–395
gastrinomas, 395
gastroenteropancreatic neuroendocrine tumors
   (GEP-NETs)
   appendiceal NETs, 395
   chemotherapy, 399
   classification, 394
   colorectal NETs, 395
   diagnostic imaging, 396–397
   diagnostic procedures, 396
   everolimus, 398

gastric NETs, 394–395
incidence, 394
liver-directed treatment, 400–401
localized tumors, 397
pancreatic, 395–396
radiolabeled SSAs, 399–400
small intestinal NETs, 394
somatostatin analogs, 397–398
sunitinib, 398–399
telotristat, 400
tumor biology and genetic syndromes, 396
tumor grade and differentiation, 394
gastrointestinal immune-related adverse events, 297
gastrointestinal stromal tumors (GISTs)
classification, 428
clinical trials, 434–435, 437–439
diagnosis, 432
epidemiology, 427–429
genomic progression, 428
immunotherapy, 439
intermediate-risk, 435–436
localized, 432–433
metastatic, 433–434
molecular characterization, 429–431
molecular targeted therapies, 426
recommendations, 439–440
risk stratification, 429
staging, 432–433
GATSBY trial, 337
gemcitabine, 152, 172
gemcitabine and capecitabine (GEMCAP), 375
gemcitabine with oxaliplatin (GEMOX), 375
genetically engineered mouse models (GEMMs), 149
genomically stable gastric cancer, 311, 312
GEP-NETs. *See* gastroenteropancreatic neuroendocrine tumors
German Rectal Cancer Study Group trial, 52
GISTs. *See* gastrointestinal stromal tumors
glucagonomas, 396
gross target volume (GTV), 411
Guillain–Barré syndrome, 298
GVAX pancreatic cancer vaccine, 212

HAART. *See* highly active antiretroviral therapy
HCC. *See* hepatocellular carcinoma
hedgehog pathway targeting, 152
hepatectomy, survivorship care, 477
hepatic artery chemotherapy (HAC), 76
hepatitis B virus infection, hepatocellular carcinoma, 224–225
hepatitis C virus infection, hepatocellular carcinoma, 225
hepatocellular carcinoma (HCC)
advanced (*see* advanced hepatocellular cancer)
alcohol-related, 226
anti-HCV therapy, 225
at-risk population, 230
cellular and molecular pathology, 233–234
curative treatments, 236
diagnosis and staging, 229–231
early-stage (*see* early-stage hepatocellular cancer)
etiology, 224
gender disparity, 224
global risk factors, 288
hepatitis B virus infection, 224–225
hepatitis C virus infection, 225
immune changes and response, 295
incidence, 230, 250
microscopic morphologic features, 229
nonalcoholic fatty liver disease, 226
nonalcoholic steatohepatitis, 226
nutritional needs, 446
prognostic indicators, 250
prognostication scoring systems, 260
screening guidelines, 229
HERACLES trial, 9
herbal supplements, cancer-related fatigue, 459
hereditary disorders, pancreatic ductal adenocarcinoma, 144, 145
hereditary nonpolyposis colorectal cancer, 145
HER2/neu amplification, 384–385
highly active antiretroviral therapy (HAART), 408
HIPEC. *See* hyperthermic intraperitoneal chemotherapy
histone deacetylase inhibitors, gastrointestinal stromal tumors, 438
HIV-positive anal carcinoma, 408
Hong Kong Liver Cancer (HKLC), 259–261
hospice care, 452–453
HSP90 inhibitor (BIIB021), 437
human epidermal growth factor receptor 2 (HER2), 9
human epidermal growth factor receptor 2 (HER2)-overexpression
esophageal adenocarcinoma, 314
gastric and esophageal cancer, 335–336
gastroesophageal junction (GEJ) adenocarcinoma, 311
metastatic colorectal cancer, 108, 124
human equilibrative nucleoside transporter 1(hENT1), 188
human papillomavirus (HPV) infection, anal cancer, 408
hyaluronidase acid (HA), 152
hyaluronidases, 152
hypergastrinemia, 395
hyperthermic intraperitoneal chemotherapy (HIPEC), 100, 101
hyperthyroidism, 298
hysterectomy, 99

IHCCA. *See* intrahepatic cholangiocarcinoma
IL-6/JAK-STAT signaling, 153
imatinib
gastrointestinal stromal tumors, 429
metastatic gastrointestinal stromal tumors, 434
immune checkpoint inhibitors
gastrointestinal stromal tumors, 439
immune-related adverse events, 297–298
indications and risk assessment, 297
nivolumab, 296
pembrolizumab, 296
immune-modulatory medications (IMMs), 297
immune-related adverse events (irAEs)
diarrhea, 297
gastrointestinal, 297
immune-modulatory medications, 297
neurologic, 298
ocular toxicities, 298
pneumonitis and renal injury, 298
skin toxicity, 298
thyroid dysfunction, 298

immunomodulators, 299
immunonutrition, 447
immunotherapy
    advanced hepatocellular cancer
        adoptive immunotherapy, 299
        clinical vignette, 299–300
        combination therapies, 298–299
        immune checkpoint inhibitors, 295–298
        immunomodulators, 299
    anal cancer, metastatic, 421–422
    biliary tract cancers (BTCs), 388–390
    gastrointestinal stromal tumors, 439
    ipilimumab, 345
    locoregional therapies, 271–272
    metastatic pancreatic cancer
        adoptive cell transfer, 212
        bispecific T-cell engagers (BiTEs), 211–212
        cancer vaccines, 212
        checkpoint agonism, 211
        checkpoint blockade, 211
        microenvironment modulation, 212–213
    molecular clues, 343–344
    MSI/dMMR mCRC
        algorithm, 134
        clinical vignette, 135–138
        consensus molecular subtypes (CMSs), 135
        microsatellite stable (MSS) population, 135
        nivolumab, 133
        objective response rate, 132–133
        pembrolizumab, 132
        progression-free survival, 132–133
        pseudoprogression, 133–134
        stromal-based approaches, 135
    nivolumab, 344, 346
    PD1 checkpoint receptor targeting, 344
    pembrolizumab, 344
    trastuzumab, 345
IMRT. *See* intensity-modulated radiation therapy
indocyanine green (ICG) clearance test, 253
inflammatory cancer-associated fibroblasts
        (iCAFs), 151
inguinal lymphadenopathy, 408
innate immune system, biliary tract cancers, 389
instrumental activities of daily living (IADLs)
        impairments, 469
intensity-modulated radiation therapy (IMRT)
    anal carcinoma, early-stage, 411
    rectal cancer, 38–39
InterAACT trial, 419
interleukin-6 (IL-6) production, pancreatic ductal
        adenocarcinoma, 151
International Duration Evaluation of Adjuvant
        Chemotherapy (IDEA) collaborative study, 27
International Rare Cancers Initiative (IRCI) trial,
        419
intra-arterial therapies, colorectal cancer, 76–82
intraductal papillary mucinous neoplasm (IMPN),
        144
intrahepatic cholangiocarcinoma (IHCCA), 350
    lymphadenectomy, 362
    surgery, biliary tract cancers (BTCs), 359
intraperitoneal chemotherapy, 22
ipilimumab, esophagogastric cancer, 345
irAEs. *See* immune-related adverse events
IRE. *See* irreversible electroporation
irinotecan-based regimens, 89
irinotecan-loaded drug-eluting beads (DEBIRIs), 77

irreversible electroporation (IRE), 76
    general anesthesia risk, 270
    hepatocellular carcinoma, 242
    hepatocellular carcinoma, LRT, 265
    procedural risk, 270

jaundice, 358
juvenile polyposis, 307

Karnofsky Performance Score (KPS), 230
Ki-67 index, gastroenteropancreatic
        neuroendocrine tumors, 394
Kirsten Ras (KRAS) mutation, 7–8
    metastatic colorectal cancer, 122–123
    pancreatic ductal adenocarcinoma, 144,
        148–149
KIT exon 11 deletion, 435
KIT mutations, gastrointestinal stromal tumors, 431
Kruppel-like factor 5 (KLF5), 150

LAP07 trial, 200
laparoscopy
    hepatectomy, 241, 254
    pancreatic cancer, 162
laser ablation, hepatocellular carcinoma, 265
lenvatinib, 288, 289
leukemia inhibitory factor (Lif), 151
linsitinib, 438
liquid biopsy, 11, 26
liver transplantation
    donor allograft utilization, 244
    GEP-NETs, 401
    Milan criteria, 243
    organ allocation and distribution policies, 243–244
    post–liver transplant recurrence, 244, 245
    technical considerations, 244
    total hepatectomy, 243
living donor liver transplantation (LDLT), 243
locally advanced pancreatic cancer
    CT findings, 202
    ECOG 4201 trial, 199
    European phase III (FFCD-SFRO) trial, 199
    first-line FOLFIRINOX, 200
    LAP07 trial, 200
    treatment algorithm, 201
locoregional therapies (LRTs)
    adverse events and management, 269–270
    bridging and downstaging therapy, 267–268
    clinical vignette, 273
    contraindications, 268–269
    curative intent ablation, 263–265
    disease recurrence/survival, 263, 268
    with immune checkpoint inhibitors, 298–299
    immunotherapeutics, 271–272
    patient selection, 259
    recovery, 268
    selection of, 270–271
    transarterial chemoembolization, 265–267
    transarterial radioembolization, 265–267
LOGiC trial, 337
lymphadenectomy, 326–327, 364
Lynch syndrome, 9

M stage, colorectal cancer, 5
magnetic resonance imaging (MRI)
    GEP-NETs, 397
    hepatocellular carcinoma, 236–237

metastatic pancreatic cancer, 204
  pancreatic adenocarcinoma, 159–160
  rectal cancer, early-stage, 46
maintenance therapy, mCRC
  algorithm, 119
  bevacizumab alone, 118
  chemotherapy-free interval, 116
  clinical trials, 117
  clinical vignette, 119–120
  erlotinib plus bevacizumab, 118
  fluoropyrimidine alone, 116
  fluoropyrimidine and bevacizumab combination, 118
malnutrition, 444
masitinib, 437
mCRC. *See* metastatic colorectal cancer
Medicare Hospice Benefit, 453
megestrol, 458
melatonin, 458
mesenchymal–epithelial transition factor (cMET), 10
mesenchymal–epithelial transition (MET) factor
  alterations, 123–124
Metabolic response evalUatioN for Individualization of neoadjuvant Chemotherapy in Oesophageal and oesophagogastric adeNocarcinoma (MUNICON) study, 315
metastasectomy, 82
metastatic anal cancer
  chemotherapy, 418–421
  clinical trials, 422–424
  HIV infected patients, 424
  immunotherapy, 421–422
  incidence, 418
  prognosis, 424
metastatic colorectal cancer (mCRC)
  antiangiogenic therapies, 107
  anti–epidermal growth factor receptor (EGFR) therapies, 107
  BRAF mutations, 108, 124–125
  clinical vignette, 111–113
  combinatorial chemotherapy, 106
  combined antiangiogenic and anti-EGRF therapies, 107–108
  EGFR mutations, 125
  fibroblast growth factor receptor (FGFR), 126
  HER2 amplification, 108, 124
  immunotherapy, 131–138
  KRAS alterations, 122–123
  maintenance therapy, 116–120
  mesenchymal–epithelial transition factor alterations, 123–124
  sample treatment algorithm, 110
  survival, 106
  systemic chemotherapy options, 109
metastatic gastric and esophageal cancer
  chemotherapy and biological therapy, 333–340
  immunotherapy, 343–346
Metastatic Pancreatic Adenocarcinoma Clinical Trial (MPACT) study, 205
metastatic pancreatic cancer
  chemotherapy, 204–207
  pancreatic ductal adenocarcinoma, 210–218
mFOLFIRINOX. *See* modified 5-fluorouracil, leucovorin, irinotecan, and oxaliplatin
micro-GISTs (GISTlets), 427
microsatellite instability high (MSI-H)
  biliary tract cancers, 388

colorectal cancer, 9, 25
gastric cancer, 311, 312
pancreatic ductal adenocarcinoma, 149, 207
microwave ablation (MWA)
  colorectal cancer, 72–74
  hepatocellular carcinoma, 242
  hepatocellular carcinoma, LRT, 264
Milan criteria, liver transplantation, 243
minimally invasive esophagectomy (MIE), 323
minimally invasive surgery (MIS)
  early-stage colon cancer, 16
  thoracotomy, 324
mirtazapine and cyproheptadine, 458
mismatch repair (MMR) deficiency, 373, 388
mitogen-activated protein kinase (MEK) inhibition, 135, 439
mitomycin C, adriamycin, and cisplatin (MAP), 419
Model of End-Stage Liver Disease (MELD) scores, 252–253
modified 5-fluorouracil, leucovorin, irinotecan, and oxaliplatin (mFOLFIRINOX), 210–211
molecular testing
  colorectal cancer
    epidermal growth factor receptor, 7–8
    mismatch repair deficiency screening, 9–10
    potentially actionable genes, 10–11
    tumor biopsy sources, 11
  gastric cancer, 311–312
MORTAVIC study, 230
MOSAIC trial, 24
MOUNTAINEER trial, 9
MRC Adjuvant Gastric Infusional Chemotherapy (MAGIC) trial, 315
MSI-H. *See* microsatellite instability high
multibipolar radiofrequency ablation (RFA), 242
multiple endocrine neoplasia type 1 (MEN1), 396
MWA. *See* microwave ablation
myofibroblastic cancer-associated fibroblasts (myCAFs), 151

N stage, colorectal cancer, 5
nab-paclitaxel, 205, 211
NAFLD. *See* nonalcoholic fatty liver disease
National Comprehensive Cancer Network (NCCN) guidelines, 189, 206
National Surgical Quality Improvement Program (NSQIP), 96
NCT02314169 clinical trial, 423
NCT02919969 clinical trial, 423
NCT03519295—SCARCE study, 423
neoadjuvant chemoradiation therapy
  early-stage gastric and esophageal cancer
    ARTIST trial, 315–316
    CALGB trial, 313, 315
    clinical vignette, 316–318
    CROSS trial, 313
    MAGIC trial, 315
    NEOSCOPE trial, 314
    PET-directed therapy paradigm, 314–315
    POET, 314
    randomized trials, 313
    RTOG 8501 trial, 313
  rectal cancer
    chemotherapy, 53–54
    clinical vignette, 54–55
    neoadjuvant therapy, 52–53
    patient selection, 52

neoadjuvant chemotherapy, oligometastatic
  colorectal cancer
  biological therapy, 63–64
  clinical vignette, 66–67
  FOLFIRI chemotherapy, 63
  FOLFOX chemotherapy, 62
  FOLFOXIRI plus bevacizumab, 64
  liver metastases, 64–65
  lung metastases, 65–66
  ovarian and peritoneal metastases, 66
neoadjuvant radiation therapy, rectal cancer
  clinical vignette, 40–41
  intensity-modulated radiation therapy, 38–39
  preoperative vs. selective postoperative
    radiation, 36
  radiotherapy-to-surgery interval, 37
  reirradiation, 39
  selective nonoperative management, 37–38
  short-course preoperative radiotherapy, 34–35
  short-course vs. standard-course postoperative
    preoperative chemoradiotherapy, 36–37
  standard-course preoperative
    chemoradiotherapy, 35–36
  treatment techniques, 40
neoadjuvant therapy, resected pancreatic cancer
  benefits, 193
  clinical studies, 194, 195
  current standard of care, 192
  definition, 192
  genomic analyses, 193
  Markov decision analysis, 193
  meta-analyses, 193–194
  preclinical studies, 193
  propensity score-matched analysis, 193
  radiation therapy, 194
  retrospective analysis, 193
NEOPAC study, 194, 195
NEPAFOX study, 194, 195
NETTER-1 trial, 399–400
neuroendocrine tumors
  GEP-NETs (*see* gastroenteropancreatic
    neuroendocrine tumors)
  nutritional needs, 447
neurofibromatosis-1 (NF1) related GISTs, 427
next-generation sequencing (NGS), 10
nilotinib, 434
nivolumab
  advanced hepatocellular cancer, 296
  anal cancer, metastatic, 421–422
  dMMR/MSI mCRC, 133
  esophagogastric cancer, 344, 346
  gastrointestinal stromal tumors, 437
N-myc downregulated gene 2 (NDRG2), 149
nonalcoholic fatty liver disease (NAFLD)
  etiologies, 226
  screening guidelines, 229
nonalcoholic steatohepatitis (NASH), 226
normal tissue complication probability (NTCP), 277
NSABP C-07 trial, 21, 24
nutritional needs
  colorectal cancer, 445
  energy and protein needs, 445
  esophageal cancer, 446
  gastric cancer, 446
  hepatocellular cancer, 446
  medical nutrition therapy, 447
  metabolic changes, 444
  nausea and vomiting, 460
  neuroendocrine tumors, 447
  nutrition screening, 444
  pancreatic cancer, 445–446
  perioperative nutrition, 447

obesity
  colorectal cancer, 3
  pancreatic ductal adenocarcinoma, 144
objective response rate (ORR), 132–133
Okuda Staging System, hepatocellular carcinoma,
  231
olaparib monotherapy, 214
olaratumab, 437
oligometastatic colorectal cancer
  adjuvant chemotherapy, 88–92
  liver metastasis
    ablation, 71–76
    intra-arterial therapies, 76–82
    liver metastasis, interventional radiology's role,
      70–71
  lungs metastasis, 82–83
  neoadjuvant chemotherapy, 62–67
  peritoneal surface disease (*see* peritoneal
    surface disease)
  surgical resection, 57–59
omentectomy, 98
onalespib, 437
Organ Procurement and Transplantation Network
  (OPTN), 243
oxaliplatin-based regimens, 20–21, 88–89
oxaliplatin-induced peripheral neuropathy (OIPN),
  479

paclitaxel monotherapy, 419
palliative care
  advance care planning, 454–455
  anorexia/cachexia management, 458
  colorectal cancer, 463
  communication, 453–454
  consultation teams, 451
  definition, 451
  depression and anxiety management, 458–459
  domains, 451
  EOL care, 455–456
  esophageal cancer, 462
  fatigue, 459
  gastric cancer, 461
  hepatocellular cancer, 462
  hospice, 452–453
  nausea and vomiting, 460
  neuroendocrine tumor, 461
  pain management, 456–458
  pancreatic cancer, 461
  recommendation, 452
pancreatectomy, 177
pancreatic cancer
  biomarker and laboratory data, 158–159
  chemotherapy, 184–185
  clinical presentation, 158
  death rates, 142
  diagnostic procedures and biopsy, 160–163
  imaging, 159–160
  incidence, 142
  locally advanced pancreatic cancer, 199–201
  metastatic (*see* metastatic pancreatic cancer)
  nutritional needs, 445–446

resected (*see* resected pancreatic cancer)
staging and resectability, 162–165
surgical treatment, 169–180
pancreatic cystic lesions, 144
pancreatic ductal adenocarcinoma (PDAC)
biologic properties and mutations, 148–150
borderline resectable pancreatic cancer, 198–199
chemotherapy, 204–207
clinical trials, 215–218
dense fibrotic stroma, 150–152
dominant pathway targeting, 152–153
genetic instability, 149
immunologic factors, 153
immunotherapy, 211–213
incidence, 142
locally advanced pancreatic cancer, 199–202
metabolic targeting, 214
modifiable and genetic risk factors, 142–145
signs and symptoms, 145
stroma and enzymatic disruption, 210–211
surgical resection, 145
survival rate, 142
targeted therapies, 213–214
pancreatic intraepithelial neoplasias (PanINs), 149
pancreatic neuroendocrine tumors, 395–396
pancreatic stellate cells (PSCs), 150
pancreatitis, 143, 149
pancreatoduodenectomy, 169, 170
panitumumab (Vectibix), 7
parenchymal-sparing techniques, 58
PD-0325901 inhibitor, 123
PDAC. *See* pancreatic ductal adenocarcinoma
PDGFRA gene mutation, 427, 430
PEGPH20, 152, 210–211
pembrolizumab
advanced hepatocellular cancer, 296
anal cancer, metastatic, 422
esophagogastric cancer, 344
metastatic colorectal cancer, 132
MSI-H/dMMR tumors, 207
peptide-based vaccines, 389
percutaneous ablation, colorectal cancer, 71, 72
perihilar cholangiocarcinoma, 359–361
peritoneal cancer index (PCI), 97
peritoneal surface disease (PSD)
aggressive regional therapeutic approach, 96
cholecystectomy, 99
clinical trials, 101–102
clinical vignette, 102–103
fascial closure, 101
hyperthermic intraperitoneal chemotherapy, 100, 101
hysterectomy, 99
omentectomy, 98
peritoneal cytoreduction, 96–98
peritonectomy, 99, 100
pyloromyotomy, 99
restorative anastomoses, 100
small bowel resection, 99
Peritoneal Surface Oncology Group International (PSOGI), 101
peritonectomy, 100
peritoniectomy, 99
pertuzumab, 9
Peutz–Jeghers syndrome, 145, 307
phosphoinositide 3-kinase (PIK3CA) mutation, 10
photon stereotactic body radiation therapy, 280

physician orders for life-sustaining treatment (POLST) forms, 454–455
PIK3CA gene mutation, 23
planning target volume (PTV), 412
platinum agents, 214
plerixafor, 212
pneumonitis, 298
poly ADP-ribose polymerase (PARP), 214
polymerase chain reaction (PCR), 10
ponatinib, 438
porcupine O-acyltransferase (PORCN) inhibitors, 126
portal hypertension, 240
portal vein embolization (PVE), 58, 241, 253
portal vein reconstruction, 244
portal vein thrombosis, stereotactic body radiation therapy, 279
positron emission tomography (PET) scan
early-stage colon cancer, 15
esophageal cancer, 314
pancreatic adenocarcinoma, 160, 161
positron emission tomography/computed tomography (PET/CT) scan
esophageal cancer, 309
gastric cancer, 309
postembolization syndrome, 400
postoperative pancreatic fistula (POPF), 177
postvagotomy diarrhea, 306
PreOperative therapy in Esophagogastric adenocarcinoma Trial (POET), 314
PRODIGE IV trial, 204, 205, 372
programmed death ligand-1 (PD-L1), 422
programmed death ligand (PD-L) receptor overexpression, 233
PROPHYLOCHIP trial, 101
PROSPECT study, 54
proton beam therapy (PBT), 279–280
proton pump inhibitors (PPIs), 395
PSD. *See* peritoneal surface disease
pyloromyotomy, 99

QUASAR study, 23

radiation cystitis, 478
radiation therapy
anal cancer, metastatic, 423–424
anal carcinoma, early-stage, 411–413
hepatocellular carcinoma
clinical vignette, 281–284
conformal radiation therapy, 277–278
hepatocellular carcinoma, 243
proton beam therapy, 279–280
radiation tolerance, 277
stereotactic body radiation therapy, 278–279
rectal cancer (*see* neoadjuvant radiation therapy, rectal cancer)
resected pancreatic cancer
with chemotherapy, 185
indications, 185
timing, 185, 188
Radiation Therapy Oncology Group (RTOG) 8501 trial, 313
radiation-induced liver disease (RILD), 278
radiobiological equivalent (RBE), 280
radioembolization
GEP-NETs, 401
oligometastatic colorectal cancer, 77, 80

radiofrequency ablation (RFA)
  colorectal cancer, 71–72
  hepatocellular carcinoma, 242, 263, 264
  NSCLC, 82
RAINBOW study, 338
ramucirumab
  advanced hepatocellular cancer, 290
  metastatic colorectal cancer, 107
RAS gene mutations, gastrointestinal stromal
    tumors, 430
RECIST. *See* Response Evaluation Criteria in Solid
    Tumors
rectal bleeding, 408
rectal cancer, early-stage
  adjuvant therapy, 52–55
  clinical vignette, 50
  diagnosis, 45
  polyps, 46–48
  presentation, 45
  radical surgical resection, 49
  standard workup, 45–46
  transanal excisions, 48–49
  treatment options scenarios, 45
REGARD study, 338
regorafenib
  advanced hepatocellular cancer, 290
  metastatic gastrointestinal stromal tumors, 434
regulatory T (Treg) cells, hepatocellular carcinoma,
    233
reirradiation, rectal cancer, 39
resected pancreatic cancer
  adjuvant therapy, 184–190
  neoadjuvant therapy, 192–195
RESORCE trial, 290
Response Evaluation Criteria in Solid Tumors
    (RECIST), 437
retaspimycin (IPI-504), 438
RETREAT prognostic scoring, 244, 245
robotic transanal minimally invasive surgery, 49
robotically assisted laparoscopic gastrectomy, 328
ROS1 gene rearrangements, 11
Roux-en-Y gastrojejunostomy (RYGJ)
    reconstruction, 327

saridegib, 152
SBRT. *See* stereotactic body radiation therapy
selective internal radiation therapy (SIRT), 77, 80
selective serotonin reuptake inhibitor (SSRI), 458
selumetinib, 123
sentinel lymph node (SLN) biopsy, gastric cancer,
    327
significantly mutated genes (SMGs), 234
single-agent fluoropyrimidines, 88
SMAD4, 188
small intestinal NETs, 394
smoking, pancreatic ductal adenocarcinoma,
    142–143
somatic mutation, sporadic well-differentiated
    NETs, 396
somatostatin analogs, 397–398
somatostatin receptor (SSTR)-based imaging, 397
sorafenib, advanced hepatocellular cancer,
    287–289, 296
Southwest Oncology Group (SWOG) S0809 trial, 371
Southwest Oncology Group (SWOG) S1505 trial,
    194, 195
SPIKES protocol, 453–454

sporadic well-differentiated NETs, 396
stereotactic body radiation therapy (SBRT)
  advanced liver disease, 279
  hepatocellular carcinoma, 243
  portal vein thrombosis, 279
  prospective trials, 278
  vs. radiofrequency ablation, 279
  toxicity, 278
steroids, cancer-related fatigue, 459
stroma, pancreatic cancer
  cancer-associated fibroblasts, 151
  extracellular matrix factors, 150
  fibrosis, 150
  hedgehog pathway targeting, 152
  hyaluronidase, 152
  IL-6/JAK-STAT signaling, 153
  immunotherapy, 152
  pancreatic stellate cells, 150–151
  PEGPH20, 210–211
stroma-targeted approach, 152
sunitinib
  gastroenteropancreatic neuroendocrine tumors,
    398–399
  metastatic gastrointestinal stromal tumors, 434
surgery-first approach, 172
surgical resection
  biliary tract cancers
    diagnosis, 354–355
    distal extrahepatic cholangiocarcinoma,
      361–362
    intrahepatic cholangiocarcinoma, 359
    lymphadenectomy, 362–364
    neoadjuvant therapy, 358
    outcomes, 364
    perihilar cholangiocarcinoma, 359–361
    preoperative biliary decompression, 358
    resectability, 358
    staging, 355–357
  early-stage esophageal cancer
    cervical incision, 324
    clinical staging, 321
    clinical vignette, 324–325
    clinical workup, 321
    en bloc resection and nodal dissection, 323
    endoscopic mucosal resection, 321–322
    esophagectomy, 322
    minimally invasive esophagectomy, 323
    neoadjuvant therapy, 322
    risk factors, 321
    risk reduction programs, 323
    squamous cell carcinoma (SCC), 321
    transhiatal approach, 322, 323
    transthoracic approach, 322
  early-stage gastric cancer
    clinical vignette, 328–329
    D2 lymphadenectomy, 326
    distal subtotal gastrectomy, 327
    endoscopic mucosal resection, 325, 326
    esophagogastroduodenoscopy, 321
    gastrectomy, 326
    incidence, 325
    laparoscopic gastrectomy, 327–328
    lymph node metastasis, 326
    lymphadenectomy, 326–327
    Roux-en-Y gastrojejunostomy reconstruction,
      327
    sentinel lymph node biopsy, 327

early-stage rectal cancer
  polyps, 46–48
  radical surgical resection, 49
  transanal excisions, 48–49
gall-bladder cancer
  diagnosis, 355
  laparoscopic cholecystectomy, 362
  lymphadenectomy, 364
hepatocellular carcinoma
  clinical vignette, 255–256
  contraindications, 251
  extrahepatic metastases, 251
  multifocal tumors, 251
  operative considerations, 253–254
  patient and hepatic characteristics, 251–253
  postoperative complication rates, 254
  tumor size and location, 251
oligometastatic colorectal cancer
  anatomic considerations, 57
  biologic resectability criteria, 58–59
  clinical vignette, 59
  liver resection, 58
  parenchymal-sparing techniques, 58
  portal vein embolization (PVE), 58
  synchronous disease, 59
pancreatic cancer
  anatomic resectability classification, 171–173
  biological detriment, 170
  borderline biology, 172–177
  borderline condition, 177–180
  distal pancreatectomy, 169
  laparoscopic and robotic approaches, 169
  metastatic progression, 170, 171
  nonmetastatic tumors, 169
  pancreatoduodenectomy, 169, 170
  removability and resectability, 170–171
survivorship care
  cardiopulmonary toxicity, 479
  central chest radiation, 478–479
  colorectal surgery, 477
  definition, 476
  gastroesophageal surgery, 476–477
  infertility, 479
  liver surgery, 477
  neuropathy, 479
  pancreatic surgery, 477
  pelvic radiation, 478
  survivorship care plan, 476
survivorship care plan (SCP), 476
Swedish Rectal Cancer Trial, 34

T stage, colorectal cancer, 5
TACE. *See* transarterial chemoembolization
TAMIS. *See* transanal minimally invasive surgery
TARE. *See* transarterial radioembolization
taxanes, 419–421
T-cell receptor (TCR) gene therapy, 423
telotristat, 400
thalidomide, 458
The Cancer Genome Atlas (TCGA), 311
thyroid dysfunction, 298
tivantinib, 290–291
TNM staging system. *See* tumor, node, and
  metastasis staging system
total hepatectomy, 243

total liver volume (TLV), 253
total mesorectal excision (TME), 34, 35
total neoadjuvant therapy (TNT), 53
total parenteral nutrition (TPN), 456
TP53 mutation, 213
transanal endoscopic microsurgery (TEM), 48–49
transanal excisions, rectal cancer, 48–49, 412
transanal minimally invasive surgery (TAMIS),
  48–49
transarterial chemoembolization (TACE)
  adverse events, 270
  Child–Pugh A or B cirrhosis, 263
  conventional form, 266
  drug-eluting beads, 266
  gelatin sponge blocks, 265
  hepatocellular carcinoma, 242
  Hong Kong Liver Cancer system, 260, 261
  nuclear medicine shunt study, 266
transarterial embolization (TAE)
  GEP-NETs, 400
  hepatocellular carcinoma, 242
transarterial radioembolization (TARE)
  adverse events, 270
  hepatocellular carcinoma, 242, 266–267
transarterial therapies, hepatocellular carcinoma,
  242
trastuzumab, 9, 336, 345
Trastuzumab for Gastric Cancer (ToGA) trial, 335
tumor, node, and metastasis (TNM) staging
  system
  anal cancer, metastatic, 418
  biliary tract cancers (BTCs), 355–357
  esophageal cancer, 309
  gastric cancer, 309
  gastrointestinal stromal tumors, 429
  hepatocellular carcinoma, 231
  pancreatic cancer, 163–164
tumor suppressor genes, gastrointestinal stromal
  tumors, 430
tumor-infiltrating lymphocyte (TIL) therapy, 423

United Kingdom Coordinating Committee on
  Cancer Research (UKCCCR) Anal Cancer
  Trial I, 410
United Network for Organ Sharing (UNOS), 268

vasoactive intestinal peptideomas, 396
vatalanib, 438
veliparib, 214
veliparib monotherapy, 214
venous thromboembolism (VTE), 378
Von Hippel–Lindau syndrome (VHL), 396
Vulnerable Elders Survey 13 (VES-13), 471

WHO analgesic ladder, 456, 457
wide local excision (WLE), anal SCC, 409
Wilms tumor 1 (WT1), 389
WJOG 4007 trial, 338
Wnt-β-catenin pathway activation, 126

XELOX regimen, 27

Y radioembolization, 241

Zollinger–Ellison syndrome (ZES), 395